Associating Liver Partition and Portal Vein Ligation for Staged Hepatectomy (ALPPS)

Jian Zhou
Editor

Associating Liver Partition and Portal Vein Ligation for Staged Hepatectomy (ALPPS)

Springer

SSTP

Editor
Jian Zhou
Liver Surgery and Transplantation
Zhongshan Hospital
Shanghai, China

ISBN 978-981-96-7366-7 ISBN 978-981-96-7364-3 (eBook)
https://doi.org/10.1007/978-981-96-7364-3

Jointly published with Shanghai Scientific and Technical Publishers

The print edition is not for sale in China (Mainland). Customers from China (Mainland) please order the print book from: Shanghai Scientific and Technical Publishers.

This Springer imprint is published by the registered company Springer Nature Singapore Pte Ltd.
The registered company address is: 152 Beach Road, #21-01/04 Gateway East, Singapore 189721, Singapore

Foreword I

Associating Liver Partition and Portal Vein Ligation for Staged Hepatectomy (ALPPS) represents a landmark innovation in hepatobiliary surgery, significantly impacting the field in recent years. Its unparalleled efficacy in inducing future liver remnant (FLR) growth and enabling tumor resection surpassed conventional methods, offering the potential for long-term survival to many patients with initially unresectable liver cancer. However, ALPPS is technically demanding and requires a high level of expertise and precision. Improper execution can lead to significant complications, compromising patient safety. Currently, a need for more standardization and uneven proficiency levels exist internationally, underscoring the need for comprehensive guidance for ALPPS. This critical gap in the literature is addressed by Professor Jian Zhou's monograph, *Associating Liver Partition and Portal Vein Ligation for Staged Hepatectomy*, the first comprehensive and systematic book dedicated to ALPPS, benefiting both clinicians and patients.

Professor Jian Zhou is a pioneering figure in the international ALPPS community. Having performed the first ALPPS in Asia in April 2013, he and his team have since conducted the largest number of ALPPS procedures for hepatocellular carcinoma globally, generating substantial research contributions. His recent advancements, including the development of "TAE-Salvaged ALPPS," further expand the application of this technique, providing curative resections and long-term survival opportunities to previously ineligible patients. The book, authored by Professor Zhou and his team, serves as an authoritative resource on ALPPS. Key contributions from Professor Hans J. Schlitt, the inventor of ALPPS, further enhance its value. Richly illustrated and meticulously integrating theory and practice, the monograph provides a systematic overview of ALPPS, detailing various procedural techniques and perioperative management strategies. Furthermore, the inclusion of the latest research findings and animal models makes it an invaluable reference for hepatobiliary surgeons and researchers alike.

Hong Kong, China
Academician of the Chinese Academy of Sciences
President of Lee Woo Sing College,
Chinese University of Hong Kong
Former President of the International
Hepato-Pancreato-Biliary Association

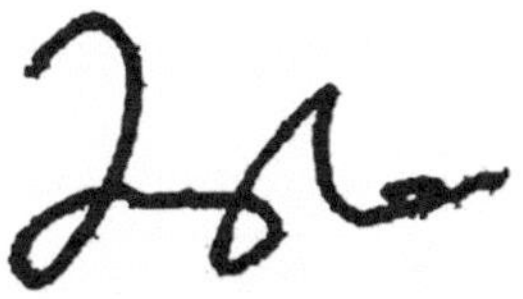

Joseph Wan Yee Lau

Winter, 2023

Foreword II

The history of liver surgery, spanning over a century since the first procedures in the West, is a compelling prologue to the present. Its evolution has been a dynamic interplay of challenges and opportunities, marked by consistent vitality and remarkable progress. Advancements have been inextricably linked to breakthroughs in fundamental sciences: aseptic techniques, anesthesiology, and blood transfusion have provided a crucial foundation; detailed surgical anatomy has fueled rapid growth; and the application of innovative technologies and materials has accelerated development. From the widespread adoption of conventional liver resection to the expansion of minimally invasive techniques and the rise of liver transplantation, the field has continually evolved through technological and conceptual innovations. The development of Associating Liver Partition and Portal Vein Ligation for Staged Hepatectomy (ALPPS) exemplifies this spirit of innovation, offering a transformative understanding of liver regeneration and achieving milestone status in the field.

In April 2013, Professor Jian Zhou of Zhongshan Hospital, Fudan University, performed China's and Asia's first ALPPS procedure. Over the subsequent decade, he has amassed the world's most extensive series of ALPPS procedures for patients with large or multifocal hepatocellular carcinoma. Significantly, Professor Zhou's contributions extend beyond technical prowess; he has also made substantial contributions to ALPPS-related basic research. I am delighted to see the publication of *Associating Liver Partition and Portal Vein Ligation for Staged Hepatectomy*, a collaborative effort between Professor Jian Zhou and Professor Hans J. Schlitt (the inventor of ALPPS), and other leading experts. This book provides the first comprehensive and systematic overview of this innovative technique, covering its origins, indications, detailed procedural requirements, potential mechanisms, and future directions. It brings together leading international ALPPS experts and scholars, seamlessly integrating theory and practice, summarizing established experiences, and sharing valuable data. This work offers crucial theoretical and technical guidance for the broader adoption of ALPPS and illuminates promising avenues for future research.

I highly recommend this book to you all. It serves not only as an indispensable reference for surgeons seeking to master ALPPS but also stands as a testament to the unwavering commitment to exploration and continuous innovation within the global hepatobiliary surgical community.

Hubei, China
Academician of the Chinese Academy of Sciences
Honorary President of Tongji Medical College,
Huazhong University of Science and Technology
Director of the Hepatobiliary and Pancreatic
Surgery Institute, Tongji Medical College,
Huazhong University of Science and Technology

Xiaoping Chen

Winter, 2023

Foreword III

The liver's remarkable regenerative capacity is central to hepatobiliary surgery, where hepatectomy remains the primary curative modality for liver malignancies. Balancing radical tumor removal with the preservation of sufficient future liver remnant (FLR) to ensure surgical safety is a critical challenge. Insufficient FLR and compromised liver function frequently preclude surgical intervention. Given the powerful regenerative potential of the liver, actively inducing rapid FLR growth to enhance surgical safety feasibility has been a major area of focus.

Technological innovation is paramount in advancing medical care. Associating Liver Partition and Portal Vein Ligation for Staged Hepatectomy (ALPPS) stands as one of the most significant surgical advancements of the twenty-first century. By combining liver partition and portal vein ligation in stage 1 operation, surgeons can induce substantial FLR hypertrophy, approximately 80% increase in 7–14 days, allowing for subsequent tumor resection within a short timeframe. ALPPS has provided a crucial opportunity for radical surgery in patients with large, multifocal, or even diffuse hepatic malignancies, offering a lifeline for many previously inoperable cases. The efficacy of ALPPS is further enhanced for patients with advanced liver cancer when combined with adjuvant therapies such as immunotherapy and targeted therapies.

Professor Jian Zhou of our hospital has been a driving force in the research and clinical application of ALPPS for liver cancer and related liver regeneration. In April 2013, he successfully carried out the first ALPPS in Asia, treating a patient with a massive hepatocellular carcinoma. In 2018, the results of the world's largest clinical study on ALPPS for hepatocellular carcinoma were published online in the *Annals of Surgery*, highlighting his contribution. Meanwhile, Professor Zhou's dedication to innovation extends to developing novel approaches; for patients where ALPPS fails to induce sufficient regeneration, he pioneered TAE-Salvaged ALPPS, enabling successful and complete radical tumor resection within 3 weeks. His ongoing research focuses on elucidating the mechanism underlying ALPPS-induced rapid liver regeneration, its impact on tumor progression, and the development of strategies to enhance its clinical applicability, bringing renewed hope for radical resection to more patients with advanced liver cancer.

The publication of *Associating Liver Partition and Portal Vein Ligation for Staged Hepatectomy*, authored by Professor Jian Zhou and a distinguished international team, marks a significant milestone. This comprehensive book provides a systematic overview of ALPPS, covering its clinical background, detailed surgical techniques, diverse applications, and the latest research advancements. It serves as an invaluable resource for hepatobiliary surgeons and researchers seeking to fully understand and further advance this transformative procedure.

I extend my warmest congratulations to the authors on this important contribution. I am confident that this monograph will prove both informative and beneficial, ultimately contributing to improved patient care.

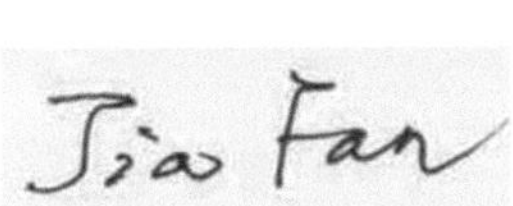

Shanghai, China
Academician of the Chinese Academy of Sciences
Honorary President of Zhongshan Hospital, Fudan University
Director of the Liver Cancer Institute, Fudan University
Winter, 2023

Jia Fan

Preface

Liver cancer presents a significant global health challenge, with China bearing a disproportionate burden, accounting for nearly half of all cases worldwide and resulting in high mortality rates. While advancements in anticancer therapies, including immunotherapy and targeted therapy, have improved prognoses for patients with advanced liver malignancies, curative surgery remains the cornerstone of treatment for achieving long-term survival and reducing tumor burden. Since the 1950s, the collective efforts of hepatobiliary surgeons globally have driven rapid advancements in surgical tech, resulting in innovative procedures and significantly improved patient outcomes. However, in China, the low rate of early diagnosis means that only 15–30% of patients are initially eligible for curative surgery, primarily due to insufficient future liver remnant (FLR). Numerous strategies to induce FLR hypertrophy and thereby increase resectability have been explored internationally, including portal vein embolization (PVE), two-stage hepatectomy (TSH), and hepatic vein embolization. However, these methods have limitations, including inefficient FLR growth, prolonged waiting times for the second-stage surgery, and the risk of tumor progression during the interval. The development of a rapid, efficient, and safe method for FLR hypertrophy remains a crucial priority in hepatobiliary surgery.

In 2007, Professor Hans J. Schlitt from the Department of Surgery, University of Regensburg in Germany, pioneered a novel approach involving liver partition and portal vein ligation in a patient with hilar cholangiocarcinoma and insufficient FLR. This procedure unexpectedly induced rapid FLR growth within 8 days, enabling successful tumor resection 10 days later. Following refinement and continuous improvement, this technique was officially announced in 2012 and named "Associating Liver Partition and Portal Vein Ligation for Staged Hepatectomy (ALPPS)," which represents a significant advancement, overcoming a major limitation in liver surgery and tremendously improving resection rates and patient survival.

In early 2013, I first encountered enthusiastic discussions about ALPPS at the Americas Hepato-Pancreato-Biliary Association Congress. At that time, ALPPS was primarily used for unresectable colorectal liver metastases (CRLM), with fewer than 100 cases reported worldwide and limited application to hepatocellular carcinoma (HCC). Inspired by its potential, I resolved to introduce this groundbreaking procedure to China. Following meticulous preoperative evaluation and planning, I successfully performed the first ALPPS in China and Asia in April 2013 on an HCC patient with a large 16 cm right lobe tumor and a 1.5 cm satellite lesion in the left lobe, rendering conventional surgery impossible. The patient was discharged successfully 18 days post-ALPPS. This successful case was published in the *Chinese Journal of Digestive Surgery* in July 2013. It was accompanied by a commentary from Academician Wan Yee Lau of the Chinese University of Hong Kong, recognizing it as "the first reported case of ALPPS in Asia" and highlighting the achievement of internationally advanced standards in Chinese liver surgery. This success significantly boosted our team's confidence and spurred further application of ALPPS in patients with advanced liver cancer, including those with liver fibrosis and cirrhosis. Our continued clinical experience has led to innovations and refinements in patient selection, surgical techniques, and perioperative management, striving for enhanced safety and efficacy.

Initially, the high complication and mortality rates associated with ALPPS presented significant challenges to its widespread adoption. However, through technical refinements and the accumulation of clinical experience, ALPPS has gained broader recognition and acceptance. Our team's extensive experience, however, underscores the technical complexity and steep learning curve inherent to ALPPS. Without proper guidance and training, attempting ALPPS without sufficient expertise can lead to unacceptably high complications and mortality rates. As the proverb says, "Giving a man a fish feeds him for a day; teaching a man to fish feeds him for a lifetime." Recognizing the importance of knowledge transfer and standardization, Professor Hans J. Schlitt and I, along with colleagues from China and abroad, agree that widespread adoption of ALPPS requires addressing the current lack of standardization and consistent procedural quality through comprehensive training and continuing education programs. We, therefore, decided to collaborate on a comprehensive academic monograph dedicated to ALPPS for the benefit of our colleagues worldwide.

This book offers a systematic and comprehensive exploration of ALPPS, covering its historical developmental, underlying mechanisms, relevant clinical anatomy, detailed procedural techniques (including both classical and modified ALPPS approaches), preoperative evaluation, patient selection criteria (indications and contraindications), surgical planning, and comprehensive postoperative management and follow-up. It also incorporates the latest research findings and results from animal model studies. The authorship team comprises renowned experts and outstanding young scholars in hepatobiliary surgery and related disciplines from leading liver surgery centers, all possessing extensive clinical or research experience with ALPPS. Professor Hans J. Schlitt, the inventor of ALPPS, has provided invaluable support, including authoring Chap. 2 and generously sharing case studies and materials from his institution. We are deeply grateful for the invaluable guidance and support from honorary editors Academician Zhaoyou Tang, Academician Wan Yee Lau, Academician Xiaoping Chen, and Chief Reviewer Academician Jia Fan, who are a pioneering and leading force of hepatobiliary surgery in China and the world.

This book aims to provide the most up-to-date theoretical and technical knowledge on ALPPS, empowering hepatobiliary surgeons to confidently and effectively perform the procedure and improve outcomes for liver cancer patients, especially those with initially unresectable tumors. It is our hope that this work will serve as a catalyst for further advancements and broader adoption of this transformative surgical technique.

The successful completion and publication of this book is a testament to the collaborative efforts and diligent contributions of experts from around the globe. However, given my own limitations and the ongoing developmental stage of ALPPS, we understand that imperfections may exist. Your insights and corrections would be invaluable to us, and we sincerely welcome any feedback or guidance you might offer.

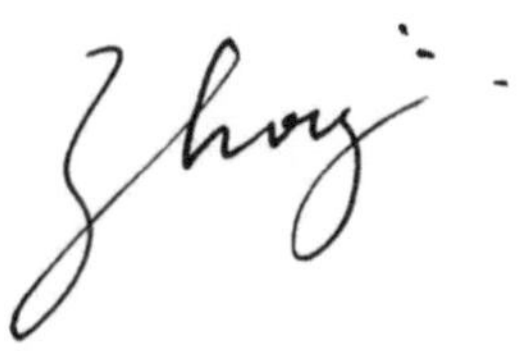

Fellow of the Academic Advisory Committee of the Chinese Academy of Medical Sciences
Shanghai, China

President of Zhongshan Hospital, Fudan University
Shanghai, China

President of the Asia-Pacific Primary Liver Cancer Expert Meeting Association (APPLE)
Shanghai, China

Jian Zhou

Winter 2023

Calligraphy

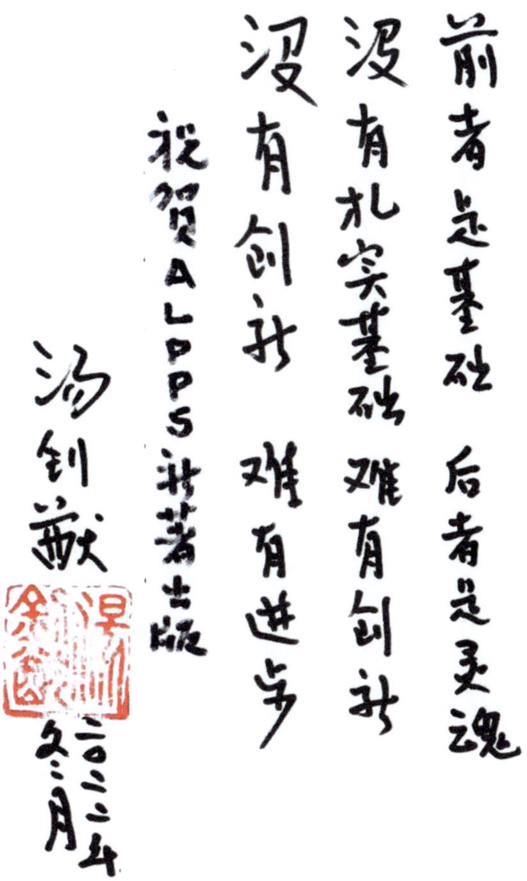

Sun Tzu said, “It is a general rule in war that the ordinary force is used to engage and the extraordinary force to win victory”. The former is the foundation, the latter is the soul. Without a solid foundation, it is difficult to innovate; without innovation, there can be no progress.

Congratulations on the publication of a new book on ALPPS.

Shanghai, China
Academician of the Chinese Academy of Engineering
Former President of Shanghai Medical University
Former Director of Liver Cancer Institute, Fudan University

Z.Y. Tang

Zhaoyou Tang

Winter 2022

Synopsis

Associating Liver Partition and Portal Vein Ligation for Staged Hepatectomy (ALPPS) is one of the most significant innovations in liver surgery over the past decade. This technique was serendipitously established by German Professor Hans J. Schlitt in 2007. ALPPS offers surgical resection opportunities in a short period for patients with liver tumors who were previously deemed unresectable due to insufficient future liver remnant (FLR), significantly improving their survival prognosis.

This book systematically introduces the development history, current status, and advancements. It provides detailed explanations of the clinical anatomy, indications, contraindications, preoperative evaluations for ALPPS, the implementation methods for the classic ALPPS and various modified techniques, and perioperative management. The book also introduces the comparisons between ALPPS and traditional two-stage hepatectomy, prevention and management of postoperative complications, follow-up management and survival prognosis, experimental models, and related mechanism studies. Additionally, it discusses the era of liver surgery with ALPPS and prospects its future.

The editorial board of this book comprises experts from many ALPPS centers. The content includes valuable experiences from the extensive clinical practice of ALPPS at the respective centers of the contributing authors, assisting hepatobiliary surgeons in performing this type of surgery rapidly and safely to benefit more patients.

This book is recommended for clinicians in the related field as a reference.

Contents

Editors and Contributors

About the Editors

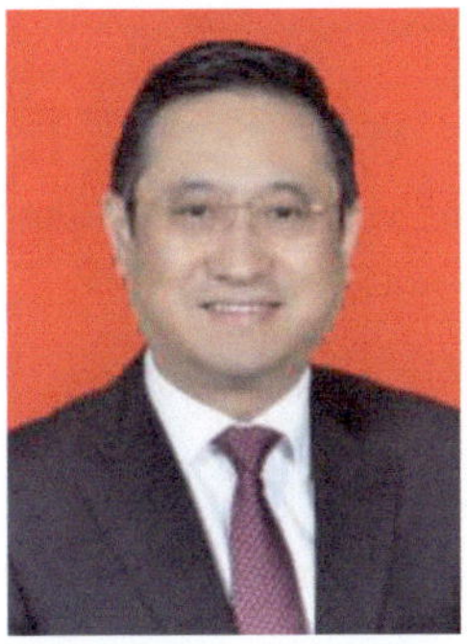

Jian Zhou

Professor of Surgery, Ph.D. & MD.
President of Zhongshan Hospital, Fudan University;
Executive Vice Director of Liver Cancer Institute, Fudan University;
Vice Director of Key Laboratory of Carcinogenesis and Cancer Invasion (Fudan University), Ministry of Education, China

Academic of the Academic Advisory Committee Position and Honors

- Fellow of the Chinese Academy of Medical Sciences;
- Winner of National Science Fund for Distinguished Young Scholars;
- Chairman Designate of Chinese Society of Oncology, Chinese Medical Association;
- President of the Asia-Pacific Primary Liver Cancer Expert Meeting Association (APPLE);
- Vice Chairman and Secretary-General of Chinese College of Surgeons;
- Vice Chairman of Chinese Society of Transplantation Immunology;
- Former Chairman of Society of Liver Cancer, China Anti-Cancer Association;
- Executive Council Member of the Asian-Pacific Association for the Study of the Liver (APASL)

Achievement
As the Professor of Department of Hepatobiliary Surgery & Transplantation, Dr. Zhou has been working on the basic and clinical studies in liver cancer for 33 years, and has clinical experience of more than 10,000 hepatectomies and 2000 orthotopic liver transplantation. He has been in charge of 26 research projects including the National Key R&D Program and Key Project of National Natural Science Foundation of China, reaching an amount of $11 million. He has published 130 scientific papers indexed in SCI as the first or correspondence author including *Journal of Clinical Oncology*, *Cell Research*, *Gastroenterology*, *Hepatology*, *Journal of Hepatology* and *Clinical Cancer Research*, etc., H-index 89. Dr. Zhou has won 5 national-level Awards for Scientific and Technological Advancement.

Chief Reviewer
Jia Fan
Zhongshan Hospital, Fudan University, Shanghai, China

Associate Editors-in-Chief
Hans J. Schlitt
University Hospital Regensburg, Regensburg, Germany
Weiping Zhou
The Third Affiliated Hospital of Naval Medical University (Eastern Hepatobiliary Surgery Hospital), Shanghai, China
Albert Chan
Queen Mary Hospital, University of Hong Kong, Hong Kong, China

Contributors

Xiujun Cai Sir Run Run Shaw Hospital, Zhejiang University School of Medicine, Zhejiang, China

Albert Chan Queen Mary Hospital, University of Hong Kong, Hong Kong, China

Feiyu Chen Zhongshan Hospital, Fudan University, Shanghai, China

Yajin Chen Sun Yat-Sen Memorial Hospital, Sun Yat-Sen University, Guangdong, China

Defei Hong Sir Run Run Shaw Hospital, Zhejiang University School of Medicine, Zhejiang, China

Jie Hu Zhongshan Hospital, Fudan University, Shanghai, China

I-Chin Lee Jiahui International Hospital Shanghai, Jiahui Health, Shanghai, China

Zhifeng Jiang Zhongshan Hospital, Fudan University, Shanghai, China

Ren'an Jin Sir Run Run Shaw Hospital, Zhejiang University School of Medicine, Zhejiang, China

Jun Li Jiahui International Hospital Shanghai, Jiahui Health, Shanghai, China

Pengpeng Li The Third Affiliated Hospital of Naval Medical University (Eastern Hepatobiliary Surgery Hospital), Shanghai, China

Kexi Liao The First Hospital Affiliated to Army Medical University (Southwest Hospital), Chongqing, China

Shuyou Peng The Second Affiliated Hospital Zhejiang University School of Medicine (SAHZU), Zhejiang, China

Yuanfei Peng Zhongshan Hospital, Fudan University, Shanghai, China

Hans J. Schlitt University Hospital Regensburg, Regensburg, Germany

Changzhen Shang Sun Yat-Sen Memorial Hospital, Sun Yat-Sen University, Guangdong, China

Guoming Shi Zhongshan Hospital, Fudan University, Shanghai, China

Huichuan Sun Zhongshan Hospital, Fudan University, Shanghai, China

Baolin Wang The First Hospital Affiliated to Army Medical University (Southwest Hospital), Chongqing, China

Xiaoying Wang Zhongshan Hospital, Fudan University, Shanghai, China

Zheng Wang Zhongshan Hospital, Fudan University, Shanghai, China

Zhiqin Xie Sun Yat-Sen Memorial Hospital, Sun Yat-Sen University, Guangdong, China

Jiayan Yan Zhongshan Hospital, Fudan University, Shanghai, China

Xinrong Yang Zhongshan Hospital, Fudan University, Shanghai, China

Lei Yu Zhongshan Hospital, Fudan University, Shanghai, China

Shuguo Zheng The First Hospital Affiliated to Army Medical University (Southwest Hospital), Chongqing, China

Jian Zhou Zhongshan Hospital, Fudan University, Shanghai, China

Weiping Zhou The Third Affiliated Hospital of Naval Medical University (Eastern Hepatobiliary Surgery Hospital), Shanghai, China

Kai Zhu Zhongshan Hospital, Fudan University, Shanghai, China

General Introduction

1

Jian Zhou and Yuanfei Peng

Liver cancer is one of the most common primary malignant tumors, and surgical resection offers the potentially curative option to achieve long-term survival [1–4]. Due to its lack of typical early symptoms, early detection of liver cancer remains challenging. Many patients are often diagnosed with large tumors or advanced tumors with invaded important vessels. Extensive liver resection is required in such cases for radical resection of the tumor. Postoperative complications such as liver function failure can occur due to insufficient future liver remnant (FLR), which may result in severe consequences, including death.

In general, these patients do not meet the inclusion criteria of liver transplantation, and meanwhile, there is a shortage of donors. Therefore, only very few patients have the opportunity to undergo liver transplantation [5, 6]. Consequently, most of them have historically been limited to non-surgical treatments, often with low survival rates. The key to improving survival for these patients lies in finding ways to convert them eligible for radical tumor resection.

Various treatment strategies have emerged with the development of liver surgery and oncology. The first involves inducing FLR regeneration, allowing sufficient liver growth and tumor removal. This method takes advantage of the remarkable and fast regenerative capacity of the liver after injury [7–9]. The second one is a down-staging strategy, which targets the tumor using treatments such as chemoembolization, intra-arterial yttrium-90 microsphere radiation, and anti-tumor drugs to achieve tumor shrinkage before surgical removal. It enables a relative increase of FLR by reducing the tumor volume and thereby decreasing the proportion of liver occupied by the tumor, compared to the absolute FLR growth induced by the first strategy. The third strategy targets both FLR and the tumor simultaneously (inducing FLR growth while treating the tumor).

These strategies aim to increase FLR (either absolute increase or relative increase of FLR), ensuring that the non-tumor-occupied FLR is sufficient before tumor removal. Currently, the first strategy (inducing FLR growth before resection) is mainstream and has enabled many patients with initially unresectable tumors to undergo surgery, improving the survival of these patients. The second strategy has historically shown poor results, but recent advancements in non-surgical treatments, especially the emergence of new target therapy and immunotherapy, have led to significant breakthroughs with rapid developments in conversion therapy [10]. Conversion therapy is currently a hot topic and represents an essential direction for the future with promising prospects, though it has yet to fully mature. The third strategy, a "two-pronged approach" addressing both FLR and the tumor, is highly aggressive and involves challenges related to patient tolerance and surgical complications. It has been less commonly used previously, but in recent years, scholars at home and abroad have begun exploring this approach actively.

Compared to other organs, the bottleneck limitation of FLR in the liver is more prominent. This is related to the need for more salvage measures. Unlike mature functional replacement technologies such as dialysis for the kidney, the development of artificial liver technology has lagged behind due to the functional complexity, resulting in poor treatment outcomes caused by post-hepatectomy liver failure (PHLF), with a mortality rate exceeding 85%. Additionally, another salvage measure, liver transplantation, is hindered by the scarcity of donors and cannot be routinely used for rescue. In general, the patients succumb to PHLF before they can receive liver transplantation [11]. Thus, FLR, as a decisive factor in liver surgery, has always been a major focus of research in hepatic surgery [12].

As early as 1879, Theodor Frerichs [13] observed that the blockage of portal vein branches could cause ipsilateral atrophy and contralateral compensatory hypertrophy. In 1920, Peyton Rous and Louise D. Larimore [14] confirmed that

J. Zhou (✉) · Y. Peng
Zhongshan Hospital, Fudan University, Shanghai, China
e-mail: zhou.jian@zs-hospital.sh.cn

J. Zhou (ed.), *Associating Liver Partition and Portal Vein Ligation for Staged Hepatectomy (ALPPS)*,
https://doi.org/10.1007/978-981-96-7364-3_1

selective portal vein ligation (PVL) could induce atrophy on the ligated side and compensatory hypertrophy on the opposite side through a rabbit model. This phenomenon is referred to as the atrophy-hypertrophy complex (portal vein ligation-induced atrophy on one side and compensatory hypertrophy on the other). Despite the early discovery in humans that portal vein occlusion could induce FLR hypertrophy, its potential value only gained attention and application in modern hepatic surgery after many years.

In the mid to late 1980s, Masatoshi Makuuchi and Hiroaki Kinoshita et al. in Japan pioneered the use of portal vein embolization (PVE) to block tumor-side portal vein branches to induce FLR increase. PVE allowed the resecting of high-burden tumors, simultaneously reducing the risk of PHLF and providing an opportunity for cure. The overall survival of patients was significantly improved [15–17]. PVE was quickly adopted by many hepatobiliary surgery centers worldwide. PVE was initially applied to tumors such as perihilar cholangiocarcinoma (PHCC) and hepatocellular carcinoma (HCC). Then, it was rapidly extended to other liver tumors, including colorectal cancer liver metastasis (CRLM), and was proven effective in preventing liver function failure after extensive liver resections [18]. With technological maturity, it became a standard method widely used to induce FLR growth before surgery in patients with large or multifocal tumors [19].

Although PVE is effective and can increase the chances of surgical resection, there are still some patients whose tumors cannot be completely and thoroughly removed in a single operation, rendering suboptimal survival benefits. This situation is particularly common in metastatic liver malignancies. In 2000, Rene Adam et al. proposed the concept of two-stage hepatectomy (TSH) for CRLM patients whose tumors could not be completely removed through a one-stage hepatectomy. During the first stage of surgery, the tumors were resected as much as they could be. If more than 60% of the liver is removed and the FLR is insufficient, PVE is performed. After a period, the second surgery is conducted to remove the remaining tumors in the liver. For patients with unresectable and multifocal metastases, two-stage hepatectomy offers the opportunity for radical or maximal tumor removal, bringing about maximum survival benefits. Rene Adam et al. reported a tumor resection rate of 81%, a median inter-stage interval of 4 months, a 3-year survival rate of 35%, and a median survival of 31 months. In comparison, systemic chemotherapy as the standard of care at that time provided these patients with unresectable tumors a median survival of no more than 12–18 months, which demonstrates that TSH combined with chemotherapy could offer significant remission for those with unresectable multifocal metastatic tumors and increase the resection rate of these patients [20].

Subsequent publications on expanded applications and long-term follow-up results showed that this strategy achieved a tumor resection rate of 69% (median inter-stage interval of 4.2 months). The 3- and 5-year overall survival rates reach 60 and 42%, respectively. The TSH offered hope for long-term survival in these unresectable extensive bilobar CRLM patients [21]. It should be noted that in Rene Adam's initial study, the primary objective was to explore the possibility of a two-stage hepatectomy. PVE was used in only a subset of patients with insufficient FLR (6 out of 13) [20].

In 2004, Daniel Jaeck and colleagues from France further assessed the effectiveness of PVE-TSH for patients with insufficient FLR. In the first stage, tumors on the left FLR were removed or treated with radiofrequency, followed by right-side PVE 3–5 weeks later. FLR increase was evaluated 5–8 weeks after PVE. The median waiting time was 2–4 months, whereas the tumor resection rate was 75.7%. The 1-year and 3-year overall survival rates of patients who completed two-stage hepatectomy reached 70.0 and 54.4%, respectively. The long-term survival rate was similar to those with initially resectable liver metastases. On the other hand, the 1-year and 3-year survival rates of patients who did not complete two-stage resection were 72.9 and 0%, respectively, which were significantly lower than those who did [22].

Daniel Jaeck et al. reported a significantly shorter inter-stage interval than before, but it still took 2 to 4 months. In 2007, Jacques Belghiti and Pierre-Alain Clavien et al. further improved TSH by performing portal vein ligation (PVL) during the first-stage surgery for tumor removal. The waiting time between the two stages was reduced to about 4 weeks [23]. In the subsequent development, other methods were combined with PVE to enhance its FLR-inducing effect, including trans-arterial embolization (TAE) and hepatic vein embolization (HVE). These methods increased FLR induction and shortened waiting times to a certain extent. However, overall improvement remained limited [24–27].

The application of PVE-TSH and PVL-TSH provided an opportunity for initially unresectable patients. However, these procedures have limitations, including a low FLR induction efficiency and long intervals between the two stages. The FLR increase rate is usually restricted to around 40% [28–31]. For patients with liver fibrosis or cirrhosis, it is even more challenging to achieve satisfactory FLR growth through the mentioned methods [32].

Classical PVE techniques require a relatively long time for FLR induction. During this waiting period, tumors often progress. Additionally, FLR growth varies significantly among patients, and the FLR growth is insufficient in some cases. These drawbacks lower the odds of surgery for many patients [33]. Early reports indicated that approximately one-third of patients undergoing PVE did not complete liver resection due to tumor progression or insufficient FLR growth during the waiting period [30, 34, 35]. A recent meta-analysis showed that the average waiting time for PVE-TSH was still as long as 45.7 days with a tumor resection rate of 78% (R0 resection rate of 37%) despite years of development and continuous improvement, leading to a significant number of patients missing the chance for curative surgery [36]. There are also issues related to the extended interval between the two stages, including excessive intra-abdominal adhesions and increased surgical difficulty [37].

In September 2007, Hans J. Schlitt at the University of Regensburg in Germany serendipitously developed a new surgical technique during a PHCC surgery: Associating Liver Partition and Portal Vein Ligation for Staged Hepatectomy (ALPPS) [38]. In the planned procedure, they intended to perform a right trisegmentectomy on a 49-year-old female PHCC patient. However, intraoperatively, they discovered that the remaining volume of the left liver was too small for tumor resection. Besides, to prevent tumor compression on the liver hilum leading to jaundice and to enhance the patient's quality of life, they decided to perform a left hepatic duct-to-jejunum anastomosis. During the anastomosis, due to difficulties in mobilizing the left hepatic duct, they dissected the liver parenchyma between the left lateral and left medial lobes along the falciform ligament, fully exposing the left hepatic duct for the anastomosis. Finally, they ligated the right portal vein, hoping to induce an increase of the left lateral lobe similar to the effect of PVE.

On postoperative day 8, the CT scan unexpectedly revealed significant growth of the left liver, with an astonishing FLR increase of over 90%, reaching 723 mL. Subsequently, they successfully performed the second-stage operation to remove the tumor. The patient, who had a risk of PHLF a week before, tolerated the resection well. Following this successful case, they applied ALPPS in various other tumor resections, including CRLM, with consistent success. This unexpected discovery and bold experimentation led Hans J. Schlitt to establish a new surgical approach that could induce rapid and significant FLR growth, allowing tumor removal in a shorter time [38, 39].

This surgical technique involves liver partition and portal vein ligation. It enables faster and more significant FLR induction and achieves higher surgical resection rates. In April 2011, at the ninth Congress of the European-African Hepato-Pancreato-Biliary Association (E-AHPBA) held in Cape Town, South Africa, Hauke Lang et al. presented three cases using this new technique (named "right portal vein ligation combined with in situ splitting" at the time) in posters, bringing international attention to the procedure [39]. In 2011, Hans J. Schlitt and Andreas A. Schnitzbauer pooled more cases and combined experiences of five German centers. They analyzed a total of 25 patients and published their findings in the *Annals of Surgery* in 2012 [40]. The median waiting time after the first-stage operation was 9 days, with the FLR volume averaging 74%, a tumor resection rate of 100%, and a 6-month overall survival rate of 86% [40]. ALPPS demonstrated rapid FLR induction and an exceptionally high surgical resection rate, significantly surpassing traditional TSH procedures. This technique was initially referred to as "right portal vein ligation combined with in situ splitting and then hepatectomy."

After the technique was formally reported in the *Annals of Surgery* in March 2012, the journal's editor-in-chief Pierre-Alain Clavien and Eduardo de Santibañes provided a commentary, introducing the procedure and naming it as "Associating Liver Partition and Portal Vein Ligation for Staged Hepatectomy" and "ALPPS" using the acronym derived from the initial letters [37]. Since then, the technique has gained widespread international recognition in hepatobiliary surgery. In the same year, an international ALPPS collaborative organization (ALPPS registry) was established, coordinated, and maintained by the Department of Surgery at the University of Zurich, Switzerland [41], with access to their experience available through www.alpps.net. Currently, over 350 centers have joined, registering more than 1228 ALPPS cases and publishing numerous essential research findings, providing crucial guidance for the application of ALPPS and significantly advancing its progress [42–52].

ALPPS has demonstrated remarkable surgical outcomes and is considered a milestone breakthrough in hepatic surgery [37, 40]. Many liver centers worldwide have enthusiastically adopted ALPPS, making it a focal point of hepatobiliary and pancreatic surgery conferences [53]. Between 2012 and 2016, there have been over 600 reported cases nationally and internationally [46]. In April 2013, Jian Zhou from Zhongshan Hospital, Fudan University, performed the first ALPPS case in Asia. A giant liver cancer (16 cm in diameter) with a lesion in the left medial lobe, which traditional surgery could not address, was removed. The FLR increased significantly from 291 mL preoperatively to 579 mL on the seventh day postoperatively, showing a 99% FLR growth. On the eighth day, they completed the extended right hemihepatectomy to remove the tumor [54, 55].

In July 2013, Jian Zhou reported this case in the *Chinese Journal of Digestive Surgery*. Academician Lau Wan Yee concurrently published a commentary highly praising the success of the surgery, stating, "To the best of my knowledge, this is the first reported ALPPS surgery in Asia. Its successful implementation also represents the leading level of liver cancer surgery in our country." Academician Lau's commentary significantly contributed to the quick acceptance and application of ALPPS by many centers in China [56]. ALPPS is an innovative surgical approach, distinguished by its in-situ split technique combined with portal vein ligation, achieving unprecedented rapid and significant

FLR growth. It allows for a two-stage liver resection in a short period, with tumor resection rates far surpassing traditional TSH. ALPPS can induce an FLR growth ranging from 58 to 110%, and even up to 200%, within a week after the first-stage operation, while PVE typically results in a 10–40% FLR growth observed between 4 and 8 weeks [29, 40, 49, 57–59].

The FLR growth rate of ALPPS is 10–11 times higher than that of PVL/PVE [52, 60]. Compared to traditional PVE-TSH, ALPPS significantly reduces waiting time, lowers the risk of tumor progression, and increases tumor resection rates, often exceeding 95%. Some centers report tumor resection rates reaching 100% [59]. A large-scale study from the ALPPS collaborative group showed that FLR growth with ALPPS ranged from 40 to 160% within 7–14 days, with a tumor resection rate of 98.3% [46]. Systematic analysis indicates that ALPPS achieves approximately 76% FLR growth, tumor resection rates between 95 and 100%, and an overall failure rate of only about 5%, attributing to insufficient FLR growth, portal vein thrombosis, and in-between deaths [44, 61].

ALPPS achieves unprecedented rapid and significant FLR growth, significantly shortening the interval between the two stages and boasting a very high tumor resection rate [44]. However, despite these numerous advantages, along with substantial benefits, it is accompanied by a high incidence of complications and mortality, raising concerns about its safety. Early reports indicated a high complication rate associated with ALPPS, particularly PHLF, bile leakage, and intra-abdominal infections [62].

In the initial report by Andreas A. Schnitzbauer and colleagues in 2012, the complication rate was as high as 68%, with a severe complication rate (Clavien-Dindo >IIIa) reaching 44% and a mortality rate of 12% [40]. While other centers, such as the Buenos Aires Hospital in Argentina, reported a postoperative mortality rate of 0% and a complication rate of only 40% in the same year, most centers showed suboptimal safety, with postoperative mortality rates ranging from 11.1 to 20% [62–64]. In 2014, the ALPPS registry published a summary of the safety and survival analysis of the first 202 ALPPS cases, revealing a 90-day postoperative mortality rate of 15%, a severe complication rate of 27%, with bile leakage and intra-abdominal infection being the major ones [49].

The high incidence of complications and mortality associated with ALPPS has sparked intense debate and scrutiny within the academic community [49, 59, 61, 64–67]. leading to concerns and criticisms about the surgery's safety. Renowned scholars, such as Jacques Belghiti, highlighted in 2014 concerns about the safety and oncological benefits (result) of the procedure. [68]. Some centers labeled the surgery as high-risk, imposing strict limitations and cautious use, with a few liver centers even ceasing to perform the procedure [41, 44, 69]. ALPPS has become a controversial surgery in the field of hepatobiliary surgery, with ongoing debates at surgical conferences.

However, the development of any new technology is not without challenges, reminiscent of the progress of past "new technologies" like liver transplantation and minimally invasive laparoscopic surgery. The drawbacks of ALPPS are not Achilles' Heels. Hepatobiliary surgeons worldwide, driven by great enthusiasm and a scientific mindset, continue accumulating experiences and lessons. Comparative studies across different centers, indications, and operative techniques, as well as pooled analyses by the ALPPS collaborative group, quickly revealed that the safety of ALPPS is associated with various factors and has significant room for improvement. For instance, advanced age and poor general condition are correlated with higher mortality rates [49]. Patients with biliary tumors have higher mortality rates compared to other tumors (CRLM, 8%; biliary tumors, 24%) [67]. Specific surgical procedures, such as ligating the right hepatic duct, can lead to a high bile leakage rate [70]. Corresponding improvement efforts were promptly initiated, covering aspects such as surgical techniques, case selection, and inter-stage management [41].

1.1 Surgical Technique Advancements

Various surgeons have proposed distinctive refinements of ALPPS, encompassing many aspects. Technological improvements primarily focus on the following facets: basic surgical techniques and skills, liver separation methods, portal vein occlusion methods, surgical approaches, and integrated enhancements of the abovementioned factors.

1.1.1 Improvements in Basic Surgical Techniques and Skills

This domain encompasses aspects such as parenchyma transection surface handling and bile leakage prevention. Early reports showed that the post-ALPPS complications and mortality were associated with bile leakage, abdominal infections, and PHLF, among others. The initial safety analysis report by the ALPPS Registry in 2014 identified bile leakage and intra-abdominal infections as major postoperative severe complications [67]. Bile leakage stands out as a crucial contributor to ALPPS complications, with an incidence ranging from 22.2 to 24%, and an even higher number of 87.5% was reported [37, 64, 70, 71]. There were numerous reasons for bile leakage, but improvements have gradually reduced these occurrences.

Firstly, bile duct ligation should be avoided in the stage 1 ALPPS operation; some centers believe ligating the right hepatic duct during the stage 1 surgery promotes sufficient FLR growth. However, the post-ALPPS bile leakage rate on the ligated side was reported as high as 87.5% by Safi Dokmak and Jacques Belghiti [70]. Fernando A. Alvarez et al. [19] early on advocated against routine ligation of the tumor-side liver duct, citing potential damage to the right hepatic artery during dissection. In 2014, R. Robles et al. compared patients with and without bile duct ligation, revealing complication rates of 40% and 8%, respectively [72]. Subsequent ALPPS procedures no longer involve bile duct ligation. Secondly, meticulous intraoperative bile leakage checks have been implemented. This is the most reliable method for the prevention of such complications. Avoiding bile leakage and abdominal infection relies not on wrapping the tumor-side liver with plastic bags but on effective measures, including thorough bile leakage checks, appropriate drainage after bile leakage, and the prophylactic use of antibiotics postoperatively. Injecting saline into the gallbladder duct, bubble testing, and injection of colorants (such as methylene blue and propofol) upon completing the stage 1 surgery, followed by cholangiography when necessary, have been proven effective in preventing bile leakage [19, 53, 73–76]. The liver surgery team at Zhongshan Hospital, Fudan University, routinely uses diluted fat emulsion injections to check for bile duct leaks, achieving an extremely low incidence of bile leakage, approaching 0% [54, 77]. Adequate drainage is ensured by placing suitable drainage tubes on the liver section at the end of the surgery [78, 79]. In addition to bile leakage checks, some scholars deploy T-tubes to reduce intra-bile duct pressure and prevent bile leakage [32].

Another concern is abdominal adhesions after the stage 1 operation. Severe adhesions may increase intraoperative bleeding and operational difficulties during the stage 2 operation. In the early years of ALPPS, plastic bags were commonly used to wrap the tumor-side liver, aiming to prevent adhesion formation and limit bile leakage, thereby reducing abdominal infections [19, 37, 40, 80]. Nonetheless, this practice led to fluid accumulation and worsened abdominal infections, causing a high incidence of post-ALPPS complications, including bile leakage [74, 81]. Moreover, as plastic bags are foreign objects, if the stage-2 operation cannot be performed, another laparotomy is required to remove them [74, 81]. Therefore, many scholars opposed their use early on [74, 81]. With the accumulation of ALPPS, it was discovered that as long as there were no complications such as bile leakage and abdominal infections, and the inter-stage interval was not long, there were rarely severe abdominal adhesions. Furthermore, many subsequent reports demonstrated that adhesions could be effectively controlled by covering the transection surface with absorbable biomaterials (such as TachoSil) and adjusting the surgical approach [74, 82–86]. Subsequent ALPPS procedures gradually abandoned the use of plastic bags. As of 2014, data from the ALPPS Registry analysis showed that only 16% of centers still used plastic bags, 35% of them did not use coverings on the raw surface after liver transection, and 26% used Tachosil [74]. Our center generally replaces plastic bags with fibrin glue and hemostatic gauze for coverage, with the addition of anti-adhesion materials (such as Chitosan) when necessary. Adhesions during the stage 2 operation are usually mild and easily separable. The anterior approach avoids dividing perihepatic ligaments, achieving excellent anti-adhesion effects [76, 78]. In addition to these techniques, using ribbons or threads to mark the portal ducts during the stage 1 surgery has been recommended as part of the standardized procedure for ALPPS stage 1, enabling easy recognition in Stage 2 operation, reducing the interference of adhesions on structural identification and shortening the operation time [19, 53, 74, 87]. In classical ALPPS procedures, segment IV is prone to ischemia, and it was advocated in the early years to resect this ischemic segment to avoid complications such as liver abscess and bile leakage [88]. Nevertheless, in practice, extensive necroses or abscesses in segment IV are rare. A survey of ALPPS Registry members showed that only 45% of surgeons observed necrosis in this segment [89]. Fernando A. Alvarez and Eduardo de Santibañes believed that segment IV resection is unnecessary in ALPPS, and routine antibiotic use after the stage 1 operation may maximally reduce problems caused by this segment [58]. Such segmentectomies are no longer performed in subsequent surgeries, except for some Japanese scholars [90]. In most cases, routine antibiotics alone, or partial division with the middle hepatic vein preserving and avoiding complete division of all Segment IV Glisson branches, are adopted, ensuring inflow and outflow of this segment.

1.1.2 Improvements in Liver Separation

Complications of ALPPS are often related to liver parenchymal transection and include bile leakage, adhesions, ischemia, and necrosis of Segment IV. A classical ALPPS involves complete transection of the liver parenchyma (up to the anterior wall of the inferior vena cava). Various improvements have been made in this regard, including partial ALPPS, replacing parenchymal transection with radiofrequency/microwave ablation, and tourniquet-ALPPS to separate left from right, giving birth to various modified procedures.

1.1.2.1 Partial ALPPS

A classical ALPPS involves complete transection of the liver parenchyma, preventing the formation of vascular collaterals between the left and right side and ensuring complete diversion of portal venous blood flow to the remnant liver. However, it poses some issues, including a large transection area and a completely ischemic segment IV. Complications after surgery are related to parenchymal transection, which can lead to bile leakage, adhesions, and necrosis caused by ischemic/reflux disorder. To address them, an early technical improvement was attempted to reduce such transection. In 2013, Henrik Petrowsky et al. [91] introduced a new strategy in their center, transitioning complete parenchymal transection to partial transection (only partition to the middle hepatic vein) in the first stage of the procedure. They found that this strategy could induce an FLR growth comparable to the classical way, with a significant decrease in postoperative complications and short-term mortality. This improvement in safety led to the establishment of partial ALPPS, as named by Henrik Petrowsky et al. [91] Concurrently, Fernando A. Alvarez et al. [92] also reported consistent findings of an FLR growth after partial ALPPS similar to complete transection, with significantly reduced complications. Comparative analysis and risk factor analysis for post-ALPPS complications showed that complete transection is an independent risk factor of postoperative complications [92]. Based on data from several major centers, partial ALPPS generates a similar FLR growth compared to classical ALPPS (50%–90%/7–15 days vs 59%–107%/6–17 days) and significantly lower rates of complications and mortality (overall complications 38.1%–60.9% vs 88.9%–90.9%, severe complications [Dindo-Clavien grade ≥ 3b] 0%–17% vs 30%–33%, 90-day mortality 0% vs 22%–27.3%) [91–95]. Nonetheless, it's worth noting that Henrik Petrowsky et al. included non-cirrhotic and non-cholestatic patients undergoing ALPPS [91, 92], and partial ALPPS in HCC patients with chronic liver disease showed different results. Albert Chan et al. [96] studied the application of partial ALPPS (50%–80% transection) in this patient population, showing contrasting findings: complete ALPPS induced larger and faster FLR growth (64.1%/7 days vs 43.1%/10.5 days), a lower severe complication rate (7.7% vs 25%), a lower 90-day mortality (0% vs 16.7%), and a shorter interval. In addition, after the second stage, patients in the complete ALPPS group recovered faster in their liver function and had lower rates of complication and mortality. Since FLR growth in patients with chronic liver disease is not as pronounced as that in those with normal livers, complete ALPPS is preferred for HCC patients with chronic liver disease to achieve optimal results [96]. Challenges of partial ALPPS are determining a sufficient transection and consequences of insufficient transection. Michael Linecker et al. conducted a dedicated study on this, revealing that at least 50% transection is needed to induce FLR regeneration comparable to complete ALPPS [93]. Insufficient transection can lead to inadequate FLR growth and prolonged waiting times [97]. Nagappan Kumar et al. [97] reported that partial ALPPS with 30%–40% liver parenchymal transection resulted in slow growth, with a median waiting time of 28 days and a median increase in liver volume of 38% (10–78%), much lower than classical ALPPS FLR growth (58–110% [57%]), and 25% of patients showed no significant growth (only 10–15%) [97]. One of the key elements of partial ALPPS is to preserve the middle hepatic vein, requiring protecting the outflow within or near the future transection line to ensure smooth blood flow and reduce complications related to the transection and ischemia/stasis of the liver segment [91]. In summary, for non-cirrhotic and non-cholestatic patients, partial ALPPS (transecting at least 50%) can induce FLR growth comparable to complete ALPPS (50–90%/7–15 days) while significantly improving safety (most centers report 0% 90-day mortality and 0–17% severe postoperative complication rate). The majority of centers recommend it as an alternative to classical ALPPS, making it the preferred option [91–95]. A decade-long review of ALPPS showed that partial ALPPS has become the most widely used modified procedure [41].

1.1.2.2 Tourniquet-ALPPS (T-ALPPS)

In 2011, Ricardo Robles Campos et al. [98] attempted to apply a tourniquet to block collateral circulation between the two lobes instead of liver parenchymal transection to induce FLR growth. Seven days postoperatively, FLR grew 150%, and the tumor was resected on postoperative day 10. The patient was followed up for 20 months and kept disease-free. Ricardo Robles Campos named this technique "Associating Liver Tourniquet and Portal Ligation for Staged Hepatectomy" (ALTPS), believing that this technique could reduce technical complexity and shorten the operation time of the first-stage surgery [98]. The technique was then expanded applications, and in 2014, R. Robles et al. [72] reported 22 cases of ALTPS surgery. Seven days postoperatively, FLR increased by 61%, with a complication rate of 63.6% (most commonly infectious fluid accumulation). The incidence of biliary complications after the second stage was 23%, and five patients experienced postoperative liver failure, resulting in a mortality of 9.1% (2/22) [72]. In 2014, Ricardo Robles Campos et al. reported further modifications to the ALTPS, termed sequential ALTPS. They combined ALTPS with delayed PVE for perihilar tumors, achieving a no-touch operation to reduce tumor spread. The sequential ALTPS involved tourniquet ligation in the first stage without portal vein ligation, followed by PVE on the fourth postoperative day. In 2019, Ricardo Robles Campos et al. [99] compared T-ALPPS and conventional TSH in 34 and 41 CRLM patients, respectively. T-ALPPS had a higher resection rate (100% vs 90.5%) and a superior volume increase (68% vs 39%) compared to TSH. There were no differences in the rates of postoperative complications and mortality. The median overall survival (OS) was 36 months and 41 months for T-ALPPS and TSH, respectively. The median disease-free survival (DFS) was 9 months for T-ALPPS and 16 months for TSH. The 1-, 3-, and 5-year OS for T-ALPPS were 76.2, 57.1, and 22.9%, while those for TSH were 81, 66.7, and 23.8%, respectively. Besides, the 1-, 3-, and 5-year DFS for T-ALPPS were 44.6, 11.1, and 11.1%, whereas those were 66.7, 9.5, and 5% for TSH, respectively. These results indicated that T-ALPPS produced results similar to TSH, making T-ALPPS a safe and effective alternative. Tourniquet-ALPPS for HCC is mainly practiced in China. In 2014, Cai Xiujun et al. [100] performed the first total laparoscopic T-ALPPS. They used a Flocare nasogastric tube composed of a guidewire for tourniquet ligation. The FLR was 35.6% before surgery and increased to 37.9% on day 10 postoperatively. No complications, such as bile leakage, occurred after the surgery. In 2015, Cai Xiujun et al. [101] summarized the results of T-ALPPS for 12 cases of hepatitis B-related HCC treated from May 2014 to June 2015. The tumor resection rate was 83.3%, and FLR growth was 28.1% on postoperative day 11. There were no postoperative bile leaks. Severe complication (≥IIIb) rates after the first and second stages were 25.0% and 40.0%, respectively [101]. Overall, the T-ALPPS method boasts many advantages and significantly reduces the occurrence of complications such as bile leaks. The tourniquet can encircle any section between the umbilical fissure plane and the Cantlie plane, but the surgical operation is more demanding, especially in laparoscopic T-ALPPS procedures. In addition to the method introduced by Cai Xiujun et al., [101] in 2022, Ciria et al. [102] from Spain also described the standard procedure for laparoscopic T-ALPPS, including hanging maneuver and Glisson transection technique. Limitations pronounce when the tumor is adjacent to the inferior vena cava (IVC), rendering it impossible to either establish an IVC tunnel or to hang the liver to perform the procedure.

1.1.2.3 Radiofrequency-Assisted ALPPS (RALPPS)

In 2014, Tamara M. H. Gall et al. [103] used radiofrequency ablation (RFA) in the first stage to create a bloodless coagulation zone, separating tumor and healthy liver tissue, replacing the classical parenchymal transection. This technique was named Radiofrequency-assisted ALPPS (RALPPS). The original intention of this technique was to overcome the high incidence of ALPPS-associated bile leakage while reducing other complications and mortality rates. RALPPS was initially applied in 5 patients with CRLM, achieving an FLR growth of 62.3%, 0 bile leakage, 0 death, and an overall complication rate of 20.0%. Compared to classical ALPPS, the incidence of postoperative complications and mortality was significantly lower [103]. Subsequently, the center conducted a randomized controlled trial (REBIRTH Trial) to further compare RALPPS and PVE-TSH. Results showed that RALPPS had superior outcomes in curative resection compared to PVE (the tumor resection rate was 92.3% vs 66.6%; the R0 resection rate was 75.0% vs 68.7%). FLR induction was better in RALPPS compared to PVE (80.7%/20 days vs 18.4%/35 days). No bile leakage was observed in the RALPPS group. There were no significant differences in complications (53.8% vs 66.7%) or 90-day mortality (3.8% vs 0%). This trial indicated that, compared to PVE, RALPPS was superior in FLR induction and R0 tumor resection, with no significant increase in complications and mortality rates [104]. Compared to conventional ALPPS in other studies (e.g., FLR growth of 68.0% in the LIGRO-RCT study [105]), FLR growth in the RALPPS group was similar but required a longer waiting time. The RALPPS study reported by Tamara M. H. Gall was associated with CRLM. The implementation of RALPPS for HCC is mainly conducted in China. Ma Kuansheng et al. systematically evaluated the safety and efficacy of RALPPS in this population. In 2016, they reported that RALPPS could achieve good results in HCC patients with liver fibrosis/cirrhosis [106]. FLR growth was 53% at 28 days, and the incidence of severe complications (Clavien-Dindo ≥IIIb) was 20%. There were no bile leaks, abdominal infections, or PHLF after the first and second stages, and the 90-day mortality rate was 10%. This suggests that in well-selected cirrhotic HCC patients with good liver function, RALPPS can achieve a satisfactory increase in FLR, albeit at the cost of a longer waiting time. RALPPS has potential advantages in eliminating severe complications associated with classical ALPPS, such as bile leakage and PHLF. Furthermore, Ma Kuansheng et al. found that in cirrhotic HCC patients with insufficient FLR growth after RALPPS, additional RFA or percutaneous ethanol injection (PEI) could further stimulate FLR increase. They proposed a salvage treatment plan for insufficient FLR growth after the first stage of RALPPS: Salvage RFA (if FLR is still insufficient 2–3 weeks after the first stage, perform percutaneous ultrasound-guided RFA/PEI to further stimulate FLR increase) [107]. In 2021, they reported the results of salvage RFA treatment in 7 cases with insufficient FLR growth after the first stage of RALPPS. FLR growth was reactivated (the highest Kinetic Growth Rate (KGR) in the first week of the first stage of RALPPS was 10%, dropping to 1.5% in the second week; after salvage RFA/PEI, KGR significantly increased to 4%). Among them, five patients successfully completed the stage 2 operation, and two patients failed, resulting in a salvage success rate of 71.4%. Except for one death after stage 2 RALPPS operation, the remaining six patients had no severe complications (Clavien-Dindo ≥IIIb) [107]. One major drawback of applying RALPPS in HCC is the longer waiting time. A systematic review by Junwei Zhang et al. showed that the average interval for RALPPS in HCC patients was 28 days, compared to an average of

11.2 days for standard ALPPS [108]. The role of RALPPS in HCC, especially its long-term effects, requires further research and evaluation.

1.1.2.4 Microwave Ablation-Assisted ALPPS

Similar to radiofrequency, Microwave Ablation (MWA) treats liver tumors by generating coagulative necrosis using electromagnetic microwaves. Its advantages lie in a wider action range, a stronger intensity, and a faster effect. In 2013, Enrico Gringeri and Riccardo Boetto introduced Laparoscopic Microwave Ablation-assisted ALPPS (LAPS) for the first time at the Italian Surgical Society video conference. Two years later, they formally reported on LAPS in HCC patients, inducing an FLR growth of 77.7% in 10 days, with minimal adhesion formation postoperatively and only mild complications (fever and mild ascites). LAPS was considered easier and faster than traditional ALPPS, reducing bile leakage, abdominal infections, and intraperitoneal adhesions, enabling quicker postoperative recovery, and a better safety profile [109]. In 2015, Umberto Cillo et al. [110] reported total laparoscopic Microwave ALPPS, showing a 90.4% increase in FLR on the ninth postoperative day with no complications. In 2016, Ugo Boggi et al. [111] also reported the application of LAPS in PHCC. Chen et al. [112] compared the safety and efficacy of laparoscopic microwave ablation and portal vein ligation for staged hepatectomy (LAPS, $n = 9$) and classical ALPPS ($n = 9$) in the treatment of HBV-related HCC. The two groups revealed a similar resection rate (88.9% vs 88.9%). The hypertrophy rate of FLR induced by classic ALPPS tended to be more rapid than that induced by LAPS. The 2-year recurrence-free survival was 0% for ALPPS and 35.7% for LAPS, whereas the 2-year overall survival for ALPPS and LAPS was 33.3 and 100.0%, respectively. The study showed that LAPS tended to induce lower morbidity and FLR hypertrophy more slowly than ALPPS, with a comparable resection rate and better long-term RFS. LAPS is currently not widely used. It was mainly reported in individual cases, and its effectiveness remains undetermined.

In summary, RFA-assisted ALPPS and MWA-assisted ALPPS use radiofrequency and microwave techniques to replace liver parenchymal transection, reducing surgical time, minimizing intraoperative blood loss, and lowering the risk of postoperative bile leakage and abdominal infections. It enhances the safety of the stage 2 operation to some extent. Nevertheless, there are several drawbacks, including weaker FLR induction, longer waiting times, a certain failure rate in HCC patients with chronic liver disease, difficulty in precise ablation, a large damage range caused by heat radiation to liver tissues, potential occupation of a significant portion of FLR parenchyma by the ablation zone when not targeting liver tumors, a threat to FLR liver ducts, and a heavier postoperative inflammatory stress response. Further research and evaluation are still needed.

1.1.3 Improvements in Portal Vein Ligation (PVL)

Typically, PVL in a classic ALPPS requires anatomical dissection of the hepatic hilum, which can lead to postoperative adhesions, affecting the second-stage surgery. For tumors involving the hepatic hilum (including PHCC and gallbladder cancer, GBC) or structures near it, dissection of the hepatic hilum violates the "no-touch" principle during the first stage, and it is not advisable. Additionally, when tumors invade the right hepatic pedicle, the right portal vein branch may not be feasible or suitable for dissection ligation. These challenges prompted some surgeons to substitute PVL with PVE to block the portal vein on the tumor side.

PVE renders dissection of the hepatic hilum unnecessary, avoiding dividing portal vein vessels. This approach not only prevents damage to arteries, bile ducts, and other structures, aligning with the "no-touch" principle for perihilar tumors but also minimizes or prevents local adhesions, reducing the adverse effects of the first-stage surgery to the maximum extent. Several techniques have been adopted, differing by the timing and method of PVE, categorized as intraoperative (Mini-ALPPS, combining with anterior approach and partial parenchymal dissection) [75] and postoperative (Hybrid ALPPS) [113]. PVE is commonly performed percutaneously through liver puncture, with interventionists accessing the FLR side into the tumor-side portal vein for embolization (as piercing through the tumor side is often challenging to bypass the tumor). However, this technique has a drawback as it may damage portal vessels of FLR and lead to complications such as bleeding and portal vein thrombosis, especially in cases with a history of tumor resection in FLR.

During intraoperative PVE, punctures can be made through the colonic veins or the inferior mesenteric vein [114, 115]. PVE is typically done with other modifications, such as liver parenchymal transection improvement (details are elaborated in the following section on combined improvements), rather than being exercised alone. This type of surgery, integrating surgical liver transection and interventional PVE, is usually performed by surgeons for parenchymal transection and interventionists for PVE. Since it is jointly performed by physicians from two disciplines, like other hybrid surgeries, this intraoperative procedure is referred to as "Hybrid ALPPS" in this book. It minimizes the impact of the first stage to facilitate rapid patient recovery, reserving the main surgical process for the second stage. Comparatively, postoperative PVE requires less equipment and personnel. The timing of PVE in clinical practice should be determined case-by-case [116]. Hybrid ALPPS is particularly suitable for perihilar tumors like PHCC and GBC, showing the potential to reduce high postoperative complications and mortality rates in ALPPS for biliary tumors.

1.1.4 Improvements in Surgical Approach

Anterior approaches and minimally invasive techniques have been applied early in ALPPS to reduce the invasiveness of the first-stage surgery, decrease postoperative complications and mortality rates, and enhance overall safety.

1.1.4.1 Anterior Approach

The anterior approach is a standard technique in general liver surgery, aiming to reduce liver and tumor mobilization during the first stage while adhering more closely to the "no-touch" principle. In 2014, based on experiences in resecting large liver tumors, Albert Chan et al. [76] introduced this approach in ALPPS. During the first stage, moderate dissection was performed at the hepatic hilum, and after ligation of the right portal vein branches, a Cavitron Ultrasonic Surgical Aspirator (CUSA) was used for in situ parenchymal transection. Ligaments on the tumor side were not detached, and no plastic bag was used for wrapping the tumor-side liver. The initial report on two cases (one hepatoblastoma, one hepatitis B-related HCC) showed minimal intra-abdominal adhesions during the second stage operation on postoperative day 10 after the first stage surgery), enabling smooth tumor resection after minimal dissection of the hepatic hilum structures, with no occurrence of bile leakage [76].

Data from the ALPPS registry in 2014 indicated that 37% (66/175) of patients underwent the anterior approach during the first stage of ALPPS (with 31% of patients having large primary liver cancers and 38% having CRLM using this approach) [74]. Approximately half of the ALPPS procedures performed at Buenos Aires, Argentina, and the University Hospital of Zurich, Switzerland, utilized the anterior approach [74]. In 2016, Albert Chan et al. [117] reported the outcomes of anterior approach ALPPS in 17 patients with hepatitis B-related HCC. Six days postoperatively, FLR increased by 48.7%, the tumor resection rate was 100%, and no significant adhesions were observed. Chan injected methylene blue to rigorously detect bile leakage, resulting in 0 cases of this complication. The rate of complications (Clavien-Dindo ≥III) was 11.8%, with an in-hospital mortality rate of 5.9%. Anterior approach ALPPS effectively induces liver hypertrophy in patients with chronic liver disease simplifies the ALPPS procedure, reduces adhesion formation, and demonstrates a comparable safety profile with other established approaches. Currently, this approach has gained widespread use, securing its role in the combined improvements of ALPPS [41]. However, it is essential to note that not all patients, especially those with CRLM, necessitate the approach.

1.1.4.2 Laparoscopic/Robotic-Assisted ALPPS (Laparoscopic/Robotic ALPPS)

Minimally invasive techniques have been employed to reduce surgical trauma, intra-abdominal adhesions, postoperative complications, and achieve better short-term postoperative outcomes [118–122]. Thanks to the potential advantages of minimizing complications and mortality, minimally invasive surgery (MIS) was introduced early in ALPPS to enhance its safety.

In 2012, Marcel Autran C Machado et al. [123] first reported laparoscopic ALPPS for CRLM. Results showed mild postoperative intra-abdominal adhesions, reduced difficulty in the second stage, and improved surgical safety [123]. Similar results were demonstrated in Claudius Conrad's study [124]. Subsequently, this technique became more widely used in major liver centers worldwide. In 2017, Marcel Autran C Machado et al. [85] pooled laparoscopic ALPPS cases and compared them with contemporaneous open ALPPS. Besides having a shorter length of stay (LOS, 11 days vs 14 days), the laparoscopic group also incurred no deaths or severe complications, while the open group had a 5% postoperative mortality rate and a 50% severe complication rate. Currently, laparoscopic techniques are increasingly applied to ALPPS [41], almost becoming a fundamental modification of ALPPS. The most common approach involves laparoscopic parenchymal transection and PVL during the first stage (Laparoscopic stage 1 ALPPS), followed by open surgery in the second stage. Fully laparoscopic ALPPS, where both stages are performed laparoscopically, is gaining momentum.

In 2019, Kawka Michal et al. [125] analyzed 1088 open ALPPS cases and 46 MIS-ALPPS cases. The latter group had a shorter between-stage interval than the former (10.3 days vs 20.1 days). MIS-ALPPS induced a higher rate of FLR hypertrophy (81.00% vs 74.49%) and a higher tumor resection rate (100% vs 98.5%). In addition, it showed a lower rate of severe complications after stage 1 operation, significantly reduced 90-day mortality (0% vs 8.45%), complication rate (0% vs 11%), bile leak rate after stage 1 operation (0% vs 4.7%), and PHLF rate after stage 2 surgery (0% vs 13.6%). The total LOS was reduced by 4.2 days in the MIS-ALPPS group (15.3 days vs 19.5 days). Although this report suggests that MIS-ALPPS may have lower complication and mortality rates and faster recovery, it is important to note that baseline characteristics were not balanced between the two groups; for example, the proportion of extended right hepatectomies was higher in the open ALPPS group (62.92% vs 38.64%) [125].

In a multicenter study in Italy in 2020, the MIS-ALPPS group had a significantly higher discharge rate after stage 1 operation compared to the open ALPPS group (78.6% vs 9.6%). After stage 2 operation, the major complication rate was 8.3% in the former group and 28.6% in the latter group. Incurring no death, MIS-ALPPS showed a significantly shorter LOS (12 days vs 22 days) [126]. The following study [127] analyzed the 268 ALPPS performed within 17 centers in Italy between 2012 and 2021. The national study showed an increased use of MIS techniques over the years and lower 90-day mortality. In 2021, Stefanie Guhra et al. [128] analyzed 510 CRLM patients from 22 ALPPS centers in the ALPPS registry from 2009 to 2019. They found that since 2015, an increasing number of patients received MIS in the first stage, leading to a significant reduction in complications after stage 2 [128]. A review of 119 mini-invasive ALPPS cases from 6 series also showed that mini-invasive ALPPS appears to be a feasible and safe procedure, with potentially better short-term outcomes in terms of blood loss, morbidity, and mortality rate if compared with those of open series [129]. Current research indicates that MIS-ALPPS reduces postoperative complications and mortality, showing promising results. However, it is crucial to note that reliable evidence regarding MIS-ALPPS is still limited. ALPPS is often used for resecting large or complex tumors (especially primary liver cancer and biliary tumors). Laparoscopic ALPPS is typically chosen for smaller, simpler tumors, while the indications for open ALPPS are much broader. Differences between participants in the study groups may lead to selection biases, thereby affecting the interpretation of comparative results. Therefore, higher-quality comparative studies, particularly randomized controlled trials (RCTs), are needed for a reliable assessment of MIS-ALPPS versus open ALPPS.

Trends towards greater use of the robotic platform are occurring in abdominal surgery. Robots are superior to conventional laparoscopy in complex fine operations such as biliary-enteric anastomosis (BEA) and vascular reconstruction. Conventional laparoscopic surgery loses the advantage of multidimensional and omnidirectional operation in open surgery due to trocar limitations, limiting the flexibility of surgeons. Nevertheless, robots can simulate manual operations to a significant extent, overcoming such limitations. In the future, robots are expected better to simulate the delicate dexterity of hands and arms and further enhance the advantages of surgeons. With technological advancement, including artificial intelligence (AI), procedures will become smarter. In 2013, Evgeny Solomonov et al. [130] reported robotic ALPPS for a 68-year-old male with right lobe HCC. Both stages of the surgery were completed with robotic assistance, and the patient recovered rapidly. In October 2014, the liver surgery team of Zhongshan Hospital, Fudan University, performed the first robotic ALPPS in Asia [131] for an HCC with portal vein tumor thrombus (PVTT), which could not be removed by traditional liver surgery. The patient has survived tumor-free for nearly 10 years postoperatively. Currently, the application of robots in ALPPS remains limited, mainly due to the scarcity of robotic resources. The high cost restricts its use to large centers and certain hepatobiliary surgeons. Additionally, conventional laparoscopy is sufficient for some MIS-ALPPS. In the early years, there was no significant difference between robotic-assisted ALPPS and conventional laparoscopic ALPPS. These factors hamper the spread of robotic ALPPS. In recent years, with the gradual popularization and updates of robotic technology, reports of stage 1 robotic-assisted ALPPS and fully robotic-assisted ALPPS (both stages performed with robotic assistance) have increased, covering various indications, including CRLM [132], HCC [133–135], intrahepatic cholangiocarcinoma (ICC) [136], and PHCC [137]. Guidetti et al. [138] reported the first study comparing full robotic ALPPS with open ALPPS. The bicentric study included open ALPPS cases from the University Hospital Zurich, Switzerland and robotic ALPPS cases from the University of Modena and Reggio Emilia, Italy from January 2015 to July 2022. The study showed that robotic ALPPS was safe and was associated with improved perioperative outcomes compared to open ALPPS in an experienced robotic center. The robotic ALPPS offers distinct advantages over the open approach, such as reduced blood loss during both ALPPS stages as well as a higher rate of inter-stage discharge, except it required a longer operation time. The surgical morbidity and mortality were comparable for the robotic ALPPS and open ALPPS. The postoperative outcomes of robotic ALPPS was similar with open ALPPS. Reports indicate that robotic ALPPS is safe and feasible, with reduced postoperative complication and mortality rates.

Nonetheless, there are still few reports on robotic ALPPS, and more research and analysis are needed. It is foreseeable that, in the near future, with the popularization, cost reduction, and miniaturization of robots, and the integration of AI, robotic ALPPS will be more widely used, especially in surgeries that require complex ductal reconstructions.

1.1.5 Combined Modifications

With the continuous improvements in ALPPS techniques and mutual exchanges of such advancement, the focus of technical enhancements has shifted from unilateral modifications (such as using radiofrequency ablation instead of liver parenchymal transection) to the combined application of various modification techniques. Liver parenchymal transection, PVE, and approach improvements are often combined to achieve optimal effects, minimize postoperative complications and mortality, and enhance safety. The most common combination includes laparoscopy, anterior approach, partial liver parenchymal transection, and PVE instead of PVL. Other fundamental technical improvements, such as rigorous bile leak detection, avoiding right hepatic duct ligation, and using absorbable hemostatic materials instead of plastic bags, are retained as basic components in every ALPPS procedure.

Most combinations were reported in Hybrid ALPPS and Mini-ALPPS [139]. Hybrid ALPPS, initially introduced by Li Jun et al., [113] has undergone continuous iteration, leading to new modified procedures. For instance, partial liver parenchymal transection is used instead of complete liver parenchymal transection, giving birth to hybrid partial ALPPS [116]. If the first stage is performed through laparoscopy, it is called laparoscopic hybrid partial ALPPS [140]. Hybrid ALPPS has the advantage of "no-touch" at the liver hilum, making it particularly suitable for tumors involving the liver hilum and/or the IVC, where PVL and liver mobilization are not feasible. Some scholars have taken further steps in combined modifications to avoid an open abdominal procedure in the first stage. Currently, the majority of ALPPS procedures require an abdominal operation (open or laparoscopic) in the first stage, subjecting patients to physiological and psychological stress associated with the surgery and general anesthesia. To avoid such procedures in the first stage, Hong Defei et al. used percutaneous microwave ablation (PMA) instead of open or laparoscopic liver parenchymal transection, combined with PVE instead of PVL, to mitigate the pain associated with the first-stage abdominal procedure. This new procedure is named percutaneous microwave ablation liver partition and portal vein embolization (PALPP) [141]. During the surgery, ultrasound-guided PMA is performed along the pre-cut surface, creating a necrotic groove from the inferior to the superior veins of the liver. PVE is then performed 3 days after PMA, leading to a 41.2% increase in FLR 10 days after embolization. On the 14th day after PVE, right trisegmentectomy and tumor resection in segment III are performed. In doing so, there is minimal intra-abdominal adhesion and no complications such as bile leak and PHLF postoperatively [141]. Alessandro Lunardi et al. reported a strategy similar to PALPP where PVE is performed first, and after 21 days, liver parenchymal transection is carried out through microwave ablation. From 2015 to 2016, three patients underwent this procedure. FLR increased by 68% to 109%, and postoperative recovery was rapid. All patients were able to stand and walk within 5 h after surgery, and the ECOG performance status remained stable between 1 and 2. No severe complications or deaths within 90 days were reported postoperatively [142].

Advancements in ALPPS surgical technique have significantly enhanced the safety of the procedure. Currently, modified procedures constitute more than 50% of all ALPPS procedures, with most centers adopting these improved techniques to varying extents [41]. Many centers have independently developed and implemented modified procedures as alternatives to the classical ALPPS, reducing complications and mortality rates. Beyond single-center data, a decade-long ALPPS registry coupled with a large-scale longitudinal analysis reveals a notable improvement in the safety of ALPPS. The 90-day mortality rate has decreased, thanks to the adoption of less invasive modified ALPPS, and surgical technique modification was independently correlated with the reduction of 90-day postoperative mortality [41].

Since the initial report of ALPPS, a plethora of modified procedures has emerged, giving rise to various ALPPS variants and introducing new terminologies. This diversity has posed challenges in conducting empirical comparisons. In February 2015, during the first expert meeting held in Hamburg, a recommendation was made to establish a universal nomenclature for these variants. Subsequently, the ALPPS registry reviewed literature related to ALPPS and the registry data, proposing a logical naming system that was submitted to the 209 centers in the registry for consensus and published in the *Annals of Surgery* [45]. The new naming system is expected to facilitate better comparisons of various ALPPS variants and promote continuous development.

1.2 Case Selection

During the initial establishment of ALPPS, hepatobiliary surgeons were enthusiastic due to its unprecedented FLR induction efficiency and high tumor resection rate. Yet some centers reported high complication and mortality rates, while others demonstrated excellent outcomes with zero death (complication rates ranging from 53 to 90% and mortality rates from 0 to 28.7%) [19, 65, 70]. The intra-center differences in patient indications and inter-center disparities in mortality and complication suggested that this procedure may not fit all. Some scholars recognized this early on and implemented case selection criteria. For instance, as early as 2014, Paulo Herman et al. [143] found that better patient selection led to improved outcomes. Important risk factors included tumor type, age, and patient's general condition. In its application of ALPPS, the center exclusively included young CRLM patients with an average age of 57 and good performance status, bringing about zero mortality and a complication rate of only 28.5% [143].

In centers with stringent case selection, zero mortality rates have been consistently reported, whereas in those without, higher rates of postoperative complications and death ensued. In 2016, 12 Italian centers reported 50 cases of ALPPS between 2012 and 2014; 20% died, and 54% suffered from severe complications. A high proportion of these patients had biliary tumors (8 ICC/11 PHCC/1 GBC), resulting in a post-ALPPS mortality rate of 40% for this indication (10% after stage 1 and 30% after stage 2). Further analysis indicated associations between postoperative 90-day mortality and biliary cancer, as well as an inter-stage peak bilirubin

>5 mg/dL. Therefore, the authors suggested suspending ALPPS for biliary cancers and terminating ALPPS in patients with elevated bilirubin during the interval [144]. Single-center data has limitations, and in the analysis of case selection, the ALPPS registry played a crucial role, making significant contributions. With the expansion of ALPPS, cases accumulated rapidly in the registry, making more reliable results possible. In 2014, the first pooled analysis of 202 ALPPS cases registered between October 2012 and December 2013 was conducted on ALPPS's safety and oncological survival [49]. The results showed a 9% mortality rate and a 27% rate of severe complications. Multivariate regression analysis identified age over 60, non-CRLM tumors, operation time of ALPPS stage 1 exceeding 300 min, and intraoperative transfusions as independent risk factors for severe complications and death. The 90-day mortality rate for CRLM patients under 60 was similar to traditional two-stage hepatectomy [49].

In 2015, with 320 accumulated cases, the ALPPS registry updated its analysis, revealing an 8.8% 90-day mortality rate. The risk factors for complications and death identified in the initial 2014 analysis held water. Additionally, liver failure after stage 1 and a MELD score > 10 before stage 2 were identified as independent predictors [50]. These safety-related factors after ALPPS were rapidly utilized to identify high-risk populations and guide surgeons in selecting appropriate candidates for ALPPS, as well as determining when or whether to perform the second-stage surgery. In the first international ALPPS consensus meeting in Hamburg in 2015, experts concluded that high complication and mortality rates in ALPPS were correlated with inappropriate case selection, proposing recommendations accordingly [145]. In 2016, the ALPPS registry further updated the analysis of adverse outcomes after ALPPS (528 patients from 38 centers) and developed two risk models, quantifying risks of short-term mortality before stage 1 and stage 2 operations [46]. The results showed a 9% short-term mortality rate. Independent predictors of short-term mortality after surgery included age $\geq$ 67 years, biliary tumors, severe complications after stage 1 operation, and elevated serum bilirubin or creatinine before stage 2. According to the pre-stage 1 model, in which age and tumor type were included as variables, 90-day mortality rates were 2.7, 4.9, 8.6, 15, 24, and 37% for scores of 0, 1, 2, 3, 4, and 5, respectively. The pre-stage 2 model included severe complications after stage 1 ($\geq$grade 3b), increased serum bilirubin, elevated serum creatinine, and cumulative pre-stage 1 risk score. In this model, 90-day mortality rates for patients with pre-stage 2 model scores of 3.9, 4.7, 5.5, and 6.9 were 5, 10, 20, and 50%, respectively [46]. Subsequently, the ALPPS registry validated the models using accumulated cases and external cohorts, confirming that age and indications remained the most critical factors in patient selection. In 2017, the ALPPS registry released a 10-year retrospective analysis, showing a significant change in case selection, shifting towards younger patients, more CRLM, and fewer biliary tumors. Adjustments in age and tumor indications reduced postoperative mortality and complication rates. Patient selection significantly impacted ALPPS safety (especially 90-day mortality and severe complications) and was identified as a key factor in improving surgical outcomes and an independent risk factor [41]. Some single-center studies also demonstrated that careful patient selection and specific surgical techniques can reduce ALPPS-associated complications and mortality rates [146].

Other risk factors were studied and included in the case selection criteria. Simultaneous ALPPS and colorectal cancer resection had a high 90-day mortality rate (15%), thus was recommended against by Kerollos Nashat Wanis et al. [52] Analysis from the ALPPS registry reported by Pierre-Alain Clavien in 2019 also indicated that concurrent colorectal liver resection was one of the risk factors [147]. Data from our center also demonstrated an association between simultaneous resection and adverse postoperative outcomes [148]. Nevertheless, inconsistent results were found in the then-largest ALPPS registry cohort (over 500 CRLM cases) in 2020 by Henrik Petrowsky et al. [149] In this analysis, resection of the primary colorectal lesion during the stage 1 surgery did not increase perioperative mortality [149]. Thus, the debate over simultaneous resection continues.

After years of development and application of ALPPS in various scenarios, along with repeated validation through different centers and the extensive data of the ALPPS registry, factors related to adverse outcomes after ALPPS have been largely identified. ALPPS cases can now be finely categorized into low-risk and high-risk patients.

In 2019, Pierre-Alain Clavien et al. [148] defined "low-risk patients" for the first time based on existing studies: CRLM patients under 67 years old without concurrent abdominal surgery who were operated in centers that have completed more than 30 ALPPS procedures. Surgical outcomes in those meeting all four criteria were comparable with patients undergoing other types of extensive liver resections. Compared to the high-risk group (non-CRLM patients over 67 years old whose surgeries were performed in low-volume centers with fewer than 30 ALPPS cases), the low-risk group had significantly lower rates of severe complications and 90-day mortality [148], yet it should be noted that the currently defined "low-risk ALPPS patients" constitute only 12% of the total ALPPS cases (120 out of 1036) who are underrepresented by this group alone. Although generally, most ALPPS patients benefit [148]. Capobianco et al. [150] developed a novel Comprehensive ALPPS Preoperative Risk Assessment (CAPRA) score. The multi-centric study analyzed whether comorbidities and patients characteristics are a risk factor in 451 ALPPS performed in 13 high-volume centers and created a score predicting 90-day mortality preoperatively. The study revealed that comorbidities play an important role in ALPPS and should be carefully considered when planning the procedure. The novel CAPRA score is calculated based on the following formula: (0.1 × age)—(2 × BSA) + 1 (in the presence of primary liver tumor) + 1 (in the presence of severe cardiovascular disease) + 2 (in the presence of moderate or severe diabetes) + 2 (in the presence of renal disease) + 2 (if classic ALPPS is planned). The predictive ability was 0.837 for the CAPRA score, 0.443 for Charlson Comorbidity Index (CCI), 0.519 for age-adjusted CCI (aCCI), 0.693 for ALPPS-RS1 and 0.807 for ALPPS-RS2. The CAPRA score showed a very good ability to predict postoperative mortality. Overall, case selection has made significant progress and has identified several risk factors for adverse outcomes after ALPPS surgery, providing substantial guidance for ALPPS case selection [42, 49, 50, 53, 61]. In 2017, the ALPPS registry's 10-year longitudinal retrospective analysis showed that case selection significantly improved the safety of ALPPS, proving to be a key factor in enhancing surgical outcomes and an independent risk factor [41]. Despite this progress, there is still a lack of robust tools to quantify individual postoperative adverse outcomes of ALPPS, and more research is needed.

1.3 Inter-stage Management in ALPPS Procedure

The importance of inter-stage management is increasingly emphasized, and with the growing body of research, the significance of a smooth inter-stage process has been repeatedly confirmed. The inter-stage course, spanning the two stages of the ALPPS procedure, plays a crucial role in determining ALPPS outcomes [46, 50, 61]. Therefore, this section is dedicated to addressing inter-stage management, which includes routine postoperative care and the decision-making process for the timing of the stage 2 surgery. Routine postoperative management aligns with that of other liver resection procedures and will not be reiterated here. A critical aspect of inter-stage management is the decision-making process for the timing of the stage-2 surgery, involving risk factor prediction and accurate assessment of FLR liver function:

1.3.1 Risk Factor Prediction

Medical teams determine whether to delay or even refuse the second-stage ALPPS surgery based on known risk factors. Stéphanie C. Truant et al. [61] analyzed 62 ALPPS procedures performed between April 2011 and September 2013 in 9 centers in France and Belgium. The results highlighted the vital role of the inter-stage course in determining ALPPS outcomes, with a 35.7% mortality rate after the stage 2 operation. Factors associated with mortality included obesity, bile leakage or ascites after stage 1, and intra-abdominal fluid infection after stage 2. The initial safety analysis by the ALPPS registry in 2014 [49] indicated that the duration of the stage 1 surgery and intraoperative transfusions were factors related to adverse outcomes after stage 2. In the 2015 update by the ALPPS registry [50] involving 320 cases, on top of the two aforementioned factors, PHLF after stage 1 and a Model for End-Stage Liver Disease (MELD) score exceeding 10 were also identified as risk factors. The mortality rate for patients meeting the International Study Group of Liver Surgery (ISGLS) criteria for PHLF after stage 1 was 20%, and that for patients with a pre-stage 2 MELD score exceeding 10 was 22% [50]. In 2016, Michael Linecker et al. [46] conducted an analysis of adverse outcome-related factors in 528 ALPPS patients from 38 centers, establishing a risk prediction model. This model was subsequently validated in 2018 with a new cohort of 258 cases [151]. The study revealed that major complications occurring after stage 1 and elevated serum bilirubin or creatinine before stage 2 were independent risk factors of 90-day mortality after stage 2 ALPPS. Additionally, pre-stage 1 risk factors (including age 67 or above and tumor type such as biliary tumors) were also identified as independent risk factors of mortality after the stage 2 surgery [46].

1.3.2 Precise Assessment of FLR Reserve Function

During inter-stage management, one of the most crucial aspects is the precise evaluation of the FLR function. The majority of postoperative deaths occur after stage 2, with PHLF being the primary cause [49, 50, 152]. Despite adjustments in surgical techniques and case selection, PHLF remains the most significant complication and the major culprit of death following ALPPS [152]. A 10-year longitudinal retrospective analysis of ALPPS procedures demonstrated that the causes of death did not significantly change over time, with PHLF continuing to be the primary reason for postoperative mortality [41].

Early observations indicated that, despite sufficient volumetric growth of the FLR before stage 2, many patients still experienced PHLF after the stage 2 operation. Subsequent practice repeatedly confirmed this phenomenon. Even in low-risk patients most suitable for ALPPS (CRLM patients aged <67 years without concurrent surgeries whose procedures were performed at centers with >30 ALPPS experiences), 5% of them experienced PHLF despite adequate physical volumetric FLR [147]. Subsequent functional studies, particularly those applying hepatobiliary scintigraphy (HBS), revealed that liver volume growth may not translate into functional gain [153]. Research indicated that FLR function did not increase in phase with physical volume, with the former growing at only about 50% of the latter [152, 154–161]. The volumetric method often overestimates liver function, and when volume regeneration outpaces function regain, it can impact the accurate timing of the stage 2 surgery. Thus, it is recommended that, in addition to achieve the required physical volume of FLR, its functional assessment should also be performed. The stage 2 surgery should only proceed when the reserve is sufficient [152].

Unfortunately, there is currently no precise method to accurately detect FLR function, and no consensus has been achieved on reliable indicators. Traditional assessments of liver functional reserve, such as indocyanine green retention rate at 15 min (ICG-R15), test the function of the entire liver (including FLR and the tumor-side liver) and do not provide information about FLR function. To date, only a few tools are available. Among them, HBS remains the preferred test because it can selectively evaluate the function of FLR [152]. In 2010, the Amsterdam group in the Netherlands used dynamic ^{99m}Tc-mebrofenin HBS to quantify FLR function. They established a marker excretion value of 2.69% min/m^2 as a safety threshold (also known as the "Amsterdam index") for predicting PHLF after extensive liver resection [162]. Patients with an FLR function below this threshold were at high risk of developing PHLF after extensive hepatectomy [162]. Fadi Rassam et al. [94] reported a significant decrease in the incidence of PHLF after the introduction of HBS functional assessment at their center since 2012. According to Kasia P Cieslak et al. [158] and Fadi Rassam et al., [94] this index can be used to assess whether the FLR is sufficient after ALPPS. Patients meeting the criteria of this index had no PHLF or death after surgery. In 2012, the Buenos Aires group established a new HBS index, the "Hospital Italiano de Buenos Aires (HIBA) index," which used dynamic planar acquisition combined with single-photon emission computed tomography (SPECT). Patients with a cut-off value <15% had an 80% risk of developing PHLF, while the others did not experience PHLF [163].

In addition to HBS functional detection, another indicator, the FLR kinetic growth rate (KGR-FLR), can also be used to predict stage 2 PHLF. Patryk Kambakamba et al. [164] from the University of Zurich in Switzerland found that a KGR > 6% per day was significantly associated with a reduced risk of PHLF, and the occurrence of PHLF was 0% in patients who met both FLR/TLV > 30% and KGR > 6% per day. However, it is important to note that the measurement time for KGR is crucial, as livers grow in a non-linear manner. The interval for assessment is vital, and the value of KGR-FLR is related to the initial FLR size before surgery.

Additionally, some other indicators and methods have been proposed: (a) Intraoperative Measurement of Portal Venous Hemodynamics: Albert Chan et al. from the University of Hong Kong reported that intraoperative measurement of portal venous hemodynamics can better assess the risk of PHLF and may offer the opportunity for flow regulation (e.g., splenic artery ligation if necessary) [117]. (b) Intraoperative indocyanine green (ICG) Measurement: Academician Wan Yee Lau [165] reported that intraoperative ICG clearance can directly assess the actual FLR function. It is suggested that the ICG clearance rate be used to determine resectability during ALPPS [166].

At present, more evidence shows that measuring only FLR and standard liver volume is insufficient to avoid PHLF. Before stage 2 surgery, functional testing of FLR should be performed [95, 160]. For many centers, local liver function assessment is far from universally applicable and clinically accessible, as it involves special drugs, and many centers are not well-equipped. The safe threshold for HBS remains controversial and requires multicenter large-sample validation, such as the Amsterdam index and HIBA index, before reaching a consensus [162, 163]. Moreover, not all detection methods fit all patients. For example, HBS testing is not suitable for patients with high bilirubin [94]; intraoperative ICG testing requires accessing the abdominal cavity to clamp the tumor-side artery. A complete block of the blood flow to the tumor side liver is a prerequisite for accurate detection.

Through unremitting efforts of hepatobiliary surgeons worldwide, great strides have been made in the technique, case selection adjustments, and reinforced intraoperative management of ALPPS since its early implementation, leading to substantial improvements in safety. The 10-year retrospective data from the ALPPS registry indicate a marked reduction in postoperative severe complications and 90-day mortality rates, now lowered to levels equivalent to massive liver resections [41]. Over time, the 90-day mortality rate decreased significantly from 17% in the early years to 4% in 2015. The percentage of patients suffering from major interstage complications decreased from 10 to 3%. A summary by Kerollos N Wanis et al., [166] covering 500 cases from 17 high-volume centers that adopted ALPPS early between 2012 and 2018, showed a decrease in both 90-day mortality and complication rates with time, indicating increased safety. Despite some variations among centers, almost all centers (except two out of 17) demonstrated the same trend. Other reports and systematic analyses also show consistent results, revealing a significant improvement in ALPPS outcomes thanks to patient selection and advancements in ALPPS technique. Its safety has now reached the level equivalent to major liver surgeries [44, 167]. This development marks a vital milestone for ALPPS [41]. However, it should be noted that, despite these notable achievements, continued improvement is needed for this procedure in terms of surgery-related safety.

The ALPPS registry and international conferences have played a crucial role in its development. The first international expert meeting on ALPPS was held in Hamburg, Germany, in February 2015, [53, 140] where many issues were discussed, and eight recommendations were proposed. The ALPPS registry consistently releases relevant analytical data, significantly propelling its advancement [53]. Gregor A Stavrou et al. [168] prospectively observed the impact of these recommendations on ALPPS outcomes, showing that the experiences and lessons from ALPPS meetings and registry centers had a profound effect on surgery results. Since the 2015 meeting, ALPPS has become safer, with a substantial reduction in complication and mortality rates, reducing severe complication rates to 16% and even achieving 0 mortality. ALPPS has successfully become an effective alternative treatment option [168]. In May 2017, the 12th E-AHPBA conference in Mainz, Germany, featured a "10-year retrospective of ALPPS," providing a systematic and in-depth review of the surgery. The discussion covered indications, perioperative management, regeneration mechanisms, and drawbacks of this novel technique, along with proposals for further advancements.

After years of development, despite the remaining controversies, ALPPS has been increasingly accepted by hepatobiliary surgeons and has become an important treatment choice. Currently, apart from Japan and the United States, ALPPS is widely practiced in most regions globally. In some centers, it has become the preferred treatment. For example, the team led by Robles-Campos at the University of Murcia in Spain [99] reported that ALPPS has taken the place of PVE-TSH, becoming the preferred technique since September 2011. In Japan, most medical centers demand a 0 mortality after liver resection and generally do not accept ALPPS [136]. Nonetheless, Salvage ALPPS (ALPPS performed after failed PVE) has been acknowledged in recent years despite overall reluctance [169]. Similarly, most liver centers in North America do not routinely adopt this innovative technology [170, 171]. As for China, in 2013, Jian Zhou at Zhongshan Hospital, Fudan University, successfully performed the first ALPPS surgery in Asia [54]. Subsequently, numerous Chinese liver centers reported multiple ALPPS cases, continuously refining the technique. Xiujun Cai established Tourniquet ALPPS (Cai-style ALPPS), and others including Defei Hong and Kuansheng Ma applied Radiofrequency-Assisted ALPPS. Our center started using laparoscopic and robotic-assisted techniques since 2014, all achieving favorable results, and many more examples exist. Chinese scholars have made significant contributions to the development of ALPPS. In particular, most ALPPS cases applied in HCC patients were carried out in China, clarifying its role in this specific population. Indications for ALPPS differ greatly between the East and the West. While Western countries primarily focus on colorectal cancer, China applies ALPPS more frequently in HCC cases, often complicated by chronic liver diseases such as fibrosis or cirrhosis, making the surgery more challenging. The ALPPS registry pooled initial data from multiple centers. The results revealed limited FLR hypertrophy when ALPPS was performed in HCC cases, resulting in a postoperative mortality rate of 31%, raising concerns and questions about this indication [42]. In 2018, Zhongshan Hospital, Fudan University, reported the results of the largest ALPPS cohort for HCC at that time, achieving an FLR hypertrophy of 56.8%, tumor resection rate of 91.1%, 90-day mortality rate of 11.1%, and significant oncological benefits. The 1-year and 3-year OS rates were 64.2 and 60.2%, respectively, and the 1-year and 3-year DFS rates were 47.6 and 43.9%, respectively. Propensity score-matched comparative analysis demonstrated that ALPPS far outperformed traditional non-surgical Transarterial Chemoembolization (TACE), and these results had been published by the *Annals of Surgery* [77]. The favorable results of these ALPPS applications in HCC played a positive role in promoting its popularization. Subsequently, to address the issue of FLR induction in HCC patients with underlying chronic liver diseases (FLR induction inversely proportional to the degree of liver fibrosis/cirrhosis), a new ALPPS procedure suitable for this population (TAE-Salvaged ALPPS) was then established. It overcame the FLR induction issue in fibrotic and cirrhotic livers, providing an opportunity for these patients to undergo stage-2 ALPPS [172]. In the subsequent expanded application, all tumors were successfully removed, with a 100% success rate [173]. As of now, the cumulative total number of ALPPS cases in China ranks among the top globally.

ALPPS has made significant progress in terms of usage, scope of application, selection of tumor types, and applicable populations. It is no longer limited to the right trisectionectomy adopted in the early days. Its principles are flexibly and fully applied, lifting the restrictions on the tumor location, resection range, liver parenchyma separation plane, and the composition, position, and number of liver segments in classical procedures. Applicable tumor locations are no longer confined to the right side. In addition, the resection range goes beyond right trisectionectomy, allowing right hemihepatectomy, extended right hemihepatectomy, left trisectionectomy, left hemihepatectomy, extended left hemihepatectomy, and combined left and right resection. Correspondingly, the FLR is not limited to the left lateral lobe; the left liver, right posterior segment, and middle segment can also be considered, and the number of liver segments has surpassed the restriction of 2, with even a single segment confirmed to be feasible for ALPPS. In addition to the application of the FLR induction principle of ALPPS, the auxiliary liver function on the tumor side is also emphasized and fully utilized. In recent years, the principles of ALPPS combined with left lateral lobe living donor liver transplantation have been used for 2-stage total liver resection to treat liver tumors that cannot be surgically removed traditionally

(Resection and Partial liver segment 2/3 transplantation with delayed total hepatectomy, RAPID) [174]. The "liver-t(w)o-heal" study including 43 CRLM patients compared the FLR increase among PVE-TSH ($n = 11$), ALPPS ($n = 23$) and living donor two-stage liver transplantation (LDLT; $n = 9$) and showed that the volume gain advantage in patients with LDLT was significant [175].

These breakthroughs have expanded the indications for ALPPS, benefiting more patients. In 2012, Eduardo de Santibanes and Pierre-Alain Clavien [37] et al. pointed out that this innovative technique should not only be applied to right trisectionectomy (segments IV, V, VI, VII, VII ± I), but also to left trisectionectomy (segments II, III, IV, V, VII ± I) and other atypical resections. Subsequent developments fully validated this statement. ALPPS is applicable to extended right hemihepatectomy and right hemihepatectomy, as long as it adheres to its core elements (liver parenchyma separation and tumor side portal vein occlusion). It enables rapid FLR hypertrophy and complete tumor resection. In the first report released by the ALPPS registry, most ALPPS procedures were standard or extended right hepatectomies [176].

In 2013, Riccardo Gauzolino et al. at the University Hospital of Poitiers in France [80] attempted to apply mesohepatectomy ALPPS with an FLR in the right liver while performing Classic ALPPS. Three years later, Tung Yu Tsui et al. in Germany [177] reported a mesohepatectomy ALPPS involving double parenchyma partition and double FLR. These surgeries were both successful. In the same year, Aiman Obed et al. formally reported and named the first case of reversal ALPPS (left trisectionectomy ALPPS is opposite to right trisectionectomy ALPPS, with the FLR on the right side, similar to a reversed classical ALPPS) [178]. In 2016, Marcel Autran C Machado et al. [179] further reported laparoscopic reversal ALPPS. Besides being used for CRLM, this technique has also been reported in HCC and PHCC [180, 181]. In China, the liver surgery team at Zhongshan Hospital, Fudan University, was the first to perform reversal ALPPS. The total number of this procedure is still relatively low. Monosegment ALPPS fully demonstrates the powerful FLR induction ability of ALPPS, pushing such operations to the limit.

The currently accepted definition of a resectable liver is one with a negative margin, retaining at least two consecutive functional segments and intact portal and arterial inflow, venous outflow, and bile drainage [182]. For routine liver resection, it is widely believed that a single-segment FLR of less than 20% renders the patient inoperable, with a very high risk of PHLF. ALPPS has been fully validated for a two-segment FLR, regardless of whether it is the left lateral lobe (segments II-III, classical ALPPS) or the right posterior segment (segments VI-VII, reversal ALPPS), and monosegment ALPPS demonstrates the regenerative limit of the liver, indicating that even a single segment is feasible for ALPPS.

In 2012, Montalvá Orón et al. in Spain [183] first reported a case of monosegment ALPPS in a 65-year-old, 68 kg female CRLM patient. After neoadjuvant chemotherapy, the tumor remained unresectable, and the volume of her segment IV was only 275 mL (19.1% of the total liver volume, FLR/patient weight = 0.42). In stage-1 operation, the left lateral lobe and the caudate lobe were resected, with the Cantlie plane transected and the right portal vein ligated. On postoperative day 7, FLR increased to 388.1 mL (29.6% of the total volume, FLR/weight = 0.59), an FLR increase of 40%. Stage-2 surgery was performed 10 days postoperatively, with a right hemihepatectomy. Grade B PHLF occurred after this stage, but later recovered. On postoperative day 28, her FLR increased to 595 mL, a relative increase of 116% compared to the preoperative value [184].

Patients undergoing monosegment ALPPS surgery are typically with a huge tumor burden (only one segment ± partial liver segment left) and a higher risk. Thus, the surgery must be performed with great caution, and the currently published studies are mainly case reports [183–188]. The largest cohort is the summary of the ALPPS registry from 2011 to 2014, reported by Erik Schadde et al. A total of 333 patients were analyzed, of which 12 underwent monosegment ALPPS at 6 centers, all for extensive bilobar CRLM. All patients were considered unresectable by conventional means. The FLR of two cases were in Segment II, 2 in Segment III, 6 in Segment IV, and 2 in Segment VI. The inter-stage interval was 13 days. The median increase rate of FLR was 160%, achieving a 100% tumor resection rate (10/12 achieved R0 resection) and zero 90-day mortality. According to ISGLS standards, 4/12 patients developed PHLF, all of which completely recovered.

Six out of 12 patients developed ascites, with 4 experiencing severe complications (> Grade IIIa), including one patient related to PHLF [189]. In 2021, Anastasia Murtha-Lemekhova et al. [184] analyzed 19 cases of monosegment ALPPS with a preoperative FLR of 15.9% (8–22%) and FLR/SLV as low as 8%. The inter-stage interval was 13 days. They found the FLR increased to 38.4% (26–53%), and 12 of the 19 cases had an increase of more than 100%. All tumors were resected without any postoperative death. PHLF was the most common complication (42%, 2 cases of Grade B PHLF, 6 cases of Grade A PHLF), and it is still a matter of concern.

The median postoperative survival of the pooled cohort was 20 months, surpassing most CRLM cohorts receiving systemic chemotherapies (FOLFOX for 7.8–19.5 months, FOLFIRI for 15.0–17.6 months) [184]. Monosegment ALPPS surgery is challenging and has high risks. Currently reported types of this procedure include S2 ALPPS, S3

ALPPS, S4 ALPPS, S6 ALPPS, and S4 + 1b ALPPS [184, 189]. Among them, the most discussed is segment IV, whose advantage lies in the partial preservation of the caudate lobe [184, 186, 187]. There are also quite a few reports of segment VI. Besides, S6 monosegment ALPPS can be performed where the inferior right hepatic vein presents [184, 190, 191]. In pediatric patients with more potent regenerative abilities, S1 ALPPS has also been performed [192].

In summary, monosegment ALPPS is a unique technique that provides curative surgical opportunities for patients with a wide range of malignant liver tumors. However, this technique is still controversial, and biases of these studies must be considered. This procedure challenges the limits of liver surgery, with potentially high surgical risks. It must be carefully performed with cautious postoperative management to prevent small-for-size syndrome (SFSS) and PHLF [183]. Overall, after years of development, ALPPS surgery has expanded its indications significantly, no longer limited to the classical right trisectionectomy of the early years. Its usage is flexible and versatile, and the scope of application has significantly extended, benefiting a larger number of patients.

Currently, ALPPS has been widely used for various liver tumors, with the most common indications being CRLM, HCC, and ICC, accounting for over 90% of ALPPS cases; the rest less than 10% are applied in other tumor types [193]. Initially applied to PHCC, ALPPS gained rapid acceptance due to its unprecedented FLR induction efficiency and high resection rates. It was soon extended to other tumors, including CRLM, GBC, HCC, and ICC [49], yet with increased application, outcomes of some indications remained suboptimal; the application in CRLM has shown favorable results, while the efficacy for biliary tumors is relatively poor, leading to a waning role of ALPPS for this patient group [53]. A ten-year retrospective analysis by the ALPPS registry [41] revealed a shift in indications, with the proportion of CRLM patients increasing from 53 to 77%, while biliary tumors decreasing from 24 to 9%. As ALPPS evolves and surgical techniques improve, along with enhanced safety, indications continue to change. For instance, modified procedures like Hybrid ALPPS and Mini-ALPPS have facilitated better application in PHCC and GBC, contributing to an increase in PHCC ALPPS cases. New procedures also expand the scope of indications, such as TAE-Salvaged ALPPS, providing more opportunities for patients with HCC and chronic liver disease prone to insufficient FLR hypertrophy and surgical failure [172, 173]. In summary, ALPPS has achieved promising results, dispelling previous doubts and reservations, leading to popularity gain. Further advancements in ALPPS safety, including technical optimizations, are expected to expand its role.

Among all ALPPS indications in liver tumors, CRLM is the most mature, with good FLR induction, low postoperative complications, and mortality rates compared to other tumors, bringing about favorable medium to long-term outcomes [53]. CRLM was the first indication recommended for ALPPS [53], and it has been specified as a treatment option in guidelines from some countries [2, 194]. Many centers, especially those with extensive ALPPS experience, increasingly use ALPPS instead of PVE to remove tumors in these patients, particularly after neoadjuvant or first-line chemotherapy [41]. The first report from the International ALPPS registry in 2014 showed that CRLM was the primary indication (70%), with lower complication and mortality rates compared to other indications (severe complication rate: 21%, 90-day mortality rate: 8%) [49]. Updated data in 2015 revealed a 5% mortality after ALPPS for CRLM, similar to reported mortality rates after major liver resection. The 1- and 2-year OS rates were 76 and 62%, respectively, while the 1- and 2-year DFS rates were 59 and 41%, respectively [195].

In 2017, Kerollos Nashat Wanis et al. reported a 3-year OS of 50% and a 3-year DFS of 13% for CRLM patients undergoing ALPPS [196]. Over time, long-term oncological results, previously lacking, have become elucidated. In 2020, Henrik Petrowsky reported the largest analysis of CRLM survival to date, involving 510 patients from 22 international ALPPS registry centers between 2009 and 2019. The 90-day mortality rate was 4.9%, with a median OS of 39 months, Cancer-Specific Survival (CSS) of 42 months, and Recurrence-Free Survival (RFS) of 15 months. The 3-year CSS, OS, and RFS were 59%, 52%, and 19%, respectively, and the 5-year rates were 33, 27, and 12%, respectively, surpassing the results of systemic chemotherapy alone. This large cohort study provided convincing evidence and meaningful conclusions on long-term oncological benefits: CRLM patients undergoing ALPPS not only have a low perioperative mortality rate but also achieve favorable long-term oncological outcomes, especially in those with good tumor biology and chemotherapy response [128, 149]. OS rates reported by other studies ranged from 28 to 54% at 3 years and 32 to 58% at 5 years [197]. For patients traditionally deemed unresectable, ALPPS significantly improves survival compared to systemic treatment [198–201].

Controversy existed for a long time regarding its comparison with traditional PVE-TSH, but recent high-level evidence, especially completed RCTs and meta-analyses of multiple single-center data, show that ALPPS has a significantly higher tumor resection rate than TSH, with comparable morbidity and mortality rates, making it an alternative to the latter. In 2017, Per Sandstrom et al. reported findings of the LIGRO Trial, a prospective multicenter RCT comparing ALPPS and PVE-TSH. For CRLM patients, ALPPS showed a higher tumor resection rate (92% vs 57%), better R0 resection rate (77% vs 57%), faster FLR induction, and shorter waiting duration, with similar complication rates (43% vs

43%) and 90-day mortality rates (8.3% vs 6.1%). Moreover, ALPPS rescued 12 cases of PVE-TSH failure (12/49), where FLR growth was insufficient. Subsequent reports in 2019 by Kristina Hasselgren et al. indicated that ALPPS had superior overall survival compared to TSH (median survival: 46 months vs 26 months), while patients with unresected tumors lived only 13 months [202]. Despite of slight variations in results from other single-center comparative studies, the conclusions generally accord [203]. A 2020 meta-analysis including eight studies and 409 patients compared the safety, efficacy, and oncological benefits of ALPPS and TSH in advanced CRLM. Data showed that ALPPS had a significantly higher tumor resection rate than the control arm (98% vs 78%), better R0 resection (66% vs 37%), and a significantly shorter waiting interval (11.6 days vs 45.7 days). The postoperative mortality and severe complication rates were comparable between groups (90-day mortality rate: 7% vs 5%; severe complication rate: 29% vs 22%), and the 1-year OS, recurrence rate, and DFS were similar (79% vs 84%, 49% vs 39%, 34% vs 39%), respectively.

The ALPPS procedure has great variations in its indications between Eastern and Western countries. In the West, it is primarily used for CRLM, while in Asian countries, HCC and other primary liver cancers are major application scenarios [176]. The first report from the ALPPS registry in 2014 indicated that HCC accounted for only 8%, much lower than CRLM's 70%. Generally, the West does not prefer ALPPS in HCC [41]. According to Jan G. D'Haese et al., from 2010 to 2015, there were only 35 HCC cases in the ALPPS registry. In contrast, in China, HCC is the primary indication. This difference reflects distinct treatment philosophies regarding this patient population in the two regions. HCC cases treated with ALPPS usually have a large tumor burden and are at a later stage. The traditional practice in the West discourages surgical treatment for such cases, while Asian countries would give it a go. Recent data from various Chinese centers have clarified the role of ALPPS in these patients. A study from 2018 in our center, applying ALPPS to Hepatitis B-related HCC, showed a tumor resection rate of 91.1%, FLR induction of 56.8%, a median inter-stage interval of 12 days, a 90-day mortality rate of 11.1%, and a complication rate of 46.5% (≥Grade 3B: 11.1%). The 1- and 3-year OS rates were 64.2 and 61.2%, respectively, and the 1- and 3-year DFS rates were 64.2 and 61.2%, respectively. Comparative analysis using propensity scores indicated that ALPPS yielded significantly better OS than non-surgical treatment (TACE) [77].

A study from 2021 by Albert Chan et al. released short-term and long-term results of ALPPS for HCC and compared them with PVE-TSH. ALPPS generated a significantly higher resection rate than PVE (97.8% vs 67.7%). There were no significant differences in major complication rates (20.7% vs 30.4%) and 90-day postoperative mortality rates (6.5% vs 5.8%). The 1-, 3-, and 5-year OS rates in the ALPPS group after tumor resection were 84.7, 60.2, and 46.8%, respectively, comparable to the control arm [204]. Weiping Zhou et al. conducted a single-center prospective RCT comparing ALPPS and TACE+PVE (TACE followed by PVE 2 weeks later). The research team found that the tumor resection rate with ALPPS was significantly higher (97.4% vs 65.8%) and FLR induction significantly better (FLR increase rate: 38%/12 days vs 39%/42 days). The 90-day postoperative mortality rates were the same (5.3% vs 5.3%). After a median follow-up of 42 months, the 3-year OS rate in the ALPPS group (65.8%) was superior to the control group (42.1%), with comparable 3-year DFS rates (48.6% vs 48%) [205]. Some other centers in China and another country have conducted studies with smaller sample sizes, showing consistent results [206–210].

In recent years, with reports from large liver cancer centers in China, the conclusion about HCC ALPPS has become expounded. With strict adherence to indications, ALPPS for HCC leads to good clinical outcomes. Its safety has greatly improved compared to earlier years, with satisfactory tumor resection rates and R0 resection rates, and good medium and long-term survival, which are superior to non-surgical treatments including TACE. These results are comparable to postoperative survival of patients with one-staged liver tumor resection and similar to or better than PVE and TACE-PVE [204, 205]. As with the application of ALPPS in CRLM, case selection and surgical techniques have a profound impact on outcomes. Case selection for ALPPS is crucial, even more so for HCC than CRLM. HCC is often associated with chronic liver disease (about 80% of these patients in China have varying degrees of liver fibrosis/cirrhosis). Liver damage from chronic liver disease significantly affects the FLR's regenerative potential and speed, making ALPPS more challenging in this indication than in CRLM, in addition to higher odds of postoperative complications.

Early data analysis from the ALPPS registry showed a negative correlation between FLR growth and the severity of liver fibrosis. Patients over 61 years of age had a notably lower survival [42]. Results from our center and some other centers show consistent conclusions [205]. ALPPS may not be as effective for HCC patients with advanced age, severe cirrhosis, and a small FLR/Standard Liver Volume (SLV) ratio. In 2015, Xiujun Cai et al. reported 12 HCC cases with cirrhosis who underwent Tourniquet-ALPPS. The severe complication rates after stage-1 and 2 were 25.0 and 40.0%, respectively. Six patients with a preoperative FLR/SLV ratio of less than 30% died of PHLF, not the other six cases with a higher FLR/SLV [101]. Junwei Zhang et al. from Peking Union Medical College Hospital reported that HCC patients with FLV/SLV <30% were prone to PHLF after ALPPS, with a severe complication rate of 21.4%. Two of these patients (one at 27% and the other at 28%) developed ISGLS Grade

C PHLF after stage 2 operation, and both died within 2 months after discharge [210]. This suggests that ALPPS should be performed in highly selected HCC patients. It is worth mentioning that ALPPS may be particularly useful in HCC patients with vein tumor thrombus, for this population is deprived of the opportunity to receive PVE or/and HVE. Due to a smaller FLR, these patients are usually not suitable for surgery and are instead referred for other non-surgical treatments, resulting in reduced overall survival. ALPPS can benefit this subgroup of patients [211, 212]. It is often used in HCC patients with type I-II PVTT (Cheng's classification), but there are also reports of its application in type III or whose tumor thrombus has invaded the FLR portal vein [213]. On the other hand, the surgical technique of ALPPS has a significant impact on the results.

Unlike ALPPS for CRLM, classic ALPPS with complete transection, rather than partial transection, works better for HCC patients. Albert Chan et al. from Hong Kong, China, showed in their research that, for HCC patients with underlying chronic liver disease, the classic ALPPS with complete transection produced better results than that with partial transection. For the studied patient population, the classic procedure should be preferred for optimal results [96]. ALPPS for HCC in our center also showed similar results. For the aforementioned indication, the classic ALPPS is usually adopted, with satisfactory FLR induction, high tumor resection rate, low postoperative severe complication rate, and low mortality rate. In 2016, Albert Chan et al. from the University of Hong Kong used an improved anterior approach for ALPPS in HCC and achieved good outcomes [76, 117, 214]. Kuansheng Ma et al. used a modified approach, RALPPS, to reduce postoperative complications and mortality [106]. In well-selected HCC patients with cirrhosis whose liver function was good, RALPPS achieved satisfactory FLR growth with a slightly longer waiting time (53%/28 days) [106–108].

Current evidence demonstrates that both classic ALPPS and appropriate modified techniques can be applied to HCC with improved treatment outcomes. Leaving aside issues of case selection and procedural selection, the main challenges for ALPPS in HCC still revolve around patients' underlying chronic liver disease, especially liver fibrosis/cirrhosis. HCC without this comorbidity is a good indication of ALPPS being easily implementable. However, those who do with it remain tricky. Firstly, the function and regenerative capacity of a liver with fibrosis/cirrhosis are challenging to assess preoperatively, and there is currently no method for precise quantification and prediction of FLR induction before surgery. Secondly, patients with cirrhosis have can but poorly tolerate complications because current artificial liver support systems are immature, prone to leading to short-term death after surgery. Although FLR growth in livers with fibrosis/cirrhosis seems faster than those without cirrhosis/cholestasis, the existing experience indicates that ALPPS remains an effective method for FLR induction in hepatitis-related HCC patients. An important advancement in recent years is the establishment of a new procedure by our team, applicable to patients with cirrhosis/severe liver fibrosis, called TAE-salvaged ALPPS, or Zhou's ALPPS [172, 173].

In 2017, when performing ALPPS on a patient with HCC and concomitant fibrosis, we found insufficient FLR growth 14 days after stage 1, and the tumor "stole" blood from the left hepatic artery. This artery of FLR was significantly narrowed compared to the preoperative one, while the supplying arteries of the large tumor in the right liver lobe became significantly wider. We performed Transarterial Embolization (TAE) to control the progression of this huge tumor. One week later, a CT examination showed that FLR growth was once again activated, reaching a sufficient volume for the stage 2 procedure. This was then expanded to nine other cases with insufficient FLR growth after stage 1 operation due to cirrhosis/fibrosis, all of which successfully completed the stage 2 surgery, establishing a new procedure: TAE-Salvaged ALPPS (Zhou's ALPPS). This procedure is expected to overcome the problem of insufficient FLR growth in patients with cirrhosis/fibrosis but requires more applications and verification. In summary, the overall survival benefit of ALPPS for HCC patients is gradually becoming clear, but there are still many issues (including safety, case selection, optimal procedural selection, and perioperative management, among others) that need further research.

Malignant biliary tumors (cholangiocarcinoma, CCC) include ICC, PHCC, and GBC. The first report from the ALPPS registry in 2014 indicated that PHCC, ICC, and GBC accounted for 5, 4, and 3% of all cases, respectively [49]. However, the surgical safety is suboptimal, with high postoperative complication and mortality rates. The 90-day mortality rates for PHCC, ICC, and GBC are significantly higher at 27%, 13%, and 33%, respectively, compared to the 8% for CRLM [49]. In 2016, a report from 12 centers in Italy on 50 ALPPS cases, including 8 ICC, 11 PHCC, and 1 GBC, showed a postoperative mortality rate of 40% (10% after stage 1 and 30% after stage 2) [144]. Univariate and multivariate analyses indicated an association between cholangiocarcinoma and increased 90-day mortality and poorer survival. Due to the high risks of complications and death, there is a recommendation against ALPPS for CCC. The ALPPS registry's pooled analysis also revealed that biliary tumors and elevated serum bilirubin levels (before stage 2) are risk factors for 90-day mortality [46].

The first ALPPS international conference in February 2015 discussed ALPPS for biliary tumors, calling for use with caution due to the reported high mortality rates [53]. However, some scholars argued that surgeries for PHCC and GBC are complex per se with inherently high complication and mortality rates even with one-staged resection. Unfortunately, studies demonstrate that even compared to one-staged resection surgery, ALPPS significantly increases complication and mortality rates. A comparative analysis of PHCC patients in 2017 by the ALPPS registry, involving 29 ALPPS cases and 257 cases of one-staged radical surgery, showed that the ALPPS mortality rate was twice that of the other group (48% vs 24%), indicating a need for caution in applying ALPPS for this population. Due to safety concerns and selective abandonment during case selection, the application of ALPPS in biliary tumors has gradually decreased. A multicenter data review by the ALPPS registry showed that the adoption in this indication decreased from 24% in the early years (before 2012) to 9% in 2015 [41]. Subsequent subgroup analysis of biliary tumors showed that the main issues were concentrated in PHCC and GBC, while ALPPS in ICC exhibited better results, making it relatively suitable for the procedure.

For ICC, a large case series based on 102 cases in the ALPPS registry reported by Jun Li et al. revealed a tumor resection rate of 97.1% (R0 resection rate 85%) with a median inter-stage interval of 11 days and a KGR of 23 mL/day [215]. The initial high complication and mortality rates have steadily decreased over the past 2 years, with a severe complication rate reduced to 29% and a 90-day mortality rate of 7%. The 3-year OS rate was 21.4%, with better outcomes in cases achieving R0 resection and with a single lesion [215]. A single-center study with 14 patients who underwent ALPPS was conducted by Jan Bednarsch et al., [216] reporting a tumor resection rate of 86%. The median OS of patients who completed ALPPS surgery was 4.2 years, and the 3-year survival rate was 64%. The median increase in FLR was 65%, major complications were 29% after the first stage, 83% after the second stage, and short-term postoperative mortality was 8%. Current data show that ALPPS for ICC yields good results and can improve the resectability rate of locally advanced ICC [215, 216]. Similar positive outcomes for ICC with ALPPS were reported by other studies. The postoperative complication and mortality rates ranged from 13.6 to 44% and 0 to 29%, respectively [217]. However, more research is needed to elucidate oncological benefits.

ALPPS as an option for surgery in the context of inadequate FLR for biliary tumors should not be dismissed lightly. Prematurely abandoning this procedure without a detailed analysis does not meet scientific requirements. For example, in PHCC, the traditional PVE is most commonly used for FLR-insufficient PHCC [218]. However, the long waiting time renders patients more prone to tumor progression and unresectability, even if the tumor is a relatively slow-growing one [219]. Until better alternative methods emerge, ALPPS should not be easily discarded. A more appropriate approach may be to use it with extreme caution while continuously improving the technique. Early reports applied classic ALPPS for the majority of cases, whose complications and mortality rates are already high. The combination of this procedure with PHCC surgery leads to a high incidence of morbidity and mortality [49]. Improvements in surgical techniques and careful case selection are expected to reduce these risks. The former include using PVE instead of PVL, anterior approach techniques, non-dissection of the hepatic hilum in stage 1, postponing bile duct reconstruction to stage 2, partial parenchymal transection, reliable intraoperative methods to detect bile leakage, and adequate drainage [83, 111, 114, 220, 221]. Hybrid modifications that incorporate various improved techniques, such as ALTIPS, mini-ALPPS, or Hybrid ALPPS, may be safer [83, 181]. Although there are currently few reported cases, they have shown a good safety improvement.

ALPPS in other liver tumors has been reported, but its overall use is relatively limited. As of February 2020, in the ALPPS registry, there were a total of 1228 cases, with only 136 cases of liver tumors ruling out common ones such as CRLM and HCC [193]. These included neuroendocrine tumor (NET) metastases and gastrointestinal stromal tumors (GIST) [222], among others. Among them, NET has been the most frequently reported. Existing studies indicate that ALPPS for NET is safe, with satisfactory long-term results [223]. An international ALPPS registry report [223] on 21 cases of bilobar NET showed sufficient FLR hypertrophy, with a median inter-stage interval of 11 days. The 1- and 2-year OS rates were 95.2 and 95.2%, respectively, while the 1- and 2-year DFS rates were 73.2 and 41.8%, respectively [223]. Another pooled analysis by Lai et al. [193] included 41 NET cases, with a median interval of 11 days between stages. The major complication rate was 33.3%. ALPPS demonstrated favorable treatment effects on NET, with 1-year OS rates ranging from 73 to 95% and 1-year DFS rates ranging from 73 to 83% [193].

ALPPS has also been reported for benign tumors [193] despite significant controversy around this. Generally, ALPPS is not recommended for patients with benign diseases, as they can wait for sufficient FLR hypertrophy to occur over time. Other methods, such as PVE or liver venous deprivation (LVD), can be applied for FLR induction. Moreover, patients with benign tumors can undergo enucleation, which, with the development of technologies, including fluorescence laparoscopy, is often easier to complete by combining such advancements and liver blood flow control.

Initially, ALPPS was applied to adults with no age restrictions. Subsequently, it was observed that the postoperative complication and mortality rates were high in elderly patients with limited FLR hypertrophy. As a result, it gradually became a preferred option for younger cases (see details in the patient selection section). Concurrently, with the development of ALPPS, it has been applied in children [203]. Nonetheless, its overall use in pediatric cases remains limited [185, 192, 193, 214–226], partly due to the extremely low incidence of malignant liver tumors in children and the limited acceptance of ALPPS in this population.

The reported age span for children undergoing ALPPS is from 54 days to 14 years [192, 226]. Despite the limited data and the small number of cases in this population, they exhibit good FLR hypertrophy and postoperative recovery capabilities. The interval between stages ranges from 8 to 16 days, with FLR hypertrophy reported between 46% and 91% [185, 192, 193, 224–227].

A notable case series by Julio Cesar Wiederkehr et al. [224] reported on five children undergoing ALPPS (two cases of hepatoblastoma, one rhabdomyosarcoma, one HCC, and one nodular regenerative hyperplasia). The average age was 9.4 ± 5.9 years (range: 2.16–17.25 years old; median: 10.25 years old), with FLR increasing by 83.8%, a median inter-stage interval of 11 days, and no complications except for asymptomatic right pleural effusion in one patient.

Most children undergoing ALPPS receive monosegment procedures. In 2019, Ruiz Figueroa et al. [185] reported one such case. A 3-year-old girl with PRETEXT IV hepatoblastoma received segment VI ALPPS (S6 ALPPS). The preoperative FLR was 21.3%, increasing to 32.57% 15 days postoperatively, with no complications other than pneumonia, and no recurrence during 3 years of follow-up [185].

In 2021, Ruiz Figueroa et al. reported another case of a 14-year-old child undergoing segment I ALPPS (S1 ALPPS) for recurrent HCC, where the caudate lobe was the sole FLR. The preoperative caudate lobe volume was only 35 mL, increasing to 288 mL 14 days after the surgery. The patient experienced Grade A PHLF and bile leak after the second stage, with no other complications and no recurrence during 6 months of follow-up [191]. In China, Yu Hui et al. [228] documented the case of a 3-year-old girl undergoing laparoscopic ALPPS for a massive mesenchymal hamartoma of the right liver, with a 78.3% FLR increase in 3 days and smooth postoperative recovery.

Currently, ALPPS in children is mainly reported through individual cases or small-sample case reports. Current data suggests that ALPPS is effective for treating large tumors in pediatric cases. However, due to the unique characteristics of this population and potential reporting biases, cautious interpretation of results and utilization are still necessary.

The controversy between ALPPS and PVE has persisted since the former was established in 2007. Prior to its dawn, PVE-TSH was the standard procedure for initially unresectable liver tumors with insufficient FLR. ALPPS demonstrated rapid and significant FLR hypertrophy, along with a high tumor resection rate and R0 resection rate, raising expectations that it could replace PVE-TSH. However, the results of its application also indicated a worrying safety profile, hence the doubt.

Subsequently, efforts were made to refine patient selection and improve surgical techniques, bringing about a substantial enhancement of its safety. Several centers compared ALPPS and PVE-TSH. In recent years, as studies completed, more reports were published, including high-level evidence generated from RCTs and long-term follow-up outcomes, clarifying the conclusion of such comparisons.

Early comparative analyses were often single-center studies with heterogeneous patient populations. As early as 2012, Wolfram Trudo Knoefel et al. [229] compared these two procedures. At that time, ALPPS was not yet named and was referred to as In Situ Liver Transection with Portal Vein Ligation (ISLT+PVL). The authors pooled 22 tumor cases (including 5 ICCs, 3 PHCCs, 2 GBCs, 1 HCC, 10 CRLMs, and 1 NET) from 2009 to 2011, comparing 7 cases of ISLT+PVL with 15 cases of PVE-TSH. The ISLT+PVL group exhibited 63% FLR hypertrophy in 3 days, with all patients completing tumor resection within 8 days (range 4–8 days), suggesting the effectiveness and reliability of this procedure to induce rapid FLR growth, even in patients with insufficient FLR increase after PVE (three PVE failure patients were successfully salvaged with ISLT+PVL).

In 2019, Long R. Jiao et al. [104] reported the REBIRTH Trial, an RCT comparing RALPPS and PVE-TSH, showing that RALPPS was superior in radical resection and FLR induction, with similar complication rates (see details above). Fadi Rassam et al. [94] reported on a single-center study of 72 cases (17 CRLM, 5 HCC, 20 PHC, 6 IHC, 2 benign tumors, 1 other tumor), including 12 cases of complete ALPPS, 9 cases of partial ALPPS, and 51 cases of PVE-TSH, whose inter-stage intervals were 8 days, 10 days, and 23 days respectively. Their severe complication rates were 30, 17, and 18%, with 90-day mortality rates of 25, 0, and 2%, respectively. Due to significant differences in postoperative complication and mortality rates among various tumor types, it is challenging to obtain reliable analytical results where confounders were unadjusted.

In recent years, there has been a gradual increase in data from single-center analyses focusing on one single tumor type, mostly on CRLM, making the comparison between ALPPS and TSH more credible. In 2017, Per Sandstrom et al. [105] published the first prospective multicenter RCT, the Scandinavian LIGRO Trial, comparing ALPPS and PVE-TSH. From 2014 to 2016, 97 CRLM patients were randomly assigned to the ALPPS group (n = 48) or the TSH group (n = 49). The ALPPS group showed a significantly higher tumor resection rate and R0 resection rate than the other group, with a similar rate of major complications. In the TSH group, 12 out of 49 patients failed to achieve sufficient FLR increase, and ALPPS was successfully used as a salvage for them. Subsequently, in 2019, Kristina Hasselgren et al. [202] reported the long-term survival results of the LIGRO study, showing a superiority of ALPPS over TSH in OS (see details above). The LIGRO study suggests that for traditionally unresectable CRLM, ALPPS is better than TSH. Results from other large-scale single-center reports are consistent [203, 230, 231]. In 2020, a meta-analysis [36] pooled 161 cases of ALPPS and 248 cases of TSH. The results indicated that ALPPS has a significantly higher tumor resection rate (98% vs 78%) and R0 resection rate (66% vs 37%) and a significantly shorter waiting time (11.6 days vs 45.7 days). The 90-day mortality (7% vs 5%) and severe complication rates (29% vs 22%) were similar. The 1-year OS rate (79% vs 84%), the 1-year recurrence rate (49% vs 39%), and the 1-year DFS rate (34% vs 39%) were comparable. Overall, for CRLM, current RCTs and single-center comparative studies show that ALPPS has a superior tumor resection rate and R0 resection rate compared to PVE-TSH. Postoperative complications and mortality rates are similar, and the long-term survival with ALPPS is either similar or superior to TSH. Patients in the TSH group whose tumors remain unresected have the lowest survival.

In addition to CRLM, there has been an increased update in data for HCC in recent years, including high-level RCT studies. Echoing the results of a single-center prospective RCT conducted by Weiping Zhou et al. [205] in 2021, Albert Chan et al. [204] reported a comparison in HCC patients between 46 cases treated with ALPPS and 102 cases with PVE-TSH. ALPPS showed a higher resection rate than PVE-TSH (97.8% vs 67.7%), with comparable rates of major complications (20.7% vs 30.4%) and perioperative mortality (6.5% vs 5.8%). The 1-, 3-, and 5-year OS rates were 84.7, 60.2, and 46.8% for ALPPS and 88.2, 73.5, and 64.1% for PVE-TSH. The 1-, 3-, and 5-year DFS rates were 63.2, 34.9, and 25.0% for ALPPS and 61.4, 41.8, and 40.7% for PVE-TSH. The short-term and long-term results of the two groups are similar for HCC, with ALPPS having a higher resection rate [204].

Comparative studies between these two procedures for other tumor types still need to be improved, and conclusions remain undecisive. Current evidence indicates the superiority of ALPPS over TSH in tumor resection rate (especially R0 resection rate) and FLR induction. While the safety of ALPPS was initially inferior to TSH, significant improvements have been made over the years through surgical technique refinement and adjustments in patient selection, narrowing the gap in this parameter. The long-term results in CRLM patients are clear, showing survival benefits of ALPPS either similar or superior to TSH. For HCC cases, the benefits are becoming elucidated, with superiority over TACE or TACE+PVE in survival and similar long-term survival as TSH. Results for other tumor types remain unclear.

ALPPS has become one of the treatment options in CRLM, superior to PVE-TSH, and can be used as the preferred choice; HCC has also become a possible indication but is still controversial and needs to be verified by more studies. The only less disputed aspect is its widely accepted role as a salvage treatment (Rescue ALPPS) in cases of PVE failure, becoming the preferred procedure for such patients [232]. Answers to other controversies, such as the preferability of ALPPS over other treatments, are expected to be tested with time. Surgeons' technical preferences, differences in treatment philosophies, and willingness to make evidence-based decisions will exceedingly impact the choice of procedure. A survey among ALPPS registry members indicated that only 84% of surgeons still consider ALPPS for indications beyond CRLM [89]. A survey of decision-making on liver augmentation techniques in 40 hospitals / hepato-pancreatico-biliary (HPB) centers in Germany, Switzerland, and Austria showed that the standard liver augmentation technique in all countries was PVE (56%), followed by ALPPS (32.1%) in Germany or PVE with HVE (33.3%) in Switzerland and Austria. Most hospitals rated the importance of PVE before resection of cholangiocarcinoma or CRLM as high, while PVE for HCC was rated as low [233]. In some centers, especially liver centers in Japan and the United States, ALPPS is not accepted by most hepatobiliary surgeons or is only considered a salvage for PVE failure. Future research should continue including more RCTs and more cases with long-term evaluations to validate the scientific and reliable nature of ALPPS in treating traditionally unresectable liver tumors.

Research on the mechanism of ALPPS is currently limited. Andreas A. Schnitzbauer et al. initially reported histological analysis on one patient during the first 25 ALPPS case series, observing increased cell proliferation in accordance with volumetric growth [40]. Early studies on its mechanism were primarily histocytological interpretations of clinical samples. Subsequently, animal models were quickly established, and research on cellular and molecular mechanisms was conducted based on both in vitro and in vivo models. Suitable ALPPS animal models are crucial for such explorations. FLR proliferation is a multifactorial process that can be simulated only in vivo rather than in vitro, considering changes in liver blood flow and systemic inflammatory responses. In 2014, Andrea Schlegel et al. created the first mouse ALPPS model [234]. Studies using this model suggested that the accelerated regeneration after ALPPS is primarily due to an "inflammatory-like response" leading to enhanced liver cell growth [234]. Libin Yao [235] and Hector Almau Trenard [236] et al. reported rat ALPPS models in the same year, followed by variants by other scholars [237–239]. These models, different in procedures, are usually named after their inventors. In addition to conventional rat ALPPS models, researchers have built rat ALPPS models with fibrotic or cirrhotic liver [240, 241].

Rodents offer several advantages for research, including ease of handling and feeding, rapid reproduction and regeneration, clear physiological and anatomical structures, and low genetic heterogeneity, allowing the collection of a large amount of data in a relatively short time. These animals boast excellent liver regeneration capabilities and high metabolic rates, enabling fast and sufficient tissue regeneration and, thus, successful completion of stage-2 surgery in a very short time [234]. Nevertheless, due to colossal differences between rodents and humans, results yielded by these models can be extrapolated neither directly nor completely onto mankind. In 2017, Mingheng Liao et al. built a medium-sized animal model using rabbits [242], but the anatomical structure of rabbit livers makes ALPPS extremely challenging.

Large animal models are more valuable in simulating and evaluating systemic responses and/or mimicking clinical conditions, providing more information. Furthermore, these models have greater similarity to human characteristics, facilitating clinical translation. In 2015, Kristopher P Croome reported a pig ALPPS model [243]. Two years later, András Budai et al. established a sheep ALPPS model [237]. However, similar to pigs, the severe vascular crossing in the liver parenchyma of sheep renders liver transection difficult. Non-human primates have significant translational potential thanks to their close physiological and anatomical resemblance to humans. Nonetheless, using such animals requires extensive expertise, well-equipped facilities, and ethical considerations. Our center has established a macaque model, but there are currently no reports of non-human primate ALPPS models abroad.

In summary, various ALPPS animal models have been established, including mice, rats, rabbits, pigs, and sheep [237]. However, an ideal model for ALPPS research is still lacking. This, to a considerable extent, has led to a delay in elucidating the mechanism of ALPPS and a cautious interpretation of the conclusions obtained in research for clinical translation. Nevertheless, research on the mechanism has made some progress, providing a better understanding of the complex process of liver regeneration in the ALPPS surgery.

Studies indicate that FLR increase after ALPPS is related to changes in liver blood flow led by PVL and local trauma-induced liver regeneration due to liver parenchymal transection. The rapid regeneration of FLR during ALPPS is primarily attributed to the following pathways [244]: ① Blood flow redistribution: According to the blood flow theory of liver regeneration [245, 246], it was early speculated that liver regeneration after ALPPS is related to portal vein pressure. PVL or PVE increases portal vein flow in FLR, increasing shear stress within the organ, thereby promoting the expression and upregulation of genes related to liver cell regeneration and initiating its proliferation. At the same time, portal blood flow diversion increases the nutritional substances within FLR, promoting rapid regeneration. Federico Tomassini et al. [161] conducted the first human study to demonstrate a significant positive correlation between portal vein flow at the end of stage-1 operation and the increase in FLR volume, although excessively high pressure may generate adverse effects [161]; ② Local trauma-induced liver regeneration due to liver parenchymal transection: Clinical practices, especially salvage ALPPS, and various established ALPPS animal studies have shown that liver parenchymal transection combined with PVO induces more robust FLR increase than PVO alone, indicating the central role of liver parenchymal transection in FLR increase [237].

A comparison of partial transection and classic complete transection ALPPS also revealed that the extent of FLR increase is related to the degree of liver parenchymal transection, especially in cases with chronic disease. Complete transection ALPPS induces more FLR increase, requires less time for induction, and has a significantly higher success rate in inducing FLR hypertrophy than partial transection [96]. Using a mouse ALPPS model, it was found that at least 50% of transection suffices enough regeneration [93]. At the cellular and molecular levels, many studies in recent years have made strides forward. The debate over the essence of FLR proliferation—an increase in the number or the size of liver cells or an expansion of the intercellular matrix—has been a focus of research from the beginning, as it is closely related to increased liver function. The actual proliferation of FLR involves an increase in the number and size of liver cells.

To differentiate between actual tissue proliferation and postoperative liver parenchymal edema, CT density analysis scans were performed as early as 2013 by Wolfram Trudo Knoefel et al., [229] who reported true parenchymal hypertrophy in FLR. Subsequent studies by other scholars used optical and electron microscopy to observe resected specimens and analyzed cellular and structural changes in FLR tissues using methods such as Ki-67 detection [40, 195]. Roberto Hernandez-Alejandro et al. [195] analyzed the Ki-67 index of biopsy tissues, finding an FLR increase from 0 to 14% after ALPPS. An animal study in mice from the University of Zurich showed that the expression of Ki-67 was significantly higher in the ALPPS group. FLR proliferation was related to liver cell proliferation and volumetric enlargement. Although data from animal models are conducive, inter-species differences in regeneration must be taken into account, and human liver cell replication typically occurs in diseased livers, which are often functionally impaired or structurally different in a severe manner. Eduardo de Santibañe et al. [247] studied changes in liver cells and molecular levels after ALPPS. FLR biopsies were obtained from patients during the first and second stages, and hematoxylin and eosin (HE) staining and immunohistochemical analysis were performed. The analysis of tissue cytology and molecular features revealed that the FLR increase is associated with liver cell proliferation [248].

Studies in rats have shown that not only liver cell replication but also cell hypertrophy is involved in liver regeneration after hepatectomy [248–250]. The rat ALPPS model studied by Ruofan Sheng et al. [251] demonstrated that the liver cells in the ALPPS group were larger, and the expression levels of Ki-67 and hepatocyte growth factor were higher compared to the PVL group and the control group. Nevertheless, clinical studies came to the opposite conclusion. Kenichi Matsuo et al. [252] performed optical and electron microscopy on FLR specimens from patients undergoing ALPPS and PVE-TSH, finding that the liver cell density in the ALPPS group was higher, whereas the liver cells were significantly smaller than in the PVE group. In the FLR, compared to the control arm, regenerating liver cells in the ALPPS group were morphologically immature. The source of liver cell proliferation (originating from either mature liver cells or progenitor cells) remains inconclusive. Some studies argued that these newly generated cells come from mature liver cells [253, 254], while others indicating anther birthplace—liver progenitor cells [255].

Clinical observations indicated that the ALPPS operation appears to promote rapid growth in liver volume rather than an increase in liver function [256]. The physical volume increase does not translate into a synchronous functional gain of FLR, as confirmed by repeated liver scintigraphy studies for liver function in clinical practices [159]. According to a study [257], the increase in FLR volume in ALPPS patients is due to effective liver cell proliferation rather than fat degeneration or edema. However, cell proliferation does not immediately lead to complete maturity [252]. Animal experiments also confirmed that liver cells after ALPPS are less mature than those after PVE [252]. Right after ALPPS, liver cells are immature, which may explain the high incidence of postoperative PHLF. Studies on the molecular mechanisms showed that liver transection promotes the production of inflammatory factors, inducing liver growth [258].

In 2014, Andrea Schlegel et al. [234] demonstrated through a mouse model that ALPPS induces rapid liver growth, and the high expression of inflammatory mediators interleukin-6 (IL-6) and tumor necrosis factor-alpha (TNF-α) is involved in this process. Serum from mice undergoing liver transection was injected into other mice undergoing only PVL (i.e., no liver parenchymal transection in stage-1 operation), causing a degree of regeneration comparable to that of a complete ALPPS procedure. This suggests that circulating inflammation and growth factors mediate liver regeneration in ALPPS. IL-6 and TNF-α were upregulated after the first stage in humans, similar to the observations in mice, indicating the activation of the IL-6-TNF-α-STAT3 pathway in the rapid increase in FLR after the stage-1 ALPPS operation [234].

Similar results were revealed in other rat ALPPS models, with upregulation of pSTAT3, nuclear NFkBp65, and YAP [259, 260]. Using protein chip detection in a rat model, Dipok Kumar Dhar et al. [261] identified 29 cytokines/chemokines, with neutrophil chemotactic factor 1 showing the strongest and earliest upregulation in the ALPPS group. IL-6, MIP-1a, IL-2, and IL-13 were upregulated within 24 h after surgery, with IL-6 showing the strongest surge [261]. Clinical specimen analysis of the liver and plasma of patients undergoing ALPPS [262] showed that mTOR-induced liver cell proliferation is related to FLR induction in ALPPS, and levels of proliferation-related cytokines IL-6, TNF-α, HGF, and EGF significantly increased. Levels of Ki-67 immunostaining and expression of cell cyclin D in the residual liver after ALPPS were also higher [262, 263], and the Hippo-YAP pathway played a role in liver structural reorganization [260]. TNF-α and IL-6 have been repeatedly confirmed to operate as a leading role in the initial stages of liver regeneration.

These two pro-inflammatory cytokines are produced by activated Kupffer cells in the liver, promoting the transition of liver cells from the G0 phase in a cell cycle to the G1 phase [264]. Transcriptomic studies identified the upregulation of Indian hedgehog (Ihh) after ALPPS, which was observed as early as 4 h after the stage-1 operation. Functional experiments showed that recombinant Ihh combined with PVL can simulate the rapid regeneration after the first stage of complete transection of ALPPS, while neutralizing Ihh can eliminate common regeneration in ALPPS. Moreover, Ihh was detected in human plasma early after the first stage, confirming its clinical relevance to this molecular pathway [265]. Magda Langiewicz and Pieter Borger et al. [266] analyzed the signal network behind the accelerated regeneration process induced by ALPPS using transcriptomics. These analyses were performed on liver tissues obtained from mouse ALPPS models, standard liver resection surgery (68% model), and other control surgeries (sham surgery, PVL, and Tx). Results revealed that ALPPS is not a simple addition of PVL plus liver parenchymal transection, but there is a significant increase and earlier activation of signaling pathways in the early stages of normal and accelerated liver regeneration [266].

A genetic analysis conducted by Kasper Jarlhelt Andersen et al. [267] in rats showed upregulation of genes involved in cell proliferation and downregulation of genes involved in cell homeostasis. The excess liver regeneration after ALPPS may be mediated by substantial parenchymal damage and subsequent release of growth stimuli, leading to the upregulation of genes involved in cell regeneration and downregulation of genes involved in cell homeostasis. Naohiko Otsuka et al. [268] established a rat ALPPS model and compared it with a PVL model, systematically analyzing liver regeneration rate, levels of inflammatory cytokines, the activation status of the JAK2/STAT3 pathway, and the expression of Reg3α and Reg3β (regenerating islet-derived, Reg). The liver regeneration rate in the ALPPS group was significantly higher than in other groups, while the levels of inflammatory cytokines were almost equal. Additional FLR increase in the

ALPPS group depended on JAK2/STAT3, and expression of Reg3α and Reg3β was observed only in the ALPPS group, indicating that the increase in inflammatory cytokines was not sufficient to describe the mechanism of rapid liver hypertrophy induced by ALPPS, and the expression of Reg3α and Reg3β may play an important role along with the activation of the JAK2/STAT3 pathway.

In conclusion, with ongoing clinical and animal research, some understanding of its underlying mechanism has been achieved. Nevertheless, its detailed mechanisms, especially the molecular mechanisms of liver regeneration, are still not completely elucidated, and further research is needed to promote better understanding and application.

Since its establishment in 2007, ALPPS has marked 15 years of rapid development. During this period, the global enthusiasm among hepatobiliary surgeons for this procedure has been soaring, with unremitting efforts invested, leading to a myriad of surgical techniques akin to a blossoming of flowers. The flexible application of its principles vividly demonstrates the fusion of surgical intellect and artistry. Groundbreaking procedures like monosegment ALPPS continuously broaden our boundaries of understanding towards liver regeneration.

The unique design of the RAPID technique, combining ALPPS with living donor liver transplantation, has opened new frontiers. The international collaborative efforts of the ALPPS registry showcase a novel model of global cooperation in modern surgery. They swiftly evaluate and address various challenges in the short term, rapidly advancing this new technology to the mature stage of technical development. ALPPS can be considered a culmination of modern surgery development and an exemplar of the evolution of new surgical techniques.

From an incidental procedure and a great discovery to rapid exploration and reporting and further global collaborative efforts, the development process of ALPPS not only exemplifies the history of technological advancement but also serves as an epitome of the latest developments in modern surgery. It provides profound insights that can greatly inspire and contribute to innovation and breakthroughs in other fields.

ALPPS has initiated a new era in the history of liver surgery and stands out as one of the greatest innovations in the field in recent decades [37]. It achieves unprecedented FLR induction and boasts a high tumor resection rate. Although initially associated with high complication and mortality rates, these have tremendously improved with technological advancements and adjustments in case selection, approaching levels comparable with those of routine extensive liver resections. Increasingly, surgeons are accepting and adopting this technique, making it one of the therapeutic choices in guidelines [2]. This new strategy provides a curative opportunity for many patients with initially unresectable liver tumors, substantially improving their survival. Simultaneously, ALPPS, to a considerable extent, alleviates surgeons' concerns about PHLF, equipping them with a powerful tool (for example, in cases where unexpected intraoperative events result in insufficient FLR, ALPPS can be performed to avoid PHLF, avoiding directly closing the abdomen and depriving patients of the opportunity for tumor resection).

Looking back at the development of ALPPS over the past decade, it has undergone an evolution from the original procedure to classic ALPPS, and various variants from right trisectionectomy ALPPS to reverse ALPPS, mesohepatectomy ALPPS, monosegment ALPPS, and various procedures with unrestricted tumor types and FLR locations. The induction of FLR by ALPPS has evolved from rapid induction to safely rapid induction. Indications have expanded from PHCC to other common malignant liver tumors such as CRLM, HCC, ICC, and rare liver tumors, including NET liver metastases and GIST liver metastases. The scope of the population has broadened from adults to children. Its application scenarios have diversified from simple FLR proliferation induction for two-stage resection to a combination of living donor liver transplantation using RAPID for total hepatectomy and salvage ALPPS after PVE failure. From initial concerns about its high complication and mortality rates, the safety profile has become less controversial, approaching levels comparable to routine extensive liver resection. There has been a transition from a lack of long-term results to the continuous publication of high-level evidence from RCTs, clarifying its efficacy, safety, and oncological benefits. Skepticism and opposition have transformed into widespread expert recognition. ALPPS has moved from being a salvage option after PVE failure to a widespread application in various scenarios.

Thanks to the enthusiasm and relentless efforts of global hepatobiliary surgeons in pursuing and exploring innovations, ALPPS has advanced significantly over a decade. Following the five stages of novel surgical technology development (IDEAL: Innovation, Development, Exploration, Assessment, and Long-term), it is currently in the Assessment phase and steadily entering the final stage [37, 149].

Looking ahead, ALPPS, as a monumental surgical innovation, is poised to make even more remarkable contributions to rescuing unresectable liver cancer patients. With the continuous improvement of ALPPS technology and its integration with multidisciplinary approaches, including conversion therapy, elucidation of liver regeneration mechanisms, and application, its scope of usage will be expanded, and safety will be further enhanced. This will provide an opportunity for curative resection for more liver cancer patients who are regarded as unresectable by traditional methods, offering them a chance for cure and long-term survival.

References

1. Alikhanov R, Dudareva A, Trigo MÁ, et al. Vascular resection for intrahepatic cholangiocarcinoma: current considerations. J Clin Med. 2021;10(17):3829.
2. Zhou J, Sun HC, Wang Z, et al. Guidelines for the diagnosis and treatment of primary liver cancer (2022 edition). Liver Cancer. 2023;12(5):405–44.
3. Clavien PA, Petrowsky H, DeOliveira ML, et al. Strategies for safer liver surgery and partial liver transplantation. N Engl J Med. 2007;356(15):1545–59.
4. Siegel R, Miller KD, Fuchs HE, et al. Cancer statistics, 2022. CA Cancer J Clin. 2022;72(1):7–33.
5. Treska V. Methods to increase future liver remnant volume in patients with primarily unresectable colorectal liver metastases: current state and future perspectives. Anticancer Res. 2016;36(5):2065–71.
6. Bruix J, Llovet JM. Prognostic prediction and treatment strategy in hepatocellular carcinoma. Hepatology. 2002;35(3):519–24.
7. Taub R. Liver regeneration: from myth to mechanism. Nat Rev Mol Cell Biol. 2004;5(10):836–47.
8. Michalopoulos GK, DeFrances M. Liver regeneration. Adv Biochem Eng Biotechnol. 2005;93:101–34.
9. Fausto N, Campbell JS, Riehle KJ. Liver regeneration. J Hepatol. 2012;57(3):692–4.
10. Sun HC, Zhou J, Wang Z, et al. Chinese expert consensus on conversion therapy for hepatocellular carcinoma (2021 edition). Hepatobiliary Surg Nutr. 2022;11(2):227–52.
11. Fernandes ESM, de Mello FPT, Andrade RO, et al. Living donor liver transplant as rescue surgery for a patient with hepatocellular carcinoma who underwent associating liver partition and portal vein ligation for staged hepatectomy (ALPPS). Am J Case Rep. 2018;19:1338–41.
12. Gruttadauria S, Vasta F, Minervini MI, et al. Significance of the effective remnant liver volume in major hepatectomies. Am Surg. 2005;71(3):235–40.
13. von Frerichs FT. A clinical treatise on diseases of the liver[M]. New York: William Wood & Co.; 2010. p. 1879.
14. Rous P, Larimore LD. Relation of the portal blood to liver maintenance: a demonstration of liver atrophy conditional on compensation. J Exp Med. 1920;31(5):609–32.
15. Makuuchi M, Thai BL, Takayasu K, et al. Preoperative portal embolization to increase safety of major hepatectomy for hilar bile duct carcinoma: a preliminary report. Surgery. 1990;107(5):521–7.
16. Makuuchi M, Takayasu K, Takuma T, et al. Preoperative transcatheter embolization of the portal venous branch for patients receiving extended lobectomy due to the bile duct carcinoma. J Jpn Pract Surg Soc. 1984;45(12):1558–64.
17. Kinoshita H, Sakai K, Hirohashi K, et al. Preoperative portal vein embolization for hepatocellular carcinoma. World J Surg. 1986;10(5):803–8.
18. Pamecha V, Levene A, Grillo F, et al. Effect of portal vein embolisation on the growth rate of colorectal liver metastases. Br J Cancer. 2009;100(4):617–22.
19. Alvarez FA, Ardiles V, Sanchez Claria R, et al. Associating liver partition and portal vein ligation for staged hepatectomy (ALPPS): tips and tricks. J Gastrointest Surg. 2013;17(4):814–21.
20. Adam R, Laurent A, Azoulay D, et al. Two-stage hepatectomy: a planned strategy to treat irresectable liver tumors. Ann Surg. 2000;232(6):777–85.
21. Wicherts DA, Miller R, de Haas RJ, et al. Long-term results of two-stage hepatectomy for irresectable colorectal cancer liver metastases. Ann Surg. 2008;248(6):994–1005.
22. Jaeck D, Oussoultzoglou E, Rosso E, et al. A two-stage hepatectomy procedure combined with portal vein embolization to achieve curative resection for initially unresectable multiple and bilobar colorectal liver metastases. Ann Surg. 2004;240(6):1037–49. discussion 1049–1051
23. Aussilhou B, Lesurtel M, Sauvanet A, et al. Right portal vein ligation is as efficient as portal vein embolization to induce hypertrophy of the left liver remnant. J Gastrointest Surg. 2008;12(2):297–303.
24. Inaba S, Takada T, Amano H, et al. Combination of preoperative embolization of the right portal vein and hepatic artery prior to major hepatectomy in high-risk patients: a preliminary report. Hepato-Gastroenterology. 2000;47(34):1077–81.
25. Yoo H, Kim JH, Ko GY, et al. Sequential transcatheter arterial chemoembolization and portal vein embolization versus portal vein embolization only before major hepatectomy for patients with hepatocellular carcinoma. Ann Surg Oncol. 2011;18(5):1251–7.
26. Vilgrain V, Sibert A, Zappa M, et al. Sequential arterial and portal vein embolization in patients with cirrhosis and hepatocellular carcinoma: the hospital beaujon experience. Semin Intervent Radiol. 2008;25(2):155–61.
27. Nagino M, Yamada T, Kamiya J, et al. Left hepatic trisegmentectomy with right hepatic vein resection after right hepatic vein embolization. Surgery. 2003;133(5):580–2.
28. Pandanaboyana S, Bell R, Hidalgo E, et al. A systematic review and meta-analysis of portal vein ligation versus portal vein embolization for elective liver resection. Surgery. 2015;157(4):690–8.
29. Hemming AW, Reed AI, Howard RJ, et al. Preoperative portal vein embolization for extended hepatectomy. Ann Surg. 2003;237(5):686–91. discussion 691–693
30. Abulkhir A, Limongelli P, Healey AJ, et al. Preoperative portal vein embolization for major liver resection: a meta-analysis. Ann Surg. 2008;247(1):49–57.
31. van Lienden KP, van den Esschert JW, de Graaf W, et al. Portal vein embolization before liver resection: a systematic review. Cardiovasc Intervent Radiol. 2013;36(1):25–34.
32. Vyas SJ, Davies N, Grant L, et al. Failure of portal venous embolization. ALPPS as salvage enabling successful resection of bilobar liver metastases. J Gastrointest Cancer. 2014;45(Suppl 1):233–6.
33. Faitot F, Soubrane O, Wendum D, et al. Feasibility and survival of 2-stage hepatectomy for colorectal metastases: definition of a simple and early clinicopathologic predicting score. Surgery. 2015;157(3):444–53.
34. Tschuor CH, Croome KP, Sergeant G, et al. Salvage parenchymal liver transection for patients with insufficient volume increase after portal vein occlusion —an extension of the ALPPS approach. Eur J Surg Oncol. 2013;39(11):1230–5.
35. Tsai S, Marques HP, de Jong MC, et al. Two-stage strategy for patients with extensive bilateral colorectal liver metastases. HPB (Oxford). 2010;12(4):262–9.
36. Zhang L, Yang ZT, Zhang SY, et al. Conventional two-stage hepatectomy or associating liver partitioning and portal vein ligation for staged hepatectomy for colorectal liver metastases? A systematic review and meta-analysis. Front Oncol. 2020;10:1391.
37. de Santibañes E, Clavien PA. Playing play-Doh to prevent postoperative liver failure: the "ALPPS" approach. Ann Surg. 2012;255(3):415–7.
38. Schlitt HJ, Hackl C, Lang SA. 'In-situ split' liver resection/ALPPS – historical development and current practice. Visc Med. 2017;33(6):408–12.
39. Baumgart J, Lang SA, Lang H. A new method for induction of liver hypertrophy prior to right trisectionectomy: a report of three cases. HPB (Oxford). 2011;13:71–2.
40. Schnitzbauer AA, Lang SA, Goessmann H, et al. Right portal vein ligation combined with *in situ* splitting induces rapid left lateral liver lobe hypertrophy enabling 2-staged extended right hepatic resection in small-for-size settings. Ann Surg. 2012;255(3):405–14.

41. Linecker M, Björnsson B, Stavrou GA, et al. Risk adjustment in ALPPS is associated with a dramatic decrease in early mortality and morbidity. Ann Surg. 2017;266(5):779–86.
42. D'Haese JG, Neumann J, Weniger M, et al. Should ALPPS be used for liver resection in intermediate-stage HCC? Ann Surg Oncol. 2016;23(4):1335–43.
43. Enne M, Schadde E, Björnsson B, et al. ALPPS as a salvage procedure after insufficient future liver remnant hypertrophy following portal vein occlusion. HPB (Oxford). 2017;19(12):1126–9.
44. Eshmuminov D, Raptis DA, Linecker M, et al. Meta-analysis of associating liver partition with portal vein ligation and portal vein occlusion for two-stage hepatectomy. Br J Surg. 2016;103(13):1768–82.
45. Linecker M, Kron P, Lang H, et al. Too many languages in the ALPPS: preventing another tower of babel? Ann Surg. 2016;263(5):837–8.
46. Linecker M, Stavrou GA, Oldhafer KJ, et al. The ALPPS risk score: avoiding futile use of ALPPS. Ann Surg. 2016;264(5):763–71.
47. Olthof PB, Coelen RJS, Wiggers JK, et al. High mortality after ALPPS for perihilar cholangiocarcinoma: case-control analysis including the first series from the international ALPPS registry. HPB (Oxford). 2017;19(5):381–7.
48. Olthof PB, Huiskens J, Wicherts DA, et al. Survival after associating liver partition and portal vein ligation for staged hepatectomy (ALPPS) for advanced colorectal liver metastases: a case-matched comparison with palliative systemic therapy. Surgery. 2017;161(4):909–19.
49. Schadde E, Ardiles V, Robles-Campos R, et al. Early survival and safety of ALPPS: first report of the international ALPPS registry. Ann Surg. 2014;260(5):829–36. discussion 836–838
50. Schadde E, Raptis DA, Schnitzbauer AA, et al. Prediction of mortality after ALPPS stage-1: an analysis of 320 patients from the international ALPPS registry. Ann Surg. 2015;262(5):780–5. discussion 785–786
51. Viganò L, Cimino MM, Adam R, et al. Improving the safety of ALPPS procedure: the optimal compromise between dropout and mortality risk. Comment on Schadde E et al prediction of mortality after ALPPS stage-1: an analysis of 320 patients from the international ALPPS registry. Ann Surg. 2015; 262: 780–786. Ann Surg. 2017;266(6):e101–2.
52. Wanis KN, Buac S, Linecker M, et al. Patient survival after simultaneous ALPPS and colorectal resection. World J Surg. 2017;41(4):1119–25.
53. Oldhafer KJ, Stavrou GA, van Gulik TM, et al. ALPPS—where do we stand, where do we go?: eight recommendations from the first international expert meeting. Ann Surg. 2016;263(5):839–41.
54. Zhou J, Wang Z, Sun J, et al. Associating liver partition and portal vien ligation for staged hepatectomy. Chin J Dig Surg. 2013;12(7):485–9.
55. Peng YF, Wang Z, Zhou J. Advances of associating liver partition and portal vein ligation for staged hepatectomy in the treatment of primarily unresectable liver cancer. Chin J Dig Surg. 2021;20(2):155–62.
56. Liu WY, Liu Stephanie HY. Comments on associating liver partition and portal vein ligation for staged hepatectomy. Chin J Dig Surg. 2013;12(7):481–4.
57. Schadde E, Schnitzbauer AA, Tschuor C, et al. Systematic review and meta-analysis of feasibility, safety, and efficacy of a novel procedure: associating liver partition and portal vein ligation for staged hepatectomy. Ann Surg Oncol. 2015;22(9):3109–20.
58. Alvarez FA, Ardiles V, de Santibañes E. The ALPPS approach for the management of colorectal carcinoma liver metastases. Curr Colorectal Cancer Rep. 2013;9(2):168–77.
59. Sala S, Ardiles V, Ulla M, et al. Our initial experience with ALPPS technique: encouraging results. Updat Surg. 2012;64(3):167–72.
60. Schadde E, Hernandez-Alejandro R, Lang H, et al. ALPPS offers a better chance of complete resection in patients with primarily unresectable liver tumors. Results of a multicentre analysis: reply. World J Surg. 2015;39(7):1850–1.
61. Truant S, Scatton O, Dokmak S, et al. Associating liver partition and portal vein ligation for staged hepatectomy (ALPPS): impact of the inter-stages course on morbi-mortality and implications for management. Eur J Surg Oncol. 2015;41(5):674–82.
62. Vicente E, Quijano Y, Ielpo B, et al. Is "small for size syndrome" a relatively new complication after the ALPPS procedure? Updat Surg. 2015;67(3):273–8.
63. Torres OJM, de Souza Martins Fernandes E, Oliveira CVC, et al. Associating liver partition and portal vein ligation for staged hepatectomy (ALPPS): the Brazilian experience. Arq Bras Cir Dig. 2013;26(1):40–3.
64. Li J, Girotti P, Königsrainer I, et al. ALPPS in right trisectionectomy: a safe procedure to avoid postoperative liver failure? J Gastrointest Surg. 2013;17(5):956–61.
65. Nadalin S, Capobianco I, Li J, et al. Indications and limits for associating liver partition and portal vein ligation for staged hepatectomy (ALPPS). Lessons learned from 15 cases at a single Centre. Z Gastroenterol. 2014;52(1):35–42.
66. Kremer M, Manzini G, Hristov B, et al. Impact of neoadjuvant chemotherapy on hypertrophy of the future liver remnant after associating liver partition and portal vein ligation for staged hepatectomy. J Am Coll Surg. 2015;221(3):717–728.e1.
67. Schadde E, Ardiles V, Slankamenac K, et al. ALPPS offers a better chance of complete resection in patients with primarily unresectable liver tumors compared with conventional-staged hepatectomies: results of a multicenter analysis. World J Surg. 2014;38(6):1510–9.
68. Figueras J, Belghiti J. The ALPPS approach: should we sacrifice basic therapeutic rules in the name of innovation? World J Surg. 2014;38(6):1520–1.
69. Kokudo N, Shindoh J. How can we safely climb the ALPPS? Updat Surg. 2013;65(3):175–7.
70. Dokmak S, Belghiti J. Which limits to the "ALPPS" approach? Ann Surg. 2012;256(3):e6. author reply e16-17
71. van den Broek MA, van Dam RM, Malagó M, et al. Feasibility of randomized controlled trials in liver surgery using surgery-related mortality or morbidity as endpoint. Br J Surg. 2009;96(9):1005–14.
72. Robles R, Parrilla P, López-Conesa A, et al. Tourniquet modification of the associating liver partition and portal ligation for staged hepatectomy procedure. Br J Surg. 2014;101(9):1129–34. discussion 1134
73. de Santibañes M, Alvarez FA, Santos FR, et al. The associating liver partition and portal vein ligation for staged hepatectomy approach using only segments I and IV as future liver remnant. J Am Coll Surg. 2014;219(2):e5–9.
74. Ardiles V, Schadde E, Santibanes E, et al. Commentary on "happy marriage or 'dangerous liaison': ALPPS and the anterior approach". Ann Surg. 2014;260(2):e4.
75. de Santibañes E, Alvarez FA, Ardiles V, et al. Inverting the ALPPS paradigm by minimizing first stage impact: the mini-ALPPS technique. Langenbeck's Arch Surg. 2016;401(4):557–63.
76. Chan ACY, Pang R, Poon RTP. Simplifying the ALPPS procedure by the anterior approach. Ann Surg. 2014;260(2):e3.
77. Wang Z, Peng YF, Hu JW, et al. Associating liver partition and portal vein ligation for staged hepatectomy for unresectable hepatitis B virus-related hepatocellular carcinoma: a single center study of 45 patients. Ann Surg. 2020;271(3):534–41.
78. Vennarecci G, Levi Sandri GB, Ettorre GM. Performing the ALPPS procedure by anterior approach and liver hanging maneuver. Ann Surg. 2016;263(1):e11.
79. Alexandrescu S, Stoica L, Grigorie R, et al. Primary hepatic lymphoma resected by ALPPS procedure (associating liver partition

and portal vein ligation for staged hepatectomy). J Transl Med Res. 2016;21(2):153.
80. Gauzolino R, Castagnet M, Blanleuil ML, et al. The ALPPS technique for bilateral colorectal metastases: three "variations on a theme". Updat Surg. 2013;65(2):141–8.
81. Ettorre G, Guglielmo N, Meniconi R, et al. Variation on a theme: alternative to plastic bag in ALPPS procedures-feasibility and clinical safety of COVA+™ membrane in ALPPS procedure. World J Surg. 2016;40(6):1532–3.
82. Brustia R, Scatton O, Soubrane O. Variation on a theme: alternative to plastic bag in ALPPS procedures. Feasibility and clinical safety of COVA+™ membrane in ALPPS procedures. World J Surg. 2016;40(6):1534.
83. Sakamoto Y, Inagaki F, Omichi K, et al. Associating liver partial partition and transileocecal portal vein embolization for staged hepatectomy. Ann Surg. 2016;264(6):e21–2.
84. Baumgart J, Jungmann F, Bartsch F, et al. Two-stage hepatectomy and ALPPS for advanced bilateral liver metastases: a tailored approach balancing risk and outcome. J Gastrointest Surg. 2019;23(12):2391–400.
85. Machado MA, Makdissi FF, Surjan RC, et al. Transition from open to laparoscopic ALPPS for patients with very small FLR: the initial experience. HPB (Oxford). 2017;19(1):59–66.
86. Olthof PB, Rassam F, van Gulik TM. The use of a NHS-PEG coated, collagen-based sealant in a patient undergoing associating liver partition and portal vein ligation for staged hepatectomy (ALPPS). Int J Surg Case Rep. 2018;47:7–10.
87. Brustia R, Scatton O, Perdigao F, et al. Vessel identifications tags for open or laparoscopic associating liver partition and portal vein ligation for staged hepatectomy. J Am Coll Surg. 2013;217(6):e51–5.
88. Andriani OC. Long-term results with associating liver partition and portal vein ligation for staged hepatectomy (ALPPS). Ann Surg. 2012;256(3):e5. author reply e16-19
89. Buac S, Schadde E, Schnitzbauer AA, et al. The many faces of ALPPS: surgical indications and techniques among surgeons collaborating in the international registry. HPB (Oxford). 2016;18(5):442–8.
90. Tanaka K, Kikuchi Y, Kawaguchi D, et al. Modified ALPPS procedures avoiding division of portal pedicles. Ann Surg. 2017;265(2):e14–20.
91. Petrowsky H, Györi G, de Oliveira M, et al. Is partial-ALPPS safer than ALPPS? A single-center experience. Ann Surg. 2015;261(4):e90–2.
92. Alvarez FA, Ardiles V, de Santibañes M, et al. Associating liver partition and portal vein ligation for staged hepatectomy offers high oncological feasibility with adequate patient safety: a prospective study at a single center. Ann Surg. 2015;261(4):723–32.
93. Linecker M, Kambakamba P, Reiner CS, et al. How much liver needs to be transected in ALPPS? A translational study investigating the concept of less invasiveness. Surgery. 2017;161(2):453–64.
94. Rassam F, Olthof PB, van Lienden KP, et al. Comparison of functional and volumetric increase of the future remnant liver and postoperative outcomes after portal vein embolization and complete or partial associating liver partition and portal vein ligation for staged hepatectomy (ALPPS). Ann Transl Med. 2020;8(7):436.
95. Truant S, El Amrani M, Baillet C, et al. Laparoscopic partial ALPPS: much better than ALPPS! Ann Hepatol. 2019;18(1):269–73.
96. Chan ACY, Chok K, Dai JWC, et al. Impact of split completeness on future liver remnant hypertrophy in associating liver partition and portal vein ligation for staged hepatectomy (ALPPS) in hepatocellular carcinoma: complete-ALPPS versus partial-ALPPS. Surgery. 2017;161(2):357–64.
97. Kumar N, Duncan T, O'Reilly D, et al. Partial ALPPS with a longer wait between procedures is safe and yields adequate future liver remnant hypertrophy. Ann Hepatobiliary Pancreat Surg. 2019;23(1):13–9.
98. Robles Campos R, Parrilla Paricio P, López Conesa A, et al. A new surgical technique for extended right hepatectomy: tourniquet in the umbilical fissure and right portal vein occlusion (ALTPS). Clin Case Cir Esp. 2013;91(10):633–7.
99. Robles-Campos R, Brusadin R, López-Conesa A, et al. Long-term outcome after conventional two-stage hepatectomy versus tourniquet-ALPPS in colorectal liver metastases: a propensity score matching analysis. World J Surg. 2019;43(9):2281–9.
100. Cai XJ, Peng SY, Duan L, et al. Completely laparoscopic ALPPS using round-the-liver ligation to replace parenchymal transection for a patient with multiple right liver cancers complicated with liver cirrhosis. J Laparoendosc Adv Surg Tech A. 2014;24(12):883–6.
101. Cai XJ, Tong YF, Yu H, et al. The ALPPS in the treatment of hepatitis B-related hepatocellular carcinoma with cirrhosis: a single-center study and literature review. Surg Innov. 2017;24(4):358–64.
102. Ciria R, Ayllón MD, Padial A, et al. Totally laparoscopic tourniquet ALPPS: technical standardization by combining the pure hanging maneuver and the approach through the sugioka gates. Ann Surg Oncol. 2022;29(4):2410–1.
103. Gall TM, Sodergren MH, Frampton AE, et al. Radio-frequency-assisted liver partition with portal vein ligation (RALPP) for liver regeneration. Ann Surg. 2015;261(2):e45–6.
104. Jiao LR, Fajardo Puerta AB, Gall TMH, et al. Rapid induction of liver regeneration for major hepatectomy (REBIRTH): a randomized controlled trial of portal vein embolisation versus ALPPS assisted with radiofrequency. Cancers. 2019;11(3):302.
105. Sandström P, Røsok BI, Sparrelid E, et al. ALPPS improves resectability compared with conventional two-stage hepatectomy in patients with advanced colorectal liver metastasis: results from a Scandinavian multicenter randomized controlled trial (LIGRO trial). Ann Surg. 2018;267(5):833–40.
106. Wang Q, Yan J, Feng XB, et al. Safety and efficacy of radiofrequency-assisted ALPPS (RALPPS) in patients with cirrhosis-related hepatocellular carcinoma. Int J Hyperth. 2017;33(7):846–52.
107. Wang Q, Chen S, Yan J, et al. Rescue radiofrequency ablation or percutaneous ethanol injection: a strategy for failed RALPPS stage-1 in patients with cirrhosis-related hepatocellular carcinoma. BMC Surg. 2021;21(1):246.
108. Zhang JW, Huang HC, Bian J, et al. Safety, feasibility, and efficacy of associating liver partition and portal vein ligation for staged hepatectomy in treating hepatocellular carcinoma: a systematic review. Ann Transl Med. 2020;8(19):1246.
109. Gringeri E, Boetto R, D'Amico FE, et al. Laparoscopic microwave ablation and portal vein ligation for staged hepatectomy (LAPS): a minimally invasive first-step approach. Ann Surg. 2015;261(2):e42–3.
110. Cillo U, Gringeri E, Feltracco P, et al. Totally laparoscopic microwave ablation and portal vein ligation for staged hepatectomy: a new minimally invasive two-stage hepatectomy. Ann Surg Oncol. 2015;22(8):2787–8.
111. Boggi U, Napoli N, Kauffmann EF, et al. Laparoscopic microwave liver ablation and portal vein ligation: an alternative approach to the conventional ALPPS procedure in hilar cholangiocarcinoma. Ann Surg Oncol. 2016;23(Suppl 5):884.
112. Chen ZB, Shen SL, Xie WX, et al. Comparison of clinical efficacy between LAPS and ALPPS in the treatment of hepatitis B virus-related hepatocellular carcinoma. Gastroenterol Rep. 2023;11:goad060.

113. Li J, Kantas A, Ittrich H, et al. Avoid "all-touch" by hybrid ALPPS to achieve oncological efficacy. Ann Surg. 2016;263(1):e6–7.
114. Balci D. Pushing the envelope in perihiler cholangiocellularcarcinoma surgery: TIPE-ALPPS. Ann Surg. 2018;267(2):e21–2.
115. Pekolj J, Alvarez FA, Biagiola D, et al. Totally laparoscopic mini-ALPPS using a novel approach of laparoscopic-assisted transmesenteric portal vein embolization. J Laparoendosc Adv Surg Tech A. 2018;28(10):1229–33.
116. Lai Q, Melandro F, Rossi M. Hybrid partial ALPPS: a feasible approach in case of right trisegmentectomy and macrovascular invasion. Ann Surg. 2018;267(4):e80–2.
117. Chan AC, Poon RT, Chan C, et al. Safety of ALPPS procedure by the anterior approach for hepatocellular carcinoma. Ann Surg. 2016;263(2):e14–6.
118. Gutt CN, Oniu T, Schemmer P, et al. Fewer adhesions induced by laparoscopic surgery? Surg Endosc. 2004;18(6):898–906.
119. Berardi G, van Cleven S, Fretland ÅA, et al. Evolution of laparoscopic liver surgery from innovation to implementation to mastery: perioperative and oncologic outcomes of 2, 238 patients from 4 European specialized centers. J Am Coll Surg. 2017;225(5):639–49.
120. Ciria R, Cherqui D, Geller DA, et al. Comparative short-term benefits of laparoscopic liver resection: 9000 cases and climbing. Ann Surg. 2016;263(4):761–77.
121. Wakabayashi G, Cherqui D, Geller DA, et al. Recommendations for laparoscopic liver resection: a report from the second international consensus conference held in Morioka. Ann Surg. 2015;261(4):619–29.
122. Jakab F. Milestones in liver surgery. Orv Hetil. 2018;159(10):375–83.
123. Machado MA, Makdissi FF, Surjan RC. Totally laparoscopic ALPPS is feasible and may be worthwhile. Ann Surg. 2012;256(3):e13. author reply e16-19
124. Conrad C, Shivathirthan N, Camerlo A, et al. Laparoscopic portal vein ligation with *in situ* liver split for failed portal vein embolization. Ann Surg. 2012;256(3):e14–5. author reply e16-17
125. Michal K, Sau M, Tamara GMH, et al. A better route to ALPPS: minimally invasive vs open ALPPS. Surg Endosc. 2020;34(6):2379–89.
126. Serenari M, Ratti F, Zanello M, et al. Minimally invasive stage 1 to protect against the risk of liver failure: results from the hepatocellular carcinoma series of the associating liver partition and portal vein ligation for staged hepatectomy Italian registry. J Laparoendosc Adv Surg Tech A. 2020;30(10):1082–9.
127. Serenari M, Ratti F, Guglielmo N, et al. Evolution of minimally invasive techniques and surgical outcomes of ALPPS in Italy: a comprehensive trend analysis over 10 years from a national prospective registry. Surg Endosc. 37(7):5285–94.
128. Guhra S, Ardelt M, Settmacher U. Long-term results after ALPPS resections in patients with colorectal liver metastases. Chirurg. 2021;92(2):169.
129. Cioffi L, Belli G, Izzo F, et al. Minimally invasive ALPPS procedure: a review of feasibility and short-term outcomes. Cancers. 2023;15(6):1700.
130. Solomonov E, Tzadok I, Stemmer S, et al. Case report: robotic ALPPS procedure for hepatocellular carcinoma in the right lobe of the liver. Front Surg. 2021;8:655683.
131. Wang XY, Gao Q, Duan M, et al. Outcomes of robot-assisted laparoscopic liver resection: a report of 142 cases. Chin J Pract Surg. 2017;37(5):548–51.
132. Machado MAC, Surjan RC, Makdissi F. Robotic ALPPS. Ann Surg Oncol. 2020;27(4):1174–9.
133. Hu MG, Wang J, Yin ZZ, et al. First two-stage robotic ALPPS in HCC patients with hepatic vein invasion: a step-by-step procedure from a clinical case. World J Surg Oncol. 2021;19(1):58.
134. di Benedetto F, Assirati G, Magistri P. Full robotic ALPPS for HCC with intrahepatic portal vein thrombosis. Int J Med Robot. 2020;16(2):e2087.
135. Fernandes ESM, de Barros F, Magistri P, et al. Total robotic ALPPS approach for hepatocellular carcinoma in cirrhotic liver. Int J Med Robot. 2021;17(3):e2238.
136. Di Benedetto F, Magistri P. First case of full robotic ALPPS for intrahepatic cholangiocarcinoma. Ann Surg Oncol. 2021;28(2):865.
137. di Benedetto F, Magistri P, Guerrini GP, et al. Robotic liver partition and portal vein embolization for staged hepatectomy for perihilar cholangiocarcinoma. Updat Surg. 2022;74(2):773–7.
138. Guidetti C, Müller PC, Magistri P, et al. Full robotic versus open ALPPS: a bi-institutional comparison of perioperative outcomes. Surg Endosc. 2024;38(6):3448–54.
139. Muñoz C, Naranjo M, Varela C, et al. Laparoscopic hybrid mini-ALPPS using transmesenteric intra-operative portal embolization for locally advanced intrahepatic cholangiocarcinoma. Cir Esp. 2024;102(1):40.
140. Oldhafer KJ, Wagner KC, Kantas A, et al. Hybrid-ALPPS followed by ante situm with cardiopulmonary bypass: rapid liver augmentation and complex surgery. Ann Surg Oncol. 2020;27(9):3341.
141. Hong DF, Zhang YB, Peng SY, et al. Percutaneous microwave ablation liver partition and portal vein embolization for rapid liver regeneration: a minimally invasive first step of ALPPS for hepatocellular carcinoma. Ann Surg. 2016;264(1):e1–2.
142. Lunardi A, Cervelli R, Volterrani D, et al. Feasibility of percutaneous intrahepatic split by microwave ablation (PISA) after portal vein embolization for hypertrophy of future liver remnant: the radiological stage-1 ALPPS. Cardiovasc Intervent Radiol. 2018;41(5):789–98.
143. Herman P, Krüger JA, Perini MV, et al. High mortality rates after ALPPS: the devil is the indication. J Gastrointest Cancer. 2015;46(2):190–4.
144. Serenari M, Zanello M, Schadde E, et al. Importance of primary indication and liver function between stages: results of a multicenter Italian audit of ALPPS 2012-2014. HPB (Oxford). 2016;18(5):419–27.
145. Donati M, Basile F, Oldhafer KJ. Present status and future perspectives of ALPPS (associating liver partition and portal vein ligation for staged hepatectomy). Future Oncol. 2015;11(16):2255–8.
146. Al Hasan I, Tun-Abraham ME, Wanis KN, et al. Optimizing associated liver partition and portal vein ligation for staged hepatectomy outcomes: surgical experience or appropriate patient selection? Can J Surg. 2017;60(6):408–15.
147. Raptis DA, Linecker M, Kambakamba P, et al. Defining benchmark outcomes for ALPPS. Ann Surg. 2019;270(5):835–41.
148. Peng YF, Chen FY, Wang Z, et al. Associating liver partition and portal vein ligation for staged hepatectomy (ALPPS) for colorectal liver metastasis (CRLM): a single-center experience and review of the literature. iLiver. 2022;1(1):25–9.
149. Petrowsky H, Linecker M, Raptis DA, et al. First long-term oncologic results of the ALPPS procedure in a large cohort of patients with colorectal liver metastases. Ann Surg. 2020;272(5):793–800.
150. Capobianco I, Oldhafer KJ, Fard-Aghaie MH, et al. Development and internal validation of the comprehensive ALPPS preoperative risk assessment (CAPRA) score: is the patient suitable for asso-

ciating liver partition and portal vein ligation for staged hepatectomy (ALPPS)? Hepatobiliary Surg Nutr. 2022;11(1):52–66.
151. Linecker M, Kuemmerli C, Kambakamba P, et al. Performance validation of the ALPPS risk model. HPB (Oxford). 2019;21(6):711–21.
152. Kang D, Schadde E. Hypertrophy and liver function in ALPPS: correlation with morbidity and mortality. Visc Med. 2017;33(6):426–33.
153. Olthof PB, van Gulik TM, Bennink RJ. Optimal use of hepatobiliary scintigraphy before liver resection. HPB (Oxford). 2016;18(10):870.
154. Sparrelid E, Jonas E, Tzortzakakis A, et al. Dynamic evaluation of liver volume and function in associating liver partition and portal vein ligation for staged hepatectomy. J Gastrointest Surg. 2017;21(6):967–74.
155. Deshayes E, Schadde E, Piron L, et al. Extended liver venous deprivation leads to a higher increase in liver function that ALPPS in early assessment: a comment to "Sparrelid, E. et al. Dynamic evaluation of liver volume and function in associating liver partition and portal vein ligation for staged hepatectomy. *Journal of Gastrointestinal Surgery* (2017)". J Gastrointest Surg. 2017;21(10):1754–5.
156. Olthof PB, Schadde E, van Lienden KP, et al. Hepatic parenchymal transection increases liver volume but not function after portal vein embolization in rabbits. Surgery. 2017;162(4):732–41.
157. Truant S, Baillet C, Deshorgue AC, et al. Drop of total liver function in the interstages of the new associating liver partition and portal vein ligation for staged hepatectomy technique: analysis of the "auxiliary liver" by HIDA scintigraphy. Ann Surg. 2016;263(3):e33–4.
158. Cieslak KP, Olthof PB, van Lienden KP, et al. Assessment of liver function using (99m)Tc-mebrofenin hepatobiliary scintigraphy in ALPPS (associating liver partition and portal vein ligation for staged hepatectomy). Case Rep Gastroenterol. 2015;9(3):353–60.
159. Olthof PB, Tomassini F, Huespe PE, et al. Hepatobiliary scintigraphy to evaluate liver function in associating liver partition and portal vein ligation for staged hepatectomy: liver volume overestimates liver function. Surgery. 2017;162(4):775–83.
160. Truant S, Baillet C, Deshorgue AC, et al. Contribution of hepatobiliary scintigraphy in assessing ALPPS most suited timing. Updat Surg. 2017;69(3):411–9.
161. Tomassini F, D'Asseler Y, Giglio MC, et al. Hemodynamic changes in ALPPS influence liver regeneration and function: results from a prospective study. HPB (Oxford). 2019;21(5):557–65.
162. de Graaf W, van Lienden KP, Dinant S, et al. Assessment of future remnant liver function using hepatobiliary scintigraphy in patients undergoing major liver resection. J Gastrointest Surg. 2010;14(2):369–78.
163. Serenari M, Collaud C, Alvarez FA, et al. Interstage assessment of remnant liver function in ALPPS using hepatobiliary scintigraphy: prediction of posthepatectomy liver failure and introduction of the HIBA index. Ann Surg. 2018;267(6):1141–7.
164. Kambakamba P, Stocker D, Reiner CS, et al. Liver kinetic growth rate predicts postoperative liver failure after ALPPS. HPB (Oxford). 2016;18(10):800–5.
165. Lau L, Christophi C, Muralidharan V. Intraoperative functional liver remnant assessment with indocyanine green clearance: another toehold for climbing the "ALPPS". Ann Surg. 2015;261(2):e43–5.
166. Wanis KN, Linecker M, Madenci AL, et al. Variation in complications and mortality following ALPPS at early-adopting centers. HPB (Oxford). 2021;23(1):46–55.
167. Dimick JB, Wainess RM, Cowan JA, et al. National trends in the use and outcomes of hepatic resection. J Am Coll Surg. 2004;199(1):31–8.
168. Stavrou GA, Donati M, Fard-Aghaie MH, et al. Did the international ALPPS meeting 2015 have an impact on daily practice? The Hamburg barmbek experience of 58 cases. Visc Med. 2017;33(6):456–61.
169. Kikuchi Y, Hiroshima Y, Matsuo K, et al. Remnant liver tumor growth activity during treatment associating liver partition and portal vein occlusion for staged hepatectomy (ALPPS). J Gastrointest Surg. 2017;21(11):1851–8.
170. Olthof PB, Schnitzbauer AA, Schadde E. The HPB controversy of the decade: 2007–2017—ten years of ALPPS. Eur J Surg Oncol. 2018;44(10):1624–7.
171. Day RW, Conrad C, Vauthey JN, et al. Evaluating surgeon attitudes towards the safety and efficacy of portal vein occlusion and associating liver partition and portal vein ligation: a report of the MALINSA survey. HPB (Oxford). 2015;17(10):936–41.
172. Wang Z, Peng YF, Sun QM, et al. Salvage transhepatic arterial embolization after failed stage I ALPPS in a patient with a huge HCC with chronic liver disease: a case report. Int J Surg Case Rep. 2017;39:131–5.
173. Peng YF, Wang Z, Qu XD, et al. Transcatheter arterial embolization-salvaged ALPPS, a novel ALPPS procedure especially for patients with hepatocellular carcinoma and severe fibrosis/cirrhosis. Hepatobiliary Surg Nutr. 2022;11(4):504–14.
174. Lim C, Turco C, Balci D, et al. Auxiliary liver transplantation for cirrhosis: from APOLT to RAPID: a scoping review. Ann Surg. 2022;275(3):551–9.
175. Ali Deeb A, Rauchfuβ F, Gaβler N, et al. Liver regeneration after two-stage liver transplantation is more effective than after other preconditioning procedures in colorectal liver metastases. J Hepatobiliary Pancreat Sci. 2023;30(5):615–24.
176. Lang H, de Santibañes E, Schlitt HJ, et al. 10th anniversary of ALPPS-lessons learned and quo Vadis. Ann Surg. 2019;269(1):114–9.
177. Tsui TY, Heumann A, Vashist YK, et al. How we do it: double *in situ* split for staged mesohepatectomy in patients with advanced gall bladder cancer and marginal future liver remnant. Langenbeck's Arch Surg. 2016;401(4):565–71.
178. Obed A, Jarrad A, Bashir A. First left hepatic trisectionectomy including segment one with new associated liver partition and portal vein ligation with staged hepatectomy (ALPPS) modification: how to do it? Am J Case Rep. 2016;17:759–65.
179. Machado MA, Surjan R, Basseres T, et al. Total laparoscopic reversal ALPPS. Ann Surg Oncol. 2017;24(4):1048–9.
180. Voskanyan SE, Rudakov VS, Shabalin MV, et al. "Reversal" ALPPS in patient with hepatocellular carcinoma and liver cirrhosis. First clinical case in Russia. Ann HPB Surg. 2021;26(3):142–8.
181. Sakamoto Y, Matsumura M, Yamashita S, et al. Partial TIPE ALPPS for perihilar cancer. Ann Surg. 2018;267(2):e18–20.
182. Shindoh J, Tzeng CW, Aloia TA, et al. Optimal future liver remnant in patients treated with extensive preoperative chemotherapy for colorectal liver metastases. Ann Surg Oncol. 2013;20(8):2493–500.
183. Montalvá Orón EM, Maupoey Ibáñez J, Bañuelos Carrillo R, et al. Monosegment ALPPS: a new variant of the techniques for rapid hepatic regeneration. Critical review of the initial results of our series. Cir Esp. 2015;93(7):436–43.
184. Murtha-Lemekhova A, Fuchs J, Schulz E, et al. Pushing the limit of liver regeneration—safety and survival after monosegment-ALPPS: systematic review and individual patient data meta-analysis. HPB (Oxford). 2022;24(3):353–8.
185. Ruiz Figueroa EF, Fernández-Placencia RM, Berrospi Espinoza FE, et al. Monosegmental ALPPS: a long-term survival alternative to liver transplant in PRETEXT IV hepatoblastoma. J Surg Case Rep. 2019;2019(5):rjz144.

186. Soggiu F, Giovinazzo F, Straiton J, et al. Monosegment ALPPS hepatectomy preserving segment 4 for colorectal liver metastases: literature review and our experience. Hepatobiliary Surg Nutr. 2018;7(2):105–15.
187. Steinbrück K, D'Oliveira M, Cano R, et al. Monosegmental ALPPS after bilateral hepatectomy. Ann Hepatol. 2017;16(5):814–7.
188. Steinbrück K, Fernandes R, Stoduto G, et al. Monosegment ALPPS for bilateral colorectal liver metastasis—one is enough. Ann Hepatobiliary Pancreat Surg. 2020;24(4):522–5.
189. Schadde E, Malagó M, Hernandez-Alejandro R, et al. Monosegment ALPPS hepatectomy: extending resectability by rapid hypertrophy. Surgery. 2015;157(4):676–89.
190. Pineda-Solís K, Paskar D, Tun-Abraham M, et al. Expanding the limits of resectability: associating liver partition and portal vein ligation for staged hepatectomy (ALPPS) using monosegment 6, facilitated by an inferior right hepatic vein. J Surg Oncol. 2017;115(8):959–62.
191. Tang JC, Suolang WJ, Yang C, et al. Monosegmental ALPPS combined with ante-situm liver resection: a novel strategy for end-stage hepatic alveolar echinococcosis. Hepatobiliary Pancreat Dis Int. 2022;21(2):186–9.
192. Ruiz E, Fernandez-Placencia R, Bustamante J, et al. Monosegment associating liver partition and portal vein ligation for staged hepatectomy: preserving segment 1 as the only liver remnant after hepatocellular carcinoma recurrence. Ann Hepatobiliary Pancreat Surg. 2021;25(4):562–5.
193. Lai Q, Mennini G, Larghi Laureiro Z, et al. Uncommon indications for associating liver partition and portal vein ligation for staged hepatectomy: a systematic review. Hepatobiliary Surg Nutr. 2021;10(2):210–25.
194. Zhou J, Sun HC, Wang Z, et al. Guidelines for diagnosis and treatment of primary liver cancer in China (2017 edition). Liver Cancer. 2018;7(3):235–60.
195. Hernandez-Alejandro R, Bertens KA, Pineda-Solis K, et al. Can we improve the morbidity and mortality associated with the associating liver partition with portal vein ligation for staged hepatectomy (ALPPS) procedure in the management of colorectal liver metastases? Surgery. 2015;157(2):194–201.
196. Wanis KN, Ardiles V, Alvarez FA, et al. Intermediate-term survival and quality of life outcomes in patients with advanced colorectal liver metastases undergoing associating liver partition and portal vein ligation for staged hepatectomy. Surgery. 2018;163(4):691–7.
197. Kambakamba P, Hoti E, Cremen S, et al. The evolution of surgery for colorectal liver metastases: a persistent challenge to improve survival. Surgery. 2021;170(6):1732–40.
198. Gallinger S, Biagi JJ, Fletcher GG, et al. Liver resection for colorectal cancer metastases. Curr Oncol. 2013;20(3):e255–65.
199. Wang JW, Li S, Liu YN, et al. Metastatic patterns and survival outcomes in patients with stage IV colon cancer: a population-based analysis. Cancer Med. 2020;9(1):361–73.
200. Bekaii-Saab T, Wu C. Seeing the forest through the trees: a systematic review of the safety and efficacy of combination chemotherapies used in the treatment of metastatic colorectal cancer. Crit Rev Oncol Hematol. 2014;91(1):9–34.
201. Foubert F, Matysiak-Budnik T, Touchefeu Y. Options for metastatic colorectal cancer beyond the second line of treatment. Dig Liver Dis. 2014;46(2):105–12.
202. Hasselgren K, Røsok BI, Larsen PN, et al. ALPPS improves survival compared with TSH in patients affected of CRLM: survival analysis from the randomized controlled trial LIGRO. Ann Surg. 2021;273(3):442–8.
203. Bednarsch J, Czigany Z, Sharmeen S, et al. ALPPS versus two-stage hepatectomy for colorectal liver metastases—a comparative retrospective cohort study. World J Surg Oncol. 2020;18(1):140.
204. Chan A, Zhang WY, Chok K, et al. ALPPS versus portal vein embolization for hepatitis-related hepatocellular carcinoma: a changing paradigm in modulation of future liver remnant before major hepatectomy. Ann Surg. 2021;273(5):957–65.
205. Li PP, Huang G, Jia NY, et al. Associating liver partition and portal vein ligation for staged hepatectomy versus sequential transarterial chemoembolization and portal vein embolization in staged hepatectomy for HBV-related hepatocellular carcinoma: a randomized comparative study. Hepatobiliary Surg Nutr. 2022;11(1):38–51.
206. Peng CH, Li C, Liu C, et al. The outcome of the HCC patients underwent ALPPS: retrospective study. Medicine. 2019;98(38):e17182.
207. Ke LX, Shen R, Fan WZ, et al. The role of associating liver partition and portal vein ligation for staged hepatectomy in unresectable hepatitis B virus-related hepatocellular carcinoma. Ann Transl Med. 2020;8(21):1402.
208. Deng ZF, Jin ZR, Qin YH, et al. Efficacy of the association liver partition and portal vein ligation for staged hepatectomy for the treatment of solitary huge hepatocellular carcinoma: a retrospective single-center study. World J Surg Oncol. 2021;19(1):95.
209. Zhang JW, Xu YY, Yang HY, et al. Application of associating liver partition and portal vein ligation for staged hepatectomy for hepatocellular carcinoma related to hepatitis B virus: comparison with traditional one-stage right hepatectomy. Transl Cancer Res. 2020;9(9):5371–9.
210. Pham AT, Truong CM, Trinh PH. Overcome intraoperative difficulties of ALPPS procedure: a single-center outcomes and technical experience. Ann Med Surg (Lond). 2024;86(7):3833–40.
211. Vennarecci G, Laurenzi A, Santoro R, et al. The ALPPS procedure: a surgical option for hepatocellular carcinoma with major vascular invasion. World J Surg. 2014;38(6):1498–503.
212. Vennarecci G, Laurenzi A, Levi Sandri GB, et al. The ALPPS procedure for hepatocellular carcinoma. Eur J Surg Oncol. 2014;40(8):982–8.
213. Cavaness KM, Majella Doyle MB, Lin Y, et al. Using ALPPS to induce rapid liver hypertrophy in a patient with hepatic fibrosis and portal vein thrombosis. J Gastrointest Surg. 2013;17(1):207–12.
214. Chan AC, Poon RT, Lo CM. Modified anterior approach for the ALPPS procedure: how we do it. World J Surg. 2015;39(11):2831–5.
215. Li J, Moustafa M, Linecker M, et al. ALPPS for locally advanced intrahepatic cholangiocarcinoma: did aggressive surgery lead to the oncological benefit? An international multi-center study. Ann Surg Oncol. 2020;27(5):1372–84.
216. Bednarsch J, Czigany Z, Lurje I, et al. The role of ALPPS in intrahepatic cholangiocarcinoma. Langenbeck's Arch Surg. 2019;404(7):885–94.
217. Lau WY, Lai EC, Lau SH. Associating liver partition and portal vein ligation for staged hepatectomy: the current role and development. Hepatobiliary Pancreat Dis Int. 2017;16(1):17–26.
218. Glantzounis GK, Tokidis E, Basourakos SP, et al. The role of portal vein embolization in the surgical management of primary hepatobiliary cancers. A systematic review. Eur J Surg Oncol. 2017;43(1):32–41.
219. Klatskin G. Adenocarcinoma of the hepatic duct at its bifurcation within the porta hepatis. An unusual tumor with distinctive clinical and pathological features. Am J Med. 1965;38:241–56.
220. Lang H, de Santibanes E, Clavien PA. Outcome of ALPPS for perihilar cholangiocarcinoma: case-control analysis including the first series from the international ALPPS registry. HPB (Oxford). 2017;19(5):379–80.
221. Balci D, Kirimker EO, Üstüner E, et al. Stage I-laparoscopy partial ALPPS procedure for perihilar cholangiocarcinoma. J Surg Oncol. 2020;121(6):1022–6.

222. Schepelew D, Reese T, Horling K, et al. Undifferentiated embryonal sarcoma of the liver treated with associating liver partition and portal vein ligation for staged hepatectomy in a young adult: a case report. Int J Surg Case Rep. 2020;66:221–7.
223. Linecker M, Kambakamba P, Raptis DA, et al. ALPPS in neuroendocrine liver metastases not amenable for conventional resection—lessons learned from an interim analysis of the international ALPPS registry. HPB (Oxford). 2020;22(4):537–44.
224. Wiederkehr JC, Avilla SG, Mattos E, et al. Associating liver partition with portal vein ligation and staged hepatectomy (ALPPS) for the treatment of liver tumors in children. J Pediatr Surg. 2015;50(7):1227–31.
225. Chan A, Chung PHY, Poon RTP. Little girl who conquered the "ALPPS'". World J Gastroenterol. 2014;20(29):10208–11.
226. Hong JC, Kim J, Browning M, et al. Modified associating liver partition and portal vein ligation for staged hepatectomy for hepatoblastoma in a small infant: how far can we push the envelope? Ann Surg. 2017;266(2):e16–7.
227. Qazi AQ, Syed AA, Khan AW, et al. Early multifocal recurrence of hepatoblastoma in the residual liver after R0 liver resection with ALPPS procedure: a case report. Ann Transl Med. 2016;4(19):375.
228. Yu H, Zheng BJ, Gao Y, et al. Total laparoscopic ALPPS in the treatment of massive liver tumor. J Clin Pediatr Surg. 2021;20(7):635–640, 657.
229. Knoefel WT, Gabor I, Rehders A, et al. *In situ* liver transection with portal vein ligation for rapid growth of the future liver remnant in two-stage liver resection. Br J Surg. 2013;100(3):388–94.
230. Adam R, Imai K, Castro Benitez C, et al. Outcome after associating liver partition and portal vein ligation for staged hepatectomy and conventional two-stage hepatectomy for colorectal liver metastases. Br J Surg. 2016;103(11):1521–9.
231. Maupoey Ibáñez J, Montalvá Orón EM, Boscà Robledo A, et al. From conventional two-stage hepatectomy to ALPPS: fifteen years of experience in a hepatobiliary surgery unit. Hepatobiliary Pancreat Dis Int. 2021;20(6):542–50.
232. Ferri JVV, Feier FH, Scaffaro LA, et al. Salvage ALPPS procedure for failed portal vein embolization. Arq Bras Cir Dig. 2023;36:e1776.
233. Yilmaz E, Torsello GF, Hosseini ASA, et al. Role of liver augmentation prior to hepatic resection—a survey on standards, procedures, and indications in Germany, Switzerland, and Austria. Langenbecks Arch Surg. 409(1):228.
234. Schlegel A, Lesurtel M, Melloul E, et al. ALPPS: from human to mice highlighting accelerated and novel mechanisms of liver regeneration. Ann Surg. 2014;260(5):839–46. discussion 846–847
235. Yao LB, Li CH, Ge XL, et al. Establishment of a rat model of portal vein ligation combined with *in situ* splitting. PLoS One. 2014;9(8):e105511.
236. Almau Trenard HM, Moulin LE, Padín JM, et al. Development of an experimental model of portal vein ligation associated with parenchymal transection (ALPPS) in rats. Cirugía Española Engl Ed. 2014;92(10):676–81.
237. Budai A, Fulop A, Hahn O, et al. Animal models for associating liver partition and portal vein ligation for staged hepatectomy (ALPPS): achievements and future perspectives. Eur Surg Res. 2017;58(3–4):140–57.
238. Dili A, Lebrun V, Bertrand C, et al. Associating liver partition and portal vein ligation for staged hepatectomy: establishment of an animal model with insufficient liver remnant. Lab Investig. 2019;99(5):698–707.
239. Shi JH, Hammarström C, Grzyb K, et al. Experimental evaluation of liver regeneration patterns and liver function following ALPPS. BJS Open. 2017;1(3):84–96.
240. Zhang B, Meng FZ, Liu Y, et al. Inhibition of TGFβ1 accelerates regeneration of fibrotic rat liver elicited by a novel two-staged hepatectomy. Theranostics. 2021;11(10):4743–58.
241. Yang XW, Yang C, Qiu YW, et al. A preliminary study of associating liver partition and portal vein ligation for staged hepatectomy in a rat model of liver cirrhosis. Exp Ther Med. 2019;18(2):1203–11.
242. Liao MH, Zhang T, Wang HC, et al. Rabbit model provides new insights in liver regeneration after transection with portal vein ligation. J Surg Res. 2017;209:242–51.
243. Croome KP, Mao SA, Glorioso JM, et al. Characterization of a porcine model for associating liver partition and portal vein ligation for a staged hepatectomy. HPB (Oxford). 2015;17(12):1130–6.
244. Nadalin S, Capobianco I. Comment on "the contribution of the deportalized lobe to liver regeneration in tourniquet-ALPPS". Ann Surg. 2020;271(3):e97.
245. Abshagen K, Eipel C, Vollmar B. A critical appraisal of the hemodynamic signal driving liver regeneration. Langenbeck's Arch Surg. 2012;397(4):579–90.
246. Michalopoulos GK. Liver regeneration after partial hepatectomy: critical analysis of mechanistic dilemmas. Am J Pathol. 2010;176(1):2–13.
247. de Santibañes M, Dietrich A, Alvarez FA, et al. Biological substrate of the rapid volumetric changes observed in the human liver during the associating liver partition and portal vein ligation for staged hepatectomy approach. J Gastrointest Surg. 2016;20(3):546–53.
248. Nagy P, Teramoto T, Factor VM, et al. Reconstitution of liver mass via cellular hypertrophy in the rat. Hepatology. 2001;33(2):339–45.
249. Miyaoka Y, Ebato K, Kato H, et al. Hypertrophy and unconventional cell division of hepatocytes underlie liver regeneration. Curr Biol. 2012;22(13):1166–75.
250. Minamishima YA, Nakayama K, Nakayama K. Recovery of liver mass without proliferation of hepatocytes after partial hepatectomy in Skp2-deficient mice. Cancer Res. 2002;62(4):995–9.
251. Sheng RF, Wang HQ, Jin KP, et al. Histogram analyses of diffusion kurtosis indices and apparent diffusion coefficient in assessing liver regeneration after ALPPS and a comparative study with portal vein ligation. J Magn Reson Imaging. 2018;47(3):729–36.
252. Matsuo K, Murakami T, Kawaguchi D, et al. Histologic features after surgery associating liver partition and portal vein ligation for staged hepatectomy versus those after hepatectomy with portal vein embolization. Surgery. 2016;159(5):1289–98.
253. Tong YF, Zhu YF, Cai XJ. The origin of newborn hepatocytes in associating liver partition and portal vein ligation for staged hepatectomy (ALPPS)-derived regeneration. Hepatobiliary Surg Nutr. 2020;9(5):687–90.
254. Mao SA, Glorioso JM, Nyberg SL. Liver regeneration. Transl Res. 2014;163(4):352–62.
255. Lin KH, Hsu HT, Teng TH, et al. Rapidly increasing liver progenitor cell numbers in human regenerating liver after portal vein ligation and liver partition. Malays J Pathol. 2017;39(3):289–91.
256. Wigmore SJ. ALPPS: the argument against. Eur J Surg Oncol. 2017;43(2):249–51.
257. Eshmuminov D, Tschuor C, Raptis DA, et al. Rapid liver volume increase induced by associating liver partition with portal vein ligation for staged hepatectomy (ALPPS): is it edema, steatosis, or true proliferation? Surgery. 2017;161(6):1549–52.
258. Moris D, Vernadakis S, Papalampros A, et al. Mechanistic insights of rapid liver regeneration after associating liver partition and portal vein ligation for stage hepatectomy. World J Gastroenterol. 2016;22(33):7613–24.
259. García-Pérez R, Revilla-Nuin B, Martínez CM, et al. Associated liver partition and portal vein ligation (ALPPS) vs selective portal vein ligation (PVL) for staged hepatectomy in a rat model. Similar regenerative response? PLoS One. 2015;10(12):e0144096.

260. Shi HW, Yang GC, Zheng TS, et al. A preliminary study of ALPPS procedure in a rat model. Sci Rep. 2015;5:17567.
261. Dhar DK, Mohammad GH, Vyas S, et al. A novel rat model of liver regeneration: possible role of cytokine induced neutrophil chemoattractant-1 in augmented liver regeneration. Ann Surg Innov Res. 2015;9:11.
262. Uribe M, Uribe-Echevarría S, Mandiola C, et al. Insight on ALPPS – associating liver partition and portal vein ligation for staged hepatectomy – mechanisms: activation of mTOR pathway. HPB (Oxford). 2018;20(8):729–38.
263. Forbes SJ, Newsome PN. Liver regeneration – mechanisms and models to clinical application. Nat Rev Gastroenterol Hepatol. 2016;13(8):473–85.
264. Schmidt-Arras D, Rose-John S. IL-6 pathway in the liver: from physiopathology to therapy. J Hepatol. 2016;64(6):1403–15.
265. Langiewicz M, Schlegel A, Saponara E, et al. Hedgehog pathway mediates early acceleration of liver regeneration induced by a novel two-staged hepatectomy in mice. J Hepatol. 2017;66(3):560–70.
266. Borger P, Schneider M, Frick L, et al. Exploration of the transcriptional landscape of ALPPS reveals the pathways of accelerated liver regeneration. Front Oncol. 2019;9:1206.
267. Andersen KJ, Knudsen AR, Jepsen BN, et al. A new technique for accelerated liver regeneration: an experimental study in rats. Surgery. 2017;162(2):233–47.
268. Otsuka N, Yoshioka M, Abe Y, et al. Reg3α and Reg3β expressions followed by JAK2/STAT3 activation play a pivotal role in the acceleration of liver hypertrophy in a rat ALPPS model. Int J Mol Sci. 2020;21(11):4077.

2 Current Status of ALPPS

Hans J. Schlitt

2.1 Background and History

ALPPS, or "*in-situ split liver resection*"—as it is still called in our center in Regensburg—has elicited a huge hype among surgeons worldwide over the last 10 years. In the year 2008, we did the first case of surgery with this new technique, more or less by accident, in a patient with perihilar carcinoma [1]. Intraoperatively, the tumor in this rather young patient appeared technically resectable, but the left lateral lobe—the prospected functional liver remnant—as definitively much too small for appropriate function. Therefore, I thought about an alternative: I came up with the idea to perform the parenchymal dissection along the falciform ligament, divide the left hepatic bile duct at the basis of the round ligament, and suture-close the central stump, which appeared tumor-free. Then I decided to divide the right portal vein (like for resection and as an intraop. Alternative to interventional embolization for hypertrophy induction) and finally performed a hepatico-jejunostomy to the dilated left-lateral bile duct. Drains were placed, and the abdomen was closed to wait for hypertrophy of the left-lateral liver lobe. Interestingly, when we performed a CT scan about 8 days after this procedure, we saw a massive hypertrophy of the left-lateral lobe and, therefore, decided to perform the second step of the operation, i.e., the completion of extended right hepatectomy already by day 10 after the first operation. The postoperative course was unproblematic, with appropriate liver function from the beginning. Misfortunately, the patient died about 1 year later due to peritoneal carcinomatosis: in the resection specimen microscopic evidence of peritoneal carcinomatosis at the lesser omentum had been found, explaining the bad oncologic outcome. In terms of technical and functional outcome, however, the operation had to be regarded as an absolute success. Subsequently, we performed this procedure on average in 2–3 patients per year (out of about 150–180 liver resections per year in our center), i.e., we saw an indication for ALLPS in only about 2% of our patients.

In parallel to the first cases performed in Regensburg, my team and I informally discussed the new approach within Germany. Some other centers adopted the technique from the year 2010 onward, with *Hauke Lang* (Mainz, Germany) formally reporting a case of surgery with this technique at a conference of the International Society of Surgery (ISS) in South Africa in 2011 [2]. Finally, it cumulated in the seminal index publication of our group, together with cases from other German centers, in *Annals of Surgery* [3] in the year 2012 with *Andreas Schnitzbauer* (currently in Frankfurt, Germany) and *Sven Lang* (currently in Aachen, Germany) as joint first authors and me (*Hans J. Schlitt*, Regensburg, Germany) as senior author. This publication was accompanied by an editorial by *Pierre Clavien* (Zurich, Switzerland) and *Eduardo de Santibañes* (Buenos Aires, Argentina), who coined the term "*Associating Liver Partition and Portal vein ligation for Staged hepatectomy (ALPPS)*" for the procedure [4]. Under this name, the procedure was then applied enthusiastically by many hepatobiliary surgical centers, particularly in Europe, Asia, and South America, while there was obviously much less enthusiasm in North America. The reason for the latter is not totally clear but may be related to more risk-aversion in complex surgery in general.

In our center—like in most other German centers—the new technique continued to be used with very strict indication and, therefore, rather rarely. However, some centers, according to their published data, have used the method very liberally—particularly in many cases where the author would not consider it necessary at all, e.g., in most cases of mere right hemihepatectomy. Of course, the very liberal use in patients with no absolute necessity to use it (i.e., with sufficient remnant functional liver mass anyway) was associated with a markedly lower rate of complications and good outcomes. In Asia, the numbers of ALPPS were also relatively high in the last 10 years, but this was, in particular, due to the

H. J. Schlitt (✉)
University Hospital Regensburg, Regensburg, Germany
e-mail: hans.schlitt@klinik.uni-regensburg.de

J. Zhou (ed.), *Associating Liver Partition and Portal Vein Ligation for Staged Hepatectomy (ALPPS)*,
https://doi.org/10.1007/978-981-96-7364-3_2

very high rate of liver tumors and, therefore, liver resections in this part of the world. Asian groups, especially the group at Shanghai Liver Cancer Center, were also the first to gain broad experience in the use of ALPPS in patients with different degrees of liver fibrosis or cirrhosis [5].

2.2 ALPPS Research and Experimental Models

In the last 10 years, since the index publication in 2012, about 750 publications on ALPPS have been published according to PubMed®—the large majority dealing with clinical issues of the method. In the last 5–6 years, about 80 publications per year on the topic have appeared; this frequency is ongoing.

So far, experimental studies on ALPPS are limited. In fact, two chapters of this book specifically look at experimental models and the mechanisms of ALPPS. In general, it remains unclear how far rodent models, particularly the mouse, for which huge amounts of reagents and genetically modified animals are available, are really informative for the human situation. Therefore, although the results are interesting, they remain of limited value. Physiologically, much closer would be a pig model, from which the first data exist, although the anatomy of the liver is somewhat different, which might again cause problems in transferability to the human situation. Nevertheless, more studies on the mechanisms of hypertrophy induction in ALPPS would be essential to better understand the molecular mechanisms involved. Here, a final goal would be to avoid the technical/surgical procedures of ALPPS and mimic them by molecular targeting of hepatocytes in the left-lateral liver lobe—probably with different targeting of cells in the extended right liver lobe, e.g., using a combination of radiological interventions and targeted drugs as preparation for single-step surgery.

2.3 Current Status of ALPPS

Making its way worldwide and through many centers with experienced hepato-biliary surgeons, many different "variations" were developed to modify the "original" ALPPS procedure. Like many new techniques coming up, there are frequently variations performed and reported, which are particularly due to the specific experiences of those surgeons or due to problems that have been observed during or after surgery. In fact, the major aim of variations is to make a procedure simpler, safer, and more suitable for specific situations. These include "Tourniquet ALPPS," "Thermic Ablation-assisted ALPPS," "Partial ALPPS," "Anterior approach ALPPS," "Laparoscopic ALPPS," "Robotic ALPPS," "Hybrid/Mini-ALPPS," [6–11] "Reversal ALPPS," [12, 13] and "TAE-salvaged ALPPS," [14, 15] which are all delineated in detail in other chapters of this comprehensive book. Of course, it currently also an important question about the role ALPPS plays in comparison to other techniques like traditional "two-staged liver resection," portal embolization or portal plus hepatic vein embolization and, maybe, even liver transplantation in cases where there is extensive tumor load in the liver.

The particular advantage of the many variations of ALPPS is that it broadens the surgical armamentarium of individually optimized surgical treatment of patients with primary liver tumors or liver metastases. This is of very high importance because only surgical removal (or destruction) of all tumor manifestations (in this case, in the liver) offers the chance of cure for these patients with advanced tumors—for whom systemic therapy, even with the advent of novel immunotherapies and targeted therapies can, in general, only delay tumor growth and, finally, death due to the tumor. Therefore, every new approach or modification of a surgical technique that helps remove the tumor(s) is helpful for the patients, and their long-term benefit must be the final goal of all surgical attempts.

The rather complex nature of ALPPS, the knowledge about the available "variations," and detailed knowledge about the wide varicty of other available techniques, as well as the technical experience and skill to apply them, makes it essential to perform treatment of patients with liver tumors only in highly specialized centers. These centers should have the whole "toolbox" of mentioned methods available, as well as interventional radiological techniques (thermic ablation, non-thermic ablation [e.g., irreversible electroporation], radioembolization [SIRT], etc.) as well as stereotactic irradiation techniques, close interaction with highly experienced medical oncologists and—ideally—the option of liver transplantation (from deceased as well as from living donors). Overall, it is not only the hepato-biliary surgical experience but the experience and skill of the whole multidisciplinary team that is important.

Therefore, the performance of ALPPS—as a highly complex treatment, technically as well as intellectually—should definitely be restricted to a few specialized centers. Only this enables its appropriate use (avoiding *overuse*, but also avoiding *underuse*, by defining its *adequate* use) and further development and refinement. Only this also allows decisions about when to use ALPPS and when rather use other techniques like conventional two-staged resection, the prior portal (± hepatic vein) embolization, or even complex one-stage resection(s).

2.4 Indications, Contraindications, Variations, and Alternative Techniques: Ideas and Clinical Examples

In particular, it is important to determine when it is adequate to use the technique. This is the most complex problem: issues to be considered are ① the underlying (oncologic) tumor type, ② the pattern of tumor distribution in the liver, ③ the quality of the non-tumor liver parenchyma (particularly in the case of fibrosis/cirrhosis in the presence of HCC), ④ abnormalities in vascular anatomy, ⑤ the experience of the surgeon/center with the method, ⑥ the advantages/disadvantages in comparison to other available advanced methods or resection in the given setting, and ⑦ the question whether it is really considered necessary vs. one-step (potentially complex) resection. Concerning the latest point, we would mostly consider it if the remnant function liver mass (with "normal" liver tissue) would be below 0.5% of the patient's body weight, but usually not above that.

Tumor indications that might be considered for ALPPS resection are colorectal metastases, intrahepatic cholangiocarcinoma (iCC), hepatocellular carcinoma (HCC), but also other rare types of liver metastasis, and—very rarely—perihilar cholangiocarcinoma (pCC, Klatskin-tumor). In fact, the technique is potentially helpful in all cases, in which liver resection would be the optimal type of tumor treatment with a potentially curative intent, and, clearly, the long-term outcome will depend more on the underlying tumor and its characteristics than on the technique as such.

As mentioned above, the ALPPS technique is not "superior" to other advanced and two-staged liver resection techniques but may be better suitable in some situations than other techniques. However, the opinion about the optimal technique to be used in a given situation may differ between surgeons—even between surgeons with similarly high experience in liver surgery. This means that—at least currently—no absolute "standard operating procedures" (SOPs) can be offered for a decision pro or against ALPPS in an individual situation. However, it has to be kept in mind that one of the advantages of (two-stage) ALPPS, e.g., in comparison to vascular embolization for hypertrophy induction, is the option of doing intraoperative (contrast-enhanced) ultrasound as the "gold-standard" imaging technique for assessing the exact number and location of liver lesions prior to starting the resection. In fact, studies in our center have shown, that intraoperative contrast-enhanced ultrasound (CEUS) leads to a modification in the surgical strategy in about 1/3 of patients scheduled for major liver resection—either due to metastases or due to HCC or iCC.

Subsequently, some cases are reported where (standard) ALPPS did not turn out to be the optimal treatment concept, had to be modified from the original approach, or required reoperation extended surgery due to complications realized intraoperatively. These are examples of how ALPPS is currently used (or not used) in our center:

Case 1: (Classical) Two-Stage Hepatectomy Instead of ALPPS

A 63-year-old male patient presented with a mid-third rectal adenocarcinoma (without functional stenosis) and multiple, large, synchronous liver metastases in both lobes (Fig. 2.1). First, he received eight courses of chemotherapy with FOLFIRI + panitumumab, leading to marked regression of tumor load (Fig. 2.2). The patient was scheduled for the ALPPS procedure.

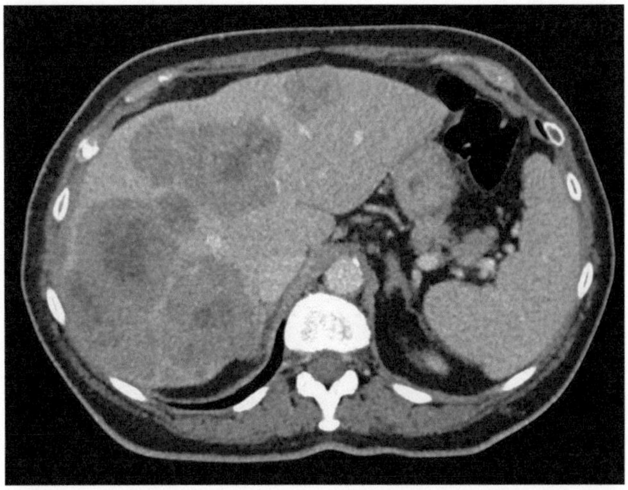

Fig. 2.1 Synchronous colorectal liver metastases at the time of diagnosis (CT-scan)

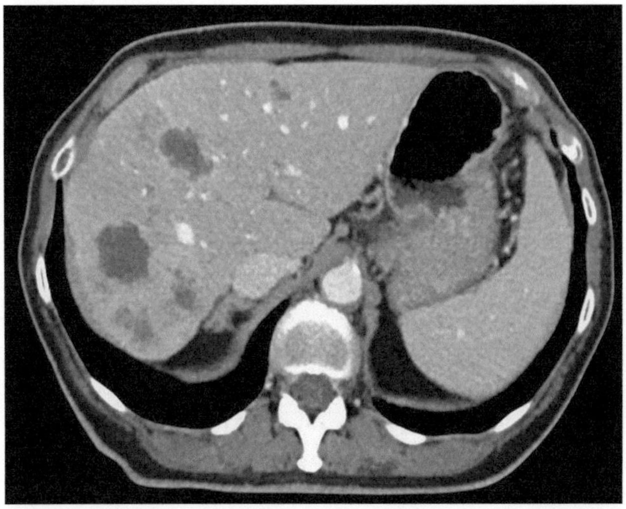

Fig. 2.2 Colorectal liver metastases after neoadjuvant chemotherapy, just before surgery

Intraoperative ultrasound revealed more and large tumor nodules in the left liver lobe, so that the decision was made not to perform ALPPS, but conventional two-stage hepatectomy. During the first operation, five subsegmental resections were performed in the left liver lobe (1 × segment II, 1 × segment II/III, 1 × segment III, and 2 × segment IVB) (Fig. 2.3), and the right portal vein branch was divided.

Eight weeks later, a CT scan showed moderate hypertrophy of the left liver lobe (Fig. 2.4), and the second surgery was performed as a slightly extended (parts of segment IVA) right hepatectomy. Another 12 weeks later, a CT scan again showed marked hypertrophy of the remaining left lobe (Fig. 2.5), and the primary tumor was resected via anterior rectum resection.

In this case, the intraoperative ultrasound findings led to a change in strategy away from the planned ALPPS procedure toward a standard two-stage hepatectomy with right portal vein division—due to a higher-than-expected tumor load in the left liver lobe requiring more extensive resections on the left side.

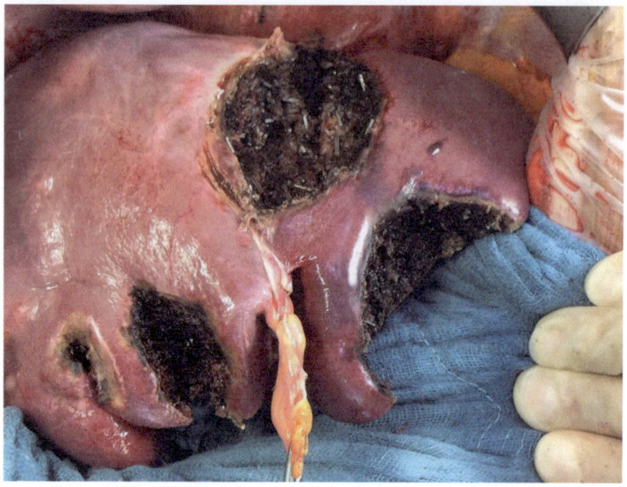

Fig. 2.3 Intraoperative view of the liver at the end of the first operation of two-stage hepatectomy with multiple subsegmental resections of the left liver lobe

Case 2: One-Stage Hepatectomy Due to Adequate Hypertrophy and Venous Congestion of the Left-Lateral Liver Lobe

A 49-year-old female patient with Echinococcus alveolaris—initially suspected as intrahepatic cholangiocarcinoma (iCC)—had a large "tumor" lesion in the right lobe of the liver with complete occlusion of the right and middle hepatic vein and stenosis of the left hepatic vein, but also occlusion of the hepatic bile duct bifurcation with jaundice (Fig. 2.6). After an unsuccessful attempt of endoscopic retrograde cholangiography (ERC) drainage of the left duct, a percutaneous transhepatic cholangio-drainage (PTCD) was performed for decompression of the bile duct. It was then discussed whether surgery should be performed as ALPPS and whether preoperative stenting of the left hepatic vein should be performed to optimize venous outflow from the left lateral liver lobe. However, it was decided against stenting for the case that a one-stage resection would be attempted with potential resection and reconstruction of the left hepatic vein.

As expected, during surgery, a markedly hypertrophied left lateral liver lobe was found with additional marked venous congestion. Intraoperative ultrasound revealed marked venous collaterals from segment IV to the left lateral lobe. Moreover, the ultrasound showed evidence of infiltration of the left hepatic vein just over 1 cm. Therefore, the decision was made to perform a one-stage extended right hepatectomy (including most of liver segments IVA and IVB and the occluded distal middle hepatic vein). Moreover, the biliary hepatic bifurcation required resection and the distal

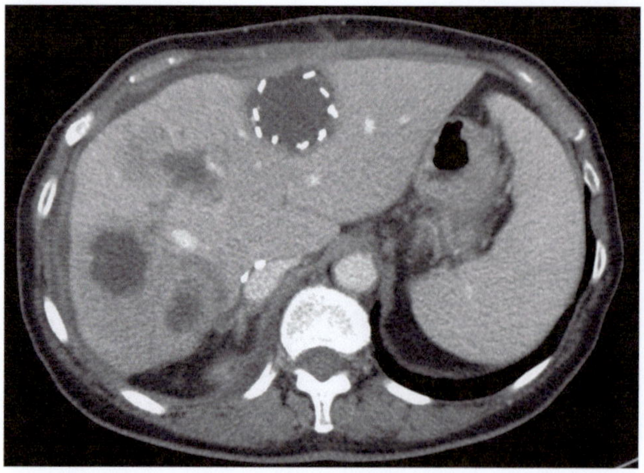

Fig. 2.4 CT scan before the second operation of the two-stage hepatectomy (partially extended right hepatectomy)

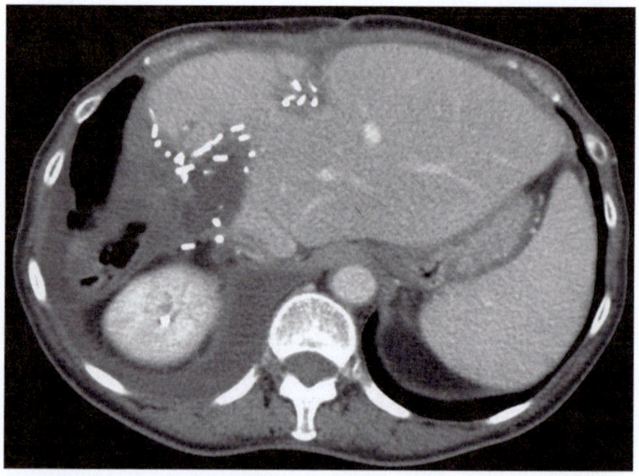

Fig. 2.5 CT scan 5 days after the second operation of the two-stage hepatectomy: tumor-free liver

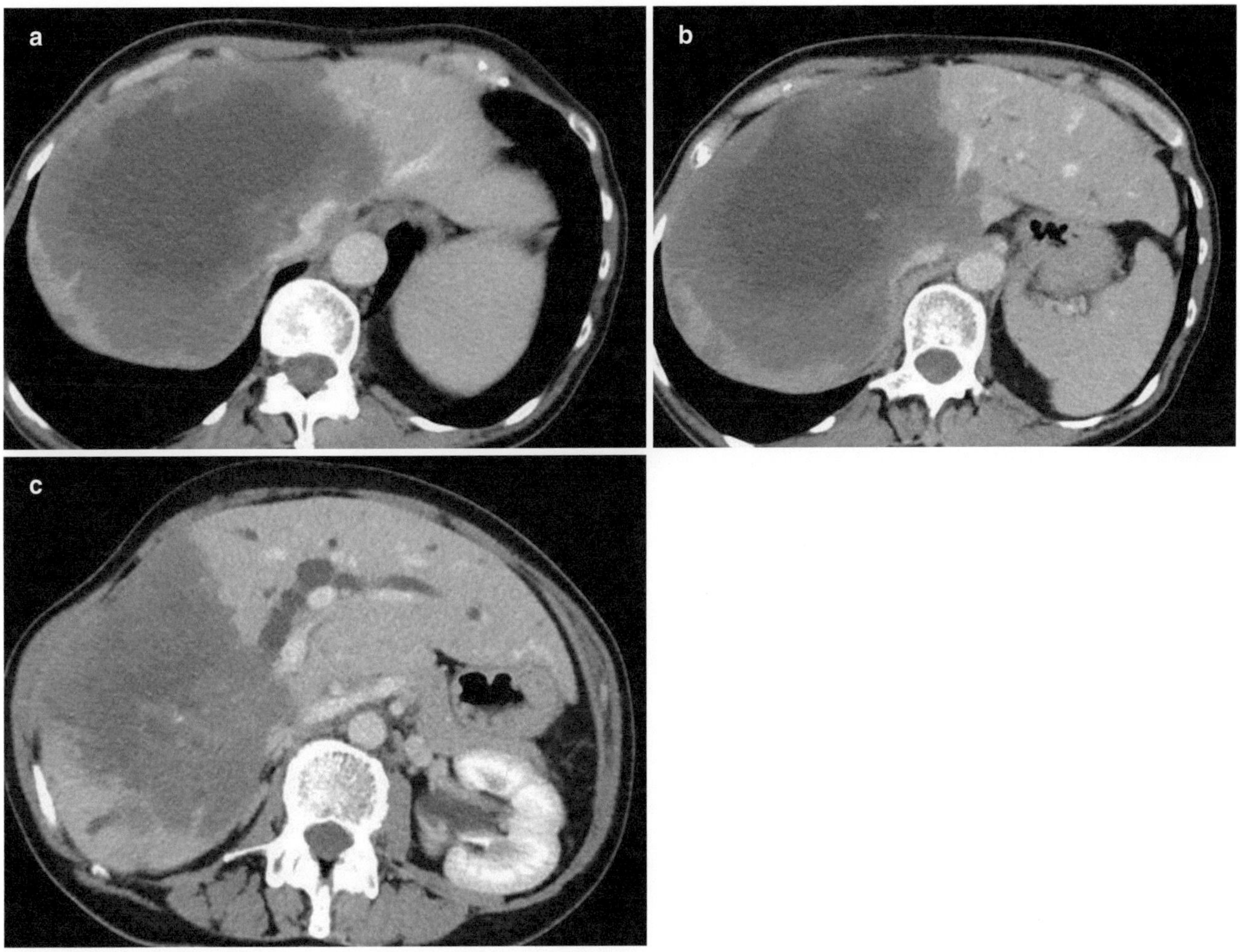

Fig. 2.6 Extensive "liver tumor" on the right side with compression of the left hepatic vein (**a**), occlusion of the right hepatic vein, and occlusion of distal middle hepatic vein (**b**) as well as compression/infiltration of bile duct bifurcation and distal left bile duct with subsequent cholestasis (**c**); CT scan

1.5 cm of the left hepatic vein with planned direct reconstruction by anastomosis. The procedure was then performed accordingly with liver inflow occlusion for about 45 min, including complete vascular occlusion for about 20 min. Finally, reconstruction by a Roux-en-Y hepatico-jejunostomy was performed. The postoperative course was uneventful, with continuously stable and good liver function (Fig. 2.7).

In this case, ALPPS—although initially considered—was not necessarily due to the already marked hypertrophy of the left lateral liver lobe and was not appropriate because of the severe venous congestion of the left lateral lobe.

Case 3: Incomplete ALPPS During the First Step Due to Avoidance of Tumor Exposure

A 59-year-old female patient had a large hepatocellular carcinoma in the right lobe of the liver, including liver segments I and IVA (Fig. 2.8). She was then scheduled to undergo ALLPS liver resection because of a low residual functional liver volume of 280 mL (= 0.4%). The tumor area in segment IVA extended to the wall of the distal left hepatic vein (Fig. 2.8a). Therefore, in case of complete parenchymal splitting, the tumor surface would have been exposed to the resection surface. For this reason, it was decided not to do a complete parenchymal dissection during the first surgery of ALPPS but to leave the cranial part undissected so that there was no potential risk of longer-term exposure of the tumor until the second stage of ALLPS with a risk of tumor cell spreading.

Thus, during the first stage of ALPPS, the parenchymal dissection included only the caudal parts of the parenchyma along the falciform ligament (Figure 2.9a), while the cranial parts were left untouched during the first operation (Fig. 2.9b). Nevertheless, appropriate hypertrophy of the left lateral liver lobe occurred so that in the second operation (after 9 days), the parenchymal dissection was then completed, and the operation was otherwise finished normally (Fig. 2.10).

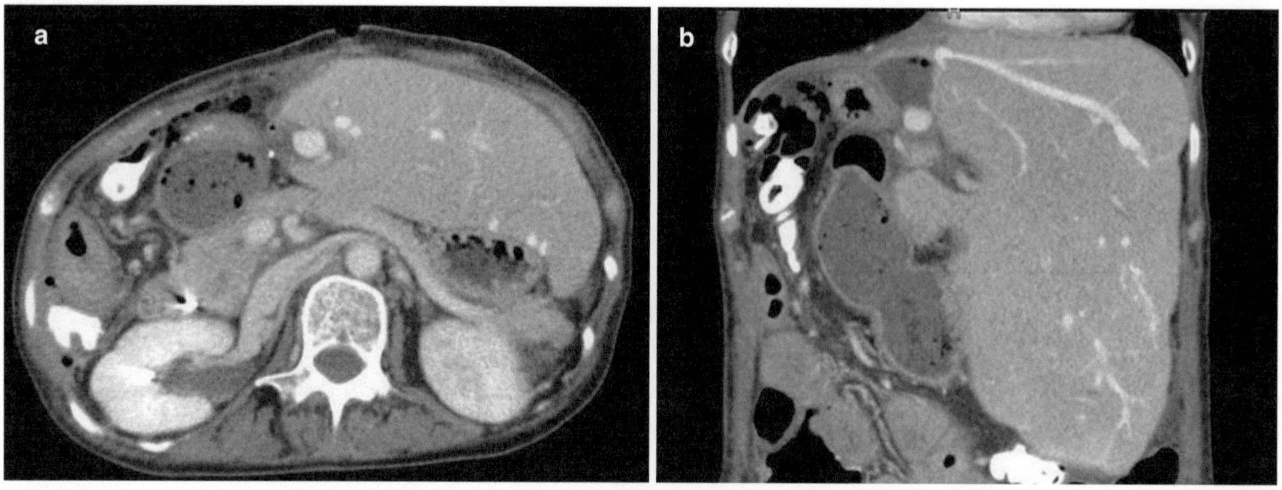

Fig. 2.7 Remnant liver (left-lateral lobe) few days after one-stage resection (axial view: **a;** coronal view: **b**) with resection and reconstruction of left hepatic vein (**b**) and hepaticojejunostomy; CT-scan

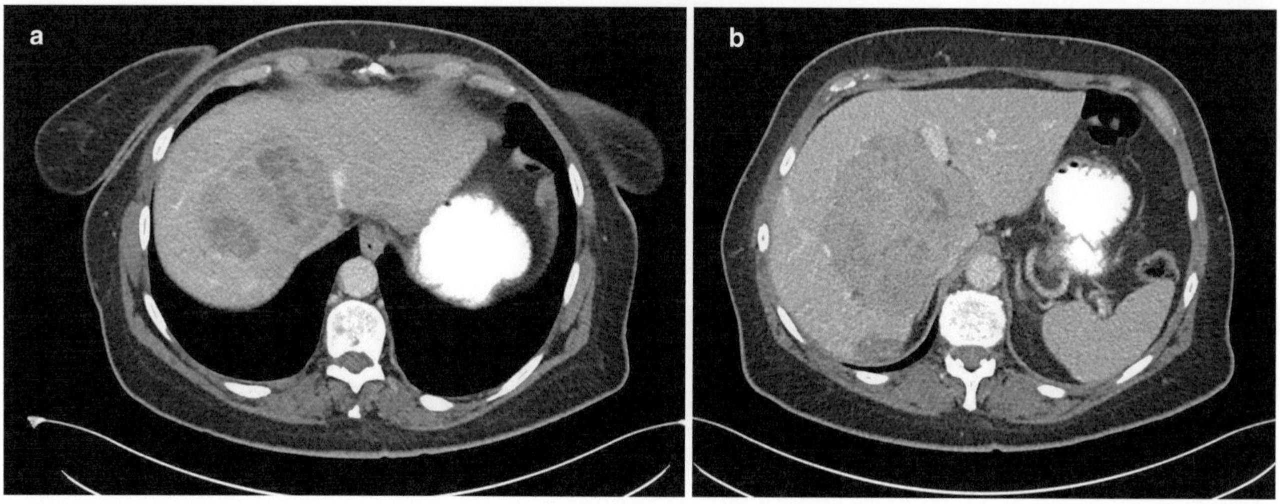

Fig. 2.8 Right-sided hepatocellular carcinoma (HCC) in a non-cirrhotic liver with compression of left hepatic vein (**a**), probably initially derived from liver segment I (**b**): CT scan just prior to surgery

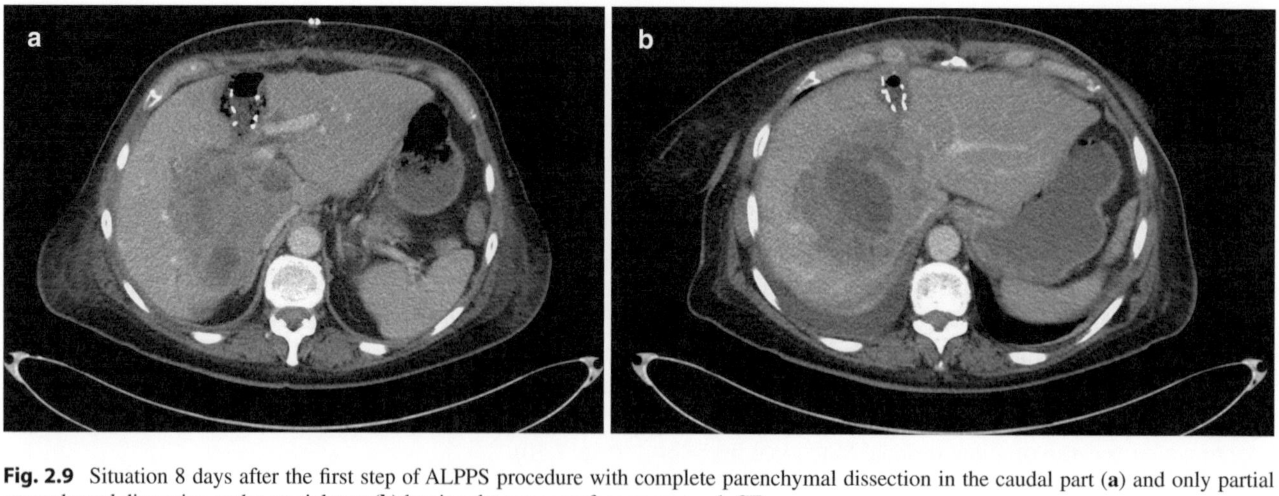

Fig. 2.9 Situation 8 days after the first step of ALPPS procedure with complete parenchymal dissection in the caudal part (**a**) and only partial parenchymal dissection at the cranial part (**b**) leaving the tumor surface unexposed; CT scan

This example shows that when a tumor extends very close to the planned resection line, we mostly choose not to perform complete parenchymal dissection for oncologic reasons but leave the area of the tumor—which might be exposed on the surface after complete dissection—untouched.

Case 4: Secondary Hepaticojejunostomy Due to Necrosis of Left Bile Duct

A 61-year-old female patient suffered from metachronous colorectal liver metastases and underwent neoadjuvant therapy with 5 cycles of FOLFIRI and bevacizumab followed by an additional 8 cycles of FOLFOXIRI and bevacizumab. The major tumor mass was in the right lobe and segment IVB and extended closely to the left portal vein as well as to the bile duct bifurcation and left bile duct (Fig. 2.11).

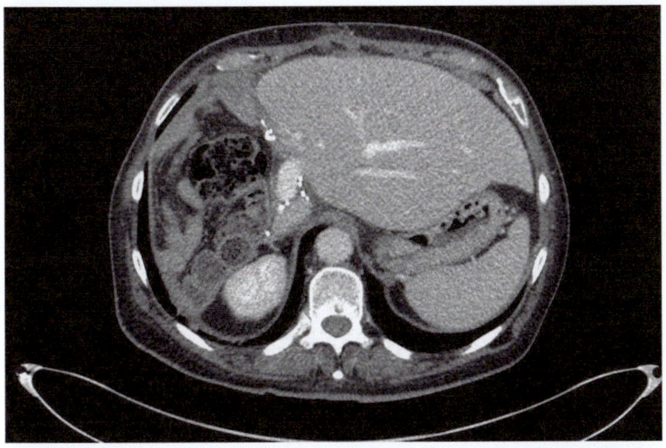

Fig. 2.10 CT scan a few days after the second step of the completed ALPPS procedure with adequate hypertrophy of the left-lateral liver lobe

The first stage of the ALPPS operation was performed generally according to standard, but the tumor was not yet dissected completely from the central left hilum—to avoid tumor exposure at the resection surface (Fig. 2.12). Appropriate hypertrophy induction occurred within 9 days when the second step of the operation was performed. After completion of parenchymal dissection and removal of the right extended lobe, a bile leakage was detected at the distal left duct just above the bifurcation. In this area, preparation directly along the bile duct wall was necessary because of the tumor localization. An attempt to close the bile leakage was unsuccessful, so the decision was made to resect the distal left duct and reconstruct the left-lateral duct by a Roux-en-Y hepaticojejunostomy (Fig. 2.13). Segment I of the liver had been left in situ in this case, and the segment I duct still drained to the main bile duct.

Postoperatively, bile leakage occurred at the hepaticojejunostomy. Therefore, a PTCD was placed for decompression (Fig. 2.14), finally healing the anastomosis.

In some cases of ALPPS—like in some cases of standard extended right hepatectomy—tumor lesions in segment IVB can come very close to the left hilum up to the round ligament over a few centimeters, even without actual compression of the bile duct and subsequent cholestasis. In these cases, tissue dissection during resection (or during the first stage of ALPPS) has to occur very closely along the structures of the left pedicle. This carries the risk of denudation of the left bile duct/bile duct bifurcation over several centime-

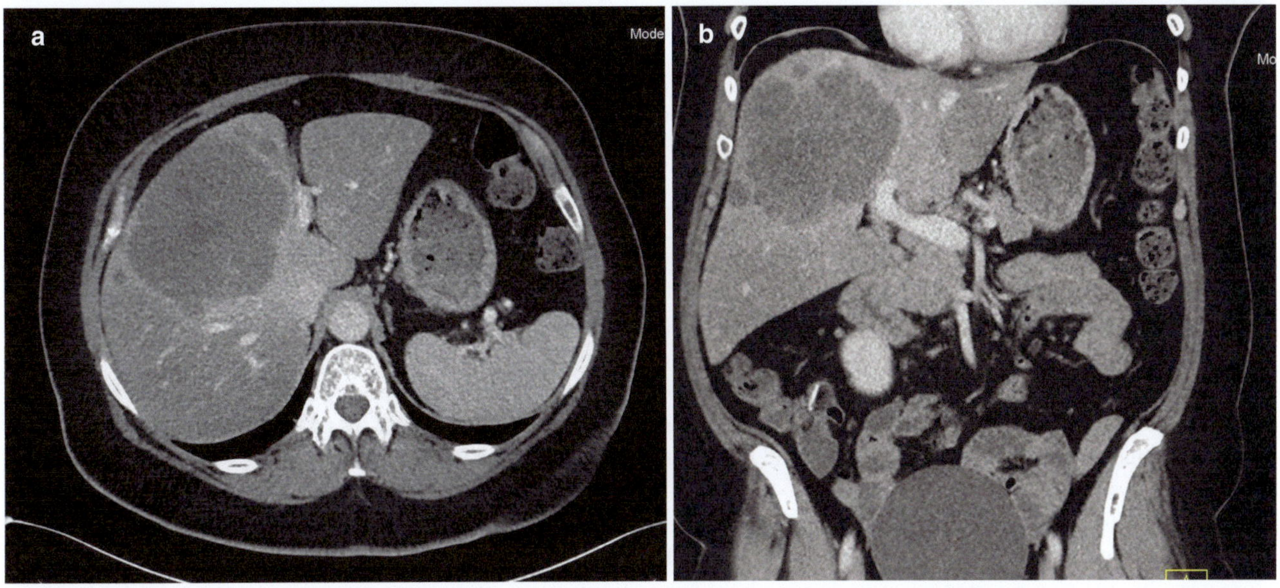

Fig. 2.11 Colorectal liver metastases after neoadjuvant chemotherapy, just before surgery; large tumor with multiple additional small nodules in the right liver lobe and liver segment IV; tumor reaching close to hilar bifurcation and left pedicle and moderately fatty change of liver parenchyma after chemotherapy; CT scan with axial (**a**) and coronal (**b**) view

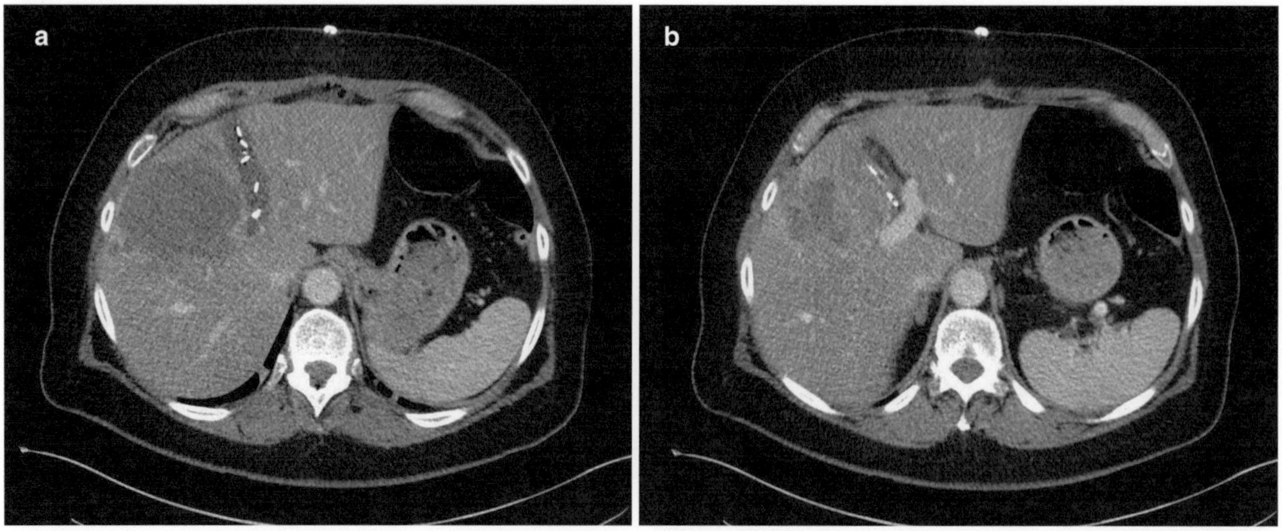

Fig. 2.12 CT-scan 8 days after the first step of ALPPS procedure (**a**) with incomplete parenchymal dissection at the left hilar pedicle (**b**)

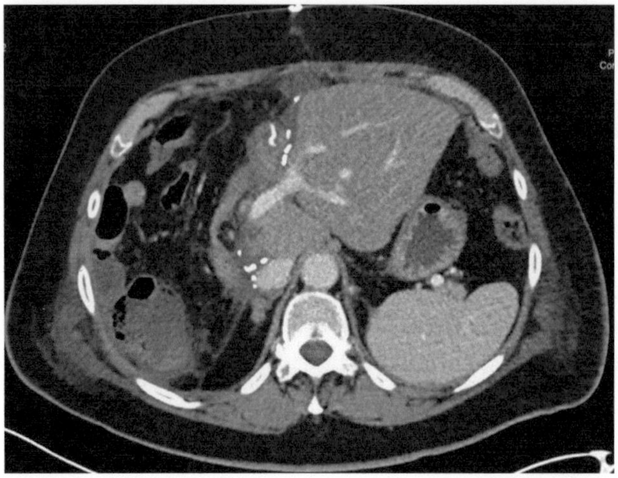

Fig. 2.13 CT scan after completion of resection (with preservation of liver segment I) and Roux-en-Y hepaticojejunostomy (anterior to left portal vein branch)

ters, which may—in the case of ALPPS, potentially only some days after the second surgery—lead to necrosis of the left bile duct wall and, finally, to bile leakage. When the wall necrosis is very limited, bile duct stenting by ERCP or—in our view, generally better—by insertion of a PPTCD can cover the leakage and may lead to regeneration of the bile duct wall. In other cases, however, resection of the necrotic duct and permanent bile drainage via a Roux-en-Y hepatico-jejunostomy is required for definite repair.

Whether prophylactic stenting or PTCD insertion can prevent bile leakage in such cases remains to be studied. Moreover, the question remains when to decide about performing a hepatico-jejunostomy already during the second stage of ALPPS surgery in high-risk situations for bile duct necrosis.

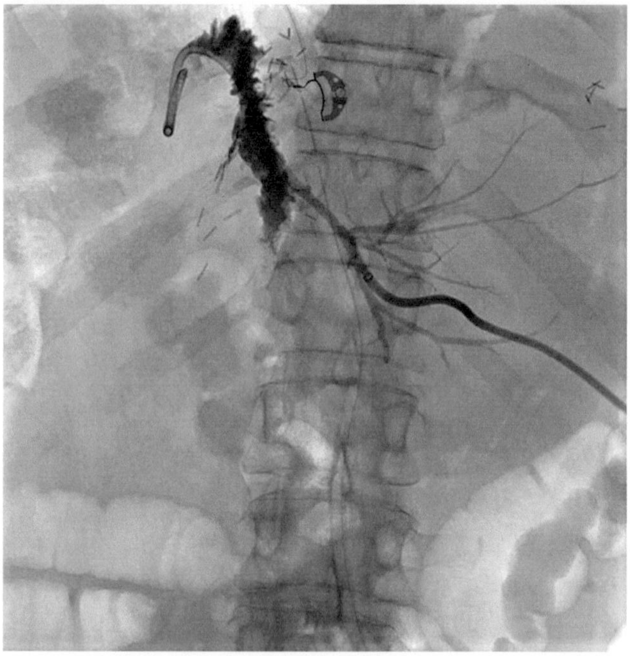

Fig. 2.14 Postoperative placement of percutaneous transhepatic cholangio-drainage (PTCD) for treatment of bile leakage at the hepaticojejunostomy

2.5 General Lessons from the "Story of ALPPS"

The "introduction" of ALPPS was one of the major new surgical techniques—or rather "strategies"—developed in the last two decades. Apart from the improvement in the treatment of patients with liver tumors, the introduction of ALPPS also provides more general information about advances in the medical/surgical field:

Surgeons should always try new things, especially in situations where something appears "unresectable." In these situations, trying new, innovative techniques is generally the only option for a cure for a patient with an advanced tumor. Of course, when introducing a new technique spontaneously, due to the lack of alternatives, as it occurred in the first case of ALPPS, formal patient consent does not exist. Nevertheless, it was considered to be ethically acceptable because the patient had clearly stated that he wanted his advanced/marginal tumor to be resected and would not want to know about the details of the surgical technique anyway. Of course, not all surgeons would think like that: many prefer clearly standardized procedures, and, particularly in the United States of America, the risk of legal consequences if they do not strictly adhere to standards might be feared. It clearly needs a highly experienced surgeon who is able to balance the risk of failure by using a new method vs. the potential chance of complete tumor removal/cure in a given situation. If an adequate balance exists, the (first) use of an innovative method should be justified. Nevertheless, there is always a remaining risk in such situations that, in the end, the risk may outweigh the chances and that a given new approach should not be used any further. However, without such "spontaneous" application of innovative techniques in given situations—and after careful evaluation by a highly experienced surgeon—many chances for advancement in surgery will be lost.

New techniques in surgery can be developed systematically, i.e., by theory and design in the beginning, and then introduced stepwise via animal experiments in the clinical setting. This is an approach that may, for example, be used to introduce new techniques or instruments for laparoscopic or robotic surgery. This is a very well-structured and systematic process that usually takes some time. These methods mostly lead to moderately innovative, small improvements in surgical techniques. However, inventing a "disruptive" new technology, e.g., ALPPS, typically occurs spontaneously "on the battlefield," i.e., in the operation room, as a sudden and innovative solution to an acute problem. Such an innovation cannot be "designed," planned, and well-prepared prior to its first use. Therefore, some unpredictable elements remain in such a situation. Only when this approach is used for a second or third time more systematic planning can occur in order to optimize it—at least preliminarily. Despite a more "unscientific" approach to such innovations, they are probably more relevant and important than those developed systematically.

Fortunately, we have—at least in Europe and probably in most non-US countries—still much less strict legal regulations for the introduction and the use of new surgical techniques as compared to new drugs, innovative medical products (IMPs, like cell therapies), and standard medical products. All these are very strictly regulated in most countries and require extensive, expensive, and time-consuming approaches to application and critical review by (mostly) several institutions, boards, and ministries. If this were also the case for new surgical techniques, basically all innovation in surgery—at least that coming from surgeons themselves—would be completely blocked. Only innovations coming through the industry would have the necessary backup support for the required application processes. Therefore, surgeons (and the medical profession as such) should ensure that the therapeutic freedom remains, at least for surgical and interventional procedures. Otherwise, surgery would—for many—just become a rather boring job.

2.6 Conclusions and Perspectives

Altogether, the first reporting of ALPPS in 2012 has been an exciting experience on how a novel surgical technique is recognized, spreads throughout the world, induces hype, and undergoes variations in techniques as well as in indication over 10 years. Since 2012, ALPPS has advanced liver surgery by introducing a new, innovative "tool" for the armamentarium of liver surgery. In the future, ALPPS is here to stay, but it still requires more exact definitions for its indications, for the most optimal techniques to be used in individual cases, and details of its delimitation from other advanced liver surgery techniques. Finally, studies of the detailed mechanisms of action are still required.

Moreover, the story shows that spontaneous decisions during surgery may have a relevant impact on the further development of surgical techniques. Therefore, such decisions must always be left open for the (experienced) operating surgeon and must not be formally regulated because this would definitely prevent progress in practical surgery for the benefit of patients.

References

1. Schlitt HJ, Hackl C, Lang SA. 'In-situ split' liver resection/ALPPS—historical development and current practice. Visc Med. 2017;33(6):408–12.
2. Baumgart J, Lang S, Lang H. A new method for induction of liver hypertrophy prior to right trisectionectomy: a report of three cases. HPB (Oxford). 2011;13(Suppl 2):71–2.
3. Schnitzbauer AA, Lang SA, Goessmann H, et al. Right portal vein ligation combined with *in situ* splitting induces rapid left lateral liver lobe hypertrophy enabling 2-staged extended right hepatic resection in small-for-size settings. Ann Surg. 2012;255(3):405–14.
4. de Santibañes E, Clavien PA. Playing play-Doh to prevent postoperative liver failure: the "ALPPS" approach. Ann Surg. 2012;255(3):415–7.
5. Wang Z, Peng YF, Hu JW, et al. Associating liver partition and portal vein ligation for staged hepatectomy for unresectable hepatitis B virus-related hepatocellular carcinoma: a single center study of 45 patients. Ann Surg. 2020;271(3):534–41.
6. Petrowsky H, Györi G, de Oliveira M, et al. Is partial-ALPPS safer than ALPPS? A single-center experience. Ann Surg. 2015;261(4):e90–2.
7. Campos RR, Paricio PP, Conesa AL, et al. A new surgical technique for extended right hepatectomy: tourniquet in the umbilical fissure and right portal vein occlusion (ALTPS). Clinical case Cir Esp. 2013;91(10):633–7.
8. Cai XJ, Peng SY, Duan L, et al. Completely laparoscopic ALPPS using round-the-liver ligation to replace parenchymal transection for a patient with multiple right liver cancers complicated with liver cirrhosis. J Laparoendosc Adv Surg Tech A. 2014;24(12):883–6.
9. Gall TM, Sodergren MH, Frampton AE, et al. Radio-frequency-assisted liver partition with portal vein ligation (RALPP) for liver regeneration. Ann Surg. 2015;261(2):e45–6.
10. Wang Q, Yan J, Feng XB, et al. Safety and efficacy of radiofrequency-assisted ALPPS (RALPPS) in patients with cirrhosis-related hepatocellular carcinoma. Int J Hyperth. 2017;33(7):846–52.
11. Gringeri E, Boetto R, D'Amico FE, et al. Laparoscopic microwave ablation and portal vein ligation for staged hepatectomy

(LAPS): a minimally invasive first-step approach. Ann Surg. 2015;261(2):e42–3.
12. Obed A, Jarrad A, Bashir A. First left hepatic trisectionectomy including segment one with new associated liver partition and portal vein ligation with staged hepatectomy (ALPPS) modification: how to do it? Am J Case Rep. 2016;17:759–65.
13. Machado MA, Surjan R, Basseres T, et al. Total laparoscopic reversal ALPPS. Ann Surg Oncol. 2017;24(4):1048–9.
14. Wang Z, Peng YF, Sun QM, et al. Salvage transhepatic arterial embolization after failed stage I ALPPS in a patient with a huge HCC with chronic liver disease: a case report. Int J Surg Case Rep. 2017;39:131–5.
15. Peng YF, Wang Z, Qu XD, et al. Transcatheter arterial embolization-salvaged ALPPS, a novel ALPPS procedure especially for patients with hepatocellular carcinoma and severe fibrosis/cirrhosis. Hepatobiliary Surg Nutr. 2022;11(4):504–14.

3 Clinical Anatomy of ALPPS

Zheng Wang and Kai Zhu

The ALPPS procedure stands as a pioneering advancement in hepatobiliary surgery over the last decade. Its critical steps include hepatic parenchymal transection/partition coupled with portal vein ligation on the resection side in the first stage, as well as the resection of tumor lesions in the second stage. The ALPPS procedure can induce rapid FLR hypertrophy, enabling the resection of a wider spectrum of liver lesions. ALPPS offers renewed hope for patients with liver tumors previously deemed unresectable [1].

A profound comprehension of liver anatomy is fundamental to successfully completing the ALPPS procedure, as it can assist in intraoperatively preventing biliary or vascular complications while maximizing the preservation of viable liver tissues and minimizing blood loss. Giant or multiple liver tumors requiring ALPPS procedure typically encompass a hemiliver or extend beyond its boundaries (requiring left or right trisegmentectomy) (Fig. 3.1). These tumors usually compress the first or second porta hepatis, resulting in alterations to the original anatomical structures. Without thorough preoperative evaluations of these alterations, inadvertent intraoperative injuries may precipitate unnecessary complications.

Z. Wang (✉) · K. Zhu
Zhongshan Hospital, Fudan University, Shanghai, China
e-mail: wang.zheng@zs-hospital.sh.cn

J. Zhou (ed.), *Associating Liver Partition and Portal Vein Ligation for Staged Hepatectomy (ALPPS)*,
https://doi.org/10.1007/978-981-96-7364-3_3

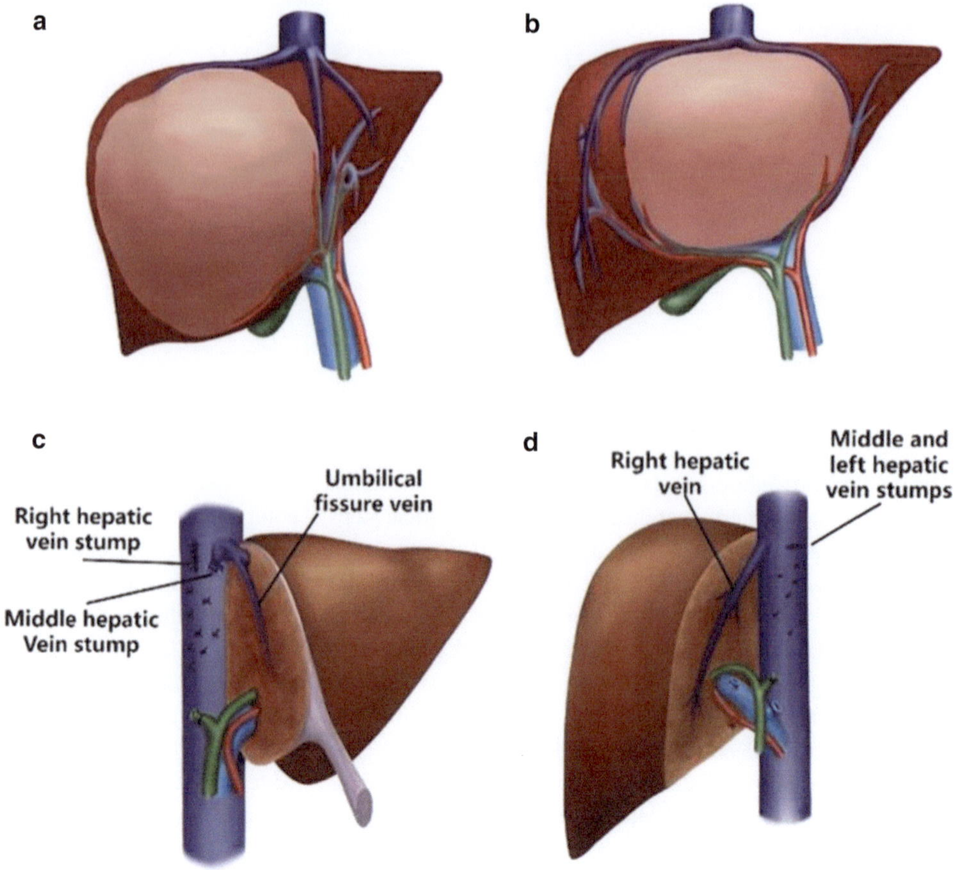

Fig. 3.1 (**a**). A giant tumor in the right lobe; (**b**). A giant tumor in the left lobe; (**c**). Right trisegmentectomy; (**d**). Left trisegmentectomy

3.1 Anatomical Division of the Liver

Couinaud created an anatomical description of the portal venous system in 1954 and established the internationally applied classification of liver anatomy [2]. Based on the portal vein distribution, the liver is categorized into eight segments (Fig. 3.2). Each segment receives a hepatic pedicle comprising a portal venous branch, a hepatic arterial branch, and a bile duct, with hepatic veins draining blood into the inferior vena cava (IVC).

The liver is anatomically divided into sections based on hepatic segments. The left hemiliver comprises segments II, III, and IV, while the right hemiliver comprises segments V, VI, VII, and VII. The left and right hemilivers are demarcated by the Rex-Cantlie line extending from the gallbladder bed to the IVC, with the middle hepatic vein coursing along the line. The left hemiliver is delineated into the left medial section (segment IV) and left lateral section (segments II and III) by the umbilical fissure, with the umbilical fissure vein coursing within this fissure. The right hemiliver is separated into the right anterior section (segments V and VII) and the right posterior section (segments VI and VII) by the course

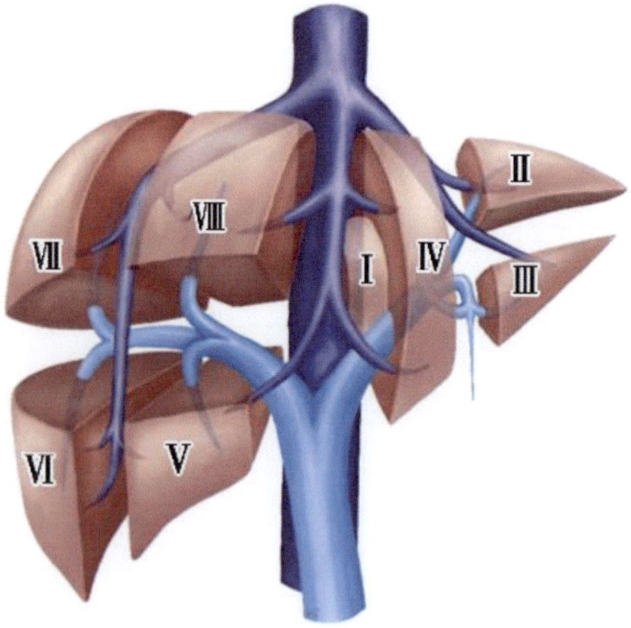

Fig. 3.2 Couinaud's segmental anatomy. Each segment (Roman numeral) receives a hepatic pedicle comprising a portal venous branch, a hepatic arterial branch, and a bile duct, with hepatic veins draining blood into the IVC

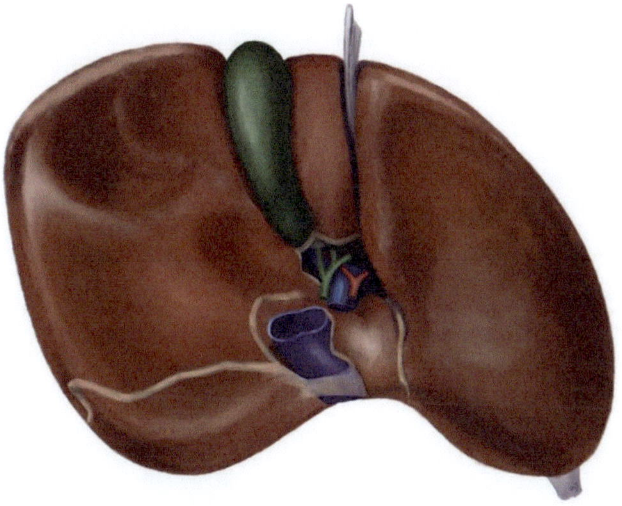

Fig. 3.3 Visceral surface of the liver

of the right hepatic vein. The caudate lobe (segment I) is subdivided into the left caudate lobe (Spiegel lobe), right caudate lobe (paracaval portion), and caudate process based on vascular supply (Fig. 3.3).

A meticulous comprehension of segmental anatomy, representing a significant advancement in hepatic surgery, underpins anatomical hepatectomy [3]. Hepatotomy may be performed along the segmental border to minimize intraoperative blood loss and postoperative necrosis of devitalized tissues. Portal vein ligation is a critical step of the ALPPS procedure. As such, a holistic comprehension of hepatic segments and anatomical hepatectomy is essential for applying ALPPS.

3.2 The First Porta Hepatis

The ALPPS procedure predominantly involves right trisegmentectomy without preserving the middle hepatic vein, and partially entails left trisegmentectomy (Fig. 3.4). During stage 1 of the ALPPS procedure, semi-hepatic portal vein ligation is necessary, while anatomizing the first porta hepatis is critical. Therefore, proficiency in the anatomy of the porta hepatis should be achieved.

The pipeline structures within and around the porta hepatis are not intuitively apparent, as they are encased within the connective tissue (i.e., Glisson's sheath) or its fusion layer. This gives rise to a three-plate structure at the porta hepatis, comprising the hilar, cystic, and umbilical plates. Specifically, the hilar plate, situated centrally, extends from segment IVb at its superior border to the hepatoduodenal ligament at its inferior border. The hilar plate courses superiorly and to the right to develop into the cystic plate, and courses to the left to become the umbilical plate. In addition, the hilar plate connects with the Arantius' duct on the left superior surface, and courses towards the root of the left hepatic vein in the direction of the second porta hepatis. Thoroughly understanding and skillfully navigating the anatomical relationship between the three-plate structure and hepatic pedicle facilitates the rapid dissection of the hepatic pedicle.

The portal vein, hepatic artery, and bile duct converge at the porta hepatis, branching off to enter the left and right hemilivers via the three-plate structure at the porta hepatis. Specifically, the hilar plate plays a particularly prominent role, as it encloses crucial structures (e.g., bile duct and portal vein bifurcations). Therefore, all vascular and bile duct branches leading to the left hemiliver can be detached from the left side of the hilar plate to the umbilical plate respectively (Fig. 3.4a). Similarly, all vascular and bile duct branches leading to the right hemiliver can be detached from the right side to the right notch of the hilar plate, respectively (Fig. 3.4b).

Managing the cystohepatic triangle (Calot's triangle) is enormously important, as the ALPPS procedure requires cholecystectomy. The cystohepatic triangle is bordered by the cystic duct laterally, the common hepatic duct medially, and the inferior surface of the liver superiorly. This triangle, through which an accessory right hepatic duct and an aberrant right hepatic artery may pass, contains lymph nodes, right hepatic artery, and cystic artery. Giant liver tumors typically exert pressure on the cholecyst to cause the compression and deformation of the cystohepatic triangle, rendering it challenging to identify the ducts within the cystohepatic triangle. This requires cholecystectomy. It is advisable to approach the cholecyst whenever feasible and avoid closely adhering to the hepatic surface during cholecystectomy. This aids in preventing an injury to the right hepatic artery and minimizing the risk of tumor rupture. In the event of accidental hemorrhage, hemostasis by electrocautery should be practiced with caution to prevent inadvertent injuries. It is advisable to immediately insert a finger into the omental foramen and make the structure within the hepatic pedicle gently squeezed between the thumb and index finger. Temporary hemostasis can be achieved by completely excluding blood flow into the liver using the Pringle maneuver. Once blood loss is mitigated, hemorrhagic spots should be meticulously identified, followed by suturing with vascular sutures to achieve hemostasis.

3.2.1 Portal Vein

A total of 70%–75% of the liver's blood supply stems from the portal vein, formed from the confluence of the splenic and superior mesenteric veins at the pancreatic neck. The portal vein collects blood from the intestinal tract to deliver nutrients to the liver, contributing to approximately 50% of

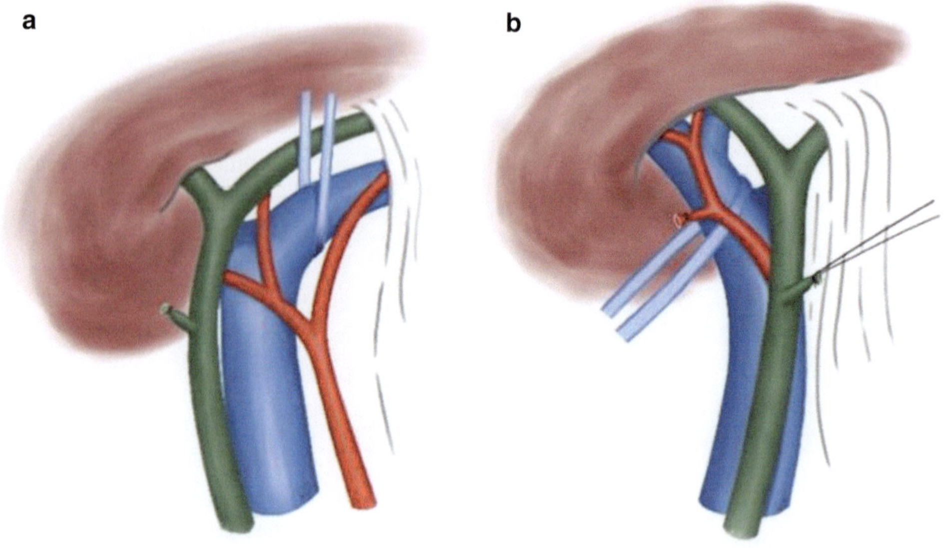

Fig. 3.4 Anatomical schematic diagram of the porta hepatis in the left hemiliver (**a**) and right hemiliver (**b**) based on ALPPS procedure

the liver's oxygen supply. The main portal vein, measuring 6.73 cm in length on average, ascends via the hepatoduodenal ligament to reach the porta hepatis, where it commonly bifurcates into left and right portal veins to enter the liver. The angle formed between the left and right portal veins is between 90° and 120°. The left portal vein, measuring approximately 2 cm in length (1.1–3.3 cm), courses horizontally to the left within the transverse sulcus, and then curves anteroinferiorly upon reaching the left sagittal sulcus, thereby forming the sagittal segment. The right portal vein, which is approximately 1.05 cm (0.6–1.8 cm) long, is shorter than the left portal vein.

The branching pattern, as well as the angles formed between the main portal vein and its branches, is paramount for implementing the ALPPS procedure. Because of numerous right portal vein variations, most international classifications are developed based on right portal vein variations. The Nakamura classification (Fig. 3.5) [4] is internationally applied. Surgical challenges vary considerably among branching patterns, with a pronounced risk of accidental injuries, necessitating meticulous preoperative evaluation. For Nakamura type B (trifurcation pattern), the right anterior and right posterior portal veins require separate ligation, as their concurrent ligation potentially leads to main portal vein stenosis. For Nakamura type C (the right posterior portal vein arising from the main portal vein) and type D (the right anterior portal vein originating from the left portal vein within the liver), it is crucial to acknowledge the presence of the right anterior portal vein. The missed ligation can result in incomplete portal vein ligation in the first stage. In particular, detaching the right anterior portal vein originating from the left portal vein within the liver is highly challenging for Nakamura type D. In this regard, attention should be devoted to safeguarding the right anterior portal vein during left hemihepatectomy for Nakamura type D.

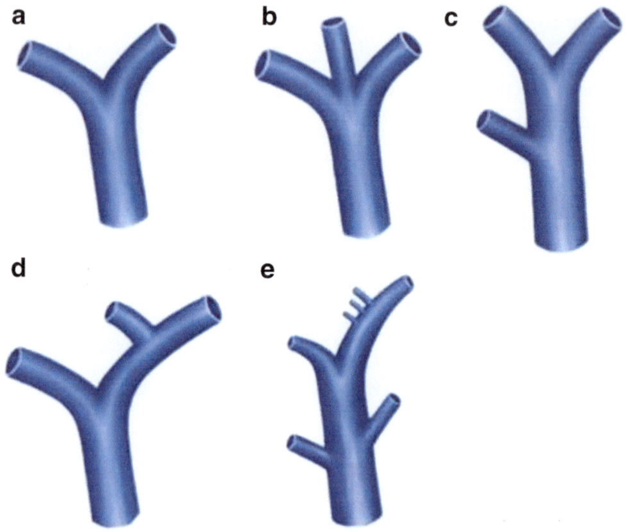

Fig. 3.5 Nakamura classification of portal vein branches. (**a**). A typical portal vein branch (92.5%); (**b**). Trifurcation (2.5%); (**c**). The right posterior portal vein arising from the main portal vein (approximately 2.5%); (**d**). The right anterior portal vein originating from the left portal vein within the liver (approximately 1.7%); (**e**). The right portal vein composed of multiple branches (0.8%)

3.2.2 Hepatic Artery

A total of 25%–30% of the liver's blood supply is derived from the hepatic artery carrying highly oxygenated blood. Because of the limited blood flow, the hepatic artery only provides 50% of the oxygen supply to the liver. From the celiac artery, the common hepatic artery courses to the right along the superior margin of the pancreas. As the common hepatic artery turns anterosuperiorly, it reaches the superior portion of the duodenal bulb, bifurcating into the proper hepatic artery and gastroduodenal artery. The

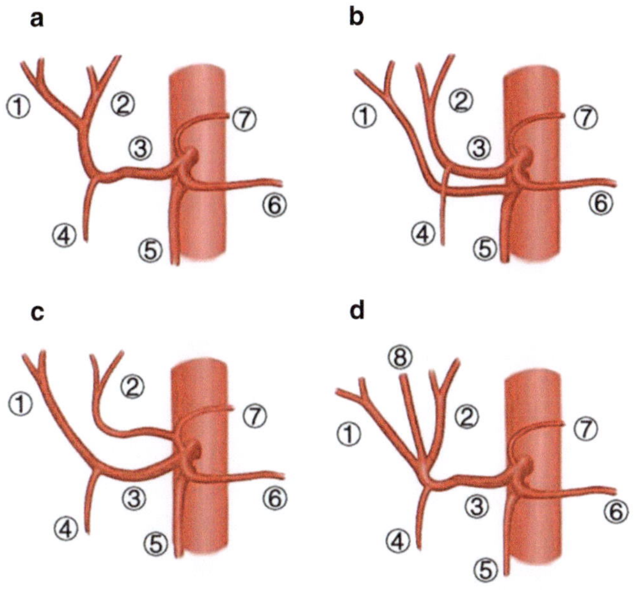

Fig. 3.6 Typical course and common variations of the hepatic artery. (**a**). Typical course of the hepatic artery; (**b**). Right hepatic artery taking origin from the superior mesenteric artery; (**c**). Left hepatic artery originating from the left gastric artery; (**d**). Left medial hepatic artery arising exterior to the porta hepatis. ① right hepatic artery; ② left hepatic artery; ③ common hepatic artery; ④gastroduodenal artery; ⑤ superior mesenteric artery; ⑥ splenic artery; ⑦ left gastric artery; ⑧ middle hepatic artery

proper hepatic artery ascends alongside the common bile duct and hepatic portal vein within the hepatoduodenal ligament, and finally divides into left and right hepatic arteries to enter the liver. The hepatic artery, situated in the most superficial layer in the hepatic hilar area, is most readily accessible during surgery. Moreover, collateral circulation pathways diminish as the hepatic artery approaches the porta hepatis, leading to compromised compensatory function. As stage 1 ALPPS procedure requires the preservation of arterial blood supply, proficiency in hepatic artery anatomy is significant for preventing intraoperative injuries.

Hepatic arterial variations are substantially present. Only two-thirds of hepatic arteries (the left and right hepatic arteries stem from the proper hepatic artery) typically course, while the remaining one-third of hepatic arteries present various course anomalies. Therefore, a meticulous preoperative evaluation is vital for confirming the presence of hepatic arterial variations. Hepatic arterial variations, which we frequently encountered, include a. common hepatic artery as well as right hepatic artery or right posterior hepatic artery taking origin from the superior mesenteric artery; b. the left hepatic artery originating from the left gastric artery; and c. the left medial hepatic artery arising exterior to the porta hepatis and specifically arising from the middle hepatic artery (Fig. 3.6).

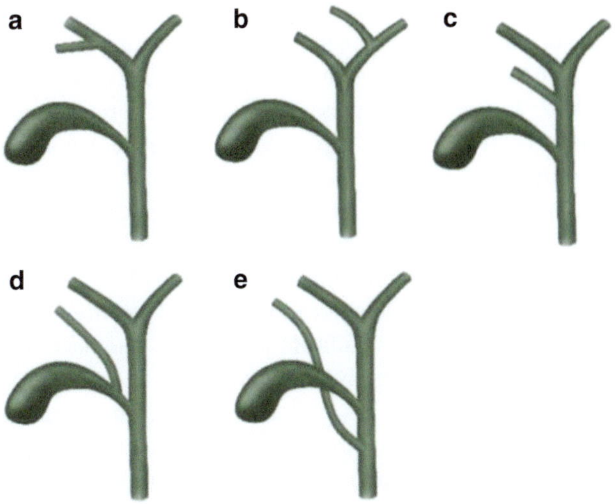

Fig. 3.7 Typical course and common variations of the bile duct. (**a**). Typical course of the bile duct; (**b**). Right posterior hepatic duct draining into the left hepatic duct; (**c**). Accessory hepatic duct draining into the common hepatic duct; (**d**). Accessory hepatic duct draining into the cystic duct; (**e**). Accessory hepatic duct draining into the common bile duct

3.2.3 Bile Duct

The hilar bile duct bifurcation, representing the most superior point within the Glisson's vascular group, courses anterosuperior to the portal vein bifurcation. The main left and right hepatic ducts measure (1.3 ± 0.5) cm and (0.7 ± 0.4) cm in length, respectively. As the intrahepatic bile duct runs alongside the portal vein, safeguarding the hepatic duct is imperative in the portal vein management in the first stage. Incorrect bile duct ligation or an injury to the bile duct can lead to bile leakage or cholestasis, ultimately compromising postoperative recovery. Furthermore, variations are present in the confluence of hepatic ducts. The most common variation is the right posterior hepatic duct draining into the left hepatic duct in approximately 22% of the population. Therefore, particular attention should be directed to such variation during left hemihepatectomy. Aside from the left and right hepatic ducts, other accessory hepatic ducts directly merge into the common hepatic duct, common bile duct, or cystic duct (Fig. 3.7). Therefore, routinely performing magnetic resonance cholangiopancreatography (MRCP) before the ALPPS procedure is necessary to understand the bile duct course.

3.3 Hepatic Vein

Hepatic veins include left, middle, and right hepatic veins and short hepatic veins draining directly into the IVC posterior to the liver. Hepatic veins lack venous valves, possess thin walls, and are embedded within the liver parenchyma.

Caution should be exercised to prevent inadvertent rupture of hepatic veins and subsequent hemorrhage, as it may lead to air embolism. Some giant liver tumors requiring ALPPS procedure typically compress the second porta hepatis. Consequently, exposing hepatic veins is challenging during liver mobilization and hepatic parenchymal transection, resulting in augmented surgical challenges. Identifying an intrahepatic tumor's relationships with Glisson's sheath and hepatic veins is essential for determining its location, relationship with the vascular location, and resectability.

Hepatic veins are significant anatomical landmarks during diagnostic imaging, liver volume measurement, determination of the scope of hepatectomy, and intraoperative determination of the transection plane. Moreover, compromising the hepatic venous reflux on the preserved side should be avoided to prevent hepatic dysfunction resulting from hepatic venous congestion during hepatic parenchymal transection.

The right hepatic vein, which enters the right wall of the IVC approximately 1–1.5 cm beneath the diaphragm, can serve as the border between the right anterior and right posterior sections, predominantly draining the right posterior section and the dorsal part of segment VII. The middle and left hepatic veins typically merge to form a common trunk before draining into the IVC. The middle hepatic vein, which typically drains segment IV, V, and the ventral part of segment VII, can divide the liver into the left and right hemilivers. In stage 1 ALPPS procedure, semi-hepatic parenchymal transection is often performed along the left side of the Rex-Cantlie line extending from the gallbladder bed to the IVC. Notably, the Rex-Cantlie line, along which viable hepatic tissues can be preserved to the greatest extent, is an irregular plane rather than a straight line. The optimal approach to defining the Rex-Cantlie line is to ligate the semi-hepatic portal vein or inject pigment (methylene blue or fluorescent staining) via the main portal vein. In addition, the middle hepatic vein, which typically courses along the Rex-Cantlie line, serves as a marker for the semi-hepatic parenchymal transection.

3.4 Hepatic Lobular Structure

The hepatic microstructures reveal hepatic lobules (Fig. 3.8). The central vein is at the center of the lobule, surrounded by a single layer of hepatocytes arranged radially in cords. Hepatic sinusoids run between these cords of hepatocytes. The sinusoidal walls are lined with hepatic macrophages, known as Kupffer cells, which possess phagocytic capabilities and are a critical component of the mononuclear phagocytic system. Between hepatic lobules is a portal area consisting of connective tissues ensheathing the hepatic artery, portal vein, and bile duct. The hepatic sinusoids represent the capillary bed of the liver, with one end linked to the small branches of the hepatic artery and portal vein and the other end connected with the central vein, facilitating the flow of blood into and out of the liver. Upon ligation of the semi-hepatic portal vein, blood flow from the contralateral portal vein communicates with the hepatic sinusoid between the left and right hemilivers to transport nutrients. Therefore, hepatic parenchymal transection or partition is necessary in stage 1 ALPPS procedure, which can block the nutritional supply to the hepatic area slated for resection.

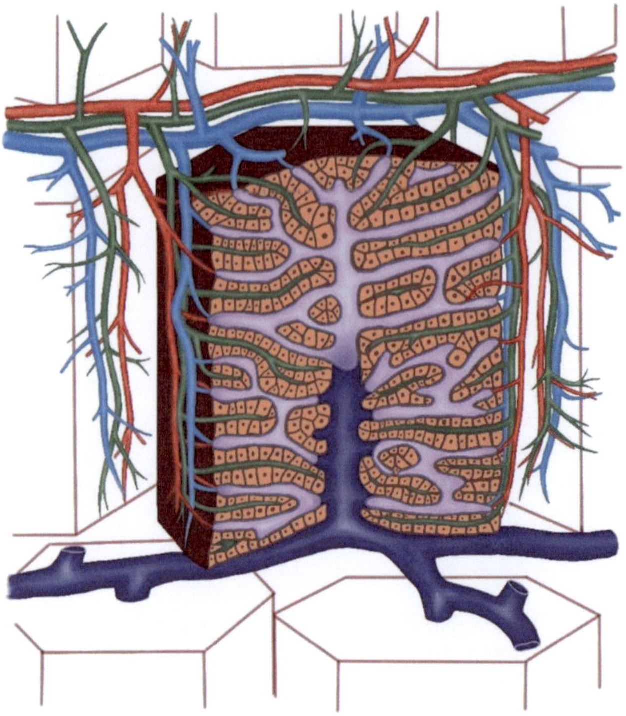

Fig. 3.8 Hepatic lobule

3.5 Perihepatic Ligament

As the hepatic serosa courses to the diaphragm and its adjacent organs, multiple ligaments are formed, including the falciform ligament, round ligament of the liver that forms part of the free edge of the falciform ligament, coronary ligament, left and right triangular ligaments, hepatorenal ligament, gastrohepatic ligament, and hepatoduodenal ligament. In the presence of a giant tumor, thick blood vessels in the perihepatic ligament often directly supply the tumor. Therefore, thorough hemostasis is imperative for the above ligaments during liver mobilization. Generally, giant tumors, situated on the diaphragmatic dome of the right liver lobe, adhere tightly to the right diaphragm and are supplied by some thick right inferior phrenic arteries, posing a risk of massive bleeding during mobilization of the diaphragmatic dome of the right liver lobe. Ligating the right inferior phrenic arteries can assist in mitigating mobilization-related hemorrhage. The ligation method is detailed as follows: Excise the lesser omentum of the stomach, and employ a retractor to pull the Spiegel lobe toward the cranial side. Then, a strip, running obliquely between the right diaphragmatic crus and the IVC, is visible, with the right inferior phrenic arteries situated in between. Irrespective of their origins, the right inferior phrenic arteries must course superiorly and to the right from their origins.

3.6 Lymphatic Vessel

The intrahepatic lymphatic vessels, located within the connective tissue of the portal canal, run parallel to the interlobular arteries, veins, and bile ducts. They can anastomose with each other, and join together to form larger lymphatic vessels that exit via the porta hepatis. The lymph from the superior surface of the liver drains into the thoracic cavity via the vena caval foramen, draining into the supradiaphragmatic lymph nodes and posterior mediastinal lymph nodes. Conversely, the lymph from the inferior surface of the liver drains into the lymph nodes at the porta hepatis. Given the presence of numerous lymphatic vessels in the perihepatic ligaments, conducting meticulous intraoperative ligation of thick lymphatic vessels is vital for preventing massive ascites resulting from postoperative lymphatic fistula from compromising postoperative recovery.

References

1. Wang Z, Peng YF, Hu JW, et al. Associating liver partition and portal vein ligation for staged hepatectomy for unresectable hepatitis B virus-related hepatocellular carcinoma: a single center study of 45 patients. Ann Surg. 2020;271(3):534–41.
2. Couinaud C. Les enveloppes vasculobiliares de foie ou capsule de Glisson. Leur interet dans la chirurgie vesiculaire, les resections hepatiques et l'abord du hile du foie. Lyon Chir. 1954;49:589–615.
3. Bismuth H. Surgical anatomy and anatomical surgery of the liver. World J Surg. 1982;6(1):3–9.
4. Nakamura T, Tanaka K, Kiuchi T, et al. Anatomical variations and surgical strategies in right lobe living donor liver transplantation: lessons from 120 cases. Transplantation. 2002;73(12):1896–903.

Indications, Contraindications, and Preoperative Evaluation

4

Zheng Wang

The intended population for ALPPS comprises colorectal liver metastasis (CRLM), hepatocellular carcinoma (HCC), intrahepatic cholangiocarcinoma (ICC), perihilar cholangiocarcinoma (PHC), gallbladder cancer, epithelioid hemangioendothelioma, and non-CRLM patients, as reported on the ALPPS registry (https://ALPPS.net). According to the ALPPS registry, CRLM, HCC, PHC, and ICC remain the most common indications for ALPPS, though ALPPS is theoretically suitable for treating nearly all primary and secondary liver tumors (Fig. 4.1). ALPPS is predominantly employed in adult patients and applied in pediatric patients [1].

Determining patients suitable for the ALPPS procedure or identifying the optimal indications for ALPPS is paramount for applying surgical techniques, particularly ALPPS. ALPPS cannot completely substitute for other techniques, such as portal vein embolization (PVE) or two-stage hepatectomy (TSH). However, experienced hepatobiliary surgeons prefer ALPPS for some patients in the absence of any other viable conventional surgical techniques.

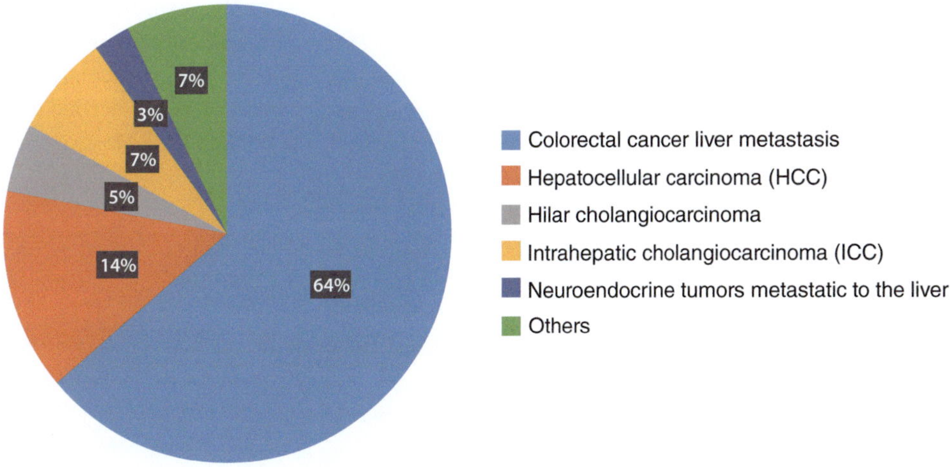

Fig. 4.1 Indications for ALPPS: The data were derived from the ALPPS registry. (Data as of May 2019; https://ALPPS.net)

Z. Wang (✉)
Zhongshan Hospital, Fudan University, Shanghai, China
e-mail: wang.zheng@zs-hospital.sh.cn

J. Zhou (ed.), *Associating Liver Partition and Portal Vein Ligation for Staged Hepatectomy (ALPPS)*,
https://doi.org/10.1007/978-981-96-7364-3_4

4.1 Indications for ALPPS

4.1.1 ALPPS for CRLM

CRLM is currently the principal indication for ALPPS procedure (constituting approximately 2/3 of the patients registered on the ALPPS registry; Fig. 4.2) [2]. ALPPS has increased the opportunity for curative treatment in CRLM patients. The tumor recurrence rate after the ALPPS procedure may be more significant as compared to that after conventional hepatectomy, predominantly because of a higher tumor burden in patients undergoing the ALPPS procedure. Nonetheless, ALPPS offers renewed opportunities and hope for intermediate to advanced CRLM patients previously deemed ineligible for surgery. A rigorous unified standard needs to be improved to curb the potential overuse of ALPPS [3]. Presently, the adequacy of such a standard lacks sufficient evidence from research on the long-term prognosis of CRLM treated with ALPPS. An early report on the treatment of CRLM with ALPPS suggested that the 1- and 2-year overall survival (OS) rates of CRLM patients were 76 and 63%, respectively [4]. These survival data needed to consider the high perioperative mortality (8%) as well as the selection bias in the presence of a high hepatic tumor burden when the ALPPS procedure was initially performed. A subsequent series study with a larger sample size indicated that the 3-year OS rate of 58 CRLM patients treated with ALPPS was 50%, with a disease-free survival rate of 13% [5]. Different studies showed that neoadjuvant chemotherapy did not adversely affect the FLR hypertrophy or the perioperative outcome following the ALPPS procedure [6].

A recent case-matched study from the ALPPS registry revealed that the historical control group receiving palliative chemotherapy was not markedly inferior to the ALPPS procedure group regarding early tumor prognosis in patients with CRLM deemed unresectable with conventional procedures [7]. It is noteworthy that the tumor burden was higher in the ALPPS procedure group as compared to the historical control group (median number of tumor-invaded liver segments: 7; median number of lesions in the liver remnant: 4). Therefore, the poor prognosis may have been attributable to the patient selection bias rather than stemming from the failure of ALPPS procedure.

Only a few articles comparing ALPPS and TSH have been published to date. Generally, ALPPS improves resectability compared with conventional TSH, with no remarkable differences in the survival rate. Adam et al. [8] reported a lower median OS following the ALPPS procedure (20 months vs 37 months). A series of studies by Ratti et al. [9] and Kambakamba et al. [10] suggested that ALPPS and TSH did not differ concerning the 1-year survival rate and 1-year disease-free survival rate. Of note, the above studies were conducted in a non-randomized and non-matched manner [11]. Recently, Roble-Campos et al. [12] published nearly identical data. A propensity score matching analysis revealed the 1-, 3-, and 5-year OS rates following tourniquet ALPPS vs conventional TSH were 81, 67, and 24% vs 76%, 57%, and 23%, respectively. Nonetheless, the long-term prognosis data were missing in almost all previous studies (Table 4.1). Further data, particularly from subsequent randomized controlled trials, are needed to evaluate the prognosis of ALPPS in treating CRLM.

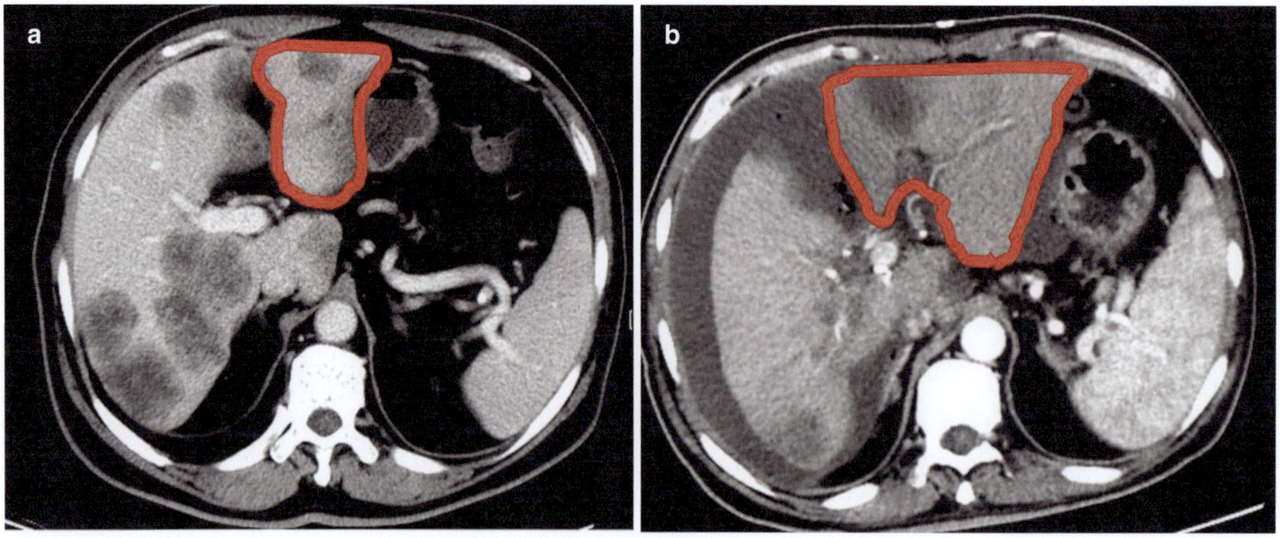

Fig. 4.2 Treatment of CLRM with ALPPS. (**a**) Image before stage 1 ALPPS procedure, showing multiple intrahepatic lesions (lesions in the left lateral lobe were resected during stage 1 ALPPS procedure); (**b**) Image before stage 2 ALPPS procedure

Table 4.1 Literature review of the survival rates following treatment of CLRM with ALPPS

Author	Year	No. of cases	1 year-survival rate (%)	2 year-survival rate (%)	3 year-survival rate (%)	5 year-survival rate (%)	Median OS (month)
Schadde et al.	2014	141	76	63	–	–	–
Oldhafer et al.	2014	7	57	–	–	–	–
Lang et al.	2015	7	–	–	64	–	–
Ratti et al.	2015	12	92	–	–	–	–
Adam et al.	2016	17	–	42	–	–	–
Björnsson et al.	2016	23	83	59	–	–	–
Kambakamba et al.	2016	41	–	–	–	–	24.7 ± 2.3
Olthof et al.	2017	70	–	62	–	–	–
Wanis et al.	2018	58	93	66	50	–	–
Robles-Campos et al.	2019	21	76	–	57	23	36
Baumgart et al.	2019	8	75	–	40	–	36.2

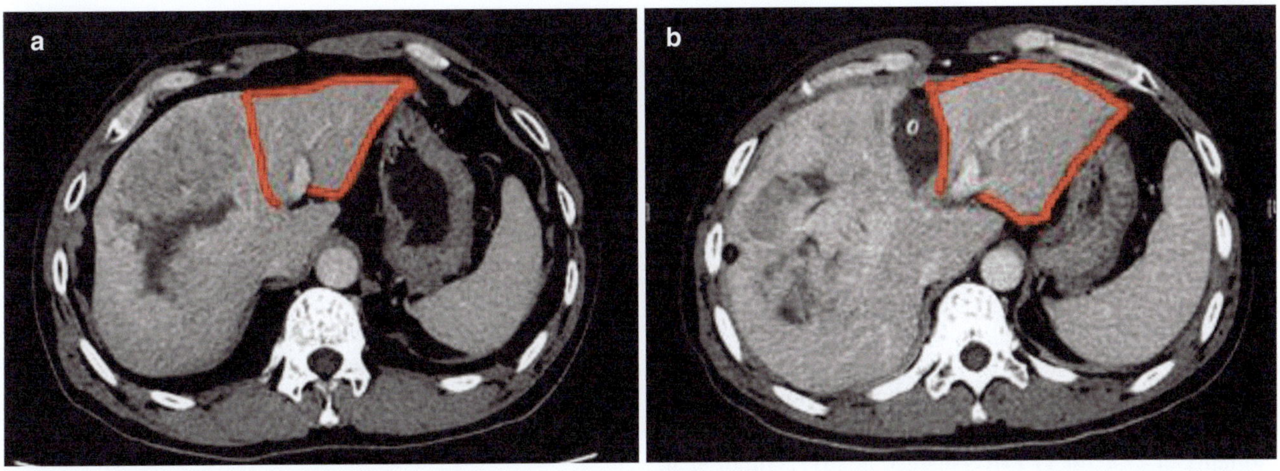

Fig. 4.3 Treatment of HCC complicated by tumor thrombus in the right branch of the portal vein with ALPPS. (**a**) Image before stage 1 ALPPS procedure; (**b**) Image before stage 2 ALPPS procedure

4.1.2 ALPPS for HCC

As HCC is typically complicated by varying degrees of liver fibrosis/cirrhosis and/or portal hypertension (PHT) and impaired liver function, performing tumor resection is more challenging in HCC patients. ALPPS improves the resectability of HCC (Figs. 4.3 and 4.4). However, the earliest report from the ALPPS registry showed that the 90-day mortality was 31% in 35 intermediate-stage HCC patients who underwent the ALPPS procedure [5]. Nevertheless, with accumulating experience and increasingly stringent case selection criteria, ALPPS has been extensively incorporated into the standards or guidelines for treating HCC deemed unresectable with single-stage surgery. The team led by Chan AC from the University of Hong Kong in China [13] developed the following criteria for HCC patients undergoing ALPPS procedure: FLR < 30% of the standardized liver volume (SLV), Child-Pugh grade A, indocyanine green retention rate at 15 min (ICG-R15) < 20%, platelet count >100/nL, and absence of thrombosis in the right branch of the portal vein. Consequently, the surgical outcomes markedly improved, reducing the 90-day mortality to 7.1%. Comparable results were also reported by Vennarecci et al. from Rome [14]. It is noteworthy that complete hepatic parenchymal transection appeared to lead to faster FLR hypertrophy as compared to partial ALPPS in patients with chronic liver disease [15].

In a recent single-center propensity score matching study in Zhongshan Hospital, Fudan University, 45 HCC patients with concurrent hepatitis B underwent ALPPS treatment were analyzed [16]. The study found a negative correlation between the severity of liver cirrhosis and the degree and rate of liver hypertrophy. The 1- and 3-year survival rates of intermediate to advanced HCC patients treated with ALPPS were 64 and 60%, respectively, notably better than those of unresectable HCC patients treated with transcatheter arterial chemoembolization (TACE).

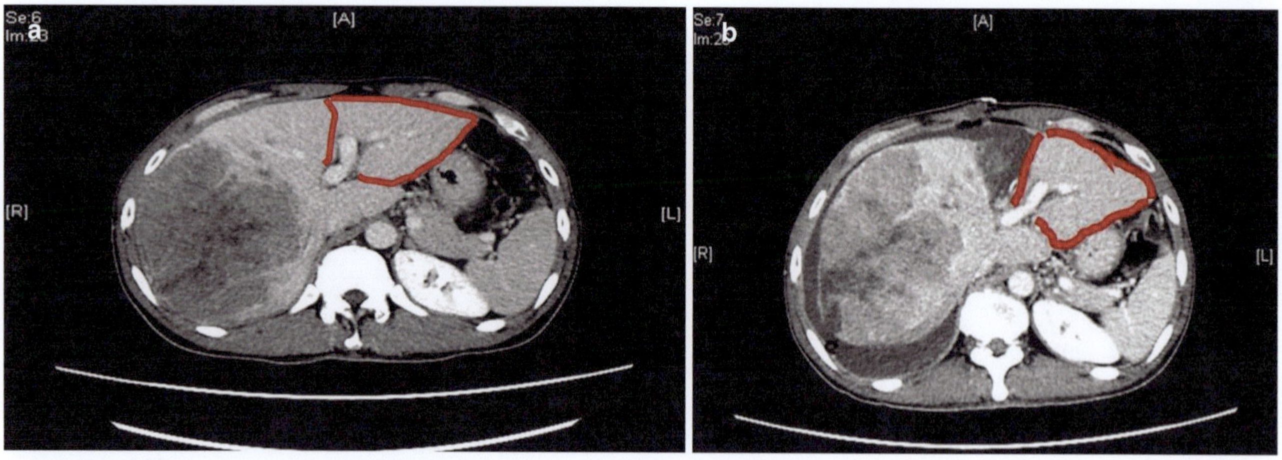

Fig. 4.4 Treatment of HCC complicated by mild liver cirrhosis with ALPPS. (**a**) Image before stage 1 ALPPS procedure; (**b**) Image before stage 2 ALPPS procedure

The aforementioned experiences from Hong Kong, Rome, and Fudan University in China collectively demonstrated that ALPPS can increase the resectability of HCC deemed unresectable with single-stage surgery in specific patients and that patients ineligible for ALPPS procedure can only opt for palliative therapy [15–17].

4.1.3 ALPPS for PHC

The ALPPS registry reported the preliminary study on treating PHC with ALPPS [4], showing a postoperative 90-day mortality of 27% for 11 PHC patients. In 2017, Olthof et al. [18] conducted a matched comparison between the outcomes of patients with PHC from the ALPPS registry and those resulting from the treatment with PVE and right trisegmentectomy. The postoperative mortality in the ALPPS group was twice as high as that in the control group (48% vs 24%), and the median survival time was merely 6 months in the ALPPS group, compared to 29 months in the control group (P = 0.048). Other reports from the ALPPS registry confirmed that biliary tumors were closely associated with deaths following the ALPPS procedure [4, 19, 20]. The application of ALPPS in patients with biliary malignancies (e.g., PHC) has a relatively high incidence of complications (e.g., bile leakage, hepatic insufficiency, severe infection, and sepsis) and mortality, especially in patients requiring biliary reconstruction [20]. It remains debated over whether PHC should be regarded as a relative contraindication to ALPPS. The analysis found that ALPPS outcomes for treating PHC were achieved using the conventional ALPPS procedure and were unsatisfactory, possibly because of a lack of surgical experience and being at the lower end of the learning curve of ALPPS in the initial stage. In order to diminish the incidence of complications and mortality while further minimizing surgical trauma in the treatment of PHC with ALPPS, several substantive improvements were made to the surgical procedure. Sakamoto et al. [21] improved the mini ALPPS concept by using ileocolic PVE rather than mesenteric PVE and achieved encouraging outcomes in three patients. Similarly, Balci et al. [22] reported the successful application of laparoscopic stage 1 ileocolic PVE in two additional patients. By refining the selection criteria for surgical patients, accurately capturing the timing of stage 2 surgery, and fine-tuning surgical techniques, ALPPS can emerge as a viable treatment alternative, allowing resection of PHC deemed unresectable with any other techniques.

4.1.4 Other Indications

Treating ICC with ALPPS has been reported but has not been investigated [23] (Fig. 4.5). In addition, patients for whom conventional PVE has failed, and those unable to undergo or deemed unsuitable for TSH with PVE (such as those with tumor thrombus in the main branches of the portal vein on the tumor side) are also indications for ALPPS (Fig. 4.6). A burgeoning body of research suggests that ALPPS is increasingly recognized as a major salvage treatment following PVE failure, as the salvage ALPPS boasts a notable success rate (92.3–100%) and exhibits comparable incidence of complications and mortality to conventional ALPPS [24, 25]. ALPPS can also be applied in patients with neuroendocrine tumors and hemangiomas (Figs. 4.7 and 4.8).

In summary, the indications for ALPPS include primary or metastatic liver cancer characterized by an inadequate FLR volume, specifically when FLR is less than 30% for a normal liver or less than 40% for a diseased liver (hepatic lesions induced by obstructive jaundice, liver fibrosis, moderate to severe fatty liver, or chemotherapy), as revealed by

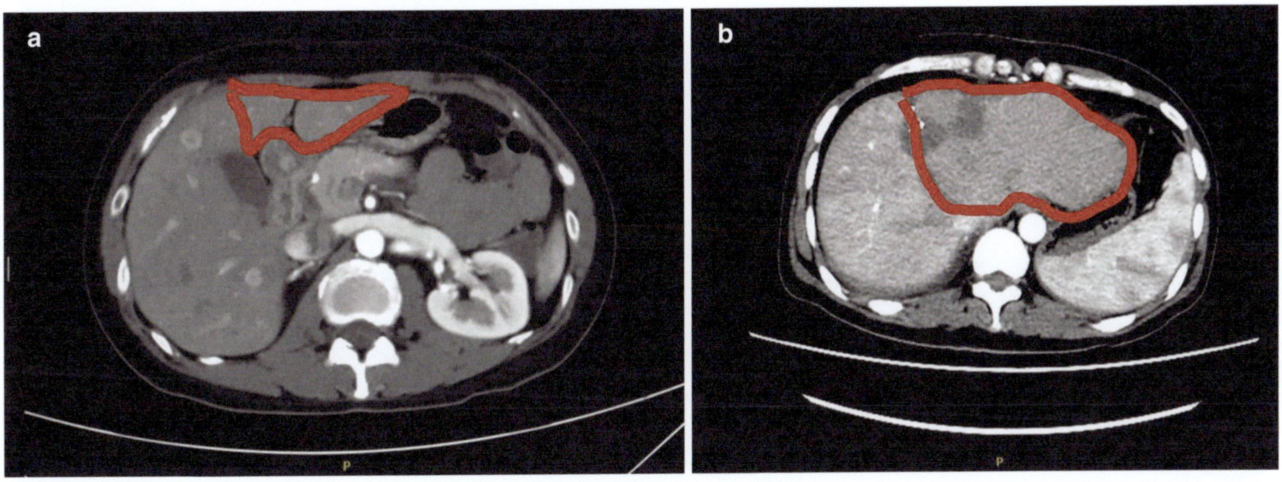

Fig. 4.5 Treatment of multiple ICC with ALPPS. (**a**) Image before stage 1 ALPPS procedure; (**b**) Image before stage 2 ALPPS procedure

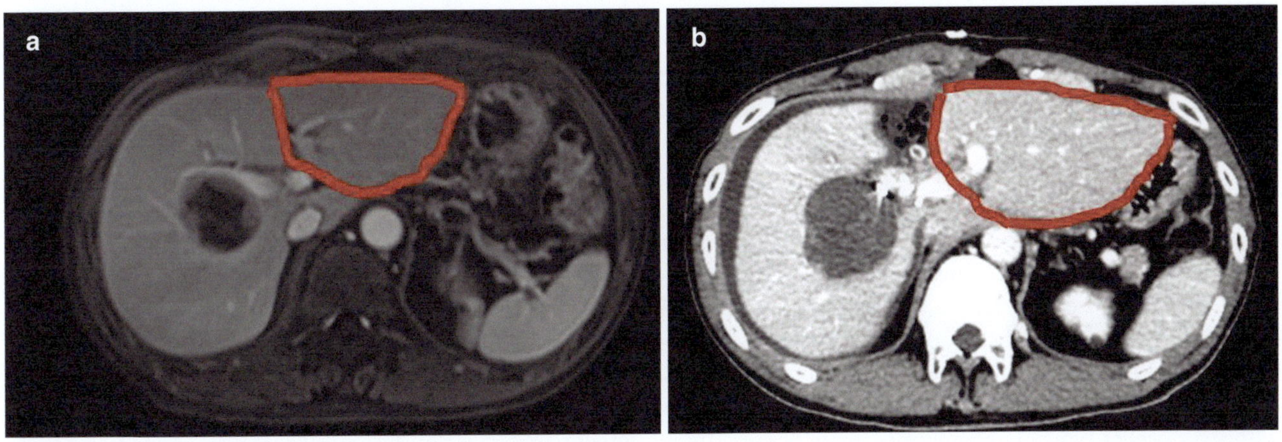

Fig. 4.6 Treatment of HCC failing PVE with ALPPS. (**a**) Image before stage 1 ALPPS procedure; (**b**) Image before stage 2 ALPPS procedure

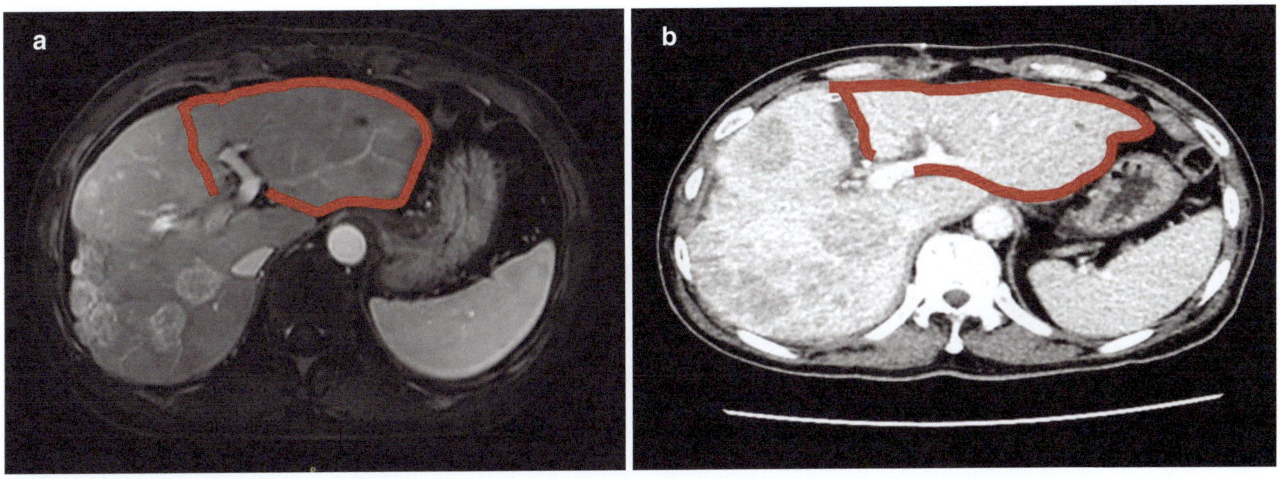

Fig. 4.7 Treatment of neuroendocrine tumors metastatic to the liver with ALPPS. (**a**) Image before stage 1 ALPPS procedure; (**b**) Image before stage 2 ALPPS procedure

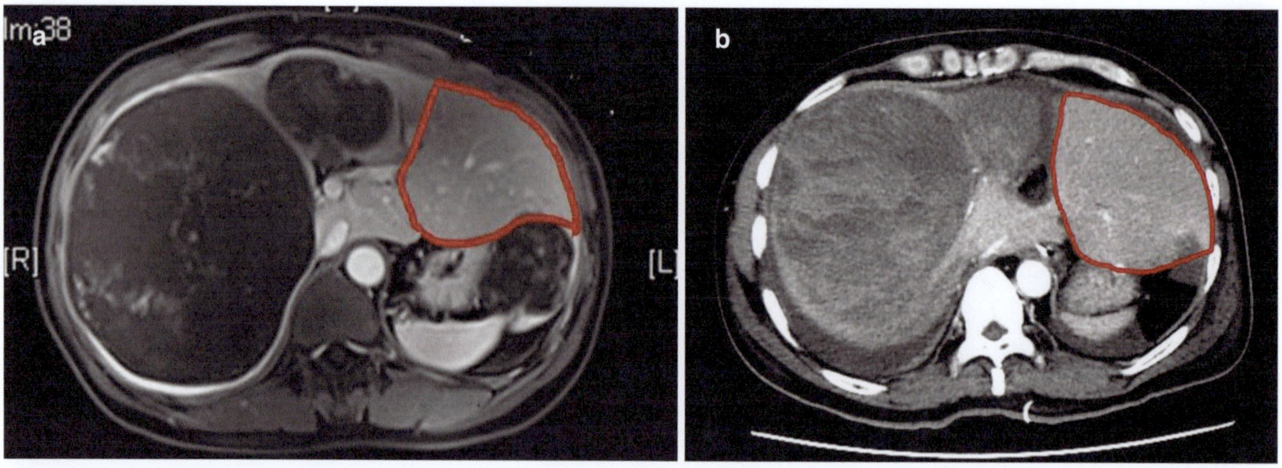

Fig. 4.8 Treatment of giant and multiple hemangioma with ALPPS. (**a**) Image before stage 1 ALPPS procedure; (**b**) Image before stage 2 ALPPS procedure

preoperative radiological evaluations. Its applicable pathological types typically include primary liver cancer or potentially resectable hilar cholangiocarcinoma with an inadequate FLR and no extrahepatic metastasis, as well as metastatic liver cancer with primary lesions that have been resected or can undergo concurrent radical resection and with no residual lesions observed extrahepatically or in the liver remnant; normal liver function or mild reversible impairment of liver function; good general conditions able to tolerate major surgery. Aside from hepatic tumors, the hepatic parenchymal status is a deterministic factor for determining the indications for ALPPS. The actual total count of functional hepatocytes (functional hepatocyte population) is lower in patients with liver cancer typically complicated by underlying liver diseases or liver injuries (e.g., viral hepatitis, liver fibrosis and cirrhosis, cholestasis, chemotherapy ± targeted therapy for liver injuries) as compared to those with a normal liver of equivalent volume. In addition, the aforementioned underlying diseases detrimentally impact FLR hypertrophy, necessitating additional time for achieving an adequate FLR. Although liver cirrhosis is not an absolute contraindication for ALPPS, meticulous preoperative evaluations before the application of ALPPS are still needed in these patients. For livers where PVE or portal vein ligation fails to induce the desired hypertrophy, ALPPS can serve as a salvage treatment.

4.2 Contraindications for ALPPS

The contraindications for ALPPS include high anesthetic risks, liver tumors for which the R0 resection cannot be achieved, poor liver function (Child-Pugh grade B or C, ICG-R15 > 20%), complications of severe PHT and/or ascites, severe liver fibrosis or cirrhosis, macrovesicular steatosis with more than 50% involvement, presence of unresectable extrahepatic metastases, poor hepatic arterial perfusion, and poor general conditions unable to tolerate major surgery. ALPPS procedure should be cautiously approached in individuals over 65 years.

4.3 Preoperative Evaluation and Case Screening for ALPPS

In 2007, Hans J. Schlitt from Regensburg, Germany, performed the world's first ALPPS procedure, and the so-called in-situ split is a novel surgical technique aimed at rapidly inducing liver hypertrophy. The research report detailing this technique in the first 25 cases was published in 2012. Nonetheless, the initial enthusiasm was dampened by the high morbidity and mortality, as well as early disease recurrence during the initial perioperative period. By refining patient selection criteria, augmenting surgical techniques to reduce the trauma associated with stage 1 surgery, and optimizing the timing of stage 2 surgery, morbidity and mortality can be further diminished, resulting in an improved prognosis following the ALPPS procedure.

Patients eligible for ALPPS procedure typically have large tumors, often accompanied by hepatitis and liver fibrosis/cirrhosis. Generally, they suffer from trauma associated with preoperative adjuvant therapies (e.g., chemotherapy, interventions, and radiofrequency) as well as ALPPS procedures. Given the complex clinical and pathological manifestations as well as the presence of hepatic anatomical variations, it is tremendously crucial to conduct precise preoperative evaluations of the FLR volume and function, accurately plan the liver partition location, and determine the optimal surgical timing. As preoperative evaluation techniques are continuously refined, the clinical evaluation approaches have become increasingly effective, enhancing surgical safety.

4.3.1 Evaluation Criteria for Post-hepatectomy Liver Failure (PHLF)

The evaluation criteria for PHLF include (a). positive 50–50 criteria: prothrombin time index<50% [or an international normalized ratio (INR) ≥1.7], serum bilirubin >50 μmol/L on postoperative day 5, predicting a mortality rate of 50%; (b) positive criteria: bilirubin concentration > 7 on postoperative day 5, serum bilirubin >70 mg/L in non-cirrhotic and non-cholestatic patients on postoperative day 5; (c) the International Study Group of Liver Surgery (ISGLS) criterion: the INR and bilirubin concentration exceeding their normal threshold values defined by the local laboratory on day 5 after hepatectomy. The presence of PHLF substantially heightens the susceptibility of patients to postoperative major complications, potentially resulting in early postoperative deaths. The quantitative evaluation criteria can be utilized to identify PHLF postoperative mortality.

4.3.2 Evaluation of FLR Volume

As most patients develop liver failure after stage 2 ALPPS procedure, it is highly crucial to evaluate the FLR volume following stage 1 ALPPS procedure. Standardization of future liver volume (FLV): The standardized FLV (SFLV) is calculated using Urata's formula [26]. Specifically, the body surface area (BSA) is calculated using body weight (kg, 0.425) × body height (cm, 0.725) × 0.007184 (m^2). Then, SLV is calculated from the formula (706.2 × BSA [m^2] + 2.4) mL. Finally, the standardized future liver volume ratio (SFLVR, i.e., FLV/SLV%) and SFLV (i.e., FLV/SLV) are calculated. The minimum cutoff values for SFLVR and SFLV essentially depend on the degree of liver cirrhosis and hepatic functional reserve. The hepatic functional reserve evaluation criteria necessary for safe resection remain essentially identical in China and beyond: for individuals with normal liver function (Child-Pugh class A and ICG-R15 < 10%), a normal liver requires SFLVR >20–30% and SFLVR should be >40% for patients with chronic liver diseases or hepatic parenchymal damage including liver cirrhosis, severe fatty liver, and chemotherapy-related liver injury; for those with impaired liver function (e.g., ICG-R15 10–20%), lager SFLV is required and SFLVR is supposed to be >50% for chronic liver disease and liver cirrhosis patients. Those who fail to meet the criteria are considered to have an inadequate FLV and should be considered for symptomatic treatments. A study from our center indicated that the severity of liver fibrosis in liver cancer patients was closely associated with the FLR hypertrophy rate. After stage 1 surgery, the median growth rate was 50.1 mL/d in patients with viral hepatitis without liver fibrosis, while the median growth rates were 19.8, 19.0, and 16.8 mL/d in patients with grades I, II, and III liver fibrosis, respectively, and that in patients with liver cirrhosis further dropped to 9.6 mL/d [16]. The data from this study provided a scientific basis for accurately calculating the FLR volume hypertrophy rate and time, contributing significantly to guide on determining the indications for ALPPS procedure. Kambakamba et al. [27] assessed the daily FLR regeneration using the kinetic growth rate (KGR) after stage 1 surgery. They concluded that a KGR of ≥6%/d is suggestive of a markedly reduced incidence of liver failure following stage 2 surgery. It is recommended that thin-slice CT scan images/MRI be used for three-dimensional liver reconstruction and that virtual surgical software be employed for virtual resection to accurately measure the FLR volume.

4.3.3 Measurement of Liver Stiffness (LS)

The ultrasonic imaging technique for measuring LS has evolved from the one-dimensional transient elastography (TE) to the two-dimensional acoustic radiation force impulse (ARFI) imaging technique, and subsequently to the current two-dimensional real-time shear wave elastography (SWE, also known as E-imaging). In measuring LS, SWE features intuitive quantification, real-time imaging, non-invasiveness, ease of operation, high accuracy, applicability to all populations, and intuitive image guidance. In addition, magnetic resonance elastography (MRE) has also been employed for LS measurement [28]. A report on the evaluation of PHLF by measuring LS with SWE showed that (a). when LS was more than 10.1 kPa, the diagnostic sensitivity and specificity for liver cirrhosis (S4) were 87.2 and 64%, respectively; (b). LS was closely associated with the incidence of PHLF, and the predicted cut-off values for PHLF and grade B or higher PHLF were 11.75 and 11.90 kPa, respectively. When LS was less than 11.9 kPa, no grade B or higher PHLF occurred, with a predictive accuracy superior to that for PHT, Child-Pugh class, or serological markers for liver fibrosis [29].

4.3.4 Evaluation of FLR Function

After stage 1 ALPPS procedure, the FLR hypertrophy progresses rapidly to achieve an adequate FLR within a short period. Nonetheless, scholars indicate that macroscopic liver volume hypertrophy does not represent the corresponding liver function improvements. Animal experiment findings identified by some scholars demonstrated that rapidly proliferating hepatocytes were mostly immature malformed cells, rendering it challenging to provide the necessary functions typical of normal hepatocytes. Apart from FLR increase, FLR function stands out as a critical influencing factor. Regular liver function test methods are as follows:

4.3.4.1 Measurement of Serum Biochemical Indicators for Liver Function

The serum biochemical indicators of liver function are measured using biochemical tests that measure hepatic uptake, synthesis, metabolism, and secretion. As the liver function is exceedingly complex, a wide array of liver function tests exist. Generally, clinicians select one or multiple panels of liver function tests based on patients' medical histories and signs identified via physical examinations. Biochemical tests for liver function are routinely performed on hospitalized patients. These tests, including total bilirubin, direct bilirubin, prothrombin time, INR of prothrombin time, serum albumin, albumin, cholinesterase, alkaline phosphatase, gamma-glutamyl transpeptidase (GGT), alanine transaminase (ALT), aspartate aminotransferase (AST), and hyaluronic acid, can reflect the overall liver function status in terms of hepatic uptake, synthesis, secretion, and metabolism. Blood samples are collected 1 day preoperatively and 1 day and 7 days postoperatively in the first stage, immediately before surgery, and 1, 7, 14, and 30 days postoperatively in the second stage. Research suggests that cholinesterase is the most dependable qualitative marker of liver function and is closely correlated with liver volume regeneration.

4.3.4.2 Special Test Methods

Child-Pugh score, Model for End-Stage Liver Disease (MELD) score, ICG-R15, breath test, lidocaine metabolism test, arterial ketone body ratio measurement, oral glucose tolerance test, and tryptophan tolerance test. The above tests can evaluate the functional reserve of the whole liver, but they may not precisely assess the FLR function. While the functional reserve of the entire liver is not identical to that of the FLR, it can serve as a reference.

Child-Pugh Score

The Child-Pugh score is determined based on readily accessible measures (e.g., albumin, bilirubin, prothrombin time, ascites, and hepatic encephalopathy). The Child-Pugh scores of 5–6, 7–9, and 10–15 points are considered Child-Pugh classes A, B, and C, respectively. In evaluating the prognosis in liver cirrhosis patients, the mortality rates associated with Child-Pugh classes A, B, and C liver failures are <5, 20, and 55%, respectively. The Child-Pugh scoring system is extensively utilized to assess and select candidates eligible for hepatectomy. Cirrhosis patients with Child-Pugh A have significantly lower rates of surgical complications and mortality compared to those with Child-Pugh B and C. In addition, hepatectomy is contraindicated in Child-Pugh class C liver cirrhosis patients. It should be approached with caution in Child-Pugh class B liver cirrhosis patients, as they demonstrate poor tolerance for hepatectomy. Notably, the Child-Pugh scoring system is unsuitable for assessing non-cirrhotic patients. The Child-Pugh scoring system suffers multiple limitations: (a) The subjective definitions of factors (e.g., ascites and hepatic encephalopathy) lead to discrepancies between Child-Pugh scores and clinical realities; (b) Although categorizing patients into classes A, B, and C, Child-Pugh scoring system exhibits considerable heterogeneity within each class; (c) Objective measures (e.g., albumin and prothrombin time) vary dramatically among laboratories, potentially confusing. Although it is found that the incidence of PHLF was noticeably higher in patients with Child-Pugh class B as compared to Child-Pugh class A (25% vs 5%), patients with Child-Pugh class A still suffer from a notable rate of liver function decompensation and a certain mortality rate post hepatectomy [30]. Therefore, the hepatic functional reserve should be further refined and evaluated in patients with a Child-Pugh score of A.

MELD Score

The MELD score is predominantly utilized to evaluate the short- and mid-term mortality rates of patients with end-stage liver disease. In surgical settings, the MELD score is principally employed to gauge the severity of liver disease among patients awaiting liver transplantation to prioritize the allocation of donor livers. A study showed that the MELD score can predict surgical risks in patients undergoing partial hepatectomy, with a MELD score of ≤10 points considered safe for hepatectomy [31]. However, a recent report suggests that the MELD score lacks accuracy in evaluating PHLF, as the incidence and mortality of PHLF remained high in patients with an MELD score of ≤11 points. This is mainly because external factors affect the MELD scoring system, which lacks correlation with the occurrence of PHLF. Differing from that, cholestasis may induce vitamin K malabsorption to cause an increased INR of prothrombin time; the creatinine level in the MELD scoring system may be elevated due to inadequate blood volume or excessive diuretic use. Therefore, the MELD scoring system is chiefly utilized to screen patients with end-stage liver disease awaiting liver transplantation. However, an analysis of 320 ALPPS patients from the ALPPS registry revealed that a MELD score of >10 points is a significant high-risk factor for postoperative 90-day mortality. It is advised that the stage 2 surgery should be postponed when patients have a MELD score of >10 points before stage 2 surgery [32] and that the MELD score can aid in evaluating the risks associated with the ALPPS procedure.

ICG-R15

Indocyanine green (ICG), completely cleared by the liver, is excreted directly into the bile without undergoing intrahepatic binding. Once ICG enters the liver, its blood level will experience an exponential drop lasting approximately 20 min. Then, approximately 97% of the dye will be excreted in the presence of a normal liver function. The ICG clearance rate can be determined by serum sampling or by noninvasively measuring the pulse dye concentration using a convenient optical sensor placed on a finger. ICG-R15 serves as a sensitive indicator of hepatic functional reserve and can be utilized to evaluate the safety margin for liver resection. Its predictive results for hepatic parenchymal cell volume are comparable to CT measurements. ICG-R15 is susceptible to interference, as it is sensitive to sampling time. Any condition causing biliary excretion disorders, such as biliary stasis, may compromise the test results. According to Fan et al. from Hongkong, China [33], ICG-R15 is the sole predictor for post-hepatectomy mortality, suggesting an ICG-R15 < 14% is considered feasible for a major hepatectomy for liver cancer, while an ICG-R15 < 23% is feasible for minor hepatectomy. Van Thiel et al. [34] indicate that the preoperative ICG-R15 < 10% is considered feasible for the resection of 2 liver segments or 30% of liver tissues in liver cancer patients; ICG-R15 of 10–20% is deemed feasible for resection of only one liver segment or up to 15% of liver tissues; when ICG-R15 is more than 20%, surgical risk remains high even with resection of one liver segment. The "Expert Consensus on Preoperative Liver Reserve Function Assessment for Liver Resection" (2011 Edition) [35] states that Child-Pugh class A patients can tolerate major hepatectomy for resection of up to 4 liver segments when the ICG-R15 is not more than 10%, major hepatectomy for resection of 2–3 liver segments when the ICG-R15 is between 10 and 19%, resection of a single segment only when the ICG-R15 is between 20 and 29%, limited hepatectomy for resection of a limited small-scale liver when the ICG-R15 is between 30 and 39%, and tumor enucleation only when the ICG-R15 is not less than 40%.

4.3.4.3 Other Techniques

Other techniques include functional tests, such as functional imaging and liver maximum capacity test. The most studied functional imaging can be categorized into nuclear medicine imaging combined with single photon emission computed tomography (SPECT)/CT examination and liver-specific contrast-enhanced magnetic resonance imaging. Research suggests that these two techniques can safely and effectively provide accurate assessments of liver function.

Technetium-99 m (^{99m}Tc)-DTPA-galactosyl human serum albumin (GSA) imaging and liver imaging with ^{99m}Tc-labeled iminodiacetic acid (IDA) derivatives are the most common representatives of hepatic radionuclide imaging. The above two techniques, developed based on different principles, can provide quantitative and intuitive imaging information of the overall and localized areas of the liver. The liver is the only site for technetium-99 m galactosyl human serum albumin (^{99m}Tc-GSA) uptake, making it an ideal agent for evaluating liver function and functional liver volume. Additionally, the hepatic uptake of ^{99m}Tc-GSA is not subject to a high serum bilirubin level, allowing its successful application even in cholestasis patients. ^{99m}Tc-GSA imaging has been extensively employed as a supplement to the ICG excretion test in Asia. Tomassini et al. [36] quantitatively evaluated the FLR function based on the hepatic uptake of ^{99m}Tc-labeled dimethyl-iminodiacetic acid within 10 min after intravenous injection, to evaluate the optimal timing for TSH in patients with the marginal SFLVR.

^{99m}Tc-labeled iminodiacetic acids (^{99m}Tc-IDA), which are a class of lidocaine analogs, undergo an uptake predominantly by hepatocytes, followed by being excreted directly into the bile duct without any biotransformation. With characteristics comparable to those of ICG, ^{99m}Tc-IDA is well suited for imaging the hepatobiliary system and diagnosing various biliary tract diseases. ^{99m}Tc-mebrofenin exhibits the lowest bilirubin replacement rate among all available IDA agents, making it the most suitable IDA for liver function assessment. The hepatic uptake of ^{99m}Tc-mebrofenin shares the same calculation method with ICG, and its uptake rate is closely correlated with the results of the ICG clearance test, effectively circumventing the uneven soft tissue distribution within the liver [37].

Gadolinium-ethoxybenzyl-diethylenetriaminepentaacetic acid (Gd-EOB-DTPA)-enhanced MRI also allows for evaluating hepatic functional reserve in humans. Motosugi et al. [38] found a significant correlation between the liver-to-spleen signal intensity ratios (LSRs) in patients undergoing Gd-EOB-DTPA-enhanced MRI scans and ICG clearance rate. Nonetheless, the employment of Gd-EOB-DTPA-enhanced MRI for liver function evaluation is marked by controversy, necessitating further investigation and evaluation.

4.4 Evaluation of PHT [39]

The causes of PHT can be categorized as prehepatic, hepatic, and posthepatic. Specifically, hepatic causes of PHT are further subdivided into pre-sinusoidal, sinusoidal, and post-sinusoidal. Post-hepatitic cirrhosis-induced PHT is typically sinusoidal or post-sinusoidal, while schistosomal liver disease-induced PHT is typically pre-sinusoidal. Methods for measuring portal venous pressure (PVP) include hepatic venous pressure gradient (HVPG) measurement and wedged hepatic venous pressure (WHVP). The former is easier to measure and thus widely used. Generally, an HVPG >10 mmHg (1 mmHg = 0.133 kPa) defines PHT, and the mean PVP is 11.9 mmHg in liver cancer patients undergoing surgery. Considering that the HVPG measurement requires an invasive examination, some scholars advocate using a non-invasive approach (i.e., the presence of esophageal varices or splenomegaly with thrombocytopenia) to diagnose clinically significant portal hypertension (CSPHT). The study found that liver cancer patients with an HVPG of >10 mmHg have a higher risk of postoperative hepatic dysfunction and poorer long-term survival outcomes. Therefore, the ALPPS procedure is not recommended for these patients.

4.5 Three-Dimensional Visualization

Three-dimensional visualization allows for three-dimensional visualization and reconstruction of the liver, providing not only a comprehensive display of the tumor location, size, morphology, and quantity but also vivid and intuitive representations of the main trunks and branches for portal vein, hepatic vein, hepatic artery, and bile duct, with accurate representations extending to tertiary branches. The 3D visualization is more intuitive than two-dimensional images, offering a more vivid and clearer representation of the three-dimensional spatial relationships between lesions and their surrounding tissues. Furthermore, this aids in significantly broadening surgeons' three-dimensional spatial perspective and effectively conducting accurate preoperative evaluations of tumor resectability, thereby minimizing the risks of intraoperative injuries to vasculature or excessive resection.

Thanks to continuous efforts and advancements made by surgeons, the safety of ALPPS procedures has been substantially improved. As with other novel surgical techniques, ALPPS suffers limitations associated with the learning curve. Initially, the morbidity and mortality of ALPPS typically remained high. With the ongoing development and refinement of the technique coupled with accumulating experience, the safety of ALPPS will be further enhanced. A recent analysis from the ALPPS registry exhibited that the incidence of major complications would decrease considerably in centers that have completed 9 successful cases [40]. Based on this, it is currently recommended that the ALPPS procedure be conducted in hepatobiliary centers with extensive liver surgery experience and strict adherence to ALPPS indications during the initial.

References

1. Hong JC, Kim J, Browning M, et al. Modified associating liver partition and portal vein ligation for staged hepatectomy for hepatoblastoma in a small infant: how far can we push the envelope? Ann Surg. 2017;266(2):e16–7.
2. Lang H, Baumgart J, Mittler J. Associating liver partition and portal vein ligation for staged hepatectomy in the treatment of colorectal liver metastases: current scenario. Dig Surg. 2018;35(4):294–302.
3. Schnitzbauer AA, Schadde E, Linecker M, et al. Indicating ALPPS for colorectal liver metastases: a critical analysis of patients in the international ALPPS registry. Surgery. 2018;164(3):387–94.
4. Schadde E, Ardiles V, Robles-Campos R, et al. Early survival and safety of ALPPS: first report of the international ALPPS registry. Ann Surg. 2014;260(5):829–36. discussion 836–838
5. Wanis KN, Ardiles V, Alvarez FA, et al. Intermediate-term survival and quality of life outcomes in patients with advanced colorectal liver metastases undergoing associating liver partition and portal vein ligation for staged hepatectomy. Surgery. 2018;163(4):691–7.
6. Hasselgren K, Malagò M, Vyas S, et al. Neoadjuvant chemotherapy does not affect future liver remnant growth and outcomes of associating liver partition and portal vein ligation for staged hepatectomy. Surgery. 2017;161(5):1255–65.
7. Olthof PB, Huiskens J, Wicherts DA, et al. Survival after associating liver partition and portal vein ligation for staged hepatectomy (ALPPS) for advanced colorectal liver metastases: a case-matched comparison with palliative systemic therapy. Surgery. 2017;161(4):909–19.
8. Adam R, Imai K, Castro Benitez C, et al. Outcome after associating liver partition and portal vein ligation for staged hepatectomy and conventional two-stage hepatectomy for colorectal liver metastases. Br J Surg. 2016;103(11):1521–9.
9. Ratti F, Schadde E, Masetti M, ct al. Strategies to increase the resectability of patients with colorectal liver metastases: a multi-center case-match analysis of ALPPS and conventional two-stage hepatectomy. Ann Surg Oncol. 2015;22(6):1933–42.
10. Kambakamba P, Linecker M, Alvarez FA, et al. Short chemotherapy-free interval improves oncological outcome in patients undergoing two-stage hepatectomy for colorectal liver metastases. Ann Surg Oncol. 2016;23(12):3915–23.
11. Baumgart J, Jungmann F, Bartsch F, et al. Two-stage hepatectomy and ALPPS for advanced bilateral liver metastases: a tailored approach balancing risk and outcome. J Gastrointest Surg. 2019;23(12):2391–400.
12. Robles-Campos R, Brusadin R, López-Conesa A, et al. Long-term outcome after conventional two-stage hepatectomy versus tourniquet-ALPPS in colorectal liver metastases: a propensity score matching analysis. World J Surg. 2019;43(9):2281–9.
13. Chan AC, Poon RT, Chan C, et al. Safety of ALPPS procedure by the anterior approach for hepatocellular carcinoma. Ann Surg. 2016;263(2):e14–6.
14. Vennarecci G, Grazi GL, Sperduti I, et al. ALPPS for primary and secondary liver tumors. Int J Surg. 2016;30:38–44.
15. Chan ACY, Chok K, Dai JWC, et al. Impact of split completeness on future liver remnant hypertrophy in associating liver partition and portal vein ligation for staged hepatectomy (ALPPS) in hepatocellular carcinoma: complete-ALPPS versus partial-ALPPS. Surgery. 2017;161(2):357–64.
16. Wang Z, Peng YF, Hu JW, et al. Associating liver partition and portal vein ligation for staged hepatectomy for unresectable hepatitis B virus-related hepatocellular carcinoma: a single center study of 45 patients. Ann Surg. 2020;271(3):534–41.

17. Vennarecci G, Ferraro D, Tudisco A, et al. The ALPPS procedure: hepatocellular carcinoma as a main indication. An Italian single-center experience. Updates Surg. 2019;71(1):67–75.
18. Olthof PB, Coelen RJS, Wiggers JK, et al. High mortality after ALPPS for perihilar cholangiocarcinoma: case-control analysis including the first series from the international ALPPS registry. HPB. 2017;19(5):381–7.
19. Schadde E, Raptis DA, Schnitzbauer AA, et al. Prediction of mortality after ALPPS stage-1: an analysis of 320 patients from the international ALPPS registry. Ann Surg. 2015;262(5):780–6.
20. Oldhafer KJ, Stavrou GA, van Gulik TM, et al. ALPPS—where do we stand, where do we go? : Eight recommendations from the first international expert meeting. Ann Surg. 2016;263(5):839–41.
21. Sakamoto Y, Matsumura M, Yamashita S, et al. Partial TIPE ALPPS for perihilar cancer. Ann Surg. 2018;267(2):e18–20.
22. Balci D. Pushing the envelope in perihiler cholangiocellularcarcinoma surgery: TIPE-ALPPS. Ann Surg. 2018;267(2):e21–2.
23. Oldhafer F, Ringe KI, Timrott K, et al. Intraoperative conversion to ALPPS in a case of intrahepatic cholangiocarcinoma. Case Rep Surg. 2015;2015:273641.
24. Ulmer TF, Jong CD, Andert A, et al. ALPPS procedure in insufficient hypertrophy after portal vein embolization (PVE). World J Surg. 2017;41(1):250–7.
25. Enne M, Schadde E, Björnsson B, et al. ALPPS as a salvage procedure after insufficient future liver remnant hypertrophy following portal vein occlusion. HPB. 2017;19(12):1126–9.
26. Urata K, Kawasaki S, Matsunami H, et al. Calculation of child and adult standard liver volume for liver transplantation. Hepatology. 1995;21(5):1317–21.
27. Kambakamba P, Stocker D, Reiner CS, et al. Liver kinetic growth rate predicts postoperative liver failure after ALPPS. HPB. 2016;18(10):800–5.
28. Lee DH, Lee JM, Yi NJ, et al. Hepatic stiffness measurement by using MR elastography: prognostic values after hepatic resection for hepatocellular carcinoma. Eur Radiol. 2017;27(4):1713–21.
29. Shen YH, Zhou CH, Zhu GD, et al. Liver stiffness assessed by shear wave elastography predicts postoperative liver failure in patients with hepatocellular carcinoma. J Gastrointest Surg. 2017;21(9):1471–9.
30. Zheng YC, Yang HY, He L, et al. Reassessment of different criteria for diagnosing post-hepatectomy liver failure: a single-center study of 1683 hepatectomy. Oncotarget. 2017;8(51):89269–77.
31. Cucchetti A, Ercolani G, Vivarelli M, et al. Impact of model for end-stage liver disease (MELD) score on prognosis after hepatectomy for hepatocellular carcinoma on cirrhosis. Liver Transpl. 2006;12(6):966–71.
32. Popescu GA, Alexandrescu ST, Grigorie RT, et al. GOOD TO KNOW: the ALPPS procedure—embracing a new technique. Chirurgia. 2017;112(3):332–41.
33. Lau H, Man K, Fan ST, et al. Evaluation of preoperative hepatic function in patients with hepatocellular carcinoma undergoing hepatectomy. Br J Surg. 1997;84(9):1255–9.
34. Van Thiel DH, Wright HI, Fagiuoli S, et al. Preoperative evaluation of a patient for hepatic surgery. J Surg Oncol Suppl. 1993;3:49–51.
35. Dong JH, Zheng SS, Chen XP, et al. Consensus on evaluation of Hepatic functional reserve before hepatectomy (2011 edition). Chin J Dig Surg. 2011;10:20–5.
36. Tomassini F, D'Asseler Y, Giglio MC, et al. Hemodynamic changes in ALPPS influence liver regeneration and function: results from a prospective study. HPB (Oxford). 2019;21(5):557–65.
37. de Graaf W, van Lienden KP, Dinant S, et al. Assessment of future remnant liver function using hepatobiliary scintigraphy in patients undergoing major liver resection. J Gastrointest Surg. 2010;14(2):369–78.
38. Motosugi U, Ichikawa T, Sou H, et al. Liver parenchymal enhancement of hepatocyte-phase images in Gd-EOB-DTPA-enhanced MR imaging: which biological markers of the liver function affect the enhancement? J Magn Reson Imaging. 2009;30(5):1042–6.
39. Sun HC, Shen YH, Li XL. Hepatic reserve function and selection of surgical procedures of hepatectomy. Chin J Practical Sur. 2018;38(4):473–6.
40. Li J, Ewald F, Kantas A, et al. Learning curve effect in ALPPS—a retrospect analysis of four years' experience. HPB. 2016;18(2):e735.

Variants of ALPPS and Terminology

5

Yuanfei Peng

In 2007, Professor Hans J. Schlitt created associating liver partition and portal vein ligation for staged hepatectomy. In 2012, Professors de Santibañes E and Pierre-Alain Clavien officially named the procedure ALPPS [1–3]. Since then, it has received widespread attention and rapidly popularized in practices [4–14]. It enables fast induction of future liver remnant (FLR) hypertrophy and a very high resection rate, giving many patients who were initially unresectable the opportunity of radical tumor resection. The principle of ALPPS is to separate the tumor-bearing part of the liver and the FLR by ligating or embolizing portal vein branches in the former and partitioning liver parenchyma, inducing FLR hypertrophy. The second stage of surgery (tumor resection) may proceed when adequate FLR growth is achieved. In the early years, classical ALPPS meant right trisectionectomy ALPPS or extended right hemihepatectomy ALPPS. In the first stage, parenchymal separation and ligation of the right portal vein are performed; Glisson branches of segment IV are completely or partially divided simultaneously; the tumor is removed in the second stage [15, 16]. Classical ALPPS induced FLR hypertrophy effectively, with a high resection rate. Nonetheless, it is relatively invasive, producing high complication and mortality rates. At the dawn of its development, the incidences of perioperative complication and 90-day mortality were as high as 68% and 12%, respectively. Its safety attracted concerns and evoked great controversy [3]. Since then, to reduce the complication and mortality rates and improve its safety, many scholars have made various improvements and derived a variety of ALPPS modifications, including Partial ALPPS, where only part of the liver parenchyma is separated in the first stage, Radiofrequency-assisted ALPPS (RALPPS), associating microwave ablation and portal vein ligation for staged hepatectomy (AMAPS) and tourniquet ALPPS (sometimes called ALTPS: associating liver tourniquet and portal ligation for staged hepatectomy where the liver partition is replaced by radiofrequency/microwave ablation or tourniquet separation, and operations performed using minimally invasive techniques (laparoscopy and robotics) [4, 16–36]. With accumulated cases, it is demonstrated that partial liver partition and separation by RFA, MWA, or tourniquet in the first stage can achieve an FLR induction similar to the classical ALPPS for patients without severe chronic liver diseases. The definition of ALPPS has also transitioned from classical liver partition to liver separation with more flexible applications, namely, the number of tumors, site of FLR, and the number of residual liver segments are no longer limited. Reversal ALPPS, mesohepatectomy ALPPS, and monosegment ALPPS drive the advancement, re-interpreting ALPPS's surgical principles while exemplifying its core components. The required site of FLR is no longer limited to the left lateral lobe or the left liver, any lobe, any segment, or even any area with independent and complete vascular structure and function, can be singled out as the FLR for hypertrophy induction [21, 37, 38]. Its indications are thus expanded prominently. These modified procedures also validate the rationale and the two core elements of ALPPS from one side of the spectrum: separation of the tumor side and FLR as well as portal vein occlusion of the tumor-side. Thanks to the unremitting exploration and joint efforts of hepatobiliary surgeons worldwide, and their continuous innovation, summary, and improvement of ALPPS, the current understanding of its surgical principles is well-established, with new procedures and flexible approaches emerging. According to the 10-year analysis by the ALPPS International Registry, the number of modified ALPPS has increased, accounting for half of all ALPPS cases [15].

However, the rapid development and popularization of ALPPS and the emergence of ALPPS variants [39] have produced many new terms, which leads to confusion and difficulties in comparing application experiences. Since many improved techniques, especially those that occur in the later period, are mostly combined modifications (integrating

Y. Peng (✉)
Zhongshan Hospital, Fudan University, Shanghai, China
e-mail: pengyuanfei@126.com

J. Zhou (ed.), *Associating Liver Partition and Portal Vein Ligation for Staged Hepatectomy (ALPPS)*,
https://doi.org/10.1007/978-981-96-7364-3_5

improvements, including access, type of parenchymal separation, and portal vein occlusion, such as mini-ALPPS), it is not easy to comprehend the essence via their abbreviated names. The consistency and clarification of ALPPS-related terms are essential to ensure exchanges and reporting. The first expert meeting held in Hamburg, Germany, in February 2015 concluded that a general surgical naming system is necessary to enable thorough comparisons and booming development of ALPPS. To this end, in 2015, the ALPPS International Registry reviewed the existing literature on ALPPS at the time, integrating studies of more than 600 ALPPS cases in 209 registered centers, and proposed a logical naming system. The system classified the then-known ALPPS procedures, putting the attributives in front of the subject ALPPS in the following order: strategy, surgical stage, access, portal vein embolization (if applicable), type of parenchymal separation, and name of hepatectomy. This naming system for ALPPS variants was subsequently submitted to each registered central for review and approval until a consensus was reached [7].

Significant progress has been made since the establishment of this naming system, yielding novel modifications. Based on all ALPPS surgeries reported as of now, this book proposes a unified naming system for better exchanges.

First, the definition and naming of ALPPS. The ALPPS was originally the first letter abbreviation of Association Liver Partition and Portal vein ligation for Staged Hepatectomy [3, 40]. In the original and classical ALPPS, parenchyma between the tumor side and the FLR is completely transected, and the portal vein is ligated. In the ensuing modifications, the complete partition has been replaced by partial partition, RFA/MWA separation, or tourniquet separation. In contrast, portal vein ligation (PVL) is sometimes replaced by portal vein embolization (PVE). The principle and connotation of ALPPS expand accordingly, rendering the original definition insufficient to cover the modifications. Therefore, the original "liver partition" is changed to "liver separation" and "portal vein ligation" to "portal vein occlusion"; the ALPPS now means "associating liver separation and portal vein occlusion for staged hepatectomy."

These modified ALPPS procedures change in several aspects compared with the classical ALPPS, which also constitute the basic variable/field of the naming system, including Access (minimally invasive/anterior approach and other alternatives instead of classical open laparotomy); type of parenchymal separation (partial partition, tourniquet separation, RFA/MWA separation alternative to complete partition); type of portal vein occlusion (PVE instead of PVL); tumor site and liver resection range (right hemihepectomy, extended right hemihepectomy, mesohepatectomy, left trisectionectomy in addition to the original right trisectionectomy); FLR and a number of the liver segment (right posterior lobe, dual lobes one from left and the other from right, monosegment alternative to the left lateral lobe); and some of the few other unique ALPPS variants (such as rescue ALPPS). Except for a small number of special modifications that require particular names, most variants can be named by integrating the variables/fields mentioned above in a standardized manner to make them clear at a glance, promoting communications.

To facilitate the comparison of ALPPS procedures with different modifications, experience sharing, and further advancement, a simple and easy-to-understand terminology naming system is developed for ALPPS variants. It must be pointed out that this is an open naming system, aiming to better communicate and promote the development of ALPPS. New surgical modifications need to be updated in a timely manner. In case of major innovations in surgical techniques, the naming rules can be revised accordingly. Different from the requirements of the International ALPPS naming system, which no longer adds new abbreviations consisting of first letters or novel words, we do not oppose or even encourage the establishment of new names for de novo ALPPS variants by their inventors. First, such inventions represent their excellent work and should be named after them. Second, names that come from many scholars are often simple, vivid, and easy to understand and memorize (just as Piggyback in liver transplantation). However, we also recommend that the authors' remarks on the new names be based on the naming rules so that readers can easily understand the changes in the novel modification. For the existing abbreviated names, we recommend respecting the outstanding contributions of their respective inventors and retaining their original names. Usually, concise and catchy surgical names are still widely used in clinical practices, and are even more popular in subspecialties. We suggest reserving these names accompanied with remarks during the application, that is, the original name of the ALPPS variant by inventor + standardized name according to naming rules. For example, mini-ALPPS (anterior approach + partial partition + PVE + right trisectionectomy ALPPS). Regarding variable/field arrangement, the order of our naming system is consistent with the international one. In front of the subject ALPPS, the following variables are placed: stage, access, PVE (an alternative of PVL, if applicable), types of separation, and type of hepatectomy [7]. Brisbane terminology of liver anatomy and surgical classification [41] is the basis of hepatectomy naming to ensure smooth international communication and better development of ALPPS.

5.1 Access

Major access modifications include the anterior and minimally invasive approaches. The access of PVO, when PVE is performed, varies, including the classical percutaneous transhepatic PVE, transileocecal PVE, and transmesenteric

PVE. The anterior approach was proposed by Professor Albert Chan from the University of Hong Kong. Minimally invasive approaches include laparoscopic ALPPS, robotic ALPPS, and hand-assisted ALPPS [24, 42–44]. In the case of large tumors and/or complicated patients, the minimally invasive approach is more often used for stage-1 surgery rather than for both stages. We recommend adding the operation stage (i.e., stage-1 and/or 2) during naming to distinguish. For example, an ALPPS with laparoscopic stage-1 operation and laparotomic stage-2 surgery is named "stage-1 laparoscopic ALPPS," whereas a whole-course laparoscopic ALPPS is named "total laparoscopic ALPPS." The simple name of robotic ALPPS, which was often used in the past referring to robotic-assisted surgeries applying robotic systems including the Da Vinci platform, cannot fully reflect the leading role of the surgeon, and is prone to misunderstanding by patients as operations done by robotics without human intervention, causing unnecessary misapprehension. Currently, it is uniformly named as robotic-assisted ALPPS. Per stages of ALPPS, their names are as follows: an ALPPS with robotic-assisted stage 1 and laparotomic stage 2 is named "stage 1 robotic-assisted ALPPS," whereas a whole-course robotic-assisted ALPPS is named "total robotic-assisted ALPPS."

5.2 Type of Parenchymal Separation

Types of parenchymal separation include the classical procedure with a complete partition (complete/total ALPPS), the partial ALPPS (p-ALPPS), radiofrequency-assisted ALPPS (RALPPS), microwave-assisted ALPPS (MALPPS), and tourniquet ALPPS [20, 23, 25, 26, 30, 35]. Partial partition is relative to complete partition in classical ALPPS. For cases with no chronic liver disease, 50–80% needs to be separated. A proportion lower than this often leads to insufficient FLR hypertrophy. The degree of partial partition varies depending on intra-operative evaluation by the surgeon. During the stage-1 operation, it often lacks effective evaluation and quantitative methods. Quantitative assessment should be explained in detail in the reports. The technique used in the author's center is as follows: 3D reconstruction and virtual resection before surgery are performed to calculate the transection surface and expected ratio of liver partition. During the stage-1 ALPPS, the parenchyma is transected according to preoperative planning. Finally, after removing the tumor side and full exposure of the transection surface during stage-2 operation, the ratio of partition area is recalculated and determined. If quantification is difficult in the real-world setting, partition to exposure of the middle hepatic vein is another option. RALPPS and MALPPS can be done percutaneously or transabdominal, which differ significantly. RALPPS or MALPPS combined with percutaneous transhepatic PVE can avoid transabdominal procedures in the first stage, minimizing the invasiveness of ALPPS operation. In our current naming system, we recommend modifying it as percutaneous RALPPS and percutaneous MALPPS. Names without the prefix of percutaneous are considered operations done transabdominally (laparotomy or laparoscopy).

5.3 Type of Portal Vein Occlusion (PVO)

PVO includes PVL used in the classical ALPPS, and PVE instead of PVL. All ALPPS cases that use PVE during the first stage are called PVE-ALPPS to distinguish them from conventional ALPPS. ALPPS without the prefix PVE refers to ALPPS procedures using PVL by default. PVE, replacing PVL, is often integrated with other modifications to form a variety of ALPPS variants, including hybrid ALPPS, mini-ALPPS, ALTPS, pre-ALPPS PVE, and sequential ALTPS [45–49]. The timing of PVE differs, concurrently during operation or separately after surgery. There are many PVE implementation methods. The default is the contralateral or ipsilateral portal vein embolization via percutaneous transhepatic puncture guided by ultrasound or CT. When the PVE is applied during stage 1 operation, in addition to the ultrasound-guided liver puncture, the portal vein can be punctured and embolized via transileocecal portal vein (transileocecal portal vein embolization, TIPE) or transmesenteric portal vein (transmesenteric portal vein embolization, TMPE) [47, 48, 50]. There are remarkable differences in these techniques. According to the international naming system, all ALPPS cases applying PVE in the first stage are called PVE-ALPPS. We recommend a more specific and refined way, adding timing and implementation methods for differentiation. Concurrent PVE (parenchymal separation and PVE intraoperatively), concurrent TIPE (parenchymal separation and TIPE intraoperatively), and concurrent TMPE (parenchymal separation and TMPE intraoperatively) correspond to hybrid ALPPS and TIPE-ALPPS in the original reports. Staged PVE-ALPPS (PVE performed several days after parenchymal separation, usually 1–3 days postoperatively) correspond to mini-ALPPS in the original publications. The specific timing of PVE (how many days after surgery) and other information should be detailed in reports.

5.4 Type and Range of Hepatectomy

ALPPS was initially applied for right trisectionectomy [2]. Afterward, the type and range of hepatectomy are expanded. At present, there are no particular restrictions on tumor site, resection range, FLR site, and liver separation plane, enabling flexible applications [51]. The range of liver resection includes right/left trisectionectomy ALPPS, extended right/left hepatectomy ALPPS, right/left hemihepatectomy ALPPS, and mesohepatectomy ALPPS

Table 5.1 Naming rules of ALPPS variants

Sequence of variables	Example
Stage of ALPPS	Stage 1
Access	Laparoscopic
Type of parenchymal separation	Partial partition
Type of PVO	Concurrent TIPE
Type and range of hepatectomy	Right trisectionectomy

[23, 37, 38, 52, 53]. The naming of hepatectomy follows the rules in Brisbane classification, Terminology of hepatic anatomy and liver resection, hemorrhage control methods, and selection principles (2nd edition) [21, 41]. Monosegment ALPPS, resection of 2 separate segments and 2 + X segment ALPPS are special variants [54, 55]. Multiple combinations of resected segments render the naming lengthy and complicated. Thus, it is named by the FLR segment (*segment X ALPPS*). For example, for monosegment ALPPS preserving only segment IV, it is called the segment IV ALPPS. When adjacent segments are preserved, for instance, segment IV + left caudal lobe, segment IV + Ia is the name. Concerning procedures preserving two discontinuous separate segments, segment X1 + segment X2 ALPPS is the name.

The finalized names for ALPPS variants arrange variables in the following order: stage of ALPPS + access + type of parenchymal separation + type of PVO + type and range of hepatectomy. This nomenclature puts the type of parenchymal separation in front of the type of PVO, which is consistent with the definition of ALPPS (associating liver separation and portal vein occlusion).

For example, a 41-year-old male patient with right intrahepatic cholangiocarcinoma (ICC) involving the right bile duct and segment IV. The first stage was carried out using laparoscopic partial parenchymal partition and concurrent TMPE. One week later, an open right trisectionectomy was performed. According to the naming rules, it was named "stage-1 laparoscopic partial partition—concurrent TMPE—right trisectionectomy ALPPS" (Table 5.1).

5.5 Special ALPPS Names

5.5.1 Rescue ALPPS

It refers to ALPPS performed to rescue failed traditional PVE-TSH, that is, apply parenchymal separation +/− PVL in cases with FLR induction failure after PVE or PVL alone. The names that have been reported are rescue ALPPS and salvage ALPPS, and now we unified the name as the former. The most common bailout is ALPPS after PVE failure. The rescue ALPPS has been widely applied and validated, showing a high success rate. Currently, rescue ALPPS has become the first choice of remedy after failed PVE. Another common scenario is a conventional staged hepatectomy for patients with colorectal liver metastasis (CRLM) during primary lesion resection. During the first stage of operation, PVL of portal branches in the affected part alone is performed (without parenchymal separation), which means that ALPPS is not jointly implemented. When PVL does not induce sufficient FLR growth, parenchymal separation proceeds to rescue FLR hypertrophy. Since the nomenclature system does not apply to this procedure, rescue ALPPS is singled out in this book, specifically referring to rescue ALPPS after PVE/PVL failure.

5.5.2 TAE-Salvaged ALPPS (Zhou's ALPPS)

This ALPPS variant was founded by Professor Jian Zhou in 2017 for patients with cirrhosis or severe liver fibrosis patients [56]. Chronic liver disease has a negative impact on FLR hypertrophy, and the degree of FLR growth was negatively correlated with the severity of liver fibrosis. Patients with cirrhosis or severe fibrosis are prone to insufficient FLR growth after stage-1 ALPPS, leading to FLR induction failure or tumor progression due to a prolonged interstage interval. In case of insufficient FLR growth 2 weeks after stage-1 ALPPS, transarterial embolization (TAE) of tumor supplying arteries is performed to reactivate fast growth of FLR, salvaging ALPPS on the brink of failure. The procedure was named TAE-salvaged ALPPS (Zhou's ALPPS). Since the nomenclature system does not apply to this procedure, we keep the original name in this book: TAE-salvaged ALPPS (Zhou's ALPPS).

References

1. Baumgart J, Lang S, Lang H. A new method for induction of liver hypertrophy prior to right trisectionectomy: a report of three cases [J]. HPB (Oxford). 2011;13(Suppl 2):71–2.
2. Schlitt HJ, Hackl C, Lang SA. "In-situ split" liver resection/ALPPS—historical development and current practice [J]. Visc Med. 2017;33(6):408–12.
3. Schnitzbauer AA, Lang SA, Goessmann H, et al. Right portal vein ligation combined with *in situ* splitting induces rapid left lateral liver lobe hypertrophy enabling 2-staged extended right hepatic resection in small-for-size settings [J]. Ann Surg. 2012;255(3):405–14.
4. D'Haese JG, Neumann J, Weniger M, et al. Should ALPPS be used for liver resection in intermediate-stage HCC? [J]. Ann Surg Oncol. 2016;23(4):1335–43.
5. Enne M, Schadde E, Björnsson B, et al. ALPPS as a salvage procedure after insufficient future liver remnant hypertrophy following portal vein occlusion [J]. HPB. 2017;19(12):1126–9.
6. Eshmuminov D, Raptis DA, Linecker M, et al. Meta-analysis of associating liver partition with portal vein ligation and portal vein occlusion for two-stage hepatectomy [J]. Br J Surg. 2016;103(13):1768–82.

7. Linecker M, Kron P, Lang H, et al. Too many languages in the ALPPS: preventing another tower of babel? [J]. Ann Surg. 2016;263(5):837–8.
8. Linecker M, Stavrou GA, Oldhafer KJ, et al. The ALPPS risk score: avoiding futile use of ALPPS [J]. Ann Surg. 2016;264(5):763–71.
9. Olthof PB, Coelen RJS, Wiggers JK, et al. High mortality after ALPPS for perihilar cholangiocarcinoma: case-control analysis including the first series from the international ALPPS registry [J]. HPB. 2017;19(5):381–7.
10. Olthof PB, Huiskens J, Wicherts DA, et al. Survival after associating liver partition and portal vein ligation for staged hepatectomy (ALPPS) for advanced colorectal liver metastases: a case-matched comparison with palliative systemic therapy [J]. Surgery. 2017;161(4):909–19.
11. Schadde E, Ardiles V, Robles-Campos R, et al. Early survival and safety of ALPPS: first report of the International ALPPS Registry [J]. Ann Surg. 2014;260(5):829–38.
12. Schadde E, Raptis DA, Schnitzbauer AA, et al. Prediction of mortality after ALPPS stage-1: an analysis of 320 patients from the international ALPPS registry [J]. Ann Surg. 2015;262(5):780–6.
13. Viganò L, Cimino MM, Adam R, et al. Improving the safety of ALPPS procedure: the optimal compromise between dropout and mortality risk. Comment on Schadde E, et al. *Prediction of mortality after ALPPS stage-1: an analysis of 320 patients from the International ALPPS Registry*. Ann Surg. 2015;262:780–6 [J]. Ann Surg. 2017;266(6):e101–2.
14. Wanis KN, Buac S, Linecker M, et al. Patient survival after simultaneous ALPPS and colorectal resection [J]. World J Surg. 2017;41(4):1119–25.
15. Zhou J, Wang Z, Sun J, et al. Associating liver partition and portal vien ligation for staged hepatectomy [J]. Chin J Dig Surg. 2013;12(7):485–9.
16. Popescu GA, Alexandrescu ST, Grigorie RT, et al. GOOD TO KNOW: the ALPPS procedure—embracing a new technique [J]. Chirurgia. 2017;112(3):332–41.
17. Vennarecci G, Levi Sandri GB, Ettorre GM. Performing the ALPPS procedure by anterior approach and liver hanging maneuver [J]. Ann Surg. 2016;263(1):e11.
18. Wang CC, Jawade K, Yap AQ, et al. Resection of large hepatocellular carcinoma using the combination of liver hanging maneuver and anterior approach [J]. World J Surg. 2010;34(8):1874–8.
19. Xiao L, Li JW, Zheng SG. Totally laparoscopic ALPPS in the treatment of cirrhotic hepatocellular carcinoma [J]. Surg Endosc. 2015;29(9):2800–1.
20. Cai XJ, Peng SY, Duan L, et al. Completely laparoscopic ALPPS using round-the-liver ligation to replace parenchymal transection for a patient with multiple right liver cancers complicated with liver cirrhosis [J]. J Laparoendosc Adv Surg Tech A. 2014;24(12):883–6.
21. Schadde E, Malagó M, Hernandez-Alejandro R, et al. Monosegment ALPPS hepatectomy: extending resectability by rapid hypertrophy [J]. Surgery. 2015;157(4):676–89.
22. Chen JX, Ran HQ, Sun CQ. Associating microwave ablation and portal vein ligation for staged hepatectomy for the treatment of huge hepatocellular carcinoma with cirrhosis [J]. Ann Surg Treat Res. 2016;90(5):287–91.
23. Petrowsky H, Györi G, de Oliveira M, et al. Is partial-ALPPS safer than ALPPS? A single-center experience [J]. Ann Surg. 2015;261(4):e90–2.
24. de Santibañes E, Alvarez FA, Ardiles V, et al. Inverting the ALPPS paradigm by minimizing first stage impact: the mini-ALPPS technique [J]. Langenbeck's Arch Surg. 2016;401(4):557–63.
25. Gall TMH, Sodergren MH, Frampton AE, et al. Radio-frequency-assisted liver partition with portal vein ligation (RALPP) for liver regeneration [J]. Ann Surg. 2015;261(2):e45–6.
26. Gringeri E, Boetto R, D'Amico FE, et al. Laparoscopic microwave ablation and portal vein ligation for staged hepatectomy (LAPS): a minimally invasive first-step approach [J]. Ann Surg. 2015;261(2):e42–3.
27. Hong DF, Zhang YB, Peng SY, et al. Percutaneous microwave ablation liver partition and portal vein embolization for rapid liver regeneration: a minimally invasive first step of ALPPS for hepatocellular carcinoma [J]. Ann Surg. 2016;264(1):e1–2.
28. Edmondson MJ, Sodergren MH, Pucher PH, et al. Variations and adaptations of associated liver partition and portal vein ligation for staged hepatectomy (ALPPS): many routes to the summit [J]. Surgery. 2016;159(4):1058–72.
29. Alvarez FA, Ardiles V, de Santibañes M, et al. Associating liver partition and portal vein ligation for staged hepatectomy offers high oncological feasibility with adequate patient safety: a prospective study at a single center [J]. Ann Surg. 2015;261(4):723–32.
30. Robles Campos R, Parrilla Paricio P, López Conesa A, et al. A new surgical technique for extended right hepatectomy: tourniquet in the umbilical fissure and right portal vein occlusion (ALTPS). Clinical case [J]. Cir Esp. 2013;91(10):633–7.
31. Vennarecci G, Grazi GL, Sperduti I, et al. ALPPS for primary and secondary liver tumors [J]. Int J Surg. 2016;30:38–44.
32. Alvarez FA, Ardiles V, Sanchez Claria R, et al. Associating liver partition and portal vein ligation for staged hepatectomy (ALPPS): tips and tricks [J]. J Gastrointest Surg. 2013;17(4):814–21.
33. Chan ACY, Chok K, Dai JWC, et al. Impact of split completeness on future liver remnant hypertrophy in associating liver partition and portal vein ligation for staged hepatectomy (ALPPS) in hepatocellular carcinoma: complete-ALPPS versus partial-ALPPS [J]. Surgery. 2017;161(2):357–64.
34. Sodergren MH, Lurje G, Edmondson M, et al. Bi-institutional case-matched comparison of short-term clinical outcomes of radiofrequency-assisted liver partition and portal vein ligation (RALPP) and associating liver partition and portal vein ligation for staged hepatectomy (ALPPS) [J]. HPB. 2016;18:e703–4.
35. Wang Q, Yan J, Feng XB, et al. Safety and efficacy of radiofrequency-assisted ALPPS (RALPPS) in patients with cirrhosis-related hepatocellular carcinoma [J]. Int J Hyperth. 2017;33(7):846–52.
36. Obed A, Jarrad A, Bashir A. First left hepatic trisectionectomy including segment one with new associated liver partition and portal vein ligation with staged hepatectomy (ALPPS) modification: how to do it? [J]. Am J Case Rep. 2016;17:759–65.
37. Machado MA, Surjan R, Basseres T, et al. Total laparoscopic reversal ALPPS [J]. Ann Surg Oncol. 2017;24(4):1048–9.
38. Oldhafer KJ, Stavrou GA, van Gulik TM, et al. ALPPS—where do we stand, where do we go?: eight recommendations from the first international expert meeting [J]. Ann Surg. 2016;263(5):839–41.
39. de Santibañes E, Clavien PA. Playing Play-Doh to prevent postoperative liver failure: the "ALPPS" approach [J]. Ann Surg. 2012;255(3):415–7.
40. Strasberg SM, Belghiti J, Clavien PA, et al. The Brisbane 2000 terminology of liver anatomy and resections [J]. HPB. 2000;2(3):333–9.
41. Chan AC, Pang R, Poon RT. Simplifying the ALPPS procedure by the anterior approach [J]. Ann Surg. 2014;260(2):e3.
42. Machado MA, Makdissi FF, Surjan RC. Totally laparoscopic ALPPS is feasible and may be worthwhile [J]. Ann Surg. 2012;256(3):e13; author reply e16–e19.
43. Michal K, Sau M, Tamara GMH, et al. A better route to ALPPS: minimally invasive vs open ALPPS [J]. Surg Endosc. 2020;34(6):2379–89.
44. Solomonov E, Tzadok I, Stemmer S, et al. Case report: robotic ALPPS procedure for hepatocellular carcinoma in the right lobe of the liver [J]. Front Surg. 2021;8:655683.

45. Li J, Kantas A, Ittrich H, et al. Avoid "all-touch" by hybrid ALPPS to achieve oncological efficacy [J]. Ann Surg. 2016;263(1):e6–7.
46. Balci D. Pushing the envelope in perihiler cholangiocellularcarcinoma surgery: TIPE-ALPPS [J]. Ann Surg. 2018;267(2):e21–2.
47. Pekolj J, Alvarez FA, Biagiola D, et al. Totally laparoscopic mini-ALPPS using a novel approach of laparoscopic-assisted transmesenteric portal vein embolization [J]. J Laparoendosc Adv Surg Tech A. 2018;28(10):1229–33.
48. Sakamoto Y, Inagaki F, Omichi K, et al. Associating liver partial partition and transileocecal portal vein embolization for staged hepatectomy [J]. Ann Surg. 2016;264(6):e21–2.
49. Sakamoto Y, Matsumura M, Yamashita S, et al. Partial TIPE ALPPS for perihilar cancer [J]. Ann Surg. 2018;267(2):e18–20.
50. Lang H, de Santibañes E, Schlitt HJ, et al. 10th anniversary of ALPPS-lessons learned and quo vadis [J]. Ann Surg. 2019;269(1):114–9.
51. Tsui TY, Heumann A, Vashist YK, et al. How we do it: double *in situ* split for staged mesohepatectomy in patients with advanced gall bladder cancer and marginal future liver remnant [J]. Langenbeck's Arch Surg. 2016;401(4):565–71.
52. Gauzolino R, Castagnet M, Blanleuil ML, et al. The ALPPS technique for bilateral colorectal metastases: three "variations on a theme" [J]. Updat Surg. 2013;65(2):141–8.
53. Hepatic Surgery Group, Surgery Branch of Chinese Medical Association. Liver anatomy and nomenclature of liver resection surgery, as well as methods and selection principles for controlling bleeding during hepatectomy (1st revision in 2017, 2nd edition) [J]. J Abdom Surg. 2017;30(2):75–8.
54. Pineda-Solís K, Paskar D, Tun-Abraham M, et al. Expanding the limits of resectability: associating liver partition and portal vein ligation for staged hepatectomy (ALPPS) using monosegment 6, facilitated by an inferior right hepatic vein [J]. J Surg Oncol. 2017;115(8):959–62.
55. Wang Z, Peng YF, Sun QM, et al. Salvage transhepatic arterial embolization after failed stage I ALPPS in a patient with a huge HCC with chronic liver disease: a case report [J]. Int J Surg Case Rep. 2017;39:131–5.
56. Peng YF, Wang Z, Qu XD, et al. Transcatheter arterial embolization-salvaged ALPPS, a novel ALPPS procedure especially for patients with hepatocellular carcinoma and severe fibrosis/cirrhosis [J]. Hepatobiliary Surg Nutr. 2022;11(4):504–14.

Classical ALPPS

6

Yuanfei Peng

6.1 Introduction

Associating liver partition and portal vein ligation for staged hepatectomy (ALPPS) was founded in 2007 by Professor Han J. Schlitt from Germany [1]. The ALPPS procedure was originally called "right portal vein ligation combined with in situ splitting." In 2012, Professors Andreas A. Schnitzbauer and Hans J. Schlitt summarized the early experience results and reported in the *Annals of Surgery* [2]. Professor de Santibañes E and Professor Pierre-Alain Clavien officially named the novel procedure "associating liver partition and portal vein ligation for staged hepatectomy" and abbreviated it as ALPPS [3]. This technique was initially associated with high perioperative complications and 90-day mortality (68% and 12%), rendering its safety controversial [2]. Subsequently, the ALPPS procedure was improved to reduce the undesirable results and increase surgical safety, giving birth to "classical ALPPS" [4–6]. On this basis, many hepatobiliary surgeons have applied various methods, making progress in multiple aspects, including surgical approach (minimally invasive/anterior approach), liver parenchymal separation methods (partial partition instead of complete separation, radiofrequency/microwave ablation and tourniquet separation instead of liver partition), and portal vein embolization (PVE) instead of PVL. These have further minimized the complication and mortality rates and optimized safety. Numerous modified ALPPS have been developed, including laparoscopic/robot-assisted ALPPS, partial ALPPS, radiofrequency ablation (RFA)/microwave ablation (MWA)-assisted ALPPS, tourniquet ALPPS, and hybrid ALPPS [4, 6, 7]. By 2015, the use of modified ALPPS procedures accounted for 52% of all ALPPS cases [6]. In addition, applications become more flexible regardless of tumor site, FLR location, and resection range. Right trisectionectomy in classical ALPPS is expanded to extended right/left hepatectomy, right/left hemihepatectomy, and mesohepatectomy [8–12]. The required number of liver segments is no longer limited to two, and single-segment ALPPS (monosegment ALPPS) has also been successfully performed [13, 14]. With the emergence of these modifications, "classical ALPPS" has become a relative concept. Meanwhile, it has been coupled with considerable improvements compared to the original procedure. Measures to ameliorate common postoperative complications (such as bile leakage) have been integrated and have become essential elements. For example, wrapping the liver with plastic bags and ligating the right bile duct have been abandoned, and strict bile leakage checks are routinely implemented. Tumor location and resection range are no longer limited to right trisectionectomy but expanded to extended right hemihepatectomy and right hemihepatectomy, and the right / extended right hemihepatectomy ALPPS have accounted for a more significant proportion in clinical practices.

Classical ALPPS contains the following elements:

6.1.1 Liver Partition: 80–100%

The liver parenchyma is separated between the tumor side and the future liver remnant (FLR) side by parenchymal partition. Cavitron ultrasonic surgical aspirator (CUSA) and/or ultrasonic dissector (such as Harmonic shear) are commonly used. The parenchyma should be completely divided to the anterior wall of the inferior vena cava (IVC) as much as possible to entirely separate the tumor side from the FLR. In cases where the tumor is adjacent to the IVC or the porta hepatis or for other reasons that render complete partition impossible in stage-1 ALPPS, at least 80% shall be partitioned. Procedures with a <80% liver partition are classified as partial ALPPS [11]. Complete partition enables the most substantial FLR induction effect and is of special significance in patients with chronic liver disease. It has been reported that partial parenchymal partition (Partial ALPPS)

Y. Peng (✉)
Zhongshan Hospital, Fudan University, Shanghai, China
e-mail: pengyuanfei@126.com

J. Zhou (ed.), *Associating Liver Partition and Portal Vein Ligation for Staged Hepatectomy (ALPPS)*,
https://doi.org/10.1007/978-981-96-7364-3_6

in patients with chronic hepatic conditions is likely to cause insufficient FLR hypertrophy, whereby a complete partition is required for this population [15]. A comparative study by Albert Chan et al. [15] showed that in hepatocellular carcinoma (HCC) patients with chronic liver disease, complete partition induced more FLR hypertrophy in a shorter time than partial partition (kinetic growth rate of FLR: 31.2 mL/d vs 17.5 mL/d) with a significantly higher success rate in facilitating FLR growth (76.9% vs 33.3%), higher stage 2 resection rate within two weeks (100% vs 58.4%), less complications (7.7% vs 25%), and lower mortality (0% vs 16.7%) [15].

6.1.2 Complete Ligation of the Tumor Side Portal Veins

All feeding portal veins on the tumor side need to be ligated, often using sutures for ligation or stitching. Hem-o-lok clips commonly applied in laparoscopic surgery can also be used to completely occlude the portal vein blood flow on the tumor side. This ligation of portal veins must be thorough and reliable, leaving no recanalization. The preoperative planning is essential. Three-dimensional (3D) reconstruction can clearly display the portal vein classification. The type of portal vein, number, and contour of the portal veins on the tumor side must be clarified before surgery. Portal veins with normal anatomy are easy to be managed. However, for patients with portal vein variations, especially Type III and IV of Cheng's classification [16] (corresponding to Type--C/D of Nakamura classification [17]), full intraoperative dissection and complete ligation with caution are required to prevent omission. Suppose portal vein branches are omitted on the tumor side. In that case, the incomplete ligation of the tumor side portal vein may lead to slow or failed FLR hypertrophy induction that demands additional PVE for salvage, increasing pain for the patient and causing difficulty in the operation. In case of any suspected residual portal vein blood supply to the tumor side during the first stage of surgery, liver CT angiography (CTA/CTV) shall be carried out shortly after the procedure in a timely manner, and PVE performed as necessary. If conducted in time, the salvage could still be successful.

6.1.3 Dissociation of Perihepatic Ligaments on the Tumor Side

Perihepatic ligaments on the tumor side should be completely or largely dissociated. This is one of the main differences between classical ALPPS (with ligament dissociation during stage-1 ALPPS) and ALPPS with an anterior approach (without ligament dissociation). They each possess pros and cons. The advantages of the former lie in that it helps liver transection surface exposure and parenchymal partition, facilitating hemostasis. In addition, after complete perihepatic ligament dissociation, the communication via blood and lymphatic vessels between the liver and its surrounding tissues is theoretically cut off, thus avoiding potential dissemination caused by tumor progression during the waiting period after the first stage surgery. On the other hand, disadvantages are adhesions caused by dissociated ligaments, which are often more severe in cases with longer interstage intervals. Additionally, huge tumors carry the risk of rupture and iatrogenic dissemination during mobilization of the liver. The interstage interval in ALPPS is usually short (1–2 weeks). Furthermore, with the advancement of techniques, the incidence of complications such as bile leakage and abdominal infection has been greatly reduced. With anti-adhesion materials and other measures, adhesion tends to impact stage 2 ALPPS operation less. There is no need to wrap the tumor side using a plastic bag after dissociating perihepatic ligaments, which was applied at the dawn of ALPPS and is currently phased out. This procedure often leads to complications, including abdominal effusion and infection. At the same time, when ALPPS fails due to insufficient FLR growth and other reasons after stage-1 ALPPS surgery, another operation is required to remove the plastic bag, which increases patients' pain.

6.1.4 Laparotomy

In a classical ALPPS, liver parenchyma partition and PVL are performed in an open manner, which is different from laparoscopic and robot-assisted ALPPS. Although the number of laparotomy has decreased in recent years with the advancement of minimally invasive technology and the emergence of improved percutaneous procedures, open surgery remains the backbone of the ALPPS family. Especially for complex and challenging cases and huge liver tumors, it plays an irreplaceable role.

Surgeries that meet the definition of ALPPS and cover the above-mentioned elements can be classified as classical ALPPS. However, it must be underscored again that classical ALPPS has become a relative concept, relative to its modifications, which are discussed in other chapters of this book (see each chapter for details).

In the ALPPS family, classical ALPPS is the mainstay with many indications, including complex cases. Its effectiveness has been well-validated with a high success rate, enabling an FLR induction of 58% to 160% or even 200% within 1 to 2 weeks after the first stage surgery and a tumor resection rate of 95% to 100% [18–22]. Although modified

ALPPS procedures emerge one after another and their applications are expanded, many of these modifications have limitations in indications. Classical ALPPS still cannot be completely replaced and remains the most important choice for ALPPS. For example, RFA/MWA ALPPS is challenging to perform when the tumor is close to the left branch of the portal vein or where related vessels are prone to injury. Tourniquet ALPPS is inappropriate when the tumor is closely adjacent to the IVC, where a tunnel before IVC cannot be established. ALPPS with partial partition for patients with liver fibrosis/cirrhosis may lead to insufficient FLR induction. Classical ALPPS and modified procedures are often compared and debated. These procedures, each possessing its pros, cons, and suitable indications, belong to the same arsenal and are not contradictory. Surgeons who perform ALPPS should be familiar with the advantages and disadvantages of each ALPPS procedure (classical ALPPS and its variants) and choose the most appropriate one on a case-by-case basis.

6.2 Indications

Indications of classical ALPPS: age < 67 years [23]; potentially resectable primary liver cancer or perihilar bile duct malignancy without extrahepatic metastasis; potentially resectable metastatic liver cancer with the primary tumor either already resected or can be radically resected concurrently, and no residual extrahepatic and FLR tumor is expected after surgery; insufficient FLR [FLR/SLV < 20%–30% in patients without chronic liver disease or liver damage, or FLR/SLV < 40% in those with chronic liver disease (liver fibrosis/cirrhosis), chemotherapy-related liver injury, cholestasis and severe steatosis]; cases with normal liver function or mild but reversible impairment [Child-Pugh class A, indocyanine green retention rate at 15 minute (ICG-R15) <15%]; patients in well performance status with normal functions in the heart, brain, lungs, kidneys, and other organs, capable of tolerating major operations without absolute contraindications for upper abdominal surgery (see Chap. 4 of this book for details).

Colorectal liver metastasis (CRLM) is the best and most widely applied indication for classical ALPPS. Postoperative complications and mortality have been reduced to levels comparable to those of extensive liver resection with promising mid-/long-term survival benefits [5, 24]. Compared with traditional PVE-based two-stage hepatectomy (PVE-TSH), it was associated with a higher resection rate and a shorter waiting time, becoming one of the options for CRLM and has been recommended as a treatment choice by some guidelines [25–30]. HCC is another major indication of classical ALPPS, especially in China. With the increasing application of partial ALPPS and other modifications in non-HCC liver tumors (such as CRLM) and the unique value of classical ALPPS in patients with chronic liver disease (see above for details), HCC has gradually become the essential indication for classical ALPPS. In recent years, the role of ALPPS for HCC has been elucidated with the accumulation of data. In highly selective patients, ALPPS enables optimal clinical outcomes. The overall safety profile has been significantly improved compared to early years, with satisfactory tumor resection and R0 resection rates. Mid-/long-term survival benefits are reassuring, far better than non-surgical treatments such as TACE, equivalent to the postoperative survival of those undergoing one-stage hepatectomy, and superior or non-inferior to PVE-TSH and TACE-PVE-TSH [31–36]. Nonetheless, the severity of underlying liver diseases and their potential impact must be carefully evaluated, and patients with severe liver cirrhosis should be treated with caution [31, 37]. Although biliary tract tumors were the initial indication for classical ALPPS, subsequent implementation results were poor, with high postoperative complication and mortality rates [5, 38, 39], leading to reduced application. Studies have showcased that classical ALPPS, when performed for biliary tumors, yielded high postoperative complication rates such as bile leakage. Thus, rigorous assessment and caution were needed [5, 39–42]; modified techniques may reduce complications and mortality to a certain extent and shall be applied as appropriate [42–49]. In addition to the type of tumor, the status of liver parenchyma is also a vital factor to be considered before classical ALPPS. Patients with liver malignancies are often afflicted by underlying liver disease or injuries (including viral hepatitis infection, liver fibrosis/cirrhosis, cholestasis, and chemotherapy +/− targeted therapy-induced liver injury), and the total number of actual functional hepatocytes is lower than that in a normal liver of the same volume. More importantly, these liver disease or liver injuries have a great impact on FLR hypertrophy. The degree of FLR growth induced by ALPPS is negatively correlated with the severity of liver fibrosis [31, 33, 37]. In patients without chronic liver diseases, many studies have confirmed that partial ALPPS can achieve a similar FLR induction to that of classical ALPPS while reducing complications and mortality, and has increasingly replaced the classical procedure [15]. Nevertheless, for those complicated by chronic liver disease, ALPPS with partial partition often induces insufficient FLR, whereas classical ALPPS can induce optimal hypertrophy. Simultaneously, studies have also demonstrated that the tumor resection rate, postoperative complication, and mortality rates of classical ALPPS were better than their partial partition counterparts. Hence, for patients with chronic liver diseases, regardless of liver tumor type (HCC, CRLM, or others), classical ALPPS is recommended [15]. For those with severe liver fibrosis and cirrhosis, more time is required to obtain sufficient FLR growth [37]. If the FLR growth remains insufficient two weeks after surgery, transarterial embolization-salvaged ALPPS (TAE-salvaged ALPPS) shall be proceeded [15, 50]. Those who have failed PVE-TSH are the absolute indication of classical ALPPS. The rescue ALPPS has a success rate between 92.3% and 100%, with comparable FLR induction efficacy, complications, and mortality rates as commonly performed ALPPS [25, 51–54]. Cases with tumor thrombus invading the main branch of the portal vein on the tumor side where PVE cannot be performed are also suitable for classical ALPPS (common in HCC). The most reported cases are those with types I-II of Cheng's classification. Applications in type III patients and even in cases where the thrombus has invaded the FLR portal vein were also presented in previous studies [55]. Nonetheless, when treating patients with tumor thrombus reaching or crossing the PVL site, ALPPS remains controversial (incisional thrombectomy may potentially cause intraperitoneal dissemination and rapid progression of distal thrombus). Another indication of classical ALPPS is cases where tumor progression or liver disease (such as severe steatosis) that are not detected preoperatively or other unexpected situations found during intraoperative exploration. If the FLR is estimated to be insufficient, ALPPS should be performed to prevent postoperative liver failure (as in the establishment process of ALPPS [1]). At present, classical ALPPS is mostly applied in adults and can also be used in children. There have been recent reports on ALPPS in pediatric patients. Due to prominent adult-child differences, prudent evaluation and procedures are required. More research is needed to this end [56].

6.3 Surgical Procedures

Classical ALPPS consists of two stages. In the first stage, the liver parenchyma is partitioned, and the right portal vein is ligated. The FLR volume is measured 5 to 7 days after stage-1 operation. If sufficient, the second stage is performed to remove the tumor (in case of insufficient FLR growth, the FLR volume is re-measured one week later; for most cases, an adequate FLR hypertrophy is achieved within 2 weeks). The schematic diagram of ALPPS is as follows (Fig. 6.1).

6.3.1 Body Position

The patient is usually in a supine position. If the transection plane is to the right, the patient can also be in a left lateral position of 30° to 45°.

6.3.2 Stage 1 ALPPS

6.3.2.1 Surgical Incision

The right subcostal incision is usually used (Fig. 6.2). In cases with huge tumors, or the porta hepatis has been involved and significantly pushed away, or when regional lymphadenectomy and biliary-enteric anastomosis are required simultaneously, a reverse "L"-shaped incision (also called "J"-shaped incision) may be used. The Benz incision is used less often.

6.3.2.2 Abdominal Exploration

The abdomen is entered layer by layer. After access, the abdominal cavity is exposed by placing a liver retractor. Full exploration is performed to exclude any extrahepatic lesions not detected by preoperative imaging and other surgical contraindications.

6.3.2.3 Mobilization of the Right Liver

The round ligament (ligament teres) and falciform ligament are divided. The root of the common trunk of the left/middle hepatic vein and the right hepatic vein are dissected, and the hepatic vein fossa is exposed and marked. The right triangular ligament, the right coronary ligament, and the hepatorenal ligament are divided. Then, the right liver is rotated to the left, the bare area and the right adrenal gland are dissociated, and the right IVC ligament and the short hepatic vein are divided. The right liver is fully mobilized.

6.3.2.4 Intraoperative Ultrasound (IOUS)

The liver is comprehensively examined using intraoperative ultrasound to confirm preoperatively diagnosed lesions and check for any other lesions, especially whether there are preoperatively undetected lesions in the FLR (Figs. 6.3 and 6.4). For CRLM, it is recommended to use Sonozoid for contrast-enhanced imaging examination to fully detect potential small

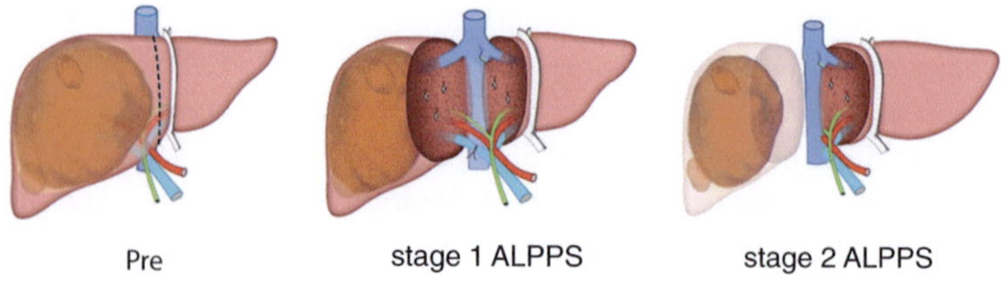

Fig. 6.1 Schematic diagram of classical ALPPS. (Note: these pictures were drawn by Yizhou He, Zhongshan Hospital, Fudan University)

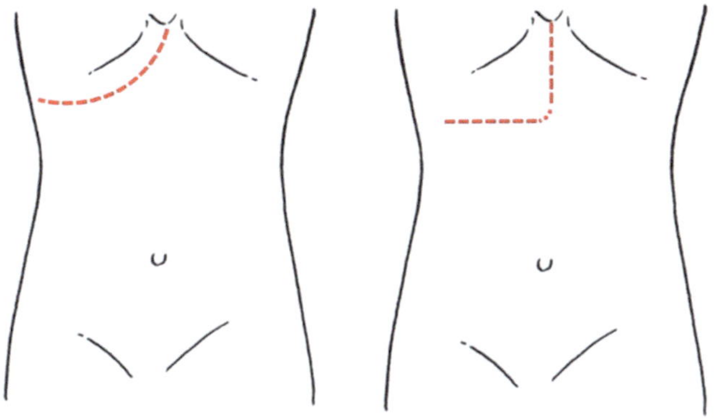

Fig. 6.2 Common incisions for classical ALPPS. Right subcostal incision or reverse "L" incision (also called "J" shaped incision)

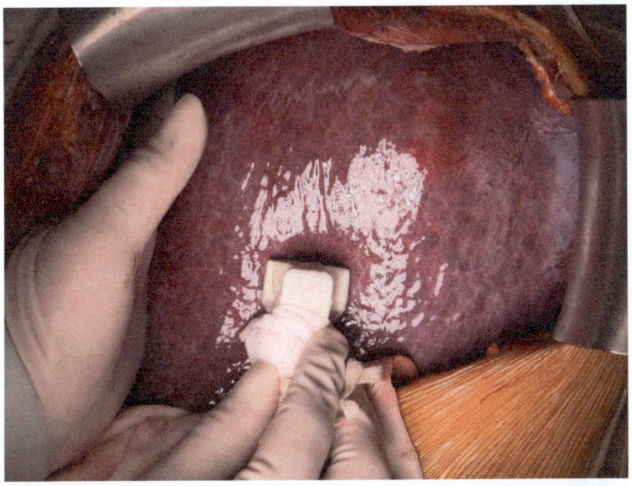

Fig. 6.3 Intraoperative ultrasound examination during stage 1 ALPPS

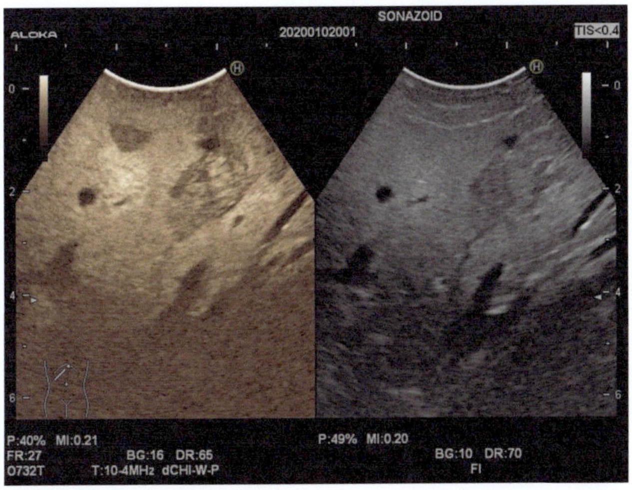

Fig. 6.4 Intraoperative ultrasonography examination of the tumor, FLR, major vessels, and their adjacent relationship (Sonozoid contrast agent was used to exclude potential lesions of the FLR)

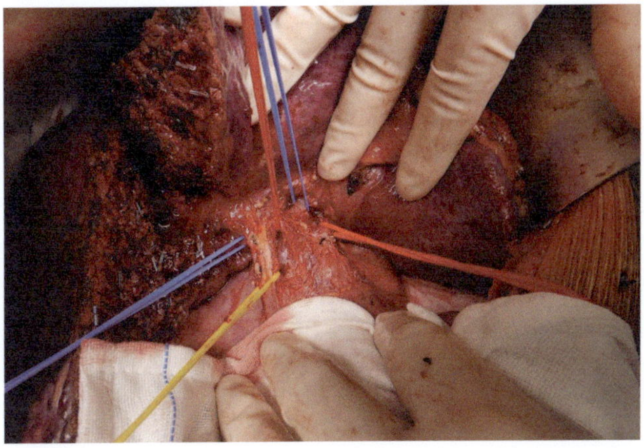

Fig. 6.5 Dissect the porta hepatis, isolate the proper hepatic artery and its left and right branches, the left and right branches of the portal vein and the common bile duct

metastases. The adjacent relationship among the tumor, FLR, and major vessels is explored and clarified. Combined with preoperative virtual surgical planning, the pre-cut line is delineated on the liver surface, and the parenchymal transection plane is determined.

6.3.2.5 Cholecystectomy

The Calot's triangle is dissected, the cystic duct and the cystic artery are exposed, ligated, and divided, and then the gallbladder is removed. If antegrade cholecystectomy is not feasible, the gallbladder can also be resected retrogradely. The cystic duct is divided close to the gallbladder side, and a certain length is reserved at the stump. After the parenchymal partition, a bile leakage check will be performed via the stump of the cyst duct by injecting a contrast agent or a color-developing agent such as fat emulsion. Anatomical variations in the bile duct are common. If bile duct variation is suspected before surgery but is not clearly shown by MRI or other examinations, contrast agents can also be injected through the cystic duct for cholangiography. ICG-based fluorescence can serve as another option. ICG can also be injected through the cystic duct to clarify the variations by fluorescence laparoscopy.

6.3.2.6 Dissection of the Porta Hepatis

The proper hepatic artery (PHA), the left (middle) and right hepatic arteries, the left and right branches of the portal vein, and the common bile duct are dissected and revealed. The right portal vein, the common bile duct, and the right hepatic artery are marked with blue, yellow, and red ribbons (Fig. 6.5). It is recommended to dissect the arteries first and then the portal vein. If the arteries are accidentally damaged, compromising arterial blood supply on the tumor side, the operation needs to be suspended in time if necessary. Liver failure can be avoided as portal vein blood flow is still preserved. If the portal vein is divided before arteries, arterial damage after PVL may lead to liver failure. This is because the auxiliary liver function of the tumor-side liver plays an important role during the waiting period for FLR growth. Studies have manifested that the tumor-side liver functioned well after PVL several days after stage-1 ALPPS and, in some cases, provided up to 60% of liver function even 6 days postoperatively [57, 58]. Recently, more attention has been oriented towards the auxiliary liver of the tumor side after stage 1 ALPPS, and it has been applied for the auxiliary liver transplantation such as the resection and partial liver segment 2/3 transplantation with delayed total hepatectomy (RAPID) procedure and other techniques [59–61]. When dissecting arteries, high-power energy equipment should be avoided as much as possible to prevent arterial damage. At the same time, it is necessary to compare the diameter of the left and right hepatic arteries. If the left hepatic artery is significantly thinner than the right hepatic artery, in cases of huge right liver tumors (HCC often occupies a large amount of arterial blood supply) where the right portal vein is ligated, dilated right hepatic artery due to the hepatic arterial buffer response (HABR) can cause "blood steal," resulting in reduced flow of the left hepatic artery, affecting FLR hypertrophy, and sometimes causing ALPPS failure. Thus, the patients' arteries change needs to be followed up after surgery. If adequate FLR is not achieved two weeks postoperatively, TAE of the arteries supplying tumors in the right liver is required to eliminate arterial blood steal, restore the blood supply to the FLR, and revoke the FLR growth (that is, TAE-salvaged ALPPS, see Chap. 15 TAE-salvaged ALPPS for details) [50]. When treating patients with intrahepatic cholangiocarcinoma or hilar cholangiocarcinoma, it is necessary to simultaneously perform skeletonization of the hepatoduodenal ligament and regional lymphadenectomy. Some surgeons prefer resect lymph nodes in the second stage surgery [1], but the abdominal inflammation, edema, and bleeding after stage-1 ALPPS render the procedures more difficult, especially after a long interstage interval.

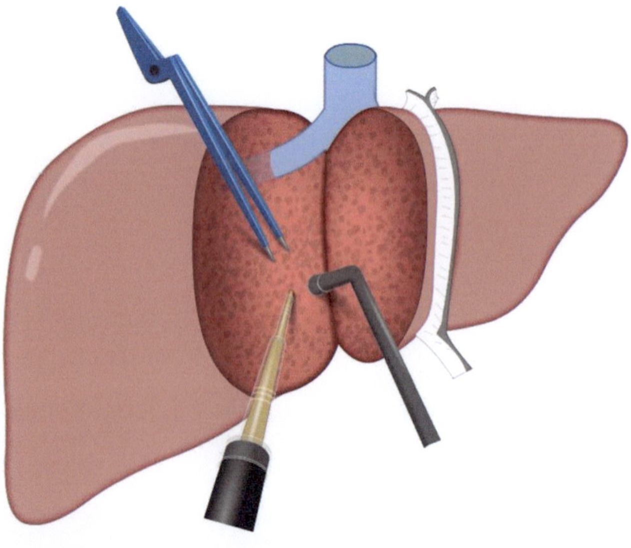

Fig. 6.6 Schematic diagram of liver parenchymal partition during stage 1 ALPPS. CUSA and bipolar electrocoagulation devices are usually used to partition the parenchyma

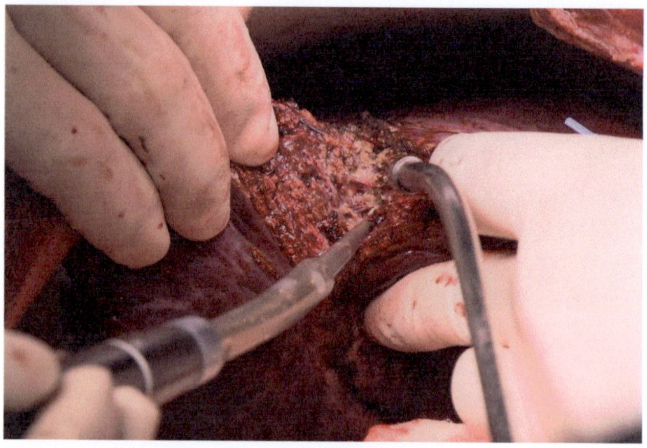

Fig. 6.7 Liver partition during stage 1 ALPPS. CUSA and bipolar electrocoagulation devices are usually used to partition the parenchyma

6.3.2.7 Parenchymal Partition

The liver parenchyma was partitioned along the precut line toward the anterior wall of the IVC. Specific manipulation may vary per surgeons' habits. Usually, CUSA and bipolar electrocoagulation devices are used for precise parenchymal transection (Figs. 6.6 and 6.7). The Glisson branches, hepatic vein branches, and other vessels encountered in the transection plane are coagulated, ligated with suture, clamped with titanium clip, or stitching. Strict hemostasis is required during this process. Ultrasonic dissectors (such as Harmonic shear) can also be applied for the transection. During the operation, the central vein pressure (CVP) shall be controlled at a low level to reduce hemorrhage through cooperation with the anesthesiologist to restrict the fluid input and administer anesthetics as deep as possible to maximally reduce the patient's tidal volume and the positive end-respiratory pressure (PEEP). If necessary, vasoactive agents (such as dobutamine and nitroglycerin) shall be given. If the above measures are not satisfactory in controlling the CVP, the body position can be adjusted to a reverse Trendelenburg position and the IVC can be partially clamped to further reduce its level. In case of severe bleeding, inflow occlusion can be used. Generally, the Pringle maneuver is used for intermittent inflow occlusion (clamp for 15 minutes, release for 5 minutes, and repeat it). Selective clamping is also an alternative. Since classical ALPPS is mostly applied for extended right hemihepatectomy or right trisectionectomy where the transected plane lies in the left lobe, selectively clamping the left blood inflow can also achieve good results. The Pringle maneuver can be safely and routinely performed in both living donor liver transplantation [62] and ALPPS. Although in early years, it was reported that this maneuver was associated with a reduction in FLR growth [38], this phenomenon has not been observed in our center or other centers in China. Belghiti's hanging maneuver and other techniques can assist the partition. Before the liver parenchymal partition, the tunnel before the anterior wall of the IVC and the Laennec capsule is accessed, a sling is inserted to suspend the liver. Then the parenchyma can be quickly partitioned to the anterior wall of the inferior cavity under the guidance, which can better ensure the complete partition.

6.3.2.8 PVL of Tumor Side Portal Veins

After liver partition, the portal vein branch on the tumor side is ligated using 4-0 polypropylene suture or silk sutures. The suture end is kept with a certain length as mark to facilitate the identification during the second stage surgery. The PVL needs to be reliable and thorough since an incomplete ligation causes residual perfusion in the tumor side, leading to surgical failure. It is recommended to use double ligation. During laparoscopy, use Hem-o-lok clip rather than titanium clip, with the tip crossing the contralateral wall of the portal vein to ensure complete and reliable clamping. The portal veins in the tumor side can also be divided first, then both stumps are sutured. Some patients possess anatomic variations in the portal vein (Cheng YF classification [16] or Nakamura classification [17] are often used). Type I cases have only the right branch of the portal vein on the right side, which is easy to handle (Fig. 6.8). For patients with other types of portal vein, attention should be paid to ligate all portal vein branches on the tumor-bearing side. Accidental omission can result in insufficient FLR growth, where prompt PVE is required for these neglected vessels. When re-evaluating the FLR volume after surgery, take notice of PVL effectiveness and whether there is perfusion of the tumor side portal vein. In case of omitted portal vein branch ligation, PVE or other remedies need to be performed in a timely manner. In addition, when dividing the right portal vein, the right caudal branch should be handled prudently to prevent bleeding.

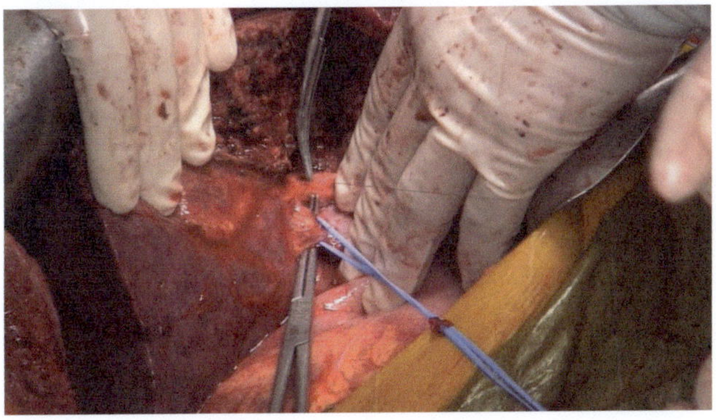

Fig. 6.8 Ligation of right portal vein (encircled by a blue ribbon) during stage 1 ALPPS the portal vein classification is Type I

6.3.2.9 Bile Leakage Check

After liver parenchymal partition, the transection surfaces should be strictly checked for bile leakage. If the vessels are handled accurately and reliably during partition and bile leakage is not expected to occur, this step can be skipped. However, it must be pointed out that bile leakage is one of the most common complications after ALPPS. In the early years, its incidence was reported as high as 22.2–24% [63–65], and even reached 87.5% when the right bile duct was ligated [66]. It has been reduced through technical improvements, and the most valuable measure being rigorous bile leakage check. Methods applied vary per center and surgeon, including pressurized injection into the cystic duct, bubble testing, injection of color-developing agents (such as methylene blue and propofol), and cholangiography when necessary [5, 67–70]. The center where the author works often uses fat emulsion injection to check for bile leakage [26, 31]. Specific steps are as follows. Open the cystic duct, clamp the common bile duct below it, use an indwelling needle to inject diluted fat emulsion from the cystic duct orifice into the bile duct, and check the existence of bile leakage on the liver transection surfaces (in case of bile leakage, the white fat emulsion will gush out from the leakage point and can be easily spotted) (Fig. 6.9). After the testing, the stumps of the cystic duct are sutured with polypropylene suture.

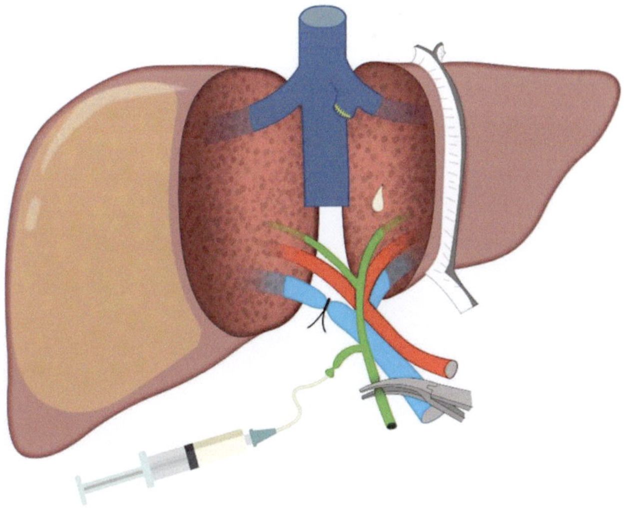

Fig. 6.9 Bile leakage check on the transection surfaces in stage 1 ALPPS. Diluted fat emulsion is injected from the cystic duct to check the existence of bile leakage on the transected surfaces (in case of bile leakage, the white fat emulsion will gush out from the transected surfaces and can be easily traced)

6.3.2.10 Mark with Colored Ribbon

Use different colored ribbon to mark the portal tracts (blue: right portal vein; yellow: common bile duct; red: proper hepatic artery) (Figs. 6.10 and 6.11) to facilitate quick identification in the second stage surgery. If these are unavailable, polypropylene suture and other sutures could be wielded to leave marks with a certain length. In cases with long interstage interval, or complicated with bile leakage, abdominal infection, or severe adhesions, the colored strings could effectively reduce the interference of adhesions on structural identification [5, 68, 71].

6.3.2.11 Management of Transection Surface

The practice of wrapping the right liver with a plastic bag was used in the early years of ALPPS and it has now been abandoned, as it is prone to abdominal fluid accumulation and infection (Fig. 6.12). In addition, if the second stage surgery cannot be performed due to insufficient FLR growth or other reasons, additional operation will be required to remove the plastic bag, increasing the patient's pain. Nowadays, in most cases transected surfaces are covered with fibrin and absorbable hemostatic gauze, showing satisfactory separation effect. After first stage surgery, many patients have abdominal effusion. The abdominal adhesions are often not serious and easy to be separated, posing limited impact on the second stage operation. In patients who have a long interstage interval with abdominal infection after surgery, adhesions are often serious and may be prone to hemorrhage during adhesion lysis.

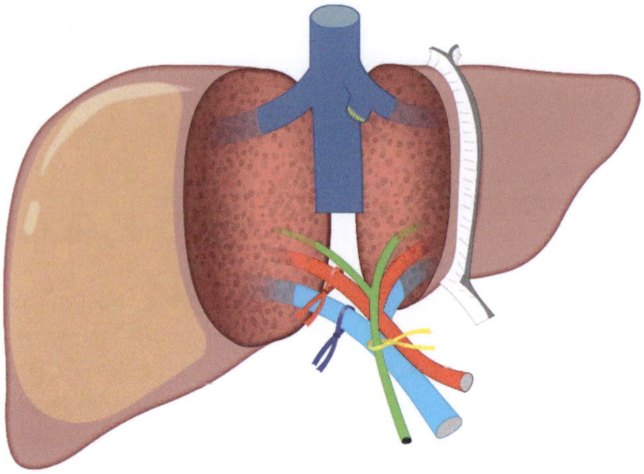

Fig. 6.10 Schematic diagram of colored ribbon marking after dissecting portal tracts (blue: the right portal vein; yellow: the common bile duct; red: the right hepatic artery)

6.3.2.12 Drainage

A drain tube (usually Jackson-Pratt drain) is placed on the transection surface. If necessary, another drainage tube can be placed under the right diaphragm. Foley catheters can be introduced in the transected surface for further drainage while preventing adhesions on both sides [72].

6.3.2.13 Coating with Anti-adhesion Materials

Coating around the liver with anti-adhesion materials can reduce abdominal adhesions and facilitate the stage 2 ALPPS surgery. The author's center usually applies chitosan to reduce abdominal adhesions after the first stage surgery.

6.3.2.14 Close the Abdomen

The abdomen is closed using absorbable sutures layer by layer. In particular, the peritoneal layer must be well-closed to ensure the smoothness of the inferior lining to reduce postoperative adhesions.

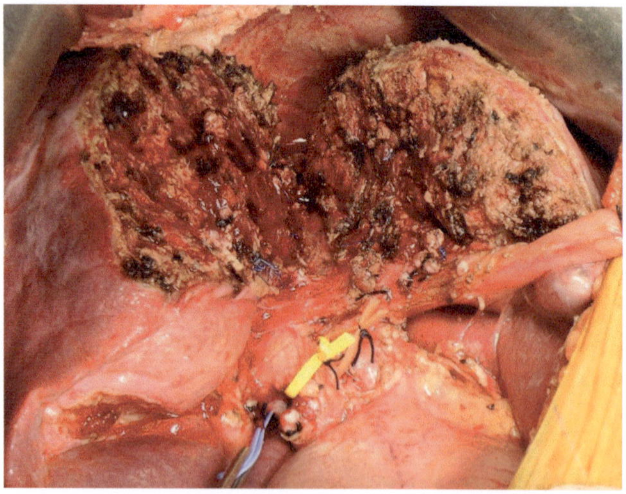

Fig. 6.11 Colored string marking after parenchymal partition and portal duct dissection in ALPPS (blue: the right portal vein; yellow: the common bile duct; red: the right hepatic artery)

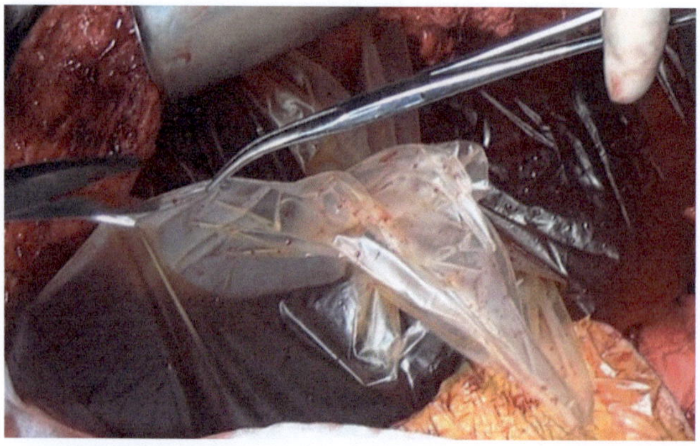

Fig. 6.12 Fluid accumulation caused by plastic bag ligation

6.3.3 Liver Volume Remeasurement After Stage 1 ALPPS

Liver volume is re-evaluated usually one week after the stage 1 ALPPS. The specific interval can be determined by the surgeon based on the actual situation. Patients with chronic liver diseases such as liver fibrosis and cirrhosis often need a longer time. When the FLR increase to the target volume, stage 2 ALPPS can be performed.

6.3.4 Stage 2 ALPPS

6.3.4.1 Re-entering the Abdomen Via the Previous Incision

There is usually a certain degree of adhesions and local congestion and edema in the abdominal cavity after the first stage surgery. When entering the abdomen, care must be taken to avoid damage to the gastrointestinal tract under the incision.

6.3.4.2 Adhesions Lysis

Most abdominal adhesions are not difficult to separate. Some patients who have a longer waiting time or who develop intra-abdominal infection after stage 1 ALPPS are complicated with severe adhesions. After adhesion lysis, the FLR is explored again and the transection surfaces and portal tracts are exposed.

6.3.4.3 Re-assessment of FLR Using IOUS

This is especially important for CRLM patients undergoing ALPPS. Examination is required to completely rule out possible residual lesions in the FLR.

6.3.4.4 Division of the Right Hepatic Artery, the Right Portal Vein, and the Right Bile Duct

There are many anatomic variations in the biliary tract, and its division is usually performed at the end, after which a biliary bougie is introduced in to confirm that the biliary tract of the FLR is intact and unobstructed. If the parenchyma is not completely partitioned during the first stage surgery, the residual parenchyma should be partitioned to the anterior wall of the IVC. During the stage 2 ALPPS operation, due to the inflammation, congestion, and edema caused by the stage 1 operation, the liver parenchyma becomes brittle, and prone to bleed during parenchymal partition. The blood loss is often significantly more than that during the first stage surgery. If necessary, the Pringle maneuver can be used to block the hepatic inflow for hemorrhage control, or using a Bulldog to clamp the portal vein trunk can usually yield promising effect. Expose and divide the hepatic veins. The stumps are sutured continuously with 4-0 polypropylene suture. Alternatively, a linear cutting stapler can be applied, making the operation faster.

6.3.4.5 Tumor Removal

If the stage 1 ALPPS is performed via an anterior approach, perihepatic ligaments on the tumor side need to be mobilized, and finally the tumor is removed.

6.3.4.6 Hemostasis and Bile Leakage Check

If the liver parenchyma is completely transected in the first stage surgery and no bile leakage is found during the stage 2 ALPPS, no need to check bile leakage on the transection surface again. However, for those with incomplete parenchyma partition in the first stage, it needs to be checked after tumor resection in the second stage. The author's center applies fat emulsion injection for bile leakage check as follow: clamp the common bile duct, use an indwelling needle to inject diluted fat emulsion from the stump orifice of the right bile duct into the bile duct of FLR, and check the existence of bile leakage in the liver transection site and hepatitis porta. After confirming no leakage, the right bile duct is closed with suturing (Fig. 6.13).

6.3.4.7 The Liver Transection Surface

The liver transection surface is sprayed with fibrin and covered with absorbable hemostatic gauze.

6.3.4.8 Drainage

A drain tube (usually Jackson-Pratt drain) is placed on the transection surface.

6.3.4.9 Closing the Falciform Ligament

The falciform ligament is sutured, and the left FLR is fixed to prevent it from twisting.

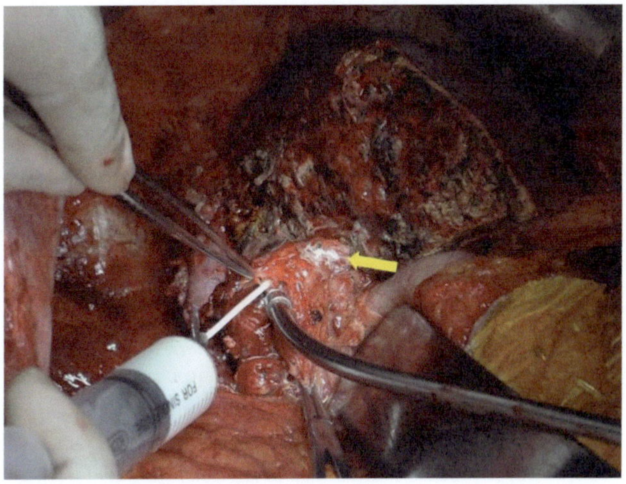

Fig. 6.13 Bile leakage check using fat emulsion injection in stage 2 ALPPS. The diluted fat emulsion is injected from the right bile duct to check for bile leakage on the liver transection surface

6.3.4.10 Closing the Abdomen Layer by Layer

Closing the abdomen layer by layer.

6.4 Pearls and Pitfalls

The key to classical ALPPS lies in the precise liver partition and complete portal venous blood flow occlusion of the tumor-side liver. During parenchymal partition, the structure and function of the FLR need to be totally preserved. In particular, the integrity of its vascular structure is the decisive factor for operation success. At the same time, it is necessary to optimize surgical margins to enable R0 resection of the tumor. The role of ultrasound during stage 1 ALPPS is critical. The portal vein in the tumor side liver needs to be ligated completely. Preoperative planning is invaluable in determining anatomic vessel variations to ensure thorough ligation intra-operatively. If there are any omissions, the tumor side portal venous blood flow is not completely blocked, which can cause ALPPS failure. Preoperative 3D reconstruction and virtual surgery planning can prevent such errors from happening. After surgery, the portal venous blood flow in the tumor side of the liver should be noticed during postoperative FLR volume re-evaluation. A salvaged PVE should be performed if needed. When separating portal tracts, arterial blood supply needs to be protected. Despite the low incidence of accidental injuries, serious consequences do follow should severe arterial damage occur, leading to liver dysfunction or direct liver failure. Pre- and intra-operatively, the anatomic variations of the arteries need to be sorted out. It is recommended to dissect arteries before portal veins and avoid using high-power energy equipment. If the arteries are unintentionally injured and cannot be reconstructed well, the ALPPS needs to be suspended when necessary. In addition, it is vital to pay attention to the blood supply of the left and right hepatic arteries. If arteries on the FLR side are too thin, "blood steal" may occur after surgery, resulting in insufficient FLR hypertrophy. In patients with severe liver fibrosis/cirrhosis and those with huge HCC, this problem is often more prominent. If necessary, TAE-salvaged ALPPS needs to be performed to prevent ALPPS failure (see Chap. 15 of this book for details). After parenchymal partition, bile leakage check is very important, since it is the most common cause of infection after ALPPS. ALPPS is highly invasive, and the postoperative liver function is in a critical state, so is the patient, often complicated with severe systemic inflammatory response and poor tolerability to infection. If bile leakage occurs after either stage of surgery, the consequences of suboptimal infection control are often detrimental. The prevention and treatment of this complication include precise liver partition, meticulous treatment of the tracts one by one, avoiding ligation of the right bile duct, and strict bile leakage check of the transected surfaces. Among them, a strict bile leakage check is the most important and shall be prioritized. The commonly used method in the author's center is fat emulsion injection, where diluted fat emulsion is injected into the intrahepatic biliary tract through the stump of the biliary duct (the orifice of the cystic duct is used for the first stage surgery, and that of the right bile duct for the second stage). Using the agent as a guide to find bile leakage, if any. More than 170 cases of ALPPS have been completed in the author's center utilizing this method, with nearly 0% bile leakage occurring. Postoperative liver failure is the most common complication and the leading cause of death after classical ALPPS, which is related to insufficient FLR functional hypertrophy [38, 73–79]. If conditions allow, hepatobiliary scintigraphy (HBS) functional liver volume measurement can be applied to better determine the timing of second-stage surgery and reduce the occurrence of liver failure [80–83]. Postoperative management of the first-stage operation is essential. If there are risk factors after the first stage, comprehensive considerations should be taken, and the stage-2 ALPPS procedure should be postponed or cancelled if necessary [20, 84]. Classical ALPPS is highly invasive and is correlated with multiple complications. Patients need to select prudently, and surgeries should be performed with caution. Despite its high success rate, related risks shall be discussed with the patient in detail before surgery, and salvaged liver transplantation or other conversion treatments must be well prepared.

References

1. Schlitt HJ, Hackl C, Lang SA. 'In-situ split' liver resection/ALPPS – historical development and current practice[J]. Visc Med. 2017;33(6):408–12.
2. Schnitzbauer AA, Lang SA, Goessmann H, et al. Right portal vein ligation combined with in situ splitting induces rapid left lateral liver lobe hypertrophy enabling 2-staged extended right hepatic resection in small-for-size settings[J]. Ann Surg. 2012;255(3):405–14.
3. Baumgart J, Lang SA, Lang H. A new method for induction of liver hypertrophy prior to right trisectionectomy: a report of three cases[J]. HPB (Oxford). 2011;13(Suppl 2):71–2.
4. Popescu GA, Alexandrescu ST, Grigorie RT, et al. GOOD TO KNOW: the ALPPS procedure – embracing a new technique[J]. Chirurgia. 2017;112(3):332–41.
5. Oldhafer KJ, Stavrou GA, van Gulik TM, et al. ALPPS—where do we stand, where do we go? : Eight recommendations from the first international expert meeting[J]. Ann Surg. 2016;263(5):839–41.
6. Linecker M, Kron P, Lang H, et al. Too many languages in the ALPPS: preventing another tower of babel?[J]. Ann Surg. 2016;263(5):837–8.
7. Lang H, de Santibañes E, Schlitt HJ, et al. 10th anniversary of ALPPS-lessons learned and quo vadis[J]. Ann Surg. 2019;269(1):114–9.

8. Tsui TY, Heumann A, Vashist YK, et al. How we do it: double in situ split for staged mesohepatectomy in patients with advanced gall bladder cancer and marginal future liver remnant[J]. Langenbeck's Arch Surg. 2016;401(4):565–71.
9. Gauzolino R, Castagnet M, Blanleuil ML, et al. The ALPPS technique for bilateral colorectal metastases: three "variations on a theme"[J]. Updat Surg. 2013;65(2):141–8.
10. Obed A, Jarrad A, Bashir A. First left hepatic trisectionectomy including segment one with new associated liver partition and portal vein ligation with staged hepatectomy (ALPPS) modification: how to do it?[J]. Am J Case Rep. 2016;17:759–65.
11. Petrowsky H, Györi G, de Oliveira M, et al. Is partial-ALPPS safer than ALPPS? A single-center experience[J]. Ann Surg. 2015;261(4):e90–2.
12. Machado MA, Surjan R, Basseres T, et al. Total laparoscopic reversal ALPPS[J]. Ann Surg Oncol. 2017;24(4):1048–9.
13. Schadde E, Malagó M, Hernandez-Alejandro R, et al. Monosegment ALPPS hepatectomy: extending resectability by rapid hypertrophy[J]. Surgery. 2015;157(4):676–89.
14. Pineda-Solís K, Paskar D, Tun-Abraham M, et al. Expanding the limits of resectability: associating liver partition and portal vein ligation for staged hepatectomy (ALPPS) using monosegment 6, facilitated by an inferior right hepatic vein[J]. J Surg Oncol. 2017;115(8):959–62.
15. Chan ACY, Chok K, Dai JWC, et al. Impact of split completeness on future liver remnant hypertrophy in associating liver partition and portal vein ligation for staged hepatectomy (ALPPS) in hepatocellular carcinoma: complete-ALPPS versus partial-ALPPS[J]. Surgery. 2017;161(2):357–64.
16. Cheng YF, Huang TL, Lee TY, et al. Variation of the intrahepatic portal vein; angiographic demonstration and application in living-related hepatic transplantation[J]. Transplant Proc. 1996;28(3):1667–8.
17. Nakamura T, Tanaka K, Kiuchi T, et al. Anatomical variations and surgical strategies in right lobe living donor liver transplantation: lessons from 120 cases[J]. Transplantation. 2002;73(12):1896–903.
18. Alvarez FA, Ardiles V, de Santibañes E. The ALPPS approach for the management of colorectal carcinoma liver metastases[J]. Curr Colorectal Cancer Rep. 2013;9(2):168–77.
19. Sala S, Ardiles V, Ulla M, et al. Our initial experience with ALPPS technique: encouraging results[J]. Updat Surg. 2012;64(3):167–72.
20. Linecker M, Stavrou GA, Oldhafer KJ, et al. The ALPPS risk score: avoiding futile use of ALPPS[J]. Ann Surg. 2016;264(5):763–71.
21. Truant S, Scatton O, Dokmak S, et al. Associating liver partition and portal vein ligation for staged hepatectomy (ALPPS): impact of the inter-stages course on morbi-mortality and implications for management[J]. Eur J Surg Oncol. 2015;41(5):674–82.
22. Eshmuminov D, Raptis DA, Linecker M, et al. Meta-analysis of associating liver partition with portal vein ligation and portal vein occlusion for two-stage hepatectomy[J]. Br J Surg. 2016;103(13):1768–82.
23. Raptis DA, Linecker M, Kambakamba P, et al. Defining benchmark outcomes for ALPPS[J]. Ann Surg. 2019;270(5):835–41.
24. Petrowsky H, Linecker M, Raptis DA, et al. First long-term oncologic results of the ALPPS procedure in a large cohort of patients with colorectal liver metastases[J]. Ann Surg. 2020;272(5):793–800.
25. Sandström P, Røsok BI, Sparrelid E, et al. ALPPS improves resectability compared with conventional two-stage hepatectomy in patients with advanced colorectal liver metastasis: results from a Scandinavian multicenter randomized controlled trial (LIGRO trial)[J]. Ann Surg. 2018;267(5):833–40.
26. Zhou J, Wang Z, Sun J, et al. Associating liver partition and portal vien ligation for staged hepatectomy[J]. Chin J Dig Surg. 2013;12(7):485–9.
27. Moris D, Ronnekleiv-Kelly S, Kostakis ID, et al. Operative results and oncologic outcomes of associating liver partition and portal vein ligation for staged hepatectomy (ALPPS) versus two-stage hepatectomy (TSH) in patients with unresectable colorectal liver metastases: a systematic review and meta-analysis[J]. World J Surg. 2018;42(3):806–15.
28. Zhou J, Sun HC, Wang Z, et al. Guidelines for diagnosis and treatment of primary liver cancer in China (2017 edition)[J]. Liver Cancer. 2018;7(3):235–60.
29. Bureau of Medical Administration, National Health and Family Planning Commission of the People's Republic of China. Standardization of diagnosis and treatment for hepatocellular carcinoma (2017 edition)[J]. Chin J Dig Surg. 2017;16(7):635–47.
30. Zhou J, Sun HC, Wang Z, et al. Guidelines for the diagnosis and treatment of hepatocellular carcinoma (2019 edition)[J]. Liver Cancer. 2020;9(6):682–720.
31. Wang Z, Peng YF, Hu JW, et al. Associating liver partition and portal vein ligation for staged hepatectomy for unresectable hepatitis B virus-related hepatocellular carcinoma: a single center study of 45 patients[J]. Ann Surg. 2020;271(3):534–41.
32. Chan A, Zhang WY, Chok K, et al. ALPPS versus portal vein embolization for hepatitis-related hepatocellular carcinoma: a changing paradigm in modulation of future liver remnant before major hepatectomy[J]. Ann Surg. 2021;273(5):957–65.
33. Li PP, Huang G, Jia NY, et al. Associating liver partition and portal vein ligation for staged hepatectomy versus sequential transarterial chemoembolization and portal vein embolization in staged hepatectomy for HBV-related hepatocellular carcinoma: a randomized comparative study[J]. Hepatobiliary Surg Nutr. 2022;11(1):38–51.
34. Zhang JW, Xu YY, Yang HY, et al. Application of associating liver partition and portal vein ligation for staged hepatectomy for hepatocellular carcinoma related to hepatitis B virus: comparison with traditional one-stage right hepatectomy[J]. Transl Cancer Res. 2020;9(9):5371–9.
35. Deng ZF, Jin ZR, Qin YH, et al. Efficacy of the association liver partition and portal vein ligation for staged hepatectomy for the treatment of solitary huge hepatocellular carcinoma: a retrospective single-center study[J]. World J Surg Oncol. 2021;19(1):95.
36. Peng CH, Li C, Liu C, et al. The outcome of the HCC patients underwent ALPPS: retrospective study[J]. Medicine (Baltimore). 2019;98(38):e17182.
37. D'Haese JG, Neumann J, Weniger M, et al. Should ALPPS be used for liver resection in intermediate-stage HCC?[J]. Ann Surg Oncol. 2016;23(4):1335–43.
38. Schadde E, Ardiles V, Robles-Campos R, et al. Early survival and safety of ALPPS: first report of the International ALPPS Registry[J]. Ann Surg. 2014;260(5):829–36.
39. Serenari M, Zanello M, Schadde E, et al. Importance of primary indication and liver function between stages: results of a multicenter Italian audit of ALPPS 2012–2014[J]. HPB. 2016;18(5):419–27.
40. Linecker M, Björnsson B, Stavrou GA, et al. Risk adjustment in ALPPS is associated with a dramatic decrease in early mortality and morbidity[J]. Ann Surg. 2017;266(5):779–86.
41. Olthof PB, Coelen RJS, Wiggers JK, et al. High mortality after ALPPS for perihilar cholangiocarcinoma: case-control analysis including the first series from the international ALPPS registry[J]. HPB. 2017;19(5):381–7.
42. Lang H, de Santibanes E, Clavien PA. Outcome of ALPPS for perihilar cholangiocarcinoma: case-control analysis including the first series from the international ALPPS registry[J]. HPB. 2017;19(5):379–80.

43. Balci D, Kirimker EO, Üstüner E, et al. Stage I-laparoscopy partial ALPPS procedure for perihilar cholangiocarcinoma[J]. J Surg Oncol. 2020;121(6):1022–6.
44. Boggi U, Napoli N, Kauffmann EF, et al. Laparoscopic microwave liver ablation and portal vein ligation: an alternative approach to the conventional ALPPS procedure in hilar cholangiocarcinoma[J]. Ann Surg Oncol. 2016;23(Suppl 5):884.
45. Sakamoto Y, Inagaki F, Omichi K, et al. Associating liver partial partition and transileocecal portal vein embolization for staged hepatectomy[J]. Ann Surg. 2016;264(6):e21–2.
46. Li J, Kantas A, Ittrich H, et al. Avoid "all-touch" by hybrid ALPPS to achieve oncological efficacy[J]. Ann Surg. 2016;263(1):e6–7.
47. Lai Q, Melandro F, Rossi M. Hybrid partial ALPPS: a feasible approach in case of right trisegmentectomy and macrovascular invasion[J]. Ann Surg. 2018;267(4):e80–2.
48. Hong DF, Zhang YB, Peng SY, et al. Percutaneous microwave ablation liver partition and portal vein embolization for rapid liver regeneration: a minimally invasive first step of ALPPS for hepatocellular carcinoma[J]. Ann Surg. 2016;264(1):e1–2.
49. Lunardi A, Cervelli R, Volterrani D, et al. Feasibility of percutaneous intrahepatic split by microwave ablation (*PISA*) after portal vein embolization for hypertrophy of future liver remnant: the radiological stage-1 ALPPS[J]. Cardiovasc Intervent Radiol. 2018;41(5):789–98.
50. Wang Z, Peng YF, Sun QM, et al. Salvage transhepatic arterial embolization after failed stage I ALPPS in a patient with a huge HCC with chronic liver disease: a case report[J]. Int J Surg Case Rep. 2017;39:131–5.
51. Tschuor CH, Croome KP, Sergeant G, et al. Salvage parenchymal liver transection for patients with insufficient volume increase after portal vein occlusion—an extension of the ALPPS approach[J]. Eur J Surg Oncol. 2013;39(11):1230–5.
52. Enne M, Schadde E, Björnsson B, et al. ALPPS as a salvage procedure after insufficient future liver remnant hypertrophy following portal vein occlusion[J]. HPB. 2017;19(12):1126–9.
53. Sparrelid E, Gilg S, Brismar TB, et al. Rescue ALPPS is efficient and safe after failed portal vein occlusion in patients with colorectal liver metastases[J]. Langenbeck's Arch Surg. 2017;402(1):69–75.
54. Ulmer TF, Jong CD, Andert A, et al. ALPPS procedure in insufficient hypertrophy after portal vein embolization (PVE)[J]. World J Surg. 2017;41(1):250–7.
55. Cavaness KM, Doyle MB, Lin Y, et al. Using ALPPS to induce rapid liver hypertrophy in a patient with hepatic fibrosis and portal vein thrombosis[J]. J Gastrointest Surg. 2013;17(1):207–12.
56. Hong JC, Kim J, Browning M, et al. Modified associating liver partition and portal vein ligation for staged hepatectomy for hepatoblastoma in a small infant: how far can we push the envelope?[J]. Ann Surg. 2017;266(2):e16–7.
57. de Santibañes E, Alvarez FA, Ardiles V. How to avoid postoperative liver failure: a novel method[J]. World J Surg. 2012;36(1):125–8.
58. de Santibañes E, Clavien PA. Playing Play-Doh to prevent postoperative liver failure: the "ALPPS" approach[J]. Ann Surg. 2012;255(3):415–7.
59. Lim C, Turco C, Balci D, et al. Auxiliary liver transplantation for cirrhosis: from APOLT to RAPID: a scoping review[J]. Ann Surg. 2022;275(3):551–9.
60. Königsrainer A, Templin S, Capobianco I, et al. Paradigm shift in the management of irresectable colorectal liver metastases: living donor auxiliary partial orthotopic liver transplantation in combination with two-stage hepatectomy (LD-RAPID)[J]. Ann Surg. 2019;270(2):327–32.
61. Balci D, Kirimker EO, Bingol Kologlu M, et al. A new approach for increasing availability of liver grafts and donor safety in living donor liver transplantation: LD-RAPID procedure in the cirrhotic setting with hepatocellular carcinoma[J]. Liver Transpl. 2021;27(4):590–4.
62. Imamura H, Takayama T, Sugawara Y, et al. Pringle's manoeuvre in living donors[J]. Lancet. 2002;360(9350):2049–50.
63. Li J, Girotti P, Königsrainer I, et al. ALPPS in right trisectionectomy: a safe procedure to avoid postoperative liver failure?[J]. J Gastrointest Surg. 2013;17(5):956–61.
64. Spetzler VN, Schepers M, Pinnschmidt HO, et al. The incidence and severity of post-hepatectomy bile leaks is affected by surgical indications, preoperative chemotherapy, and surgical procedures[J]. Hepatobiliary Surg Nutr. 2019;8(2):101–10.
65. van den Broek MAJ, van Dam RM, Malagó M, et al. Feasibility of randomized controlled trials in liver surgery using surgery-related mortality or morbidity as endpoint[J]. Br J Surg. 2009;96(9):1005–14.
66. Dokmak S, Belghiti J. Which limits to the "ALPPS" approach?[J]. Ann Surg. 2012;256(3):e6;author reply e16–e17.
67. Ardiles V, Schadde E, Santibanes E, et al. Commentary on "happy marriage or 'dangerous liaison': ALPPS and the anterior approach"[J]. Ann Surg. 2014;260(2):e4.
68. Alvarez FA, Ardiles V, Sanchez Claria R, et al. Associating liver partition and portal vein ligation for staged hepatectomy (ALPPS): tips and tricks[J]. J Gastrointest Surg. 2013;17(4):814–21.
69. de Santibañes M, Alvarez FA, Santos FR, et al. The associating liver partition and portal vein ligation for staged hepatectomy approach using only segments I and IV as future liver remnant[J]. J Am Coll Surg. 2014;219(2):e5–9.
70. Chan ACY, Pang R, Poon RTP. Simplifying the ALPPS procedure by the anterior approach[J]. Ann Surg. 2014;260(2):e3.
71. Brustia R, Scatton O, Perdigao F, et al. Vessel identifications tags for open or laparoscopic associating liver partition and portal vein ligation for staged hepatectomy[J]. J Am Coll Surg. 2013;217(6):e51–5.
72. Alexandrescu S, Stoica L, Grigorie R, et al. Primary hepatic lymphoma resected by ALPPS procedure (associating liver partition and portal vein ligation for staged hepatectomy)[J]. J Transl Med Res. 2016;21(2):153.
73. Schadde E, Raptis DA, Schnitzbauer AA, et al. Prediction of mortality after ALPPS stage-1: an analysis of 320 patients from the international ALPPS registry[J]. Ann Surg. 2015;262(5):780–5.
74. Kang D, Schadde E. Hypertrophy and liver function in ALPPS: correlation with morbidity and mortality[J]. Visc Med. 2017;33(6):426–33.
75. Sparrelid E, Jonas E, Tzortzakakis A, et al. Dynamic evaluation of liver volume and function in associating liver partition and portal vein ligation for staged hepatectomy[J]. J Gastrointest Surg. 2017;21(6):967–74.
76. Deshayes E, Schadde E, Piron L, et al. Extended liver venous deprivation leads to a higher increase in liver function that ALPPS in early assessment: a comment to "Sparrelid, E. et al. Dynamic evaluation of liver volume and function in associating liver partition and portal vein ligation for staged hepatectomy. *Journal Of Gastrointestinal Surgery* (2017)"[J]. J Gastrointest Surg. 2017;21(10):1754–5.
77. Olthof PB, Schadde E, van Lienden KP, et al. Hepatic parenchymal transection increases liver volume but not function after portal vein embolization in rabbits[J]. Surgery. 2017;162(4):732–41.

78. Truant S, Baillet C, Deshorgue AC, et al. Drop of total liver function in the interstages of the new associating liver partition and portal vein ligation for staged hepatectomy technique: analysis of the "auxiliary liver" by HIDA scintigraphy[J]. Ann Surg. 2016;263(3):e33–4.
79. Cieslak KP, Olthof PB, van Lienden KP, et al. Assessment of liver function using (99m)Tc-mebrofenin hepatobiliary scintigraphy in ALPPS (associating liver partition and portal vein ligation for staged hepatectomy)[J]. Case Rep Gastroenterol. 2015;9(3):353–60.
80. Rassam F, Olthof PB, van Lienden KP, et al. Comparison of functional and volumetric increase of the future remnant liver and postoperative outcomes after portal vein embolization and complete or partial associating liver partition and portal vein ligation for staged hepatectomy (ALPPS)[J]. Ann Transl Med. 2020;8(7):436.
81. Truant S, Baillet C, Deshorgue AC, et al. Contribution of hepatobiliary scintigraphy in assessing ALPPS most suited timing[J]. Updat Surg. 2017;69(3):411–9.
82. de Graaf W, van Lienden KP, Dinant S, et al. Assessment of future remnant liver function using hepatobiliary scintigraphy in patients undergoing major liver resection[J]. J Gastrointest Surg. 2010;14(2):369–78.
83. Tomassini F, D'Asseler Y, Linecker M, et al. Hepatobiliary scintigraphy and kinetic growth rate predict liver failure after ALPPS: a multi-institutional study[J]. HPB (Oxford). 2020;22(10):1420–8.
84. Linecker M, Kuemmerli C, Kambakamba P, et al. Performance validation of the ALPPS risk model[J]. HPB. 2019;21(6):711–21.

7 Tourniquet ALPPS (Cai's ALPPS)

Xiujun Cai and Ren'an Jin

7.1 Introduction

ALPPS is hailed as a breakthrough and innovative procedure in hepatobiliary surgery in the twenty-first century. It combines the essence of portal vein embolization and conventional two-staged liver resection, enabling the increase of FLR in a short period. The procedure was unintentionally created in 2007 by Professor Hans J. Schlitt in Regensburg, Germany. When he operated on a patient with hilar cholangiocarcinoma, the bile duct branches of the right three lobes of the liver were invaded, where extended right hemihepatectomy and left lateral hepatic lobe cholangiojejunostomy were needed. However, since the patient's left lateral lobe was too small to tolerate such an operation, an unconventional surgery was performed in which liver parenchyma was separated along the falciform ligament, and the right branch of the portal vein was ligated. On the CT scan 8 days after the operation, it was surprising to find that the patient's left lateral lobe was significantly enlarged. Subsequently, an extended right hemihepatectomy was successfully performed, which was also named "in situ splitting (ISS) liver resection" [1]. In 2012, a study including 25 patients from 5 centers in Germany with primary liver tumors preoperatively appeared to be marginally resectable but had a tumor-free left lateral lobe was performed with a two-staged hepatectomy was published in Annals of Surgery. After a median waiting period of 9 days (range = 5–28 days), the volume of the left lateral lobe had increased to 536 mL (range = 273–881 mL), representing a median volume increase of 74% (range = 21–192%) [2]. In the same year, Pierre-Alain Clavien, editor-in-chief of *Annals of Surgery*, and Argentinian Professor Eduardo de Santibanes officially named this procedure as associating liver partition and portal vein ligation for staged hepatectomy (ALPPS) [3].

Since then, this new approach of ALPPS has been explored and spread quickly worldwide, and the International ALPPS Registry (www.alpps.net) has been established after that. However, at the dawn of its application, the issue of low safety and reliability was unsatisfactory, with high rates of complication and mortality (the incidence of complications after operation from 22% to 87.5% and mortality from 12% to 28.7% [2, 4, 5]). How to improve the feasibility and safety of ALPPS has been a thorny scientific question, thus promoting its technical progress and innovation. In addition to classical ALPPS (Chap. 6 of this book for details), there are multiple modified ALPPS procedures [6]. Bleeding, infection, bile leakage, and postoperative liver failure were the main complications of ALPPS in early case series. Modified ALPPS procedures aim to reduce surgical trauma, decrease complication incidence, and improve surgery safety. At present, the main point of innovation of the modified ALPPS procedures focuses on liver separation techniques, including tourniquet, radiofrequency ablation, microwave ablation, and partial liver parenchymal transection. Surgical methods have also evolved from traditional laparotomy to laparoscopy and da Vinci robotic surgery. In 2013, Machado et al. [7] reported the application of the first case of total laparoscopic ALPPS on a patient with colorectal cancer liver metastases. More minor surgical trauma and milder abdominal adhesions not only reduced the difficulty of the surgery in the second stage but also improved the safety of the operation. The authors also recommended against using bioactive plastic bags for residual liver wrapping to avoid infection caused by foreign bodies. These exquisite operational methods have prompted more and more hepatobiliary surgeons to explore the clinical value of total laparoscopic ALPPS for patients with liver tumors. By generating a clear surgical field of view with detailed hepatic portal anatomical structures, laparoscopic ALPPS enables precise liver transection, reducing postoperative adhesions and the difficulty in the

X. Cai (✉) · R. Jin
Sir Run Run Shaw Hospital, Zhejiang University School of Medicine, Zhejiang, China
e-mail: srrsh_cxj@zju.edu.cn

J. Zhou (ed.), *Associating Liver Partition and Portal Vein Ligation for Staged Hepatectomy (ALPPS)*,
https://doi.org/10.1007/978-981-96-7364-3_7

second stage. Despite its advantages of less trauma and quick recovery, surgeons are required to have a richer experience and better skills.

Professor Xiujun Cai from Sir Run Run Shaw Hospital, Zhejiang University School of Medicine, drew upon the merits of laparoscopy and conventional liver hanging maneuver to further ameliorate total laparoscopic ALPPS, solving the problems of bile leakage and infection that is prone to occur after liver parenchyma transection in the first stage of ALPPS [8]. Both stages of the operation were performed under a laparoscope. For patients with liver cirrhosis and liver cancer, a nasogastric tube with a guide wire was applied to ligate the left and right liver parenchyma at the pre-cut line instead of in situ separation, thereby blocking intralobular ducts on both sides and completely preventing the occurrence of bile leakage. Patients recovered rapidly, and the FLR increased quickly shortly after the first stage. Adhesions were milder, as were observed during the second stage. During liver parenchyma transection, the insulation effect induced by external cannulas can diminish perihepatic tissue damage, effectively compensating for the disadvantages of a high complication rate and slow postoperative recovery of the transection. This modified ALPPS was then named Tourniquet-ALPPS (Cai's ALPPS).

7.2 Indications

The case selection of Cai's ALPPS is not significantly different from that of conventional laparoscopic ALPPS, with rigorous pre-operative evaluation criteria for the patient's general condition, liver function grade, FLR, and liver functional reserve. We calculate standard liver volume using the existing general formula, that is, SLV = 706.2 × BSA (m^2) + 2.4, BSA (m^2) = weight (kg) $^{0.425}$× height (cm) $^{0.725}$ × 0.007,184. Based on experiences at home and abroad, the generally accepted safety bottom line for liver resection is FLR no less than 25% to 30% of SLV for patients without parenchymal liver disease or cirrhosis; for parenchymal diseased or cirrhotic patients, the FLR shall be no less than 40% of SLV. ALPPS is suitable for patients whose tumors are potentially resectable but with insufficient FLR to achieve the safety of one-staged liver resection. The evaluation of liver reserve function is also an important aspect; Child-Pugh A and ICG-R15 < 10% are required. Regarding disease selection, it is mostly appropriate for primary or metastatic liver tumors without extrahepatic distant metastasis. Currently, the main indication of ALPPS is CRLM, and ALPPS has gradually become one of the optional treatments for CRLM. Additionally, existing data show that ALPPS is feasible for HCC with meticulous evaluation of the existence, severity, and potential impact of underlying chronic liver disease. ALPPS in those with severe liver cirrhosis should be performed with caution [9, 10]. For ICC patients with insufficient FLR, ALPPS could be one of the treatment options. However, because of the high rate of postoperative complications and mortality, such as biliary leakage, liver insufficiency, severe infection, and sepsis, ALPPS should be used with caution, especially in patients requiring biliary duct reconstruction [6].

In addition, patients who have previously been inconvenient or ineligible for two-staged PVE and resection (complicated with tumor thrombus in the tumor-side portal vein branch, highly malignant tumor, and it is expected to progress rapidly during the waiting period for PVE) are also indicated for ALPPS. Failure of FLR hyperplasia induced by traditional PVE is also an indication that ALPPS salvage ALPPS can be performed. Nevertheless, ALPPS should be carried out with great caution in patients with severe liver cirrhosis, an advanced age, gallbladder cancer, and hilar cholangiocarcinoma.

7.3 Surgical Procedures

Tourniquet-ALPPS (Cai's ALPPS) can be completed under total laparoscopy (stage 1 and stage 2 are total laparoscopies).

7.3.1 Position

Patients are usually put in a supine position, with the right side elevated 35°-40°. When lying down and the head is elevated higher than the feet, the right side should also be elevated 35°–40°. Place two layers of sandbags on the right side of the lower back to keep the patient in a recumbent position. At the same time, attention should be paid to shoulder and hip restraints to prevent accidental fallings. In this position, the patient's left side (left shoulder included) is under pressure, and soft objects need to be placed to guard against local pressure sores or pain after surgery.

7.3.2 Surgical Procedures for Stage 1 ALPPS

7.3.2.1 Surgical Incisions

A 4-portal Trocar layout is usually chosen (Fig. 7.1a). Using a 10 mm Trocar, the observation portal is located two finger-widths above and two finger-widths on the right side of the umbilicus. Using a 12 mm Trocar, the main operating portal is situated under the right costal margin above the observation portal. The auxiliary portals can be positioned under endoscopy as far posterior and superior as possible. One is located under the costal margin of the right midaxillary line,

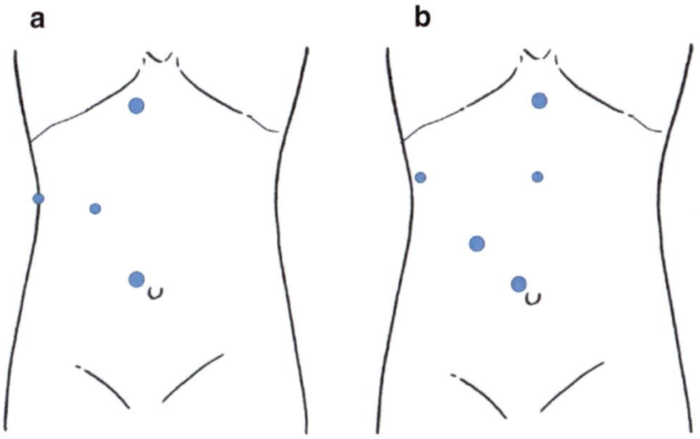

Fig. 7.1 Trocar layout of Cai's ALPPS. (**a**) Four-portal trocar layout; (**b**) Five-portal trocar layout

using a 5 mm Trocar, and the other on its medial plane, at the midclavicular line, using a 12 mm Trocar. A 5-portal Trocar layout is an alternative (Fig. 7.1b). The observation portal sits two finger-widths above and two finger-widths on the right side of the umbilicus, using a 10 mm Trocar. The main operating portal is located 5 cm below the ribs on the outer edge of the right rectus abdominis with a 12 mm Trocar. A 12 mm Trocar and a 5 mm Trocar are set on the midline cranially to caudally, and a 5 mm Trocar sits in the anterior axillary line under the right costal margin.

7.3.2.2 Laparoscopic Exploration

Establish pneumoperitoneum via carbon dioxide and maintain its pressure at 12–15 mmHg. Introduce a laparoscope and explore the abdominal cavity for any extrahepatic lesions not detected by preoperative imaging to rule out surgical contraindications.

7.3.2.3 Cholecystectomy

Use a laparoscopic Peng's multifunctional operative dissector (LPMOD) to dissect Calot's triangle. Separate, clamp and divide the cystic duct and cystic artery, and remove the gallbladder in an antegrade manner.

7.3.2.4 Dissect the First Porta Hepatis (Hilus Hepatis)

Dissect the Glisson sheath using the curettage and aspiration dissection technique, dissect the proper hepatic artery, the left hepatic artery, and the right hepatic artery (Fig. 7.2), and suspend them with silicone bands to facilitate traction (Fig. 7.3). Use dissection forceps to dissect the common bile duct on the left side of the proper hepatic artery (Fig. 7.4), and suspend it with a silicone band (Fig. 7.5) to help retract the common bile duct to the left and expose the portal vein posterior to it. Dissect the portal vein with separation forceps and LPMOD to expose the main trunk, left

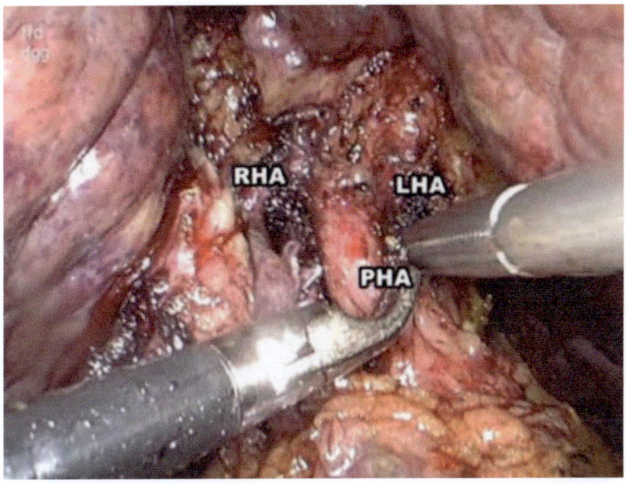

Fig. 7.2 The porta hepatis is dissected by the curettage and aspiration dissection technique, separating the proper hepatic artery, the left hepatic artery, and the right hepatic artery. PHA: proper hepatic artery; LHA: left hepatic artery; RHA: right hepatic artery

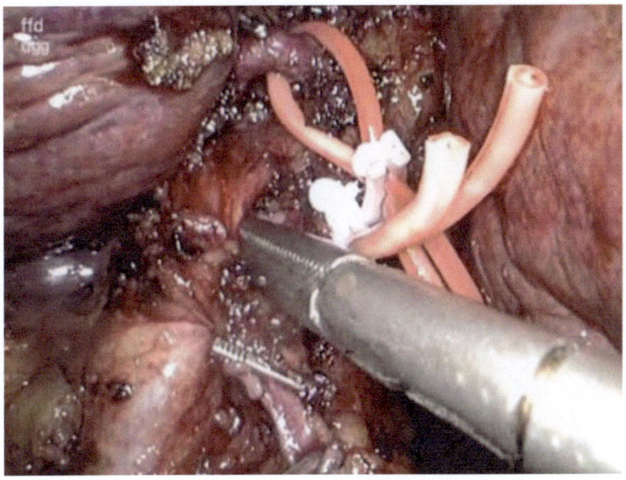

Fig. 7.3 Suspend the proper hepatic artery and right hepatic artery with a silicone band

and right branches of the portal vein, and their confluence (Fig. 7.6). During the process of separating its right branch, large right-angle forceps shall be wielded with patience and care to part the anterior and the posterior repeatedly without using excessive force so that portal vein tearing and massive bleeding can be avoided. Goldfinger dissectors could also be used to penetrate from behind the right branch of the portal vein to enable its complete separation (Fig. 7.7). Use silk suture to ligate the root of this branch of the portal vein (Fig. 7.8), and then utilize Hem-o-lok to clamp both the distal and proximal ends before dissection (Fig. 7.9). The right hepatic artery is marked with silk suture or Prolene to enable quick positioning during the second stage (Fig. 7.10).

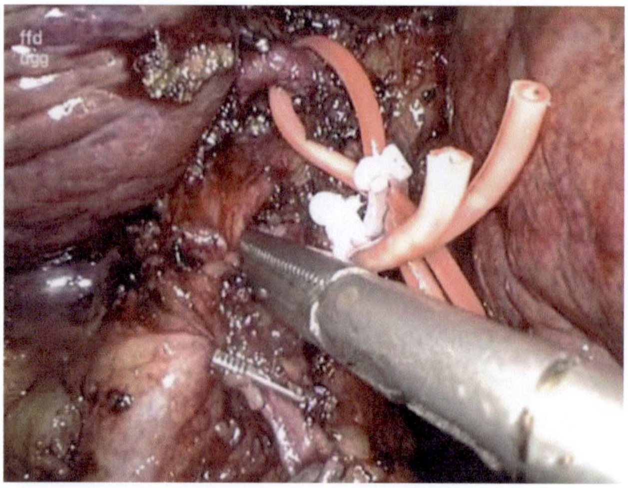

Fig. 7.4 Use dissection forceps to dissect the common bile duct on the left side of the proper hepatic artery

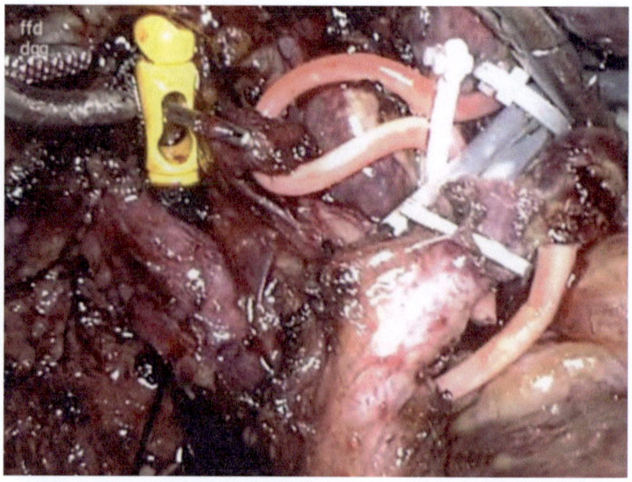

Fig. 7.7 The Goldfinger dissector passes behind the right branch of the portal vein

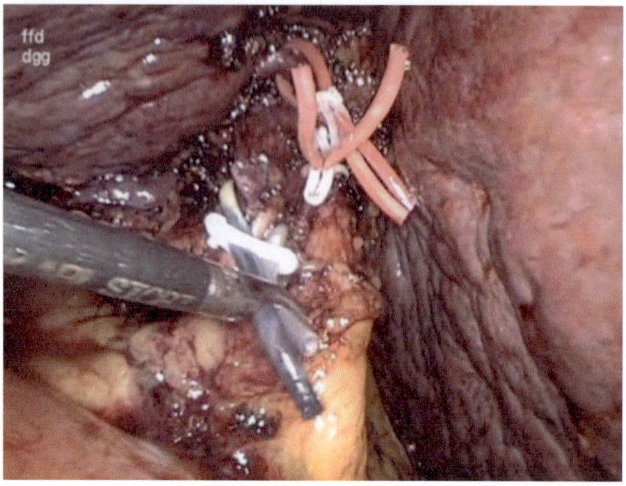

Fig. 7.5 Suspend the common bile duct

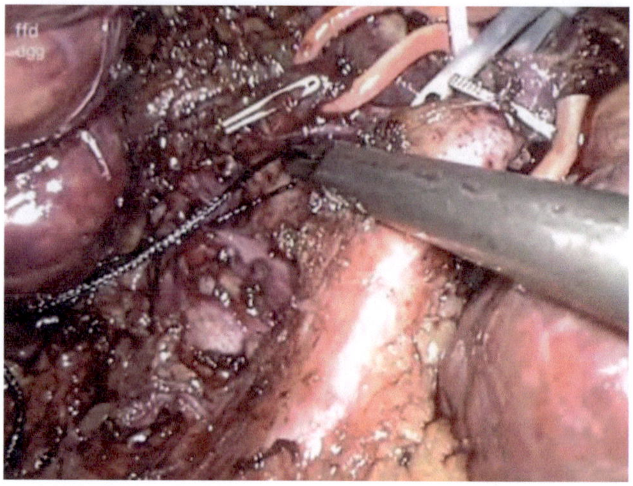

Fig. 7.8 Use silk suture to ligate the root of the right branch of the portal vein

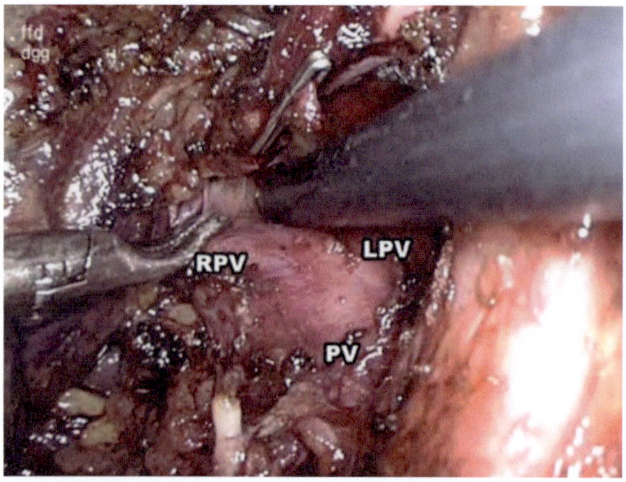

Fig. 7.6 Dissect the portal vein to reveal the main trunk, left and right branches of the portal vein, and their confluence. PV: portal vein; LPV: left branch of portal vein; RPV: right branch of portal vein

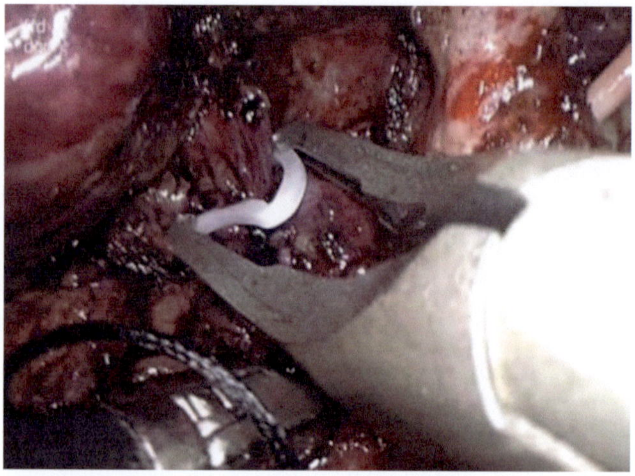

Fig. 7.9 Hem-o-lok clamping of the right branch of the portal vein

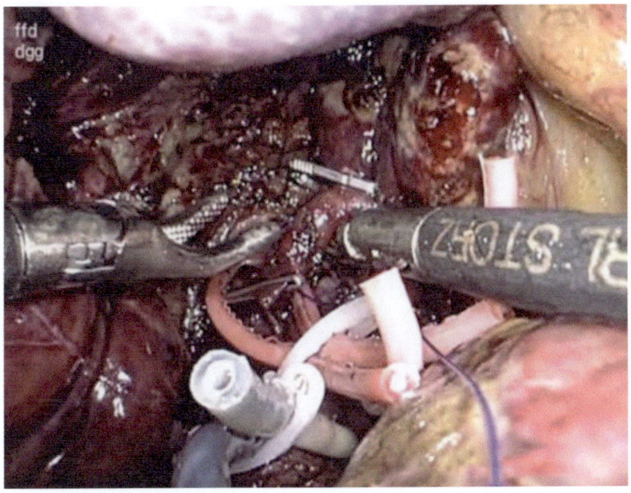

Fig. 7.10 The right hepatic artery is marked with Prolene

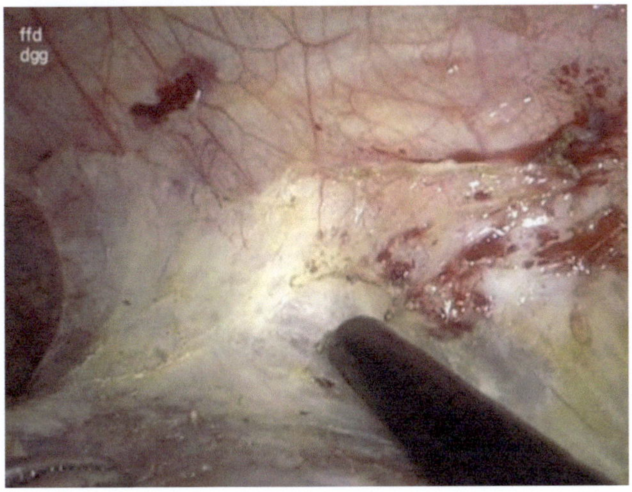

Fig. 7.11 Expose the hepatic vein fossa

7.3.2.5 Dissociate the Right Side of the Liver

Sever the ligament teres and falciform ligament, separate the superior and inferior vena cava in the front, and expose the hepatic vein fossa (Fig. 7.11). Dissect the right triangular ligament, coronary ligament, and hepatorenal ligament, flip the liver over, separate the bare area and the right adrenal gland, and dissociate the short hepatic veins (Fig. 7.12) and the right inferior vena cava ligament. A tunnel is established behind the liver parenchyma and in the avascular area on the right side of the inferior vena cava until the confluence of the right hepatic vein and the inferior vena cava is exposed (Fig. 7.13). Now, the right liver is completely freed.

7.3.2.6 Tourniquet Indwelling

After freeing the right liver, the right hepatic vein is dissected at the confluence of hepatic vein and inferior vena cava (the second porta hepatis) (Fig. 7.14) and marked with silk suture

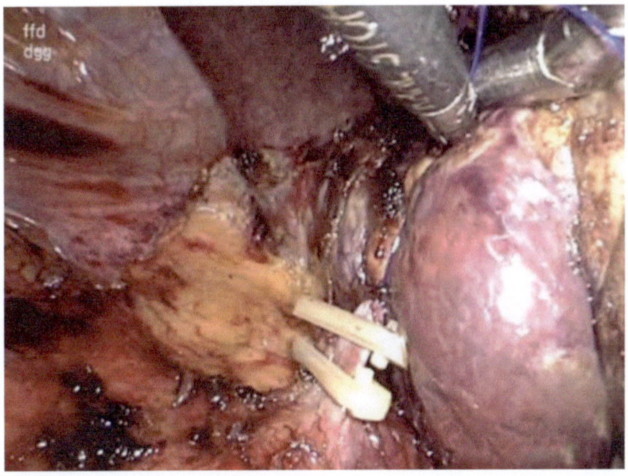

Fig. 7.12 Dissociate the short hepatic veins

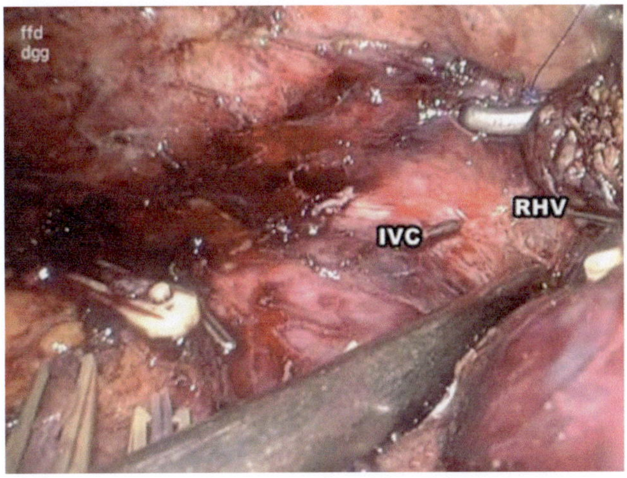

Fig. 7.13 Expose the confluence of the right hepatic vein and inferior vena cava. IVC: inferior vena cava; RHV: right hepatic vein

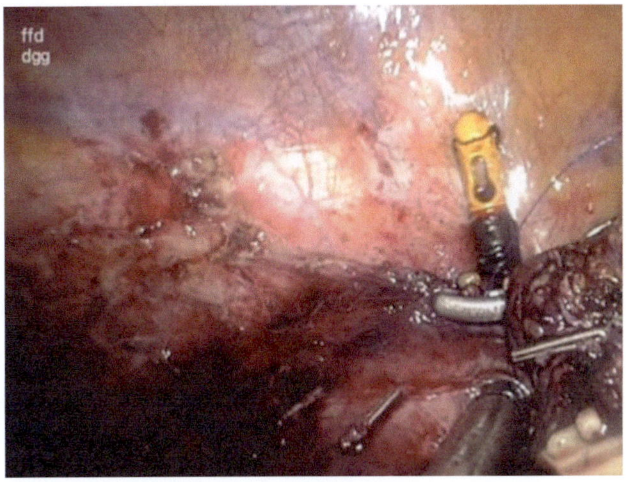

Fig. 7.14 Dissect the right hepatic vein at the confluence of hepatic vein and inferior vena cava (the second porta hepatis)

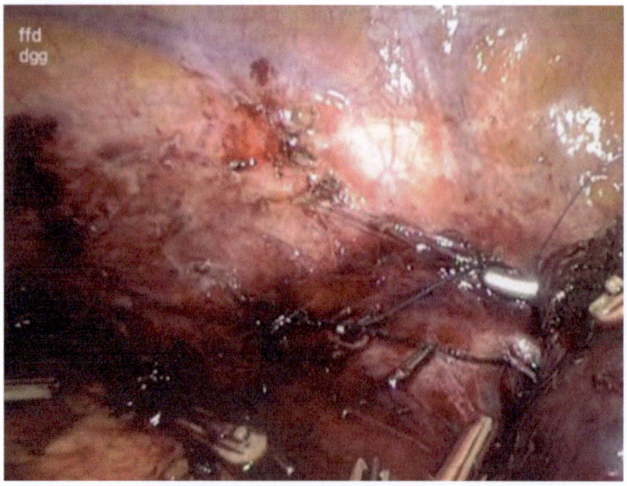

Fig. 7.15 Mark the right hepatic vein with Prolene

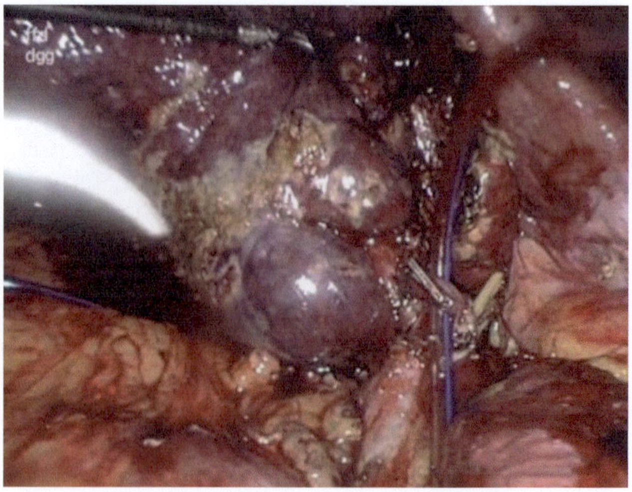

Fig. 7.17 The tourniquet should avoid the right hepatic artery

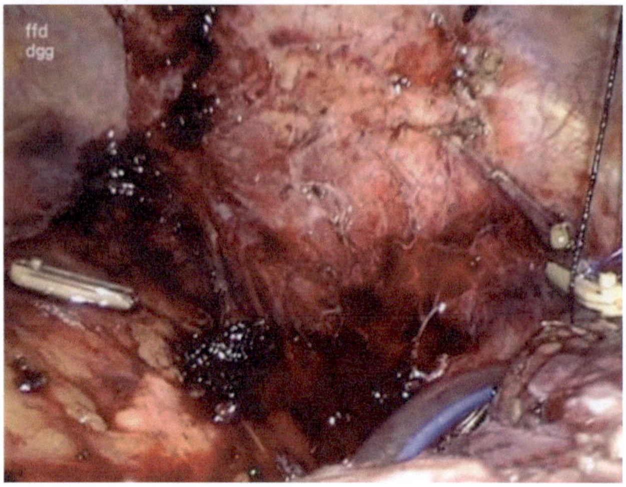

Fig. 7.16 Tourniquet indwelling

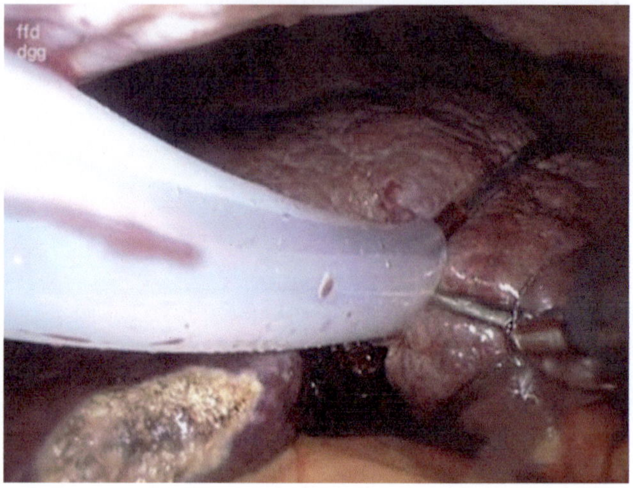

Fig. 7.18 Tourniquet tightening-up

or Prolene (Fig. 7.15). Use a guided nasogastric tube to pass through the left side of the right hepatic vein (Fig. 7.16), close the caudate lobe posteriorly and the inferior vena cava anteriorly, and then go around to the anterior of the retrohepatic tunnel, avoid the posterior of the right hepatic artery (Fig. 7.17) close to the root of the right liver pedicle and wrap it anterior to the liver, bring the two ends of the tourniquet around the liver together, and pull it out of the patient through a portal in the abdominal wall at the right midclavicular line. Put on a 36 Fr chest tube as a pressure external cannula, tighten the tourniquet (Fig. 7.18), push it in the cannula, and clamp it with a hemostat (Fig. 7.19). Before tightening, intraoperative ultrasound is used to confirm that the tumor sits on the right side of the tourniquet, ensuring that the blood flow between the left and right of the liver is completely blocked.

7.3.2.7 Drainage Tube Placement

Place an abdominal drainage tube in the porta hepatis.

7.3.2.8 Close the Incisions

Close the fascia at Trocar sites. Generally, 5/8c curved suture needles (fishhook needles) are used for suturing, and fascial incisions can also be closed using fascial closure devices and endoscopic inversion sutures. Some patients have large amounts of ascites after the first stage of ALPPS. Closing Trocar sites can prevent ascites from leaking in case of poor abdominal drainage.

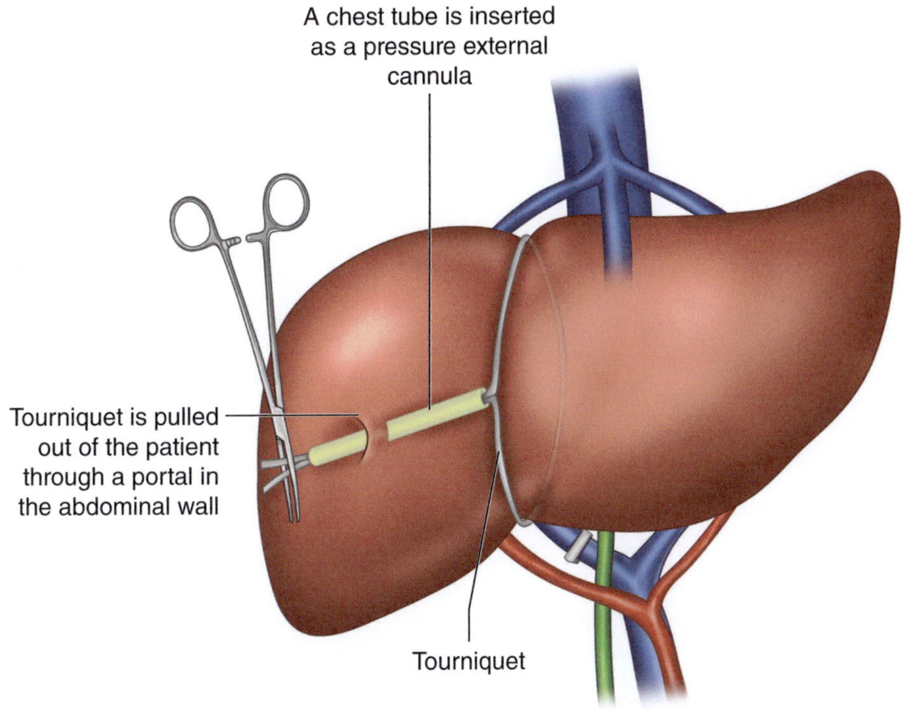

Fig. 7.19 Schematic diagram of Tourniquet ALPPS

7.3.3 Volume Remeasurement After the First Stage of ALPPS

During the interval, liver imaging examinations are generally performed 7 to 10 days after the first stage, and three-dimensional reconstruction of the liver is carried out to calculate FLR sufficiency for the second stage. If FLR is deemed insufficient, the second-stage surgery needs to be postponed, and liver imaging examinations and volume assessments will be implemented once a week.

7.3.4 Surgical Procedures for Stage 2 ALPPS

7.3.4.1 Surgical Incisions

Enter the abdomen through the original portals and establish pneumoperitoneum via CO_2.

7.3.4.2 Exploration of the Abdominal Cavity

Laparoscopic exploration to observe the existence of ascites, bleeding, and bile leakage in the abdominal cavity.

7.3.4.3 Separate Abdominal Adhesions

Carefully separate abdominal adhesions and expose the positions of the porta hepatis and the confluence of the hepatic vein and inferior vena cava.

7.3.4.4 Intraoperative Ultrasonography

Intraoperative ultrasonography examines the blood supply of the pre-preserved liver and the existence of suspicious hepatic nodules.

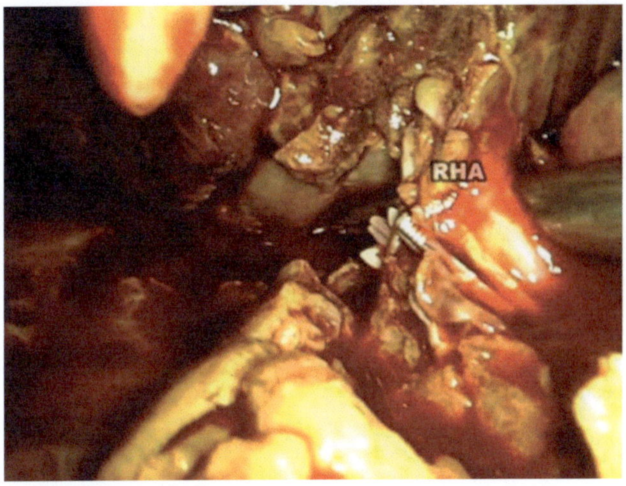

Fig. 7.20 Find the marked right hepatic artery, clamp and divide it

7.3.4.5 Dissection of the Right Hepatic Artery

Find the marked right hepatic artery at the porta hepatis, ligate it with silk sutures, clamp with absorbable clips or Hem-o-loks before dissociation (Fig. 7.20).

7.3.4.6 Liver Parenchyma Division

The assistant lifts the tourniquet outside the abdominal wall, and uses LPMOD to separate the liver parenchyma by curettage and aspiration (Fig. 7.21). Use LPMOD to cut the liver envelope, incise the liver parenchyma 3–5 mm, and then start curetting the liver tissue in a direction parallel to the tangent line. When encountering thin vessels, electrocoagulation is performed; for thick vascular structures, switch curetting

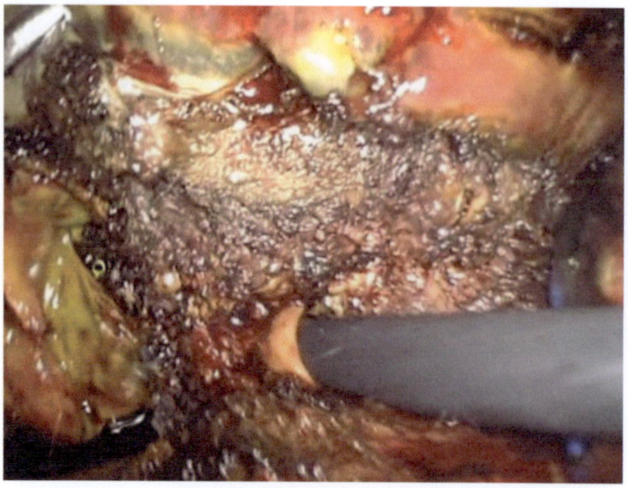

Fig. 7.21 Use LPMOD to divide liver parenchyma by curettage and aspiration

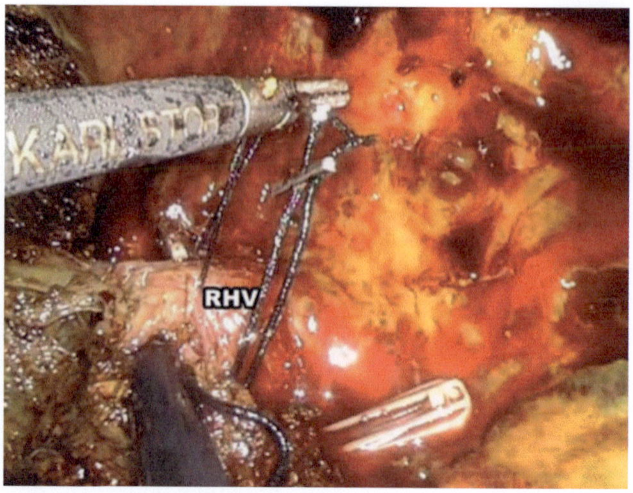

Fig. 7.23 Find the marked right hepatic vein

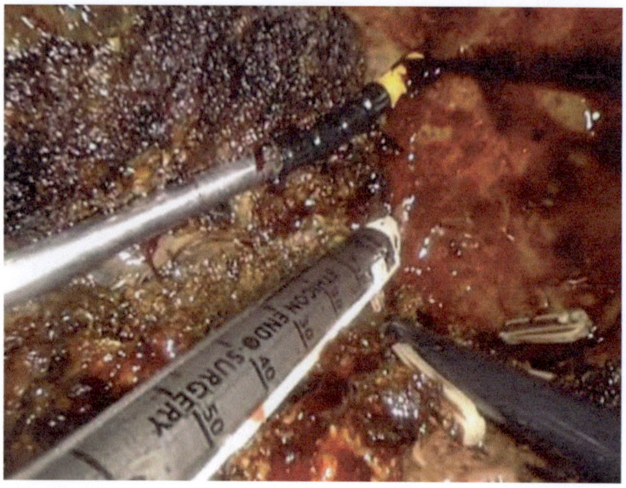

Fig. 7.22 Use a linear cutting stapler to divide the right hepatic pedicle

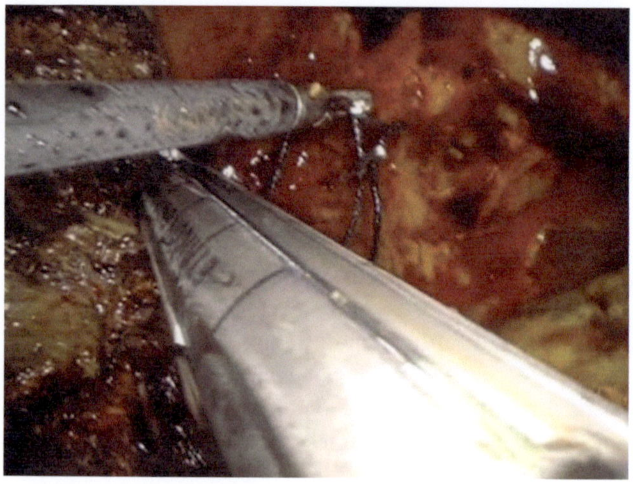

Fig. 7.24 Use a straight cutting stapler to divide the right hepatic vein

direction so that it is parallel to the tunnel, reveal a section of the path, and then apply absorbable clamps or Hem-o-loks for clamping. A linear cutting stapler can be used to assist in isolating the right hepatic pedicle (Fig. 7.22). To the confluence of the right hepatic vein and the inferior vena cava, locating the marked right hepatic vein (Fig. 7.23), use a straight cutting stapler for division (Fig. 7.24), and remove the specimen. In the process of liver dissection, the electrical coagulation can be strengthened directly against the tourniquet due to its insulating effect. There is no need to worry about injuring the deep tissues, especially the inferior vena cava inferior to the liver, which makes the process of liver transection safe and reliable.

7.3.4.7 Liver Wound Management

Drain the accumulated blood and flush the wound with clean water. Monopolar or bipolar electrocoagulation devices can be used for hemostasis in regions with small bleeding. In areas with unmanageable bleeding or bile leakage, prolene sutures need to be applied. After proper treatment, bioprotein glue or other hemostatic materials could be applied per personal preference.

7.3.4.8 Drainage Tube Placement

Place 1 drainage tube on the liver transection area. Close the incisions.

7.4 Pearls and Pitfalls of the Surgery

Traction of the tourniquet around the liver after the first stage of surgery may cause ischemia, atrophy, and necrosis of the tied-up liver tissue, and the tourniquet may become loose. It needs to be tightened 5–6 days after the operation to achieve better bundling results. Cai's ALPPS uses a tourniquet to replace conventional liver transection, avoiding bile leakage after the first stage of surgery. At the same time, it blocks the blood flow of the liver parenchyma, so that the portal vein blood flow can be redistributed, the preserved liver grows rapidly in a short period of time.

The use of laparoscopic tourniquet instead of liver parenchyma transection boasts the following advantages. First, the binding of the liver blocks the blood flow between the left and right parenchyma, contributing to the rapid increase of FLR. Second, replacing liver parenchymal transection by Tourniquet avoids bile leakage after the first stage while reducing the incidence of perioperative complications and mortality. Third, when LPMOD is applied for liver transection during the second stage, thanks to the traction of the tourniquet, there is no need to worry about damaging deep tissues, especially the inferior vena cava behind the liver, making the transection safe and reliable. Fourth, during liver transection, the Belghiti lifting technique is combined with the tourniquet to maintain a certain tension on the transected surface, which is conducive to quick and accurate division.

When performing ALPPS procedures, it is vital to protect the blood flow running out of the liver. Otherwise, it will inflict intrahepatic congestion, hepatocyte swelling, and necrosis. In particular, the treatment of the middle hepatic vein is essential. If there are no contraindications, this vein should be preserved as much as possible during the operation. During the process of tourniquet placement and upward-pulling, it is easy to cause the bile duct to be excessively stretched and angulated, leading to postoperative obstructive jaundice. Therefore, it is recommended to avoid the liver pedicle when bundling. It is best to lower the hepatic hilar plate, free the gap between the liver and the plate, and pass the tourniquet in the middle to avoid squeezing the pedicle and reduce the incidence of postoperative obstructive jaundice.

When dissecting the porta hepatis, the portal vein on the side of the lesion is ligated, the hepatic artery is freed and marked, and the right hepatic vein dissected at the confluence of hepatic vein and inferior vena cava should also be marked for identification during the second stage.

References

1. Lang SA, Loss M, Schlitt HJ. "In-situ split" (ISS) liver resection: new aspects of technique and indication[J]. Zentralbl Chir. 2014;139(2):212–9.
2. Schnitzbauer AA, Lang SA, Goessmann H, et al. Right portal vein ligation combined with in situ splitting induces rapid left lateral liver lobe hypertrophy, enabling 2-staged extended right hepatic resection in small-for-size settings[J]. Ann Surg. 2012;255(3):405–14.
3. de Santibañes E, Clavien PA. Playing Play-Doh to prevent postoperative liver failure: the "ALPPS" approach[J]. Ann Surg. 2012;255(3):415–7.
4. Li J, Girotti P, Königsrainer I, et al. ALPPS in right trisectionectomy: a safe procedure to avoid postoperative liver failure?[J]. J Gastrointest Surg. 2013;17(5):956–61.
5. Nadalin S, Capobianco I, Li J, et al. Indications and limits for associating liver partition and portal vein ligation for staged hepatectomy (ALPPS). Lessons learned from 15 cases at a single centre[J]. Z Gastroenterol. 2014;52(1):35–42.
6. Oldhafer KJ, Stavrou GA, van Gulik TM, et al. ALPPS—where do we stand, where do we go?: eight recommendations from the first international expert meeting[J]. Ann Surg. 2016;263(5):839–41.
7. Machado MA, Makdissi FF, Surjan RC. Totally laparoscopic ALPPS is feasible and may be worthwhile[J]. Ann Surg. 2012;256(3):e13.
8. Cai XJ, Tong YF, Yu H, et al. The ALPPS in the treatment of hepatitis B-related hepatocellular carcinoma with cirrhosis: a single-center study and literature review[J]. Surg Innov. 2017;24(4):358–64.
9. D'Haese JG, Neumann J, Weniger M, et al. Should ALPPS be used for liver resection in intermediate-stage HCC?[J]. Ann Surg Oncol. 2016;23(4):1335–43.
10. Wang Z, Peng YF, Hu JW, et al. Associating liver partition and portal vein ligation for staged hepatectomy for unresectable hepatitis B virus-related hepatocellular carcinoma: a single center study of 45 patients[J]. Ann Surg. 2020;271(3):534–41.

8 Radiofrequency/Microwave Ablation-Assisted ALPPS

Defei Hong and Shuyou Peng

8.1 Introduction

ALPPS is primarily used for the treatment of metastatic liver cancer (such as those from colorectal cancer and pancreatic neuroendocrine tumor) and primary hepatobiliary carcinoma (such as hepatocellular carcinoma, intrahepatic cholangiocarcinoma, and hilar cholangiocarcinoma) with insufficient future liver remnant (FLR). The significant advantages of ALPPS include the promotion of FLR hypertrophy by 47% to 110% approximately two weeks after the first stage surgery and a two-stage hepatectomy success rate of more than 95%. However, ALPPS has significant drawbacks: The postoperative morbidity and mortality rate were reported to be as high as 13.44% to 44% and 0 to 30%, respectively, because of two major surgeries with short intervals; ALPPS is against the "no touch" principle of tumor treatment, while some surgeons even regard it as an "all touch technique" that could increase the theoretical risk of cancer metastasis. The long-term efficacy of tumor treatment with ALPPS is still under observation, as the one-year recurrence rate is reported to be as high as 40%. With 70% of ALPPS procedures being done for metastatic liver cancer, clinical data of ALPPS application is relatively limited in the cases of primary liver and biliary tumors, such as hepatocellular carcinoma (HCC) and hilar cholangiocarcinoma, in patients with underlying conditions such as hepatitis B viral infection, liver fibrosis, and cirrhosis [1–6]. According to the data of the international ALPPS registry, D'Haese et al. compared the clinical outcomes of ALPPS in 35 cases of primary liver cancer and 225 cases of metastatic liver cancer. The results showed that the average FLR hypertrophy rate was 47% for primary liver cancer and 74% for metastatic liver cancer; the 90-day mortality rate was 31% for primary liver cancer and 7% for metastatic liver cancer. Statistically significant, these differences indicate variations in clinical efficacy between the two groups [6]. Major severe perioperative complications of ALPPS include biliary fistula, hepatic failure, and abdominal infection secondary to biliary fistula, with incidence up to 20%, 23%, and 24%, respectively. These complications mainly result from the physical partition of hepatic parenchyma during the first-stage surgery and the significant trauma from the ensuing second-stage surgery. Therefore, finding ways to reduce surgical trauma, minimize perioperative morbidity and mortality, and explore innovative solutions have been the focus of research in the field of ALPPS.

To prevent complications from liver transections in first-stage surgery, hepatobiliary surgeons worldwide have developed non-partition hepatic parenchymal separation techniques, which include (a) open liver separation with tourniquet modification (Robles R) [7] and laparoscopic round-the-liver ligation (Cai X) [8]. (b) radio-frequency-assisted liver partition technique reported by Tamara M.H. Gall et al. in 2015 [9], and associated microwave ablation and portal vein ligation technique by Chen Jianxun in 2015 [10]. Although these techniques have reduced the morbidity and mortality associated with ALPPS to some extent, an ensuing second liver surgery is still required. In 2016, Hong Defei and Peng Shuyou described the percutaneous microwave/radio-frequency ablation liver partition and portal vein embolization (PALPP) [11, 12] and the terminal branches portal vein embolization (TBPVE) techniques [13]. These two techniques achieve liver parenchymal partitioning or blockade of collateral circulation utilizing interventional methods, demonstrating FLR regeneration efficiency comparable to the first stage of ALPPS. They transform the two-staged ALPPS liver surgery into a single-stage procedure and realign ALPPS with the principles of a typical hepatobiliary surgical procedure.

D. Hong (✉)
Sir Run Run Shaw Hospital, Zhejiang University School of Medicine, Zhejiang, China
e-mail: hongdefei@zju.edu.cn

S. Peng
The Second Affiliated Hospital Zhejiang University School of Medicine (SAHZU), Zhejiang, China

J. Zhou (ed.), *Associating Liver Partition and Portal Vein Ligation for Staged Hepatectomy (ALPPS)*,
https://doi.org/10.1007/978-981-96-7364-3_8

8.2 Indications

In recent years, the combination of systemic therapy (namely targeted therapy and immunotherapy) and locoregional treatments (such as TACE) has set the stage for the downstaging of HCC and tumor biological transformation. To increase the long-term survival rate of patients with intermediate to advanced-staged HCC with insufficient FLR, Hong Defei and others have advocated a dual strategy that prioritizes tumor downstaging or biological transformation followed by FLR regeneration. Because a "time window" is required for HCC tumor downstaging or transformation, portal vein embolization (PVE) or its modified techniques, such as PALPP and TBPVE, are the first choice for FLR regeneration. At the same time, classical ALPPS or liver transplantation serves as the last resort [14].

8.3 Surgical Procedures

8.3.1 Radio-Frequency-Assisted (or Microwave-Assisted) Liver Separation

8.3.1.1 Open Radio-Frequency-Assisted (or Microwave-Assisted) Liver Separation with Portal Vein Ligation

In 2015, Tamara M.H. Gall et al. [9] reported the use of radio-frequency-assisted liver partition with portal vein ligation (RALPP) as an alternative to the first stage of ALPPS. A matched controlled study was conducted with five cases of RALPP compared to five cases of PVE in patients with colorectal cancer liver metastasis. The results showed 62.3% (ranging from 53.1% to 95.4%) average FLR regeneration at (21.8 ± 9.4) days after the first step of RALPP, and 24.6% (ranging from 8.4% to 35.4%) at (55.4 ± 15.6) days after PVE. Both groups had no postoperative severe complications such as bile leakage, bleeding, intra-abdominal infection, or deaths during 90-day follow-up. In 2016, Chen Jianxun et al. [10] reported a case of open associating microwave ablation and portal vein ligation for staged hepatectomy (AMAPS) in a patient with hepatocellular carcinoma and liver cirrhosis. Two and three weeks after the first-stage surgery, the future liver remnant to standard liver volume ratio (FLR/SLV) increased from 29.1% preoperatively to 40.9% and 51.2%, respectively. The right hepatectomy was performed three weeks after the first-stage surgery, with no adhesion identified during the procedure, 200 mL intraoperative blood loss, and 100 minutes of surgical time. The patient experienced no surgical morbidities and was discharged seven days after surgery.

8.3.1.2 Laparoscopic or Robotic Liver Separation with Microwave (or Radio-Frequency) Ablation

In 2015, Enrico Gringeri et al. [15] reported a case of laparoscopic microwave ablation and portal vein ligation for staged hepatectomy (LAPS). The patient was a 66-year-old male with a 20 cm right liver mass (postoperative pathology confirmed hepatocellular carcinoma, grade G_1) that invaded the right hepatic vein and middle hepatic vein. In the first stage of operation, intraoperative ultrasound identified a tumor margin 3 cm away from the ablation surface, then liver parenchymal partitioning with microwave ablation and ligation of the right branch of the portal vein. Nine days after that, the FLR increased from 390 mL to 693 mL (an increase of 77.7%). A right hepatectomy was performed on the 10th day, and the patient was discharged on the 12th day after the second procedure. In the same year, Umberto Cillo et al. [16] reported a case of LAPS in a patient with liver metastasis of colon cancer where the FLR increased by 90.4% on the 15th day after the first-stage procedure. No perioperative complications or deaths were documented following liver resection.

In 2016, Long R. Jiao et al. [17] and Ugo Boggi et al. [18] reported individual cases of success with laparoscopic radiofrequency-assisted liver partition with portal vein ligation (LRALPP) in treating patients with colon cancer liver metastasis and hilar cholangiocarcinoma without any complications or deaths. Long R. Jiao et al. have been known to have managed more than 20 cases of insufficient FLR in liver cancer using LRALPP, with successful and favorable outcomes.

8.3.1.3 Percutaneous Microwave/Radio-Frequency Ablation Liver Separation

The two-stage hepatectomy techniques, namely open or laparoscopic liver parenchymal separation with the use of round-the-liver tourniquet maneuver and open or laparoscopic radiofrequency/microwave liver parenchymal separation, have to some extent reduced the morbidity and mortality associated with the ALPPS procedure. However, patients still have to endure the risks, pain, and medical expenses of the ensuing second liver surgery. In 2016, based on preclinical animal experiments, Hong Defei et al. reported the first percutaneous microwave/radiofrequency ablation liver partition and portal vein embolization (PALPP) technique for the treatment of large or multiple hepatocellular carcinoma and hilar cholangiocarcinoma with insufficient FLR [9, 10]. The procedure consists of two steps. The first step constitutes percutaneous microwave or radiofrequency liver parenchymal partitioning, followed by the second step two days later, which involves percutaneous portal venography to establish collateral vessel occlusion before the tumor-side portal vein is embolized with coils and gelatin sponges. Two weeks after PALPP, when FLR and liver function become eligible, the hepatectomy to remove the liver tumor is to be conducted. After three cases of success, the authors modified the procedure by performing concomitant first and second steps. This means that after percutaneous microwave or radiofrequency liver parenchymal partitioning, the portal vein of the tumor side is embolized during the same procedure (Figs. 8.1, 8.2, 8.3, 8.4, 8.5, 8.6, 8.7, and 8.8). Patients with hilar cholangio-

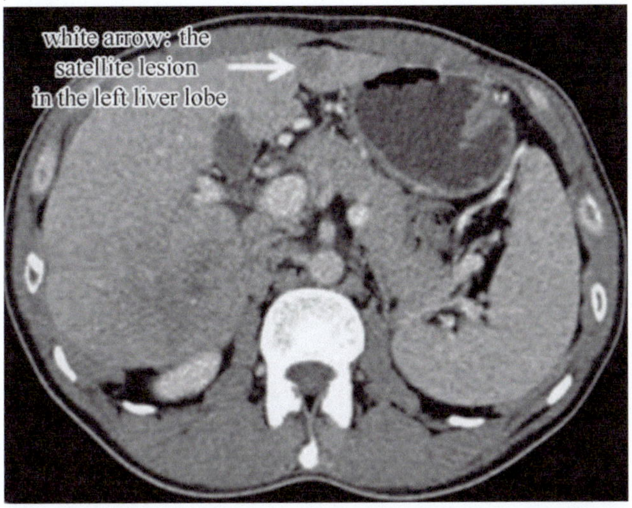

Fig. 8.1 A massive liver cancer in the right liver lobe with a satellite lesion in the left liver lobe on contrast-enhanced CT

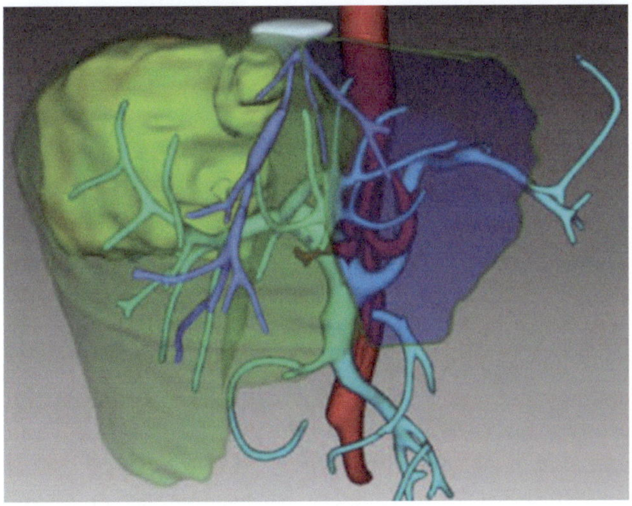

Fig. 8.2 The planning of right trisegmentectomy of the liver. CT three-dimensional reconstruction calculating SLV at 1231.2 mL and FLR 355.6 mL, FLR/SLV 28.9%

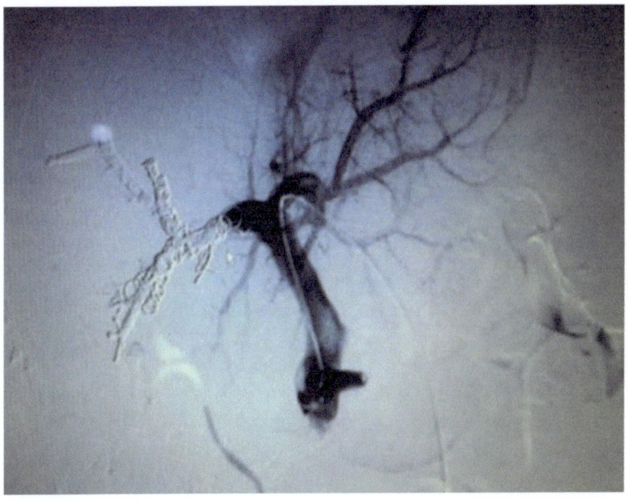

Fig. 8.3 The right portal vein is embolized using coils and a gelatin sponge

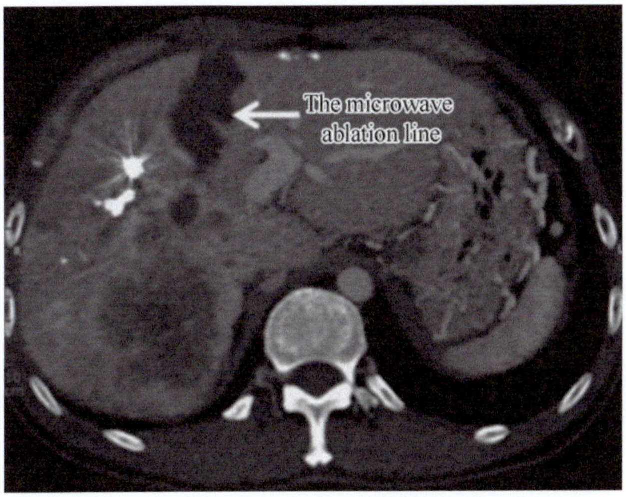

Fig. 8.4 A significant increase in the FLR (the left lateral lobe) on CT examination one week after the PALPP procedure (with concomitant percutaneous injection of absolute alcohol into the satellite lesion in the left liver lobe)

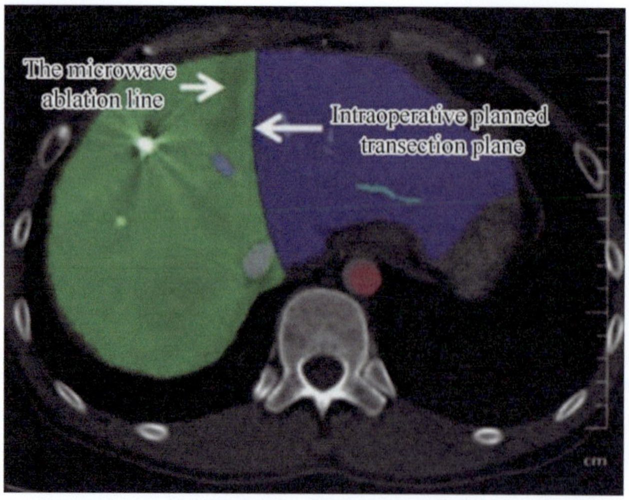

Fig. 8.5 CT three-dimensional reconstruction to calculate the volume of the left lateral lobe two weeks after the PALPP procedure. FLR (blue area) measured 502.1 mL, FLR/SLV 40.8%, an increase of 41.2%

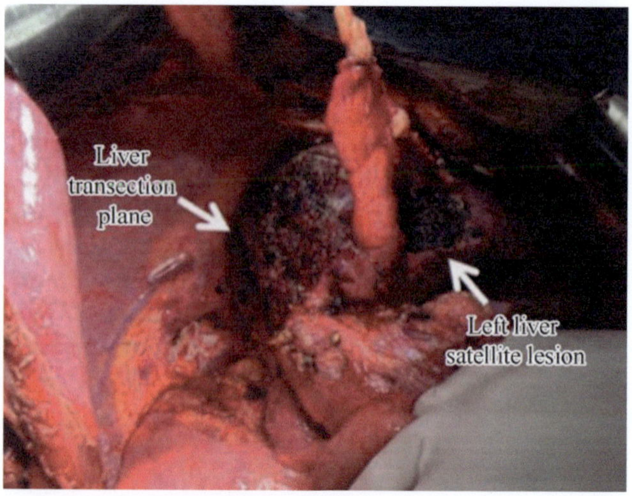

Fig. 8.7 Intraoperative view after the right trisegmentectomy and local resection of the satellite lesion in the left liver

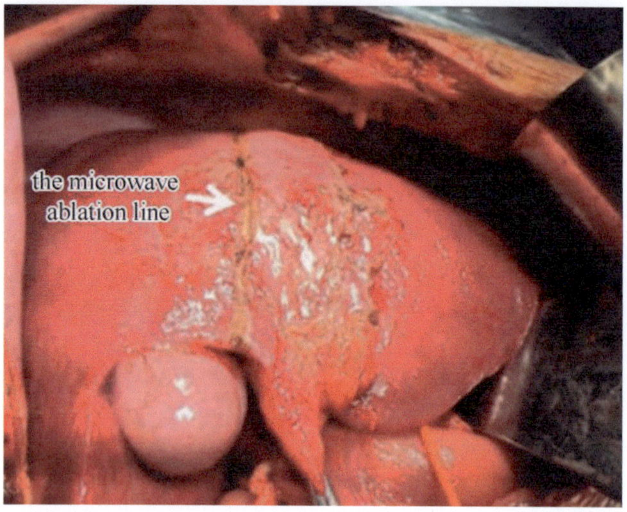

Fig. 8.6 Image from the liver resection surgery where the microwave ablation plane is identified, free of significant perihepatic adhesion

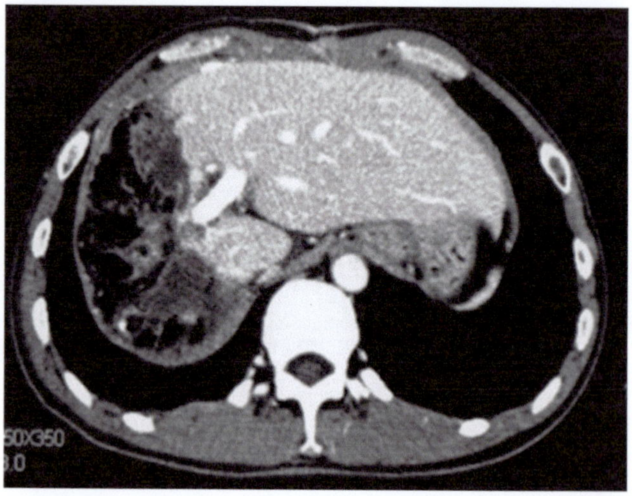

Fig. 8.8 Continued enlargement of the lateral lobe of the left liver one week after the right trisegmentectomy

carcinoma often present with jaundice. In severe cases, percutaneous transhepatic cholangial drainage (PTCD) can be performed to reduce jaundice before the PALPP procedure.

PALPP, a modification of the ALPPS procedure, replaces the first stage operation of ALPPS with percutaneous microwave or radiofrequency ablation liver parenchymal partitioning. This approach avoids the liver mobilization, flipping, and compression of liver tumors in the first stage of ALPPS, and the bile leakage and bleeding caused by physical liver parenchymal partitioning. It also prevents the development of peritoneal adhesion caused by the surgical separation or abdominal infection in ALPPS stage 1, thereby reducing the risks associated with the second stage of surgery. PALPP maximizes the minimally invasive nature of the liver parenchymal partitioning in ALPPS stage one, transforming the two-stage ALPPS procedure into a single surgery. By promoting rapid regeneration of the FLR in a short time, PALPP resolves the fundamental causes of severe morbidity and mortality associated with ALPPS and facilitates the second stage of liver resection surgery. By ensuring the "no touch" principle during liver tumor resection, PALPP may improve the theoretical long-term survival rates (Fig. 8.9).

From January 2016 to July 2018, 20 patients with primary liver cancer, metastatic liver cancer, and hilar cholangiocarcinoma with insufficient FLR underwent PALPP treatment.

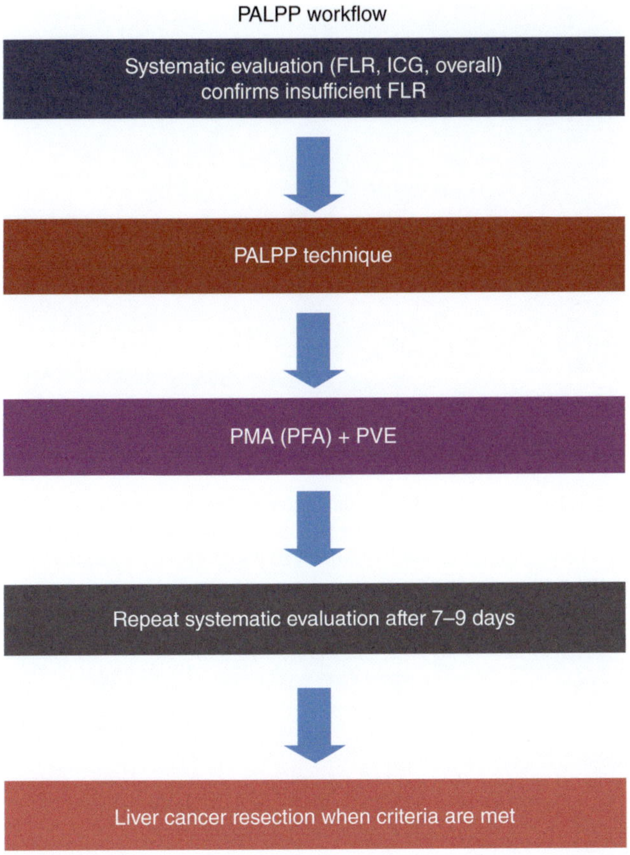

Fig. 8.9 PALPP workflow (PMA: percutaneous microwave ablation liver partition; PFA: percutaneous radio-frequency ablation liver partition)

Among the 20 patients, the average age was (56 ± 5.4) years, with a male-to-female ratio of 9:1. Of them, 13 had hepatocellular carcinoma (HCC), 3 hilar cholangiocarcinoma, and 4 liver metastasis from colorectal cancer. Of the 20 patients, 16 underwent hepatectomy while 4 did not, 2 due to inadequate compensatory liver volume after PALPP, and the other 2 poor post-PALPP liver function recovery (hypoalbuminemia). Among the 16 patients who underwent hepatectomy, the average preoperative FLR was 362.53 mL, accounting for 30.77% of the Standardized Liver Volume (SLV). The average interval between PALPP and hepatectomy was 9.33 days, and the average increase in FLR was 51.02%. Among the 16 hepatectomy cases, 2 experienced hepatic insufficiency, 1 bile leakage, and 5 pleural effusions after surgery, all of which were treated conservatively. No deaths were documented within 90 days after surgery. Some cases received adjuvant transcatheter arterial chemoembolization (TACE) and/or sorafenib. During a follow-up period of 5 to 28 months, 72.7% of patients experienced intrahepatic recurrence and lung metastasis, or both, but 80.2% of the patients remained alive with tumor presence. Those who did not undergo liver resection survived for more than 14 months, and one of them received a liver transplantation.

In contrast to ALPPS, PALPP has the following advantages in addition to promoting rapid FLR growth within two weeks: Firstly, PALPP eliminates severe complications such as perilesional adhesions and bile leakage, allowing more flexibility in the timing of the liver resection surgery. In contrast, ALPPS posts a strict time limit for the second-stage liver resection surgery (ideally within two weeks) to prevent significant adhesion. Secondly, the in situ liver parenchymal partitioning with microwave or radiofrequency ablation and PVE on the tumor side is consistent with the "no touch" principle, avoiding tumor dissemination due to liver mobilization and tumor flipping in ALPPS stage one. When metastatic lesions are present in the remnant liver, temporary control through alcohol injection or microwave or radiofrequency ablation can be applied simultaneously. Thirdly, since the vascular communication along the liver partition has been disrupted by ablation, liver resection along the ablation plane significantly reduces bleeding and bile leakage. Fourthly, the inflammatory mediators produced by microwave or radiofrequency ablation enter the bloodstream, accelerating FLR growth. In addition, PALPP significantly reduces complications and medical costs, making it a routine liver resection procedure with high patient acceptance. It can also be applied to the resection of large liver tumors with undesirable predicted margins, thereby improving the R0 resection rate for liver cancer. Lastly, the first step involves interventional techniques, exerting minimal impact on liver function or the occurrence of severe complications. Since no foreign objects are left in the patient's body, even if the patient declines liver resection for various reasons or if the remnant liver function does not meet the criteria for liver resection, the patient's quality of life is not compromised. The embolization of the tumor side portal vein and the thermal partitioning of the liver using microwave or radiofrequency are also beneficial for controlling liver cancer growth and preventing metastasis to the healthy side. Targeted therapies and immunotherapies alone or with other approaches, such as TACE, can be selected to control the tumor, thereby improving the patient's quality of life and survival benefits. However, the drawback is that percutaneous ablation of liver parenchymal partitioning is technically demanding, and caution should be exercised to avoid injury to the hepatic veins and bile ducts of the remnant liver side [11, 12].

To avoid injury to the inferior vena cava, percutaneous microwave or radiofrequency ablation, the liver parenchymal partitioning technique cannot completely separate the liver like the first stage of ALPPS surgery. Liver parenchyma within 1 cm of the inferior vena cava defies ablation and separation, but leaving it during the procedure does not affect the FLR growth efficiency. In this study of 20 cases, 16 underwent liver resection, and the average FLR increased by 51.02% after 9 days. In 2015, Henrik Petrowsky et al. compared 18 cases of partial liver partitioning ALPPS (p-ALPPS) with 18 cases of classical ALPPS (all cases were liver metastasis from colon cancer). In the p-ALPPS group, 50% to 80% of the liver parenchyma was separated. The FLR increased by 60% and 61% respectively after the first stage of surgery. The p-ALPPS group had no in-hospital deaths, while the ALPPS group had a mortality rate of 22% (4/18), including one case of heart failure and three cases of liver failure leading to multi-organ failure [19].

8.3.2 Terminal Branches Portal Vein Embolization and Liver Partitioning

In 2016, Peng Shuyou et al. [11] reported the use of terminal branches portal vein embolization (TBPVE) for the treatment of hepatocellular carcinoma with insufficient FLR in the presence of liver cirrhosis. TBPVE effectively blocks the communication between liver segments at the peripheral portal vein level. The procedural steps are as follows: based on a three-dimensional imaging model of the portal vein, the embolization plan is developed, and various puncture points into the liver segments are selected based on the location of portal vein embolization. After that, the planned puncture points are administered with local anesthesia before being accessed with a 21G Chiba liver puncture needle. A small amount of contrast agent is injected when the needle tip reaches the predetermined site to confirm the portal vein branch. A guidewire is then introduced, and a percutaneous transhepatic biliary drainage catheter is exchanged through the liver puncture and advanced into the portal vein trunk before being exchanged for a 5F catheter. A 5F angiographic catheter is used to perform portal vein angiography and pressure measurement near the mesenteric vein. Then, a microcatheter is exchanged and advanced into the selected branch for embolization. Under fluoroscopy, an appropriate amount of surgical adhesive (α-cyanoacrylate) mixed with ethiodized oil emulsion (at a ratio of 1:4) is slowly injected for embolization. Peripheral portal veins are embolized first, followed by gradual embolization of the main branches of the portal vein until blood flow in the target vessels stops. To complete the procedure, coils are used as appropriate to embolize the right/left main branch of the portal vein. During PVE in the first step, embolic agents are applied to the peripheral portal veins of segments 5 and 8 (or segment 4). Then the right main branch/left main branch of the portal vein is embolized with coils, achieving blockage of the communication between the left and right sides and driving all portal vein blood into the tumor-free side of the portal vein (Figs. 8.10 and 8.11) [20].

In 2021, Peng Shuyou et al. reported the results of a study involving 150 cases of TBPVE for the treatment of HCC with insufficient FLR. The results are as follows: within 2 weeks after TBPVE, 100% of the cases recovered FLR and reached the resection criteria. Among the 53 cases who underwent liver resection, 20.8% had postoperative complications, such as ascites. One case (1.9%) experienced bleeding and subsequent hepatic failure and death. The 1-year and 3-year survival rates were 87.5% and 64.5%, and the disease-free survival rates were 64.7% and 40.6%, respectively. Subgroup analysis of patients who received TACE before liver resection showed that the 1-year and 3-year survival rates and disease-free survival rates were 87.5%, 65.0%, 75.0%, and 42.1% for the TACE group, and 85.2%, 60.0%, 62.0%, and 25.7% for the non-TACE group. The 3-year survival rate and 1-year and 3-year disease-free survival rates between the two groups were significantly different ($P < 0.05$). Among the 97 patients who underwent TBPVE

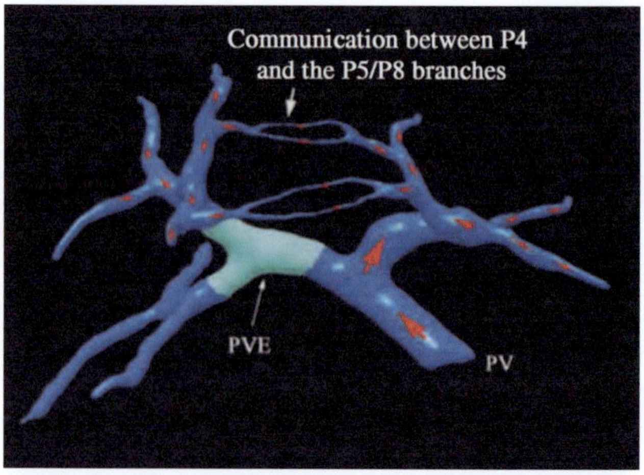

Fig. 8.10 In traditional PVE, only the right/left branches of the portal vein are embolized, and it is not possible to embolize the communication between P5, P8, and P4 [20]. PVE: portal vein embolization; PV: portal vein

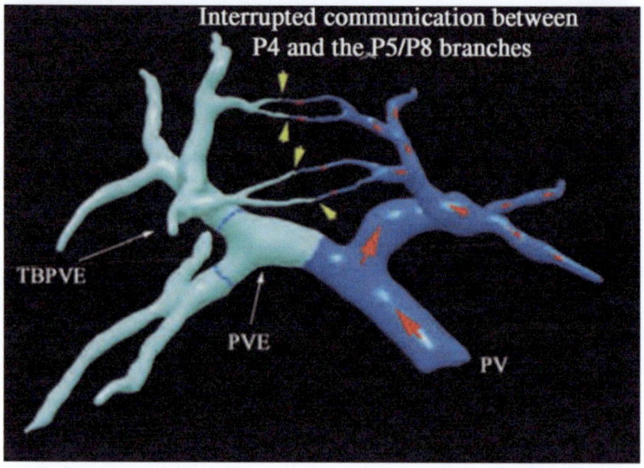

Fig. 8.11 Blockade of the communication between P5, P8, and P4 by TBPVE, as well as the right branch of the portal vein [20]. TBPVE: terminal branches portal vein embolization; PVE: portal vein embolization; PV: portal vein

combined with TACE but did not undergo liver resection, the 1-year and 3-year survival rates were 80.1% and 53.7% (some also received targeted and immune therapy). These findings indicate that TBPVE can safely and effectively promote rapid regeneration of FLR to meet the requirements for surgical resection. Furthermore, the combination of TBPVE and TACE can further improve patient prognosis, confirming the importance of downstaging in the treatment of liver cancer [21].

The advantages of the TBPVE parenchymal separation technique are as follows: As it eliminates the need for the classical ALPPS stage-one procedure, it avoids complications such as bile leakage, bleeding, and abdominal infection that can occur after the classical ALPPS stage-one procedure, and minimizes surgical insult and economic burden of patients. Nevertheless, the disadvantages include a possible ectopic embolization, and the inability to address cases with tumor thrombus in the right or left branches of the portal vein, as the guidewire may dislodge the tumor thrombus. The authors believe that TBPVE is currently the least invasive, safest, and most cost-effective technique for FLR induction.

Currently, ALPPS is rarely performed for biliary tumors because studies revealed higher rates of morbidity and mortality, such as bile leakage, hepatic failure, and severe abdominal infection. Research results from the international ALPPS registry and others have shown its 90-day mortality rates for hilar cholangiocarcinoma, intrahepatic cholangiocarcinoma, and gallbladder cancer were 27%, 13%, and 33%, respectively. A matched comparison study of 29 cases undergoing ALPPS and radical surgery for hilar cholangiocarcinoma showed that the 90-day mortality rate in the ALPPS group was twice that of the radical surgery group (48% vs 24%), with the median overall survival of 6 and 27 months, respectively [21–23]. Our team has achieved favorable results using TBPVE in patients with hilar cholangiocarcinoma and intrahepatic cholangiocarcinoma with insufficient FLR (Figs. 8.12, 8.13, and 8.14).

In conclusion, ALPPS is a revolutionary but cost-intensive technique. The innovative techniques of non-partitioning parenchymal separation are as revolutionary as ALPPS in the rapid FLR regeneration while significantly reducing the heavy cost of high-grade morbidity and mortality associated with ALPPS. In particular, techniques such as PALPP and TBPVE require only one intervention and one hepatic sur-

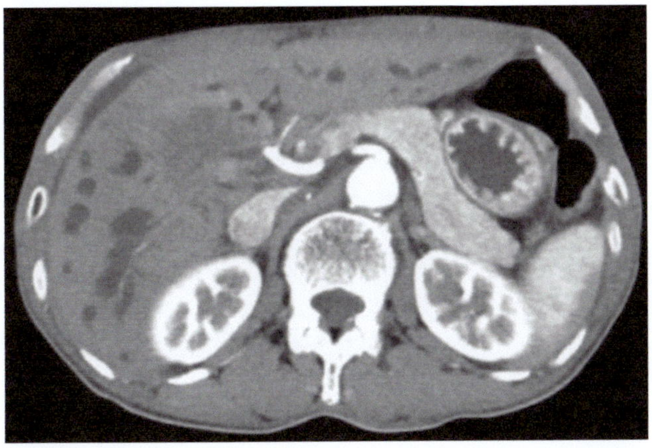

Fig. 8.12 Hilar cholangiocarcinoma revealed in preoperative enhanced CT. A right trisegmentectomy is planned

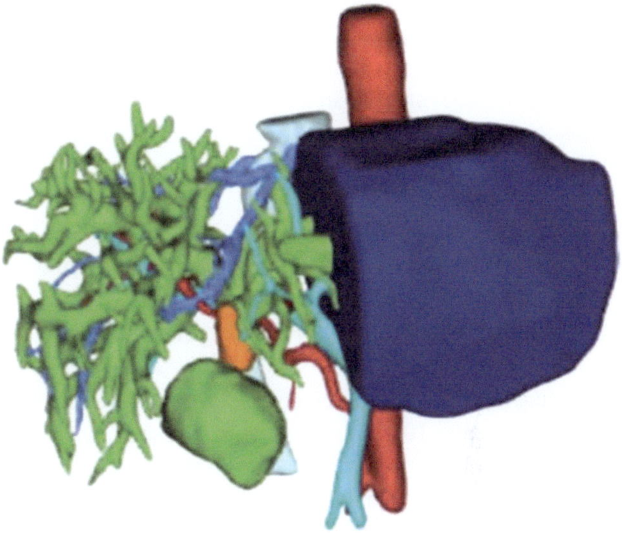

Fig. 8.13 Volume of the left lateral lobe (FLR) at 503 mL, SLV 1702 mL, and the FLR/SLV ratio 29.6% on three-dimensional CT reconstruction

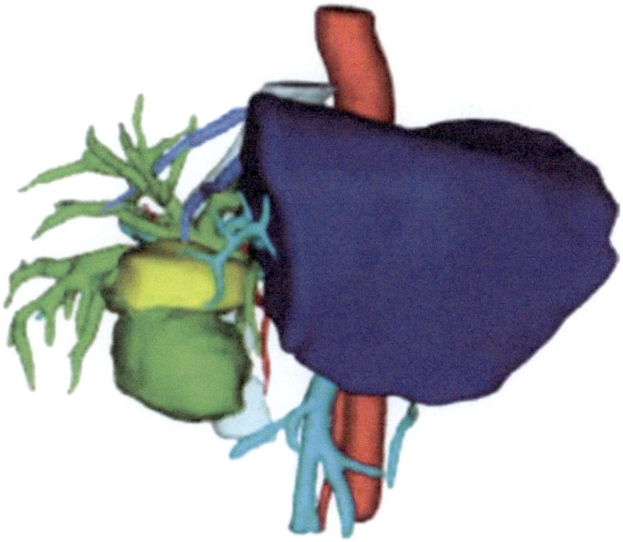

Fig. 8.14 FLR (left lateral lobe) at 610 mL, SLV 1383 mL, and the FLR/SLV ratio 44.1% two weeks after TBPVE

gery to accomplish the surgical resection of advanced-stage liver cancer and hilar cholangiocarcinoma with insufficient FLR. This reflects the modern surgical concept that prioritizes patients and fully utilizes the wisdom, skills, and teamwork of multidisciplinary experts. It is worth discussing how we can maximize patient benefit by applying 3D digital reconstruction and selecting justifiable non-separation parenchymal partitioning techniques based on different stages of disease (mainly the presence or absence of portal vein tumor thrombus), characteristics and locations of liver and biliary tumors, and the technical competence in various hospitals. Additionally, hepatobiliary surgeons and experts worldwide should investigate and address several topics: multi-center studies on non-separation parenchymal partitioning techniques and research on FLR regeneration mechanisms and their impact on the biological behavior of liver tumors.

8.4 Advocating for a Dual Strategy Where Tumor Biology Conversion Takes Precedence Over FLR Regeneration

Analyzing the clinical efficacy of ALPPS in the treatment of HCC over the past 10 years, we recognized a shift away from a pessimistic outlook. However, perioperative morbidity and mortality rates remain relatively high. The 3-year overall survival rate is higher than that of transcatheter arterial chemoembolization (TACE), but the 5-year survival rate is not improved compared to two-stage hepatectomy after portal vein embolization (PVE) [24–28]. The reason behind this is that HCC with insufficient FLR is a typical advanced disease predisposed to recurrence and metastasis. ALPPS only achieves surgical resection but does not achieve biological resection. Previous studies have shown that for intermediate and advanced HCC, downstaging with TACE or selective internal radiation therapy followed by resection can result in a 5-year survival rate comparable to that of early-stage HCC resection [29, 30]. TACE only achieves resection in less than 20% of liver cancer patients after downstaging, but in recent years, significant progress in combined targeted therapy and immunotherapy for HCC has provided an opportunity for downstaging or conversion, which will undoubtedly revolutionize the traditional two-stage hepatectomy based on "tumor downstaging or conversion" without relying on the ALPPS-induced rapid FLR regeneration [31–33]. Therefore, in order to improve long-term survival rates for intermediate and advanced HCC with insufficient FLR, the authors recommend a dual strategy with a focus on tumor downstaging and biological conversion, followed by FLR regeneration, the preferred methods for FLR regeneration are TBPVE, PALPP, or PVE (Figs. 8.15, 8.16, 8.17, 8.18, 8.19, and 8.20), the classical ALPPS or liver transplantation considered as the last resort [14].

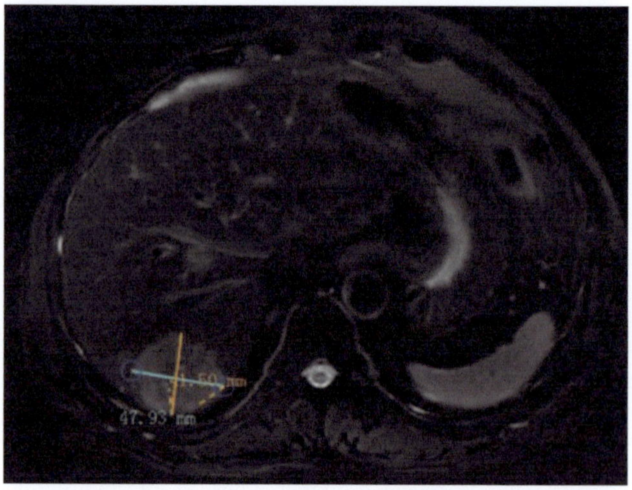

Fig. 8.15 Enhanced liver MR revealing multiple lesions in the right liver (metastatic foci from hepatic central veins), consistent with intrahepatic cholangiocarcinoma. Liver biopsy and immunohistochemistry report intrahepatic cholangiocarcinoma

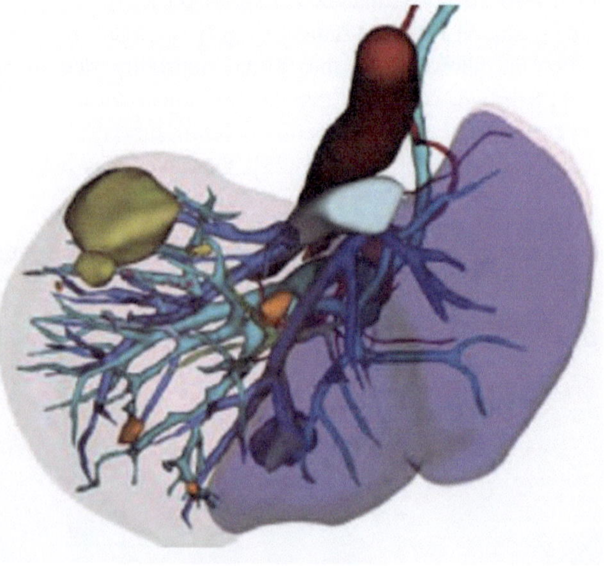

Fig. 8.16 FLR (left liver lobe) volume at 427 mL, with an FLR/SLV ratio of 31.54% on CT three-dimensional reconstruction

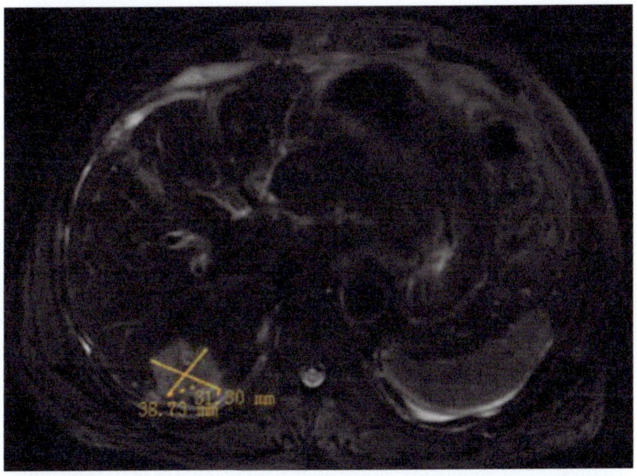

Fig. 8.17 After 2 cycles of GEMOX chemotherapy combined with targeted immunotherapy (camrelizumab and apatinib), a follow-up MR examination showed size reduction in the multiple malignant tumor lesions in the right liver and the elimination of the lesions adjacent to the hepatic central veins, evidence of established biological transformation resulting in FLR regeneration

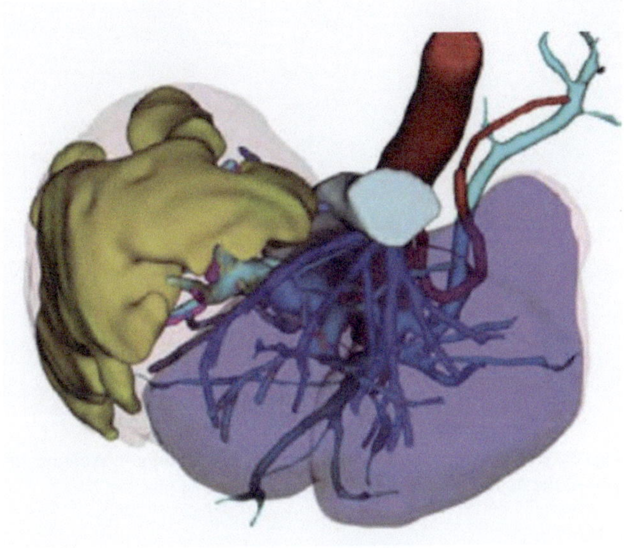

Fig. 8.19 FLR volume at 582 mL, with an FLR/SLV ratio of 43.1% on CT three-dimensional reconstruction

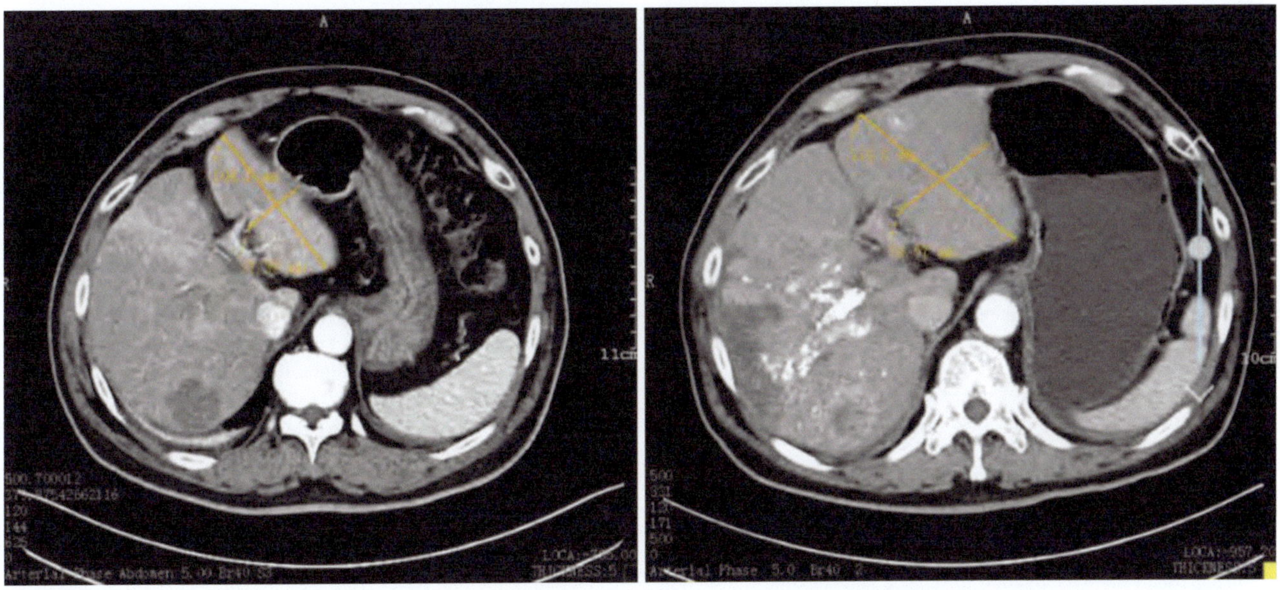

Fig. 8.18 A significant increase in the size of the FLR in the left hepatic lobe on CT reevaluation three weeks after TBPVE combined with TACE

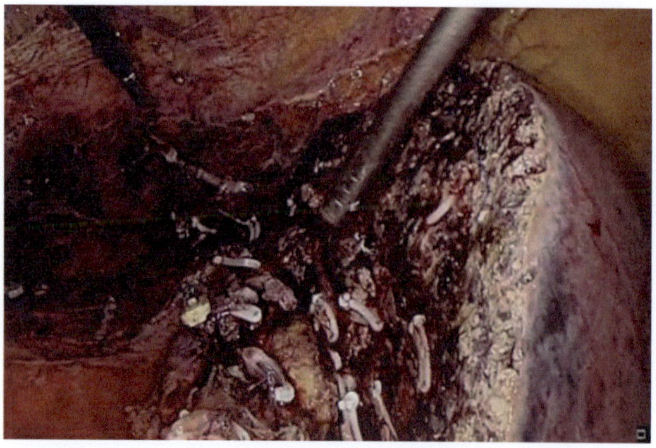

Fig. 8.20 Laparoscopic anatomical right hepatectomy + skeletonization of the hepatoduodenal ligament

References

1. Wu H, Pan G. Associating liver partition and portal vein ligation for staged hepatectomy[M]/Operative Techniques in Liver Resection. Dordrecht: Springer Netherlands; 2015. p. 249–54.
2. Lau WY, Lai EC, Lau SH. Associating liver partition and portal vein ligation for staged hepatectomy: the current role and development[J]. Hepatobiliary Pancreat Dis Int. 2017;16(1):17–26.
3. Schadde E, Ardiles V, Robles-Campos R, et al. Early survival and safety of ALPPS: first report of the International ALPPS Registry[J]. Ann Surg. 2014;260(5):829–38.
4. Troja A, Khatib-Chahidi K, El-Sourani N, et al. ALPPS and similar resection procedures in treating extensive hepatic metastases: our own experiences and critical discussion[J]. Int J Surg. 2014;12(9):1020–2.
5. Schadde E, Ardiles V, Slankamenac K, et al. ALPPS offers a better chance of complete resection in patients with primarily unresectable liver tumors compared with conventional-staged hepatectomies: results of a multicenter analysis[J]. World J Surg. 2014;38(6):1510–9.
6. D'Haese JG, Neumann J, Weniger M, et al. Should ALPPS be used for liver resection in intermediate-stage HCC?[J]. Ann Surg Oncol. 2016;23(4):1335–43.
7. Robles R, Parrilla P, López-Conesa A, et al. Tourniquet modification of the associating liver partition and portal ligation for staged hepatectomy procedure[J]. Br J Surg. 2014;101(9):1129–34.
8. Cai XJ, Peng SY, Duan L, et al. Completely laparoscopic ALPPS using round-the-liver ligation to replace parenchymal transection for a patient with multiple right liver cancers complicated with liver cirrhosis[J]. J Laparoendosc Adv Surg Tech A. 2014;24(12):883–6.
9. Gall TM, Sodergren MH, Frampton AE, et al. Radio-frequency-assisted liver partition with portal vein ligation (RALPP) for liver regeneration[J]. Ann Surg. 2015;261(2):e45–6.
10. Chen JX, Ran HQ, Sun CQ. Associating microwave ablation and portal vein ligation for staged hepatectomy for the treatment of huge hepatocellular carcinoma with cirrhosis[J]. Ann Surg Treat Res. 2016;90(5):287–91.
11. Hong DF, Zhang YB, Peng SY, et al. Percutaneous microwave ablation liver partition and portal vein embolization for rapid liver regeneration: a minimally invasive first step of ALPPS for hepatocellular carcinoma[J]. Ann Surg. 2016;264(1):e1–2.
12. Zhang YB, Hong DF, Fan XM, et al. Percutaneous microwave/radiofrequency ablation liver partition and portal vein embolization for planned hepatectomy for colorectal liver metastases with insufficient future liver remnant[J]. Chin J Oncol. 2017;39(7):545–6.
13. Peng SY, Huang CY, Li JT, et al. Terminal branches portal vein embolization for planed hepatectomy[J]. Chin J Surg. 2016;54(9):664–8.
14. Hong DF, Peng SY, Wanyee YY. Ten-year retrospect of ALPPS in the treatment of hepatocellular carcinoma: an eternal concept with cautious technologic choice[J]. Zhonghua Wai Ke Za Zhi. 2022;60(2):113–6.
15. Gringeri E, Boetto R, D'Amico FE, et al. Laparoscopic microwave ablation and portal vein ligation for staged hepatectomy (LAPS): a minimally invasive first-step approach[J]. Ann Surg. 2015;261(2):e42–3.
16. Cillo U, Gringeri E, Feltracco P, et al. Totally laparoscopic microwave ablation and portal vein ligation for staged hepatectomy: a new minimally invasive two-stage hepatectomy[J]. Ann Surg Oncol. 2015;22(8):2787–8.
17. Jiao LR, Hakim DN, Gall TM, et al. A totally laparoscopic associating liver partition and portal vein ligation for staged hepatectomy assisted with radiofrequency (radiofrequency assisted liver partition with portal vein ligation) for staged liver resection[J]. Hepatobiliary Surg Nutr. 2016;5(4):382–7.
18. Boggi U, Napoli N, Kauffmann EF, et al. Laparoscopic microwave liver ablation and portal vein ligation: an alternative approach to the conventional ALPPS procedure in hilar cholangiocarcinoma[J]. Ann Surg Oncol. 2016;23(Suppl 5):884.
19. Petrowsky H, Györi G, de Oliveira M, et al. Is partial-ALPPS safer than ALPPS? A single-center experience[J]. Ann Surg. 2015;261(4):e90–2.
20. Peng SY, Wang XA, Huang CY, et al. Evolution of associating liver partition and portal vein ligation for staged hepatectomy: simpler, safer and equally effective methods[J]. World J Gastroenterol. 2017;23(23):4140–5.
21. Peng SY, Huang CY, Wang XA, et al. The clinical value of terminal branches portal vein embolization for hepatocellular carcinoma with insufficient future liver remnant[J]. Chin J Surg. 2021;59(10):829–35.
22. Lang H, de Santibanes E, Clavien PA. Outcome of ALPPS for perihilar cholangiocarcinoma: case-control analysis including the first series from the international ALPPS registry[J]. HPB (Oxford). 2017;19(5):379–80.
23. Olthof PB, Coelen RJS, Wiggers JK, et al. High mortality after ALPPS for perihilar cholangiocarcinoma: case-control analysis including the first series from the international ALPPS registry[J]. HPB. 2017;19(5):381–7.
24. Cai XJ, Tong YF, Yu H, et al. The ALPPS in the treatment of hepatitis B-related hepatocellular carcinoma with cirrhosis: a single-center study and literature review[J]. Surg Innov. 2017;24(4):358–64.
25. Xiang F, Hu ZM. Chance and challenge of associating liver partition and portal vein ligation for staged hepatectomy[J]. Hepatobiliary Pancreat Dis Int. 2019;18(3):214–22.
26. Chan A, Zhang WY, Chok K, et al. ALPPS versus portal vein embolization for hepatitis-related hepatocellular carcinoma: a chang-

ing paradigm in modulation of future liver remnant before major hepatectomy[J]. Ann Surg. 2021;273(5):957–65.
27. Li PP, Huang G, Jia NY, et al. Associating liver partition and portal vein ligation for staged hepatectomy versus sequential transarterial chemoembolization and portal vein embolization in staged hepatectomy for HBV-related hepatocellular carcinoma: a randomized comparative study[J]. Hepatobiliary Surg Nutr. 2022;11(1):38–51.
28. Wang Z, Peng YF, Hu JW, et al. Associating liver partition and portal vein ligation for staged hepatectomy for unresectable hepatitis B virus-related hepatocellular carcinoma: a single center study of 45 patients[J]. Ann Surg. 2020;271(3):534–41.
29. Fan J, Tang ZY, Yu YQ, et al. Improved survival with resection after transcatheter arterial chemoembolization (TACE) for unresectable hepatocellular carcinoma[J]. Dig Surg. 1998;15(6):674–8.
30. Zhao HT, San XT, Rui JA, et al. Clinical efficacy of hepatectomy after down-staging treatments in patients with unresectable advanced primary liver cancer[J]. Acta Acad Med Sin. 2009;31(4):503–5.
31. Kudo M, Ueshima K, Chan S, et al. Lenvatinib as an initial treatment in patients with intermediate-stage hepatocellular carcinoma beyond up-to-seven criteria and child-pugh A liver function: a proof-of-concept study[J]. Cancers. 2019;11(8):1084.
32. Alliance of Liver Cancer Conversion Therapy, Committee of Liver Cancer of the Chinese Anti-Cancer Association. Chinese expert consensus on conversion therapy for hepatocellular carcinoma (2021 edition)[J]. Chin J Practical Surg. 2021;41(6):618–32.
33. Lau WY, Ho SK, Yu SC, et al. Salvage surgery following down-staging of unresectable hepatocellular carcinoma[J]. Ann Surg. 2004;240(2):299–305.

Partial ALPPS

9

Zheng Wang and Jie Hu

9.1 Introduction

Associating liver partition and portal vein ligation for staged hepatectomy (ALPPS), representing a revolutionary approach in the realm of liver cancer treatment over the last decade, can induce rapid future liver remnant (FLR) hypertrophy within a brief timeframe, offering renewed resection opportunities for patients with liver tumors (e.g., giant liver tumors) previously deemed unresectable because of an inadequate FLR volume and providing survival benefits to these patients [1]. Nonetheless, the mortality and complication rates are greater following the ALPPS procedure as compared to the conventional hepatic surgery. When initially implemented [2], the ALPPS procedure confers high rates of major complications (44%) and mortality (12%), hindering its widespread adoption and application.

As surgical techniques are continuously refined and case inclusion criteria become increasingly stringent, the incidence of complications declines. A retrospective study, which enrolled 202 patients undergoing ALPPS procedure, demonstrated that despite dropping to 9% and 28%, respectively [3], the rates of in-hospital mortality and Grade 3b or higher [4] complications were markedly greater than those observed following the conventional hepatectomy. In this regard, multiple surgical modifications were introduced. Partial ALPPS (p-ALPPS) was first proposed by Fernando A. Alvarez [5], who is an Argentine surgeon. The conventional ALPPS procedure involves complete hepatic parenchymal transection extending from the capsule on the ventral surface of the liver to the ventral side of the inferior vena cava, thereby reducing the portal venous supply to the resection side to expedite the future liver remnant (FLR) hypertrophy. In contrast, the p-ALPPS procedure entails transecting only 50–80% of the hepatic parenchyma. For instance, the p-ALPPS procedure, involving the preservation of the left hemiliver, necessitates transecting the hepatic parenchyma extending from the capsule on the liver surface to the ventral side of the middle hepatic vein (Fig. 9.1). This facilitates rapid hepatic hypertrophy while circumventing liver injuries associated with complete parenchymal transection, thereby mitigating the risk of complications (e.g., bile leakage).

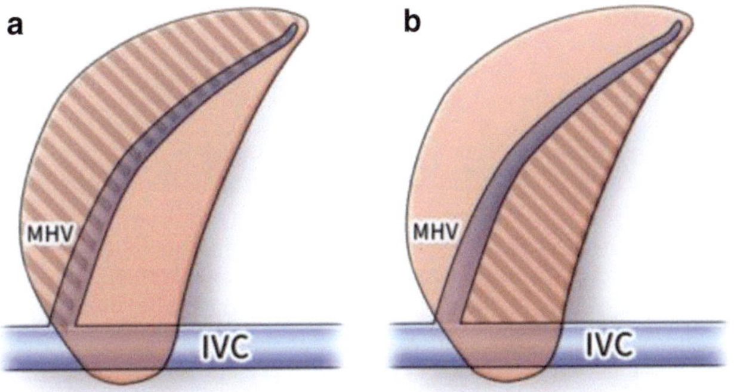

Fig. 9.1 p-ALPPS procedure involving the preservation of the left hemiliver. (**a**) Stage 1 p-ALPPS procedure entails transecting the parenchyma from the projection of the middle hepatic vein on the liver surface to the horizontal caudal border of the middle hepatic vein (dashed area); (**b**) Stage 2 p-ALPPS procedure necessitates transecting the plane from the middle hepatic vein to the inferior vena cava (dashed area) along the transection line finished in stage 1 p-ALPPS procedure, culminating in the resection of the right hemiliver

9.2 Indications

The indications for the p-ALPPS procedure do not include all patients slated for the ALPPS procedure. The eligibility for the p-ALPPS procedure should be evaluated considering oncological and anatomical factors. Patients with tumors on the resection side being in close proximity to the transection plane should preferably undergo the conventional ALPPS procedure involving complete hepatic parenchymal transection, thereby precluding enlarged tumors from invading the

Z. Wang (✉) · J. Hu
Zhongshan Hospital, Fudan University, Shanghai, China
e-mail: wang.zheng@zs-hospital.sh.cn

J. Zhou (ed.), *Associating Liver Partition and Portal Vein Ligation for Staged Hepatectomy (ALPPS)*,
https://doi.org/10.1007/978-981-96-7364-3_9

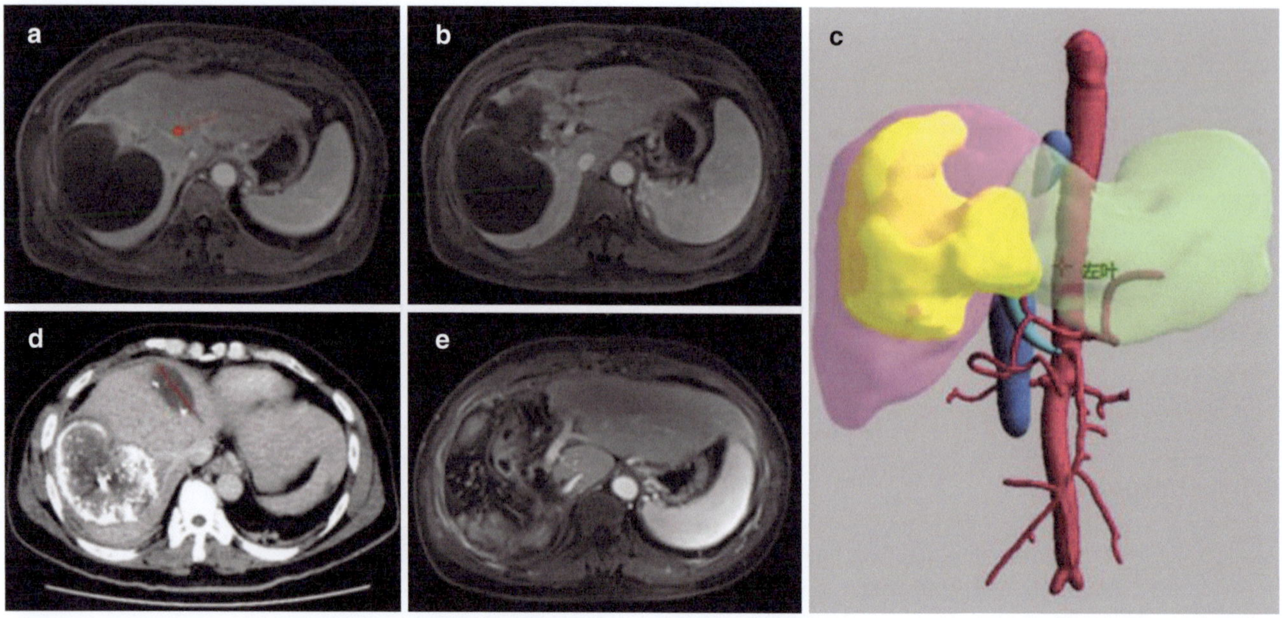

Fig. 9.2 ALPPS procedure involving the preservation of the left lateral section is performed following conversion therapy for the giant tumor invading segment IVb in the right lobe. (**a**) The transection plane, where the tumor invades segments VII and VII in the right lobe, is positioned at a considerable distance from the middle hepatic vein; (**b**) The tumor in the right lobe invades segment IVb by transgressing segment V; (**c**) Three-dimensional reconstruction demonstrates the relationships between the tumor and the left and right hemilivers; (**d**) Laparoscopic ALPPS procedure is performed utilizing the hepatic vein between segments II/III and IV as a landmark to complete hepatic parenchymal transection; (**e**) Imaging findings following right trisegmentectomy in stage 2 surgery

liver on the preservation side or metastasizing to the FLR via portal venous communications within the hepatic parenchyma while awaiting FLR hypertrophy following stage 1 surgery (Fig. 9.2).

Suppose preoperative routine three-dimensional reconstruction reveals the presence of abundant portal venous communications between the preservation and resection sides. In that case, the conventional ALPPS procedure involving complete hepatic parenchymal transection should take precedence to block the portal venous supply to the tumor-bearing side, thereby inducing rapid hypertrophy of the contralateral liver. If three-dimensional reconstruction exhibits an anatomical variation (i.e., the portal venous supply to the dorsal side of segment V originates from the portal venous branch in segment IV) in patients with giant tumors in the right hemiliver and an inadequate left liver volume, implementing the conventional ALPPS procedure involving complete hepatic parenchymal transection should be considered (Fig. 9.3). It merits emphasis that the p-ALPPS procedure may induce a sluggish volumetric increase of the FLR in such patients, resulting in the failure to achieve an anticipated FLR volume.

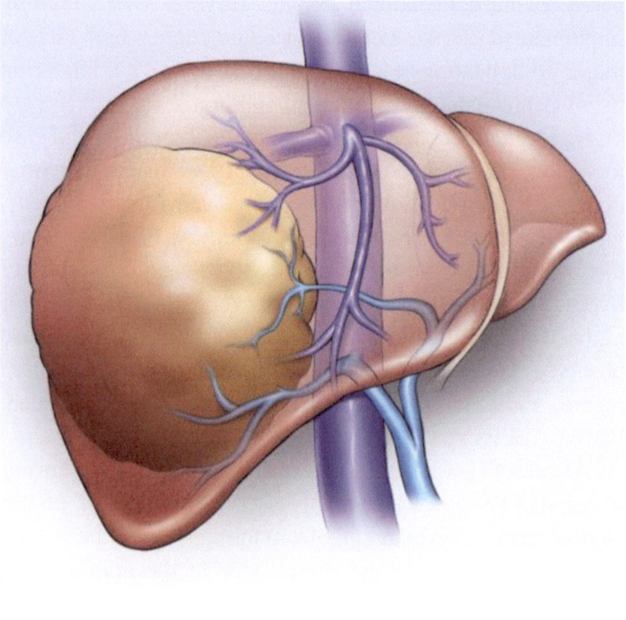

Fig. 9.3 Portal venous anatomical variations (i.e., the portal venous supply to the hepatic parenchyma in segment V partially originates from the portal venous branch in segment IV, while the portal venous supply to the tumor in the right lobe is partially derived from a branch originating from the sagittal segment of the left portal vein in segment IV, which enters segment V from the dorsal side of the middle hepatic vein). Patients exhibiting such anatomical variations are deemed ineligible for p-ALPPS procedure, as partial transection cannot effectively block the portal venous supply to the right lobe

9.3 Surgical Maneuvers

The maneuvers of the p-ALPPS procedure are comparable to those of the conventional ALPPS procedure. Specifically, stage 1 surgery entails portal vein ligation and partial hepatic parenchymal transection. This is followed by awaiting FLR hypertrophy to achieve an adequate FLR volume that falls within the safety margin. Subsequently, stage 2 surgery commences to resect the liver on the tumor-bearing side. The p-ALPPS procedure encompasses stage 1 surgery implemented via an open or laparoscopic approach. Patients without prior surgical history and no contraindications to laparoscopy should preferably undergo stage 1 laparoscopic p-ALPPS procedure, as this procedure can induce minimal trauma and facilitate postoperative recovery.

Patients presenting with tumors in both the left and right hemilivers should undergo the simultaneous resection or ablation of liver tumors on the preservation side during stage 1 surgery. This can prevent the enlargement or metastases of tumors in the FLR during FLR hypertrophy, thereby circumventing the need for a more extensive hepatic resection to resect any tumors within the FLR during stage 2 surgery. During stage 1 surgery, localized enucleation of hepatic tumors within the FLR may be performed, provided that an adequate resection margin is ensured. If the evaluation reveals a negligible loss of the functional liver volume within the portal venous territory harboring the tumors in the FLR, anatomic resection may be performed.

Stage 1 surgery encompasses cholecystectomy, mobilization, and ligation of the right portal vein, and hepatic parenchymal transection extending from the projection line of the middle hepatic vein on the liver surface to the ventral side of the middle hepatic vein (Fig. 9.4). The transection plane is delineated based on ischemic demarcation line-based guid-

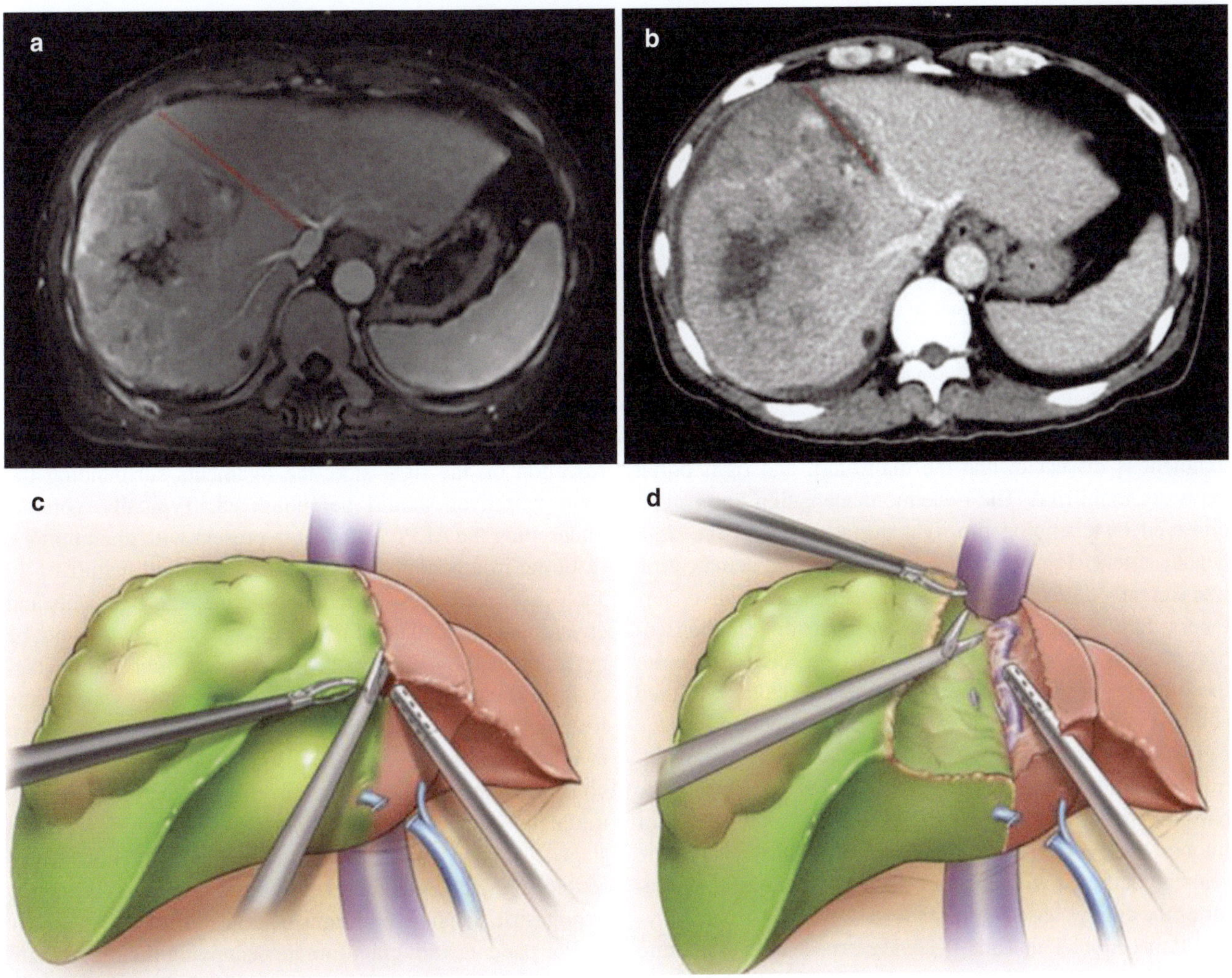

Fig. 9.4 Planning of the hepatic parenchymal transection line during stage 1 laparoscopic p-ALPPS procedure. (**a**) Preoperative image of a giant tumor in the right hemiliver, depicting that the intended hepatic parenchymal transection plane is guided by the course of the middle hepatic vein. The red dotted line denotes the plane along which the middle hepatic vein courses; (**b**) Postoperative image one week after stage 1 laparoscopic p-ALPPS procedure, demonstrating the completion of hepatic parenchymal transection on the ventral side of the middle hepatic vein. The red dotted line denotes the transection plane; (**c**) ICG fluorescence navigation is employed to delineate the transection line between the left and right hemilivers; (**d**) The depth of hepatic parenchymal transection extends from the liver surface until the level of the middle hepatic vein during stage 1 laparoscopic p-ALPPS procedure

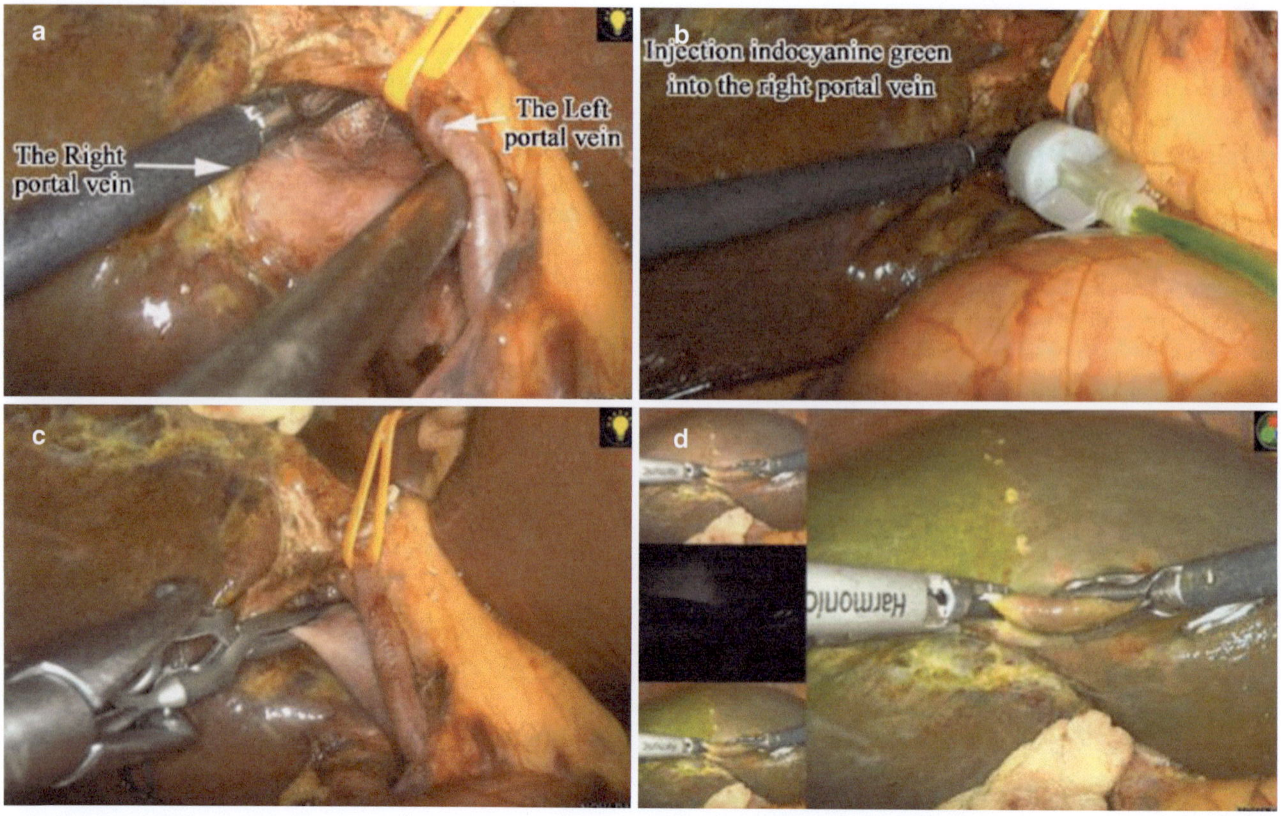

Fig. 9.5 The transection line between the left and right hemilivers is delineated by the ischemic demarcation line or fluorescence navigation (provided by Professor Xiaoying Wang). (**a**) The main portal vein is mobilized at the first porta hepatis to expose the left and right portal veins; (**b**) The right portal vein is punctured, followed by injection of a diluted solution of ICG; (**c**) The right portal vein is clamped, rendering the ischemic demarcation line in the right hemiliver discernible; (**d**) The hepatic parenchyma is transected based on fluorescence guidance

ance or laparoscopic fluorescence navigation to delineate the transection line between the left and right hemilivers (Fig. 9.5a). Following cholecystectomy, the hepatoduodenal ligament is dissected, and the main, left, and right portal veins are mobilized. The ischemic demarcation line can be observed by clamping the right portal vein and the right hepatic artery (Fig. 9.5c). While the ischemic demarcation line can only delineate the transection plane on the liver surface, it fails to provide guidance for navigating the transection plane in the hepatic parenchyma. To precisely delineate the transection plane in the hepatic parenchyma, a diluted solution of indocyanine green (ICG) can be injected into the right portal vein (Fig. 9.5b). The green fluorescence can distinctly delineate the left and right hemilivers, allowing for partial hepatic parenchymal transection along the course of fluorescence (Fig. 9.5d). It is advisable to employ a harmonic scalpel combined with a cavitron ultrasonic surgical aspirator as the energy-based surgical device for hepatic parenchymal transection. This can effectively expose the vasculature to maintain a well-defined hepatectomy plane, thereby lessening the risk of postoperative complications. The transection may proceed in caudal-to-cephalic and ventral-to-dorsal directions until the transection plane reaches the level of the middle hepatic vein.

If a plastic bag is utilized to envelop the liver slated for resection on the right side, the ligaments surrounding the right hemiliver should be mobilized. Typically, patients undergoing the ALPPS procedure present with giant tumors, resulting in a confined space around the right hemiliver. In such cases, forcefully mobilizing perihepatic ligaments and enveloping the ipsilateral liver with a plastic bag may not be essential, as the majority of recent reports indicated the discontinued use of plastic bags. Following stage 1 surgery, the liver volume should be radiologically measured weekly to evaluate the FLR hypertrophy. Immediately after the FLR volume reaches the safety margin, stage 2 surgery should be initiated. Considering that a large liver specimen is resected, stage 2 surgery is typically executed via an open or laparoscopic approach, with the liver specimen extracted through a hypogastric incision to minimize surgical trauma.

For patients with giant tumors occupying the right posterior section, right anterior section, and left medial section, a p-ALPPS procedure involving the preservation of the left lateral section only may be indicated. In such cases, the absence of the middle hepatic vein as a landmark for the transection plane necessitates the utilization of the hepatic vein between segments II/III and IV as the positioning landmark for the transection plane to achieve partial parenchymal transection. In cases where p-ALPPS procedure is indicated because of a tumor location precluding the delineation of the transection plane along anatomical hepatic segment boundaries, the depth of hepatic parenchymal transection can be evaluated, with 50–80% of the hepatic parenchymal transection area as the criterion.

9.4 Complication and Mortality Rates Associated with p-ALPPS

The p-ALPPS procedure, which necessitates the transection of reduced hepatic parenchyma, confers lower rates of postoperative complications (e.g., bleeding and bile leakage) and mortality compared to the conventional ALPPS procedure. A prospective single-center study, which enrolled 30 patients undergoing ALPPS procedure, demonstrated that the extent of hepatic parenchymal transection was significantly correlated with the incidence of postoperative complications ($P = 0.049$); the complication rate was noticeably lower following p-ALPPS procedure as compared to complete ALPPS procedure; the volumetric increases of the FLR did not differ considerably between patients undergoing partial and complete ALPPS procedures ($P = 0.45$) [5].

A meta-analysis, which included 124 patients undergoing ALPPS procedure, revealed that the FLR hypertrophy rates and the intervals between stages 1 and 2 surgeries did not differ statistically between patients undergoing the partial and conventional ALPPS procedures ($P = 0.09$ vs $P = 0.57$); however, the complication rate was markedly lower following p-ALPPS procedure as compared to the conventional ALPPS procedure (OR = 0.38; $P = 0.03$); p-ALPPS procedure conferred a lower perioperative mortality rate compared to the conventional ALPPS procedure (4.9% vs 18.9%), with the difference deemed not statistically significant [6]. The findings of a study indicated that the p-ALPPS procedure was safer and exhibited a comparable FLR hypertrophy rate in non-cirrhotic patients compared to the conventional ALPPS procedure [7].

Another retrospective study compared the impacts of portal vein embolization (PVE), conventional ALPPS, and p-ALPPS procedures on FLR hypertrophy and postoperative complications. The findings signaled that the ALPPS procedures were markedly superior to PVE in inducing a volumetric increase of the FLR; the p-ALPPS procedure and conventional ALPPS procedure demonstrated comparable roles in inducing a volumetric increase and functional restoration of the FLR; laparoscopic p-ALPPS procedure conferred remarkably lower rates of complications and mortality [8].

While transecting reduced hepatic parenchyma (30–40%) and dissecting fewer portal venous branches necessitates an extended interval for FLR hypertrophy in the p-ALPPS procedure as compared to the conventional ALPPS procedure, this ultimately facilitates achieving an adequate FLR volume for completing stage 2 surgery while conferring a significant reduction in surgical complication risks and eliminating mortality [9].

A study suggested that p-ALPPS conferring no advantages in patients with a background of chronic liver disease, conventional ALPPS procedure can induce rapid FLR hypertrophy without elevating perioperative risks compared to the p-ALPPS procedure [10].

In summary, the majority of studies reveal that the p-ALPPS procedure exhibits a comparable FLR hypertrophy rate and confers lower complication and mortality rates compared to the conventional ALPPS procedure. Nonetheless, a handful of studies suggest that the conventional ALPPS procedure induces a comparable perioperative risk and a more rapid volumetric increase of the FLR compared to the p-ALPPS procedure. Due to the limited number of cases and the absence of precise long-term oncological benefit assessments, the benefits and drawbacks of the p-ALPPS procedure over the conventional ALPPS procedure await confirmation through large-scale randomized controlled studies [11].

References

1. Zhou J. Revolutionary ALPPS surgery in the treatment of patients with unresectable huge liver cancer *via* traditional surgery[J]. Chin Arch Gen Surg (Electron Ed). 2020;14(6):420.
2. Schnitzbauer AA, Lang SA, Goessmann H, et al. Right portal vein ligation combined with in situ splitting induces rapid left lateral liver lobe hypertrophy, enabling 2-staged extended right hepatic resection in small-for-size settings[J]. Ann Surg. 2012;255(3):405–14.
3. Schadde E, Ardiles V, Robles-Campos R, et al. Early survival and safety of ALPPS: first report of the International ALPPS Registry[J]. Ann Surg. 2014;260(5):829–36. discussion 836–8
4. Clavien PA, Barkun J, de Oliveira ML, et al. The Clavien-Dindo classification of surgical complications: five-year experience[J]. Ann Surg. 2009;250(2):187–96.
5. Alvarez FA, Ardiles V, de Santibañes M, et al. Associating liver partition and portal vein ligation for staged hepatectomy offers high oncological feasibility with adequate patient safety: a prospective study at a single center[J]. Ann Surg. 2015;261(4):723–32.
6. Wu XK, Rao JW, Zhou XZ, et al. Partial ALPPS versus complete ALPPS for staged hepatectomy[J]. BMC Gastroenterol. 2019;19(1):170.
7. Huang HC, Bian J, Bai Y, et al. Complete or partial split in associating liver partition and portal vein ligation for staged hepatectomy: a systematic review and meta-analysis[J]. World J Gastroenterol. 2019;25(39):6016–24.

8. Rassam F, Olthof PB, van Lienden KP, et al. Comparison of functional and volumetric increase of the future remnant liver and postoperative outcomes after portal vein embolization and complete or partial associating liver partition and portal vein ligation for staged hepatectomy (ALPPS)[J]. Ann Transl Med. 2020;8(7):436.
9. Kumar N, Duncan T, O'Reilly D, et al. Partial ALPPS with a longer wait between procedures is safe and yields adequate future liver remnant hypertrophy[J]. Ann Hepatobiliary Pancreat Surg. 2019;23(1):13–9.
10. Chan ACY, Chok K, Dai JWC, et al. Impact of split completeness on future liver remnant hypertrophy in associating liver partition and portal vein ligation for staged hepatectomy (ALPPS) in hepatocellular carcinoma: complete-ALPPS versus partial-ALPPS[J]. Surgery. 2017;161(2):357–64.
11. Petrowsky H, Györi G, de Oliveira M, et al. Is partial-ALPPS safer than ALPPS? A single-center experience[J]. Ann Surg. 2015;261(4):e90–2.

10 Anterior Approach ALPPS

Albert Chan

10.1 Introduction

Insufficient future liver remnant (FLR) is a common limitation that prevents patients from undergoing extensive hepatectomy. Recent studies have shown that an FLR of less than 20% is strongly associated with postoperative liver failure and increased mortality rates. Consequently, to enhance the safety of extensive liver resection, it is imperative to identify strategies to augment FLR.

Portal vein embolization (PVE) is regarded as the gold standard for inducing hepatic growth. The predominant embolization route is the transhepatic approach on either the ipsilateral or contralateral side of the portal vein, contingent upon the portal vein's anatomy and the tumor's location. Nonetheless, PVE is not devoid of risks. Recent studies have indicated that the overall complication rate ranges from 5% to 12%. Of greater concern are severe complications such as thrombosis of the portal vein trunk, incomplete portal vein embolization, and migration of emboli, which can result in the failure of FLR hypertrophy, hence the inability or postponement of surgery. Based on the author's experience over the past several decades, 30% of PVE patients were ineligible for hepatectomy due to insufficient liver augmentation or tumor progression. Consequently, there is an exigent need to explore new alternatives to elevate FLR hypertrophy success rates.

10.1.1 Initial Development of ALPPS

In its early stages, ALPPS faced skepticism about its effectiveness in promoting liver regeneration and was criticized for its high rates of surgical complications and short-term mortality. Nevertheless, the creation of an international ALPPS registry [1] and progress in surgical techniques has led to improved short-term results, with the 90-day mortality rate dropping from 10% to 3% and the complication rate decreasing from 17% to 4% [2]. Even with these advancements, most ALPPS research in existing studies has focused on bilobar colorectal liver metastases (CRLM) [3, 4] or liver tumors not associated with hepatitis [5, 6]. The experience with employing ALPPS in chronic liver disease and hepatocellular carcinoma (HCC) remains limited. There are persisting doubts about whether ALPPS can effectively induce rapid FLR growth in patients with chronic liver disease. Some hypotheses have emerged suggesting that the so-called liver proliferation may merely be a manifestation of tissue edema, or that the regenerating tissue might not be functional. At the time, these arguments lacked high-quality evidence, and there appeared to be no logical reason why ALPPS could not be utilized in patients with hepatitis-related HCC. Consequently, the author began studying the role of ALPPS in this indication in 2013.

10.1.2 The Author's First Adult HCC Patient in Hong Kong University

The inaugural ALPPS experience at the author's center involved a 6-year-old child diagnosed with hepatoblastoma. Following the successful outcome of this surgery, I proceeded to perform the first ALPPS on an adult patient in December 2013. This case involved a 62-year-old male with hepatitis B virus-associated HCC.

Before initiating this complex and challenging procedure, a critical consideration was whether to use a plastic bag to encase the right liver to prevent adhesions and manage potential bile leakage, as described by Andreas A. Schnitzbauer et al. [5] However, a potential issue is that intraperitoneal fluid and infection might accumulate within the plastic bag, necessitating a second laparotomy if the FLR does not proliferate adequately. To address this challenge, based on our center's experience with resecting large liver

A. Chan (✉)
Queen Mary Hospital, University of Hong Kong,
Hong Kong, China
e-mail: acchan@hku.hk

J. Zhou (ed.), *Associating Liver Partition and Portal Vein Ligation for Staged Hepatectomy (ALPPS)*,
https://doi.org/10.1007/978-981-96-7364-3_10

tumors, we adopted an "anterior approach" to perform in situ parenchyma partition [7]. This patient was diagnosed with a HCC in the right lobe, measuring 10 cm in diameter, along with cirrhosis and classified as Child-Pugh Class A. The preoperative Indocyanine Green Retention Rate at 15 minutes (ICG-R15) was 17.8%, and the left liver volume was 286.2 mL, representing 26.6% of the estimated standard liver volume (ESLV). Following the ligation of the right portal vein branch, a Cavitron Ultrasonic Surgical Aspirator (CUSA) was employed to separate the liver tissue. The intraparenchymal ducts were revealed, and both the left and right sides were secured with titanium clips, tied off, and subsequently cut. The left hepatic pedicle was looped within the parenchyma and pulled caudally to facilitate parenchymal transection cephalad from the inferior vena cava (IVC). After the parenchymal division, the full path of the middle hepatic vein was revealed and subsequently severed at its starting point. The Pringle maneuver was not used during the procedure, and the right liver remained unmobilized in the early phase of the surgery. A bile leakage test was performed by injecting methylene blue dye into the cystic duct. No drainage was inserted following the operation.

On postoperative day 7 (POD7), the volume of the left liver augmented by 26%, reaching 360 mL, equivalent to 33.5% of ESLV. By POD10, the second stage was conducted, revealing only some delicate adhesions within the abdominal cavity and no bile leak in the liver transection plane. Following the division of the right hepatic artery, right hepatic duct, and right hepatic vein, the extended right hepatectomy was effortlessly completed, and only then was the right liver mobilized and excised. Postoperative pathological examination confirmed chronic active hepatitis with grade 2 liver fibrosis (Batts and Ludwig classification). Immunohistochemical staining demonstrated a significant increase in the proportion of Ki67 and VEGF-positive cells in the left FLR, rising from 1% to 20% and from 10% to 100%, respectively. This suggests vigorous cellular regeneration following the first-stage ALPPS operation, which refutes the assertion that ALPPS merely induces "tissue edema." With the growing fascination in this new surgical technique among medical professionals, it is expected that additional information on this topic will emerge shortly.

Our preliminary experience indicates that ALPPS is viable in patients with chronic liver disease. Nonetheless, intraperitoneal plastic bags still present a risk of intra-abdominal infection. The anterior approach provides a remedy by allowing for full parenchymal separation to the IVC without needing to mobilize the right liver beforehand. Consequently, significantly fewer adhesions in the perihepatic and para-IVC regions are anticipated. Additionally, this method lowers the chance of inadvertently causing tumor rupture during the mobilization of the right liver, a surgical risk that can make the second stage more difficult. Skilled use of the CUSA also allows for precise exposure and management prior to cutting the intraparenchymal duct. Combined with methylene blue testing, these steps decrease the risk of bile leakage without needing plastic bags. Consequently, the surgeon faces significantly reduced pressure about the length of the Stage 2 procedure.

10.2 Indications and Selection Criteria

Since ALPPS is a surgery related to hepatic augmentation, the indications for ALPPS in HCC align with those for PVE, as outlined below: (1) FLR < 40%, (2) ICG-R15 < 20, (3) Liver function Child-Pugh Class A, (4) Platelet count $\geq 100 \times 10^9$/L, (5) The right branch of the portal vein remains patent and there is no cancerous thrombus completely obstructing the portal vein blood flow.

Exclusion criteria include full right portal vein tumor thrombosis (PVTT), a serum platelet count below 100×10^9/L, clinical evidence of portal hypertension like ascites or abdominal varices, and the existence of distant metastases. The FLR volume will be evaluated using an enhanced CT scan, with the ESLV determined by the Urata formula [8].

10.3 Functional Evaluation of FLR

Routine evaluation of FLR function is conducted by measuring ICG-R15. This assessment is performed at various time points preoperatively and intraoperatively using the LiMON device (Pulsion Medical Systems, Munich, Germany). The intravenous dosage of ICG administered both before and during surgery is 0.5 mg/kg. The preoperative ICG-R15 is measured within two weeks before the initial stage of the procedure. To mimic a right-sided hepatectomy and evaluate the function of the future liver remnant (FLR), this index is measured following temporary clamping of the right portal vein and hepatic artery at this stage. Based on our experience, an ICG-R15 of less than 40% indicates sufficient proliferation in the subsequent 7–14 days, accompanied by significant improvement in FLR function, rendering the second-stage procedure feasible.

10.4 Steps of the Anterior Approach ALPPS

10.4.1 Stage 1 ALPPS

The abdomen is entered through a right subcostal incision extending to the midline. Intraoperative ultrasound is utilized to confirm the tumor's location, assess the patency of the left hepatic vasculature, and exclude the presence of a tumor in

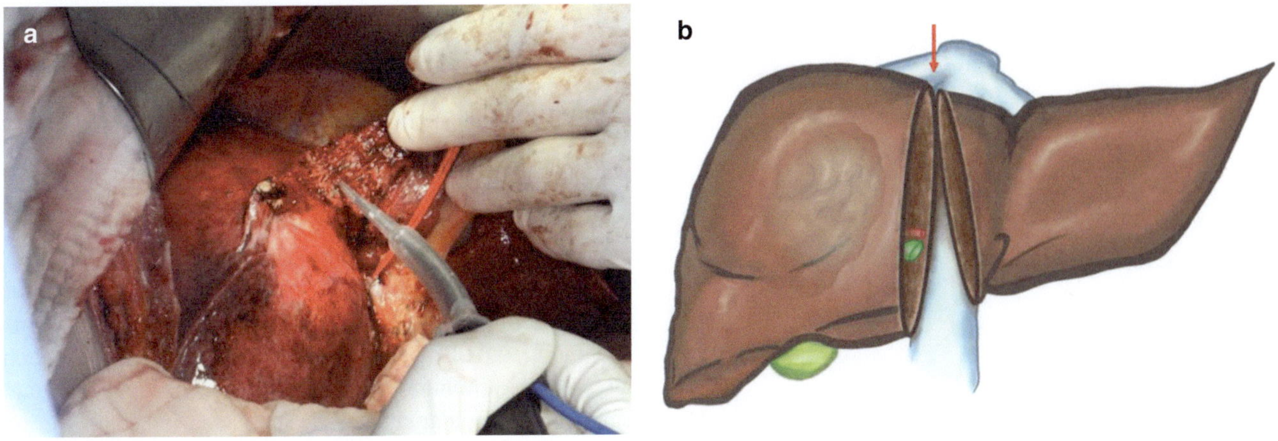

Fig. 10.1 (**a**) Anterior approach, with parenchymal transection starting from the caudal part of the liver. (**b**) The groove between the root of the right hepatic vein and middle hepatic vein on the anterior surface of the IVC (red arrow) is dissected and identified

the left liver. Then, portal dissection is carried out, wherein the right hepatic artery is encircled with a ribbon, and the right branch of the portal vein is ligated and transected. The hepatic transection plane is subsequently delineated along the ischemic line induced by the temporary clamping of the right hepatic artery. The fundamental steps of in situ parenchymal split are subsequently described.

Initially, the lower portion of the liver is carefully dissected with the CUSA device (Valleylab, Boulder, CO, USA) until the hilar plate and right hepatic duct are revealed (Fig. 10.1a). Precise sharp dissection is carried out to locate the venous groove separating the origin of the right hepatic vein from the origin of the middle hepatic vein, situated anterior to the inferior vena cava (IVC) (Fig. 10.1b, red arrow). The upper section of the liver is removed to widen the gap between the two transection planes, making it easier to expose and isolate the right hepatic duct (Fig. 10.2). The left and right caudate lobes are divided, the retrohepatic inferior vena cava (IVC) is uncovered, and the avascular groove located in front of the IVC is subsequently located (Fig. 10.3, black arrow). Elevating the liver along the posterior avascular plane with a right-angle tool can speed up the division of the deeper liver tissue while protecting the front surface of the inferior vena cava (IVC) (Fig. 10.4). In a right-sided hepatectomy, the liver parenchyma is dissected upward to reach the venous groove separating the right and middle hepatic veins. For a right trisegmentectomy, the origin of the middle hepatic vein is severed, and the dissection line is adjusted to favor the venous groove between the right and middle hepatic veins. Fully divide the liver parenchyma up to the front surface of the inferior vena cava (IVC) located behind the liver (Fig. 10.5).

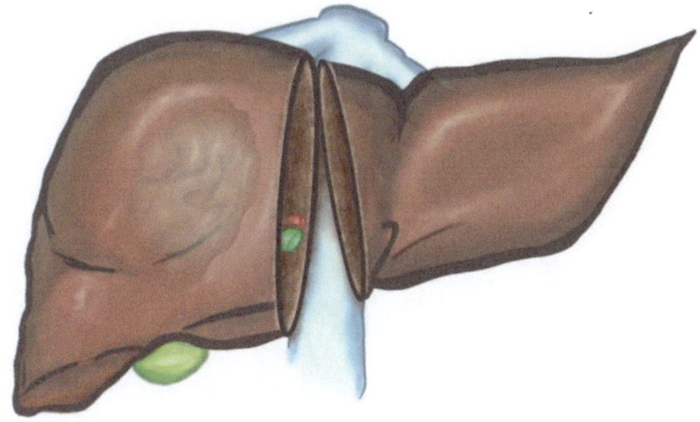

Fig. 10.2 The cranial part of the liver is transected

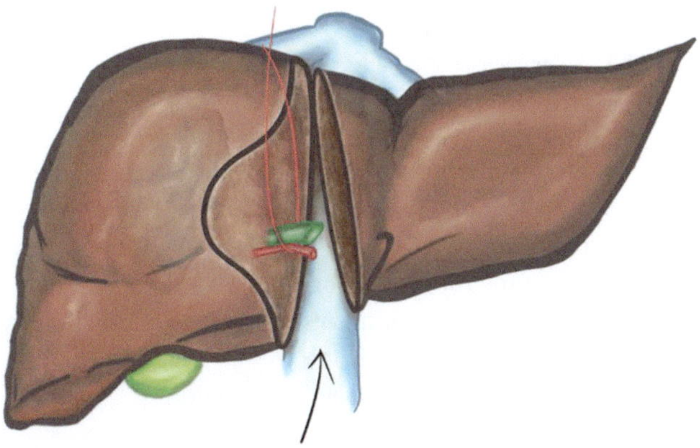

Fig. 10.3 The left and right caudate lobes are split to expose the retrohepatic IVC and identify the avascular retrohepatic groove anterior to the IVC (black arrow)

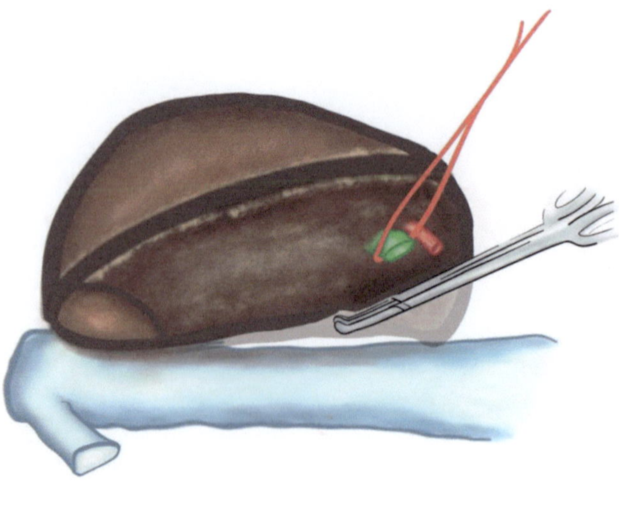

Fig. 10.4 The liver is lifted by right-angle forceps along the avascular retrohepatic plane to expedite deep parenchymal transection and safeguard the anterior surface of the IVC

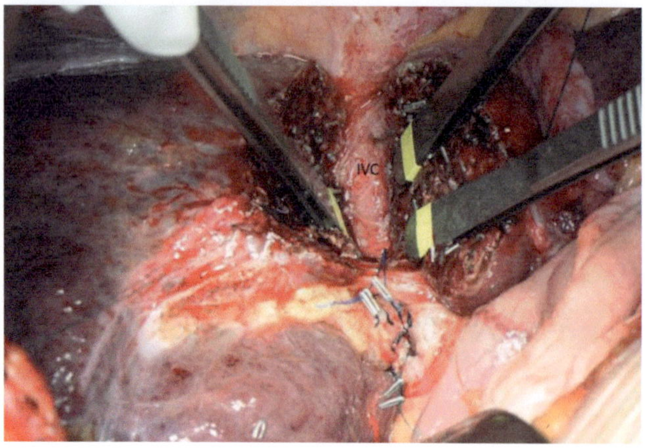

Fig. 10.5 A complete split is performed down to the IVC

Intraoperative ultrasound is used to verify the openness of the right hepatic artery, followed by a bile leak test. The right hepatic artery and bile duct are marked with colored non-absorbable sutures for later recognition. No drainage tubes, plastic bags, anti-adhesion agents, or hemostatic materials are inserted. Prior to closing, the wound is infused with a local anesthetic (0.5% levobupivacaine solution).

10.4.2 Stage 2 ALPPS

The right hepatic artery and hepatic duct are tied off separately, the right hepatic vein is divided, and the right liver is disconnected from the diaphragm and retroperitoneum. Afterward, the right liver is taken out, and the specimen is retrieved.

10.5 Is the Anterior Approach the Better Approach?

ALPPS, akin to any novel surgical innovation, is continually being pursued for enhancement. The anterior approach reduces adhesion formation in the right retroperitoneal region and surrounding liver surfaces, thereby preventing iatrogenic tumor rupture during the initial-stage mobilization. Our previous experience with the anterior approach for the resection of large tumors motivated us to apply the same technique to ALPPS [7]. In contrast to the anterior approach used in conventional right hepatectomy, the right bile duct and right hepatic artery are preserved and left intact during the single-stage procedure. Excessive or repeated clamping of the right hepatic artery should be avoided during the in situ division of the liver parenchyma to prevent thrombosis or dissection. The technique for intrahepatic control and exposure of the right hepatic duct is similar to the method used to expose the bile duct before right liver resection in living donor liver transplantation. We observed that fully encircling the right bile duct with a non-absorbable single-strand suture (e.g., 2-0 Prolene) aids in its later identification and, more significantly, reduces adhesion formation in this region, which could otherwise pose challenges in the second stage. During the in situ transection, a right-angle instrument is inserted into the avascular retrohepatic tunnel to lift the deep parenchyma, accelerating separation while safeguarding the right hepatic pedicle and the anterior wall of the retrohepatic IVC (Fig. 10.4). This "suspension" technique was initially described by Belghiti et al [9] The advantage of employing this instrument lies in its capacity to facilitate a small and gradual separation of the liver parenchyma, in contrast to attempting to pass the band directly through this plane during the suspension procedure. This approach aids in preventing accidental injury to the deeper and cranial regions during the band's passage through the retrohepatic IVC or its branches, which would be challenging to manage if the right liver remained attached to the retroperitoneum. Additionally, after dividing the left and right caudate lobes, the visibility of this plane improves considerably, enabling full separation as the dissection of the liver parenchyma progresses toward the vein separating the right and middle hepatic veins (Fig. 10.3).

By employing the aforementioned technical methods, the FLR volume in ALPPS increased by 48%, and the FLR/ESLV ratio increased by an additional 12.3% within six days post-surgery. The between-stage interval was seven days [10].

The effect of fully segmenting cirrhotic livers in situ on the degree of FLR hypertrophy is still unclear [11]. From a technical standpoint, completely isolating the IVC guarantees that blood flow is fully redirected to the FLR, even if sufficient liver growth does not take place. This is particularly vital for patients with limited liver function reserve, for whom hepatectomy may be their sole curative option.

10.6 Complete Split or Partial Split

Recent findings indicate that for non-cirrhotic and non-cholestatic livers, partial split (50–80% of total transection) is comparable to complete split concerning FLR hypertrophy (Fig. 10.6) while exhibiting reduced postoperative morbidity and mortality [11]. Nonetheless, information pertaining to the impact of partial transection on FLR growth in chronic liver disease remains insufficient.

According to our findings, complete separation results in significantly greater FLR growth compared to partial separation [12]. The complete transection group showed a larger increase in absolute liver volume (187.1 mL vs. 132.6 mL, $P = 0.022$) and a higher daily proliferation rate (31.2 mL/day vs. 17.5 mL/day, $P = 0.002$), leading to an improved FLR/ESLV ratio (42.1% vs. 33.9%, $P = 0.019$). Additionally, this group was more likely to reach the FLR/ESLV threshold of 35% for liver resection within 10 days (76.9% vs. 33.3%, $P = 0.024$). As a result, patients with complete separation were more likely to proceed to second-stage surgery within 14 days of the initial procedure (100.0% vs. 58.3%, $P = 0.009$), which ultimately shortened their hospital stay (17.5 days vs. 22 days, $P = 0.016$).

When grouped by liver condition, our results showed that complete transection led to more significant FLR growth in cases linked to chronic hepatitis compared to partial transection, as evidenced by both the daily proliferation rate and the improvement in the FLR/ESLV ratio [10]. Additionally, the results indicated that ALPPS can stimulate FLR growth in cirrhotic livers within a short timeframe. Although complete separation exhibited a tendency to accelerate FLR augmentation more rapidly than partial separation in cases of cirrhosis (proliferation rate: 32.2 mL/day vs. 16.9 mL/day, $P = 0.086$), the difference was not statistically significant (FLR/ESLV% increase: 14.8% vs. 11.0%, $P = 0.668$). Conversely, in chronic hepatitis, the discrepancy was statistically significant (FLR/ESLV% increase: 18.1% vs. 11.3%, $P = 0.042$) [10].

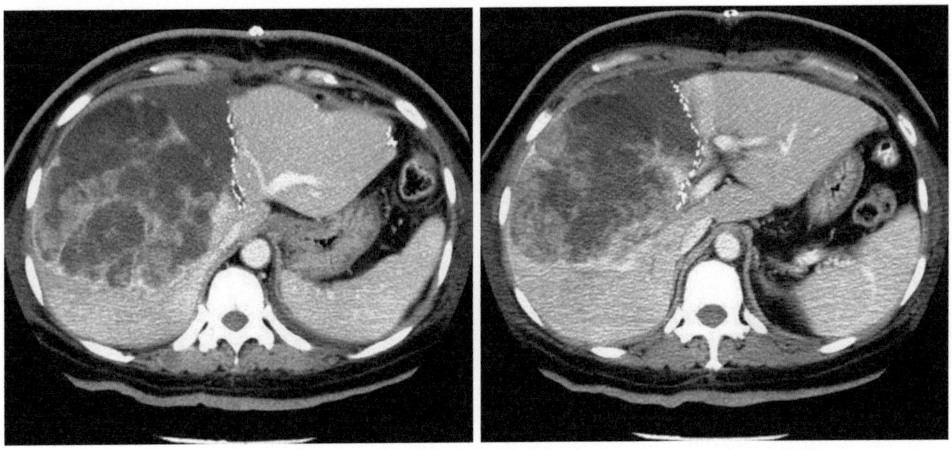

Fig. 10.6 Complete split

10.7 Recovery of Liver Function After Stage 1 and Stage 2 Surgery

Serum bilirubin levels returned to near-normal levels prior to the second stage of surgery in both the complete and partial transection groups. However, the complete split group experienced higher serum bilirubin levels from the first to the fourth day after the initial procedure, yet these levels normalized much more quickly between the second and fifth days following the second-stage surgery [12]. Conversely, in the partial split group, liver function recovered more swiftly after Stage 1. Nevertheless, there was a significant increase in serum bilirubin levels on the fourth and fifth days after surgery, accompanied by elevated serum aspartate transaminase (AST) levels from the first to the third day and again on the sixth day following the second-stage procedure [12].

Given that FLR tissue growth is reduced in chronic hepatitis livers compared to non-cirrhotic livers, identifying factors that affect FLR hypertrophy is essential. From a surgical perspective, determining whether the degree of parenchymal transection influences outcomes is critical, as it shapes the resection approach during surgery and the scheduling of the second-stage procedure. Our findings indicated that complete transection promoted more substantial FLR growth than partial transection, required an earlier second-stage surgery, and led to faster recovery of liver function after Stage 2. Despite the greater FLR growth, complete transection proved to be as safe as partial transection, with no increase in complications or mortality.

In fact, complete transection possesses several advantages. First, from a technical perspective, the "complete" portal vein shunt is successfully achieved in a 1-stage operation, ensuring effectiveness even without sufficient FLR proliferation. Second, the second-stage operation becomes safer, avoiding hemi-transection plane re-examination, with faster liver function recovery, including earlier normalization of serum bilirubin and AST levels. More significantly, a greater FLR volume is attained rapidly, improving the safety buffer for extensive hepatectomy against postoperative liver failure and circumventing technical difficulties associated with a delayed Stage 2 procedure.

It remains ambiguous whether the learning curve impacted ALPPS outcomes. Partial transection, more frequently conducted in the initial stages of our ALPPS cases, exhibited a more pronounced bleeding tendency than complete resection in terms of the second-stage procedure and mortality. Nevertheless, since the liver parenchymal transection technique employing CUSA in ALPPS parallels conventional hepatectomy, we attribute the bleeding to the incomplete transection plane following the trauma from the first-stage operation, rather than immature techniques. Additionally, the two deaths in partial split ALPPS occurred at varied times, indicating the learning curve likely didn't impact short-term outcomes, mainly affecting complete transection strategy and second-stage timing.

We posit that the timing of the second-stage surgery is pivotal in determining its technical complexity. It stands to reason that a prolonged between-stage interval exacerbates the difficulty of adhesion separation and liver parenchymal transection. Due to sluggish FLR proliferation, the two transection planes in one patient with partial split ALPPS in this cohort even fused together when the second-stage surgery was conducted 70 days post-first stage. Furthermore, a notably larger percentage of patients in the complete transection group attained sufficient FLR growth and qualified for Stage 2 within 14 days after the initial stage. Given that significant FLR expansion is critical for ensuring liver function recovery after surgery, complete transection should be favored whenever possible.

While complete transection provides potential advantages, it may not always be practical due to technical difficulties. For example, a large tumor in the right anterior segment pressing against the middle hepatic vein during an in situ split for an extended right hepatectomy could lead to significant venous bleeding. Similarly, tumors near the IVC or caudate lobe might make full transection to the IVC unfeasible. In these cases, a partial split may be more suitable, though it comes with the expectation of a delayed Stage 2 due to slower FLR proliferation.

In summary, complete transection ALPPS stimulates faster FLR proliferation compared to partial split, without escalating the perioperative risk in chronic liver disease. Given that FLR augmentation in chronic liver disease is less pronounced than in normal liver, complete transection is recommended for hepatitis-related HCC to attain optimal outcomes.

10.8 Postoperative Outcomes of ALPPS

Alterations in portal vein hemodynamics during ALPPS yield effect on FLR function. To date, ALPPS research has predominantly centered on colorectal liver metastases or other non-primary liver tumors [2–4]. Short-term outcomes of ALPPS for hepatitis-related HCC are rarely documented, and this condition merits recognition as a separate category, as liver hypertrophy in chronic liver disease is less robust than in healthy livers after ALPPS [13]. There is limited information on possible changes in portal vein hemodynamics during ALPPS.

The effect of increased sinusoidal shear stress on the FLR when portal vein flow rises significantly after contralateral portal vein ligation (PVL) and hepatic parenchymal transection remains unclear [14–16]. This question initially arose as our main concern, based on our clinical observations of small-for-size syndrome in living donor liver transplantation [17, 18]. Our findings elucidate this question, demonstrating that despite a rapid escalation in portal vein pressure post-PVL and a nearly threefold increase in FLR portal vein flow, the elevation in hepatic parenchymal transection was not linked with a substantial rise in portal vein flow (Fig. 10.8). This observation further substantiates the notion that the role of parenchymal separation is predominantly to trigger the release of hepatic growth factors [19], rather than solely a matter of flow dynamics. Additionally, the augmentation in FLR blood flow following PVL markedly enhances the delivery efficiency of these growth factors, resulting in accelerated hepatic regeneration.

Drawing from our experience with living donor liver transplantation, we understand that heightened portal flow can be a double-edged sword in cases of chronic hepatitis or cirrhosis. The issue of a "small liver" resulting from increased portal flow may arise due to endothelial damage induced by sinusoidal shear stress. To mitigate this problem, as evidenced by our data, portal flow is autonomously regulated to revert to baseline levels while awaiting stage 2 surgery [10]. Overall hepatic function remained intact, as the tumor-side liver, sustained solely by the hepatic artery, continued to offer some functionality (as evidenced by ^{99m}Tc hepatic scintigraphy of the liver pre- and post-ALPPS), while the FLR underwent regulation during the interim period.

Moreover, an inability to independently manage FLR portal flow under conditions of increased portal pressure could be harmful and should act as a warning sign that might prevent the successful completion of hepatectomy. In these situations, additional measures to regulate portal flow, such as splenic artery ligation or embolization, should be considered [20, 21], or the second-stage surgery should be postponed until adequate FLR growth is observed [22, 23].

Despite the rapid growth of the FLR, it is still unclear whether ALPPS simultaneously improves FLR function. Recently, Biller-Andorno and Jüni. demonstrated the value of hepatic scintigraphy in assessing FLR function after ALPPS in noncirrhotic livers [24], but there is limited data on its application in chronic liver disease. Our experience suggests that while ALPPS boosts both FLR function and volume in chronic hepatitis, its impact on function in cirrhosis seems minimal. This finding is consistent with growing evidence that the functional recovery of these immature, regenerating hepatocytes in the expanding FLR trails behind the rapid volume increase [22, 23, 25], with this recovery being particularly delayed in cirrhosis. Clinically, this suggests that patients with cirrhosis need a longer interval before Stage 2 to allow hepatocytes sufficient time for full functional restoration.

10.9 Surgical Complications of ALPPS

The most frequently documented complications of ALPPS are bile leaks and sepsis [1, 26], posing significant risks for patients with cirrhosis, as sepsis-induced bile leaks are infamously associated with liver failure [27, 28]. As a result, when ALPPS was first conducted at our center, we took every precaution to reduce the chances of bile leaks. Liver parenchymal transection utilizing CUSA proves particularly advantageous, as it facilitates clear identification and ligation of individual bile ducts, while bile leakage testing on reliable liver transection planes can detect and eradicate occult bile leaks. As a result, no bile leaks occurred in our series post-ALPPS. All complications following the first-stage surgery were minor and did not impede the execution of the second-stage surgery. Furthermore, employing an anterior approach prevents extensive mobilization in the subhepatic and para-IVC regions, thereby reducing the formation of severe adhesions and avoiding iatrogenic tumor rupture during the first-stage surgery [7, 29]. These measures contribute to the maximum preservation of the untouched area, facilitating the second-stage surgery.

From a clinical perspective, it is essential for surgeons to recognize perioperative factors that can forecast adequate FLR hypertrophy, enabling more accurate prediction of the timing for Stage 2. Chronic hepatitis, an ICG value of $\leq$39.5% during the first-stage surgery, and the absence of postoperative complications all positively influence FLR augmentation. Notably, the occurrence of stage 2-related complications has been demonstrated to impact FLR growth. In essence, inadequate FLR augmentation predisposes patients to postoperative risks during stage 2, necessitating the postponement of the surgery until sufficient regeneration is attained. When all advantageous conditions were met, Stage 2 surgery was successfully completed within an average of 7.5 days (ranging from 7 to 19 days) with no in-hospital deaths. Among these factors, intraoperative ICG-R15 measurement stands out as a valuable clinical tool that assists clinicians in determining the optimal timing for the two-stage procedure. Intraoperative ICG testing is simple and straightforward to conduct, delivering real-time insights into FLR function and, most importantly, providing critical data on whether the FLR is sufficient. Hepatic scintigraphy-detected FLR function changes strongly correlate with intraoperative ICG value shifts between first- and second-stage surgeries [10]. Intraoperative ICG measurement offers a clinical alternative to hepatic scintigraphy for evaluating FLR function. It presents a more economical and accessible option compared to radionuclide scintigraphy for numerous centers globally. Consequently, we advocate for its routine implementation in evaluating FLR function during the first stage of ALPPS. In cases of chronic hepatitis with intraoperative ICG-R15 values below 39.5%, adequate proliferation of the FLR is anticipated, permitting the second stage to be scheduled approximately one week after the initial stage. However, in patients with cirrhosis or intraoperative ICG-R15 exceeding 39.5%, a prolonged waiting period (at least two weeks) is necessary before proceeding with the next stage. The limitation of this measurement is that it necessitates exposure of the hepatic hilum and inflow vessels, potentially complicating the second stage due to adhesion formation. Therefore, we routinely ligate the right portal vein after suture ligation to avoid further manipulation of this area and encircle the right hepatic artery with a non-absorbable suture for identification and division during the second stage.

10.10 Perioperative Outcomes

All complications and mortality rates associated with ALPPS are documented in Table 10.1. The incidence of complications post-stage 1 was 21.7%, while post-stage 2 it was 19.6%. All stage 1 complications were classified as Clavien-Dindo Grade 1 or 2. The mean hospitalization duration for patients in the ALPPS group was 18 days. Among the three surgical fatalities in the ALPPS cohort (patients numbered 10, 16, and 34), the median age was 69 (67–74) years. Patients 10 and 34 developed ascites after the initial surgery. The causes of death for these cases are detailed in Table 10.1. Although no statistically significant risk factor for mortality was identified in multivariate analysis, severe refractory ascites post-stage 1 surgery is considered a critical warning sign in our center. Two-thirds of the patients who succumbed shortly after stage 2 surgery experienced this complication prior to the second procedure. Consequently, due to this preventative measure adopted by the author, one patient (number 48) was spared from undergoing stage 2 surgery, thereby averting death.

Table 10.1 ALPPS-related complications [10]

Grade	Stage I	Stage II
I	Pleural effusion without drainage (*n* = 5)	
II	Mild ascites (<500 mL), relieved by diuretics (*n* = 3) Gross ascites, not relieved by diuretics (*n* = 2)	Mild ascites, relieved by diuretics (*n* = 5)
III		Intestinal obstruction due to adhesions requiring surgical resolution (*n* = 1)
IV		
V		Liver failure after reoperation due to bleeding (*n* = 1) Liver failure due to dysfunction (*n* = 1) Sepsis with multiple organ failure (*n* = 1)

10.11 Oncological Outcomes

The primary source of tumor blood supply in HCC is the hepatic artery [30]. Consequently, a significant concern regarding the oncological feasibility of ALPPS is the abrupt interruption of portal vein blood flow during the initial stage of surgery, coupled with the augmented hepatic arterial blood flow due to the buffering effect, and the resultant alterations in the tumor microenvironment during the interim period [31]. Recent studies have demonstrated that the overexpression of PD-L1 and alpha-fetoprotein (AFP) in tumors is correlated with early recurrence and poor survival prognosis [32, 33]. Tumor expression of VEGF has also been correlated with tumor aggressiveness and prognosis in HCC [34, 35]. Nevertheless, our study confirmed that none of these markers were overexpressed in ALPPS compared to the control group, indicating that this procedure did not have a significant stimulatory effect on tumor growth compared to PVE or primary hepatectomy.

More importantly, irrespective of tumor stage, the long-term disease-free survival (DFS) and overall survival (OS) for ALPPS were analogous to those for PVE, with no significant difference in the tumor recurrence pattern between the two groups. Therefore, ALPPS should be considered viable tumor surgery and incorporated into the standard algorithm for HCC surgical treatment in patients with insufficient FLR. From a surgeon's perspective, ALPPS ensures the complete diversion of portal vein blood flow to the FLR and mitigates the risk of incomplete surgery seen in PVE, such as portal vein reintubation or partial portal vein blood flow obstruction [36, 37]. Additionally, this procedure circumvents the risk of contralateral portal vein thrombosis or major portal vein thrombosis due to the migration of embolic material during PVE [37].

Nonetheless, ALPPS remains a major procedure involving two separate extensive surgeries performed under general anesthesia and should be reserved for patients with inadequate FLR who require a substantial volume increase within a defined timeframe or in patients with partial portal vein tumor thrombosis where PVE poses a risk of displacing tumor thrombus to the contralateral branch. Consequently, we recommend ALPPS for HCC patients with FLR/ESLV <30%, while PVE should be utilized for HCC patients with FLR/ESLV between 30% and 40%.

10.12 FLR Hypertrophy Effect: ALPPS vs. PVE

The experience at the author's center indicates that within a fixed period, ALPPS-induced proliferation is 4–5 times faster than PVE. Consequently, the hepatectomy timeline for ALPPS is significantly earlier than that for PVE, typically occurring within 2–4 weeks [10]. Factors such as non-cirrhosis, ICG-R15 < 39% during the initial surgery, and absence of postoperative complications are conducive to sufficient hypertrophy. FLR can proliferate at a rate exceeding FLR/ESLV >1% per day [10].

In summary, our findings demonstrate that ALPPS is a safe and effective approach for inducing liver regeneration in patients with chronic liver disease, with comparable risks of complications and mortality to PVE. However, due to the complexity of the procedure, ALPPS must be performed by experienced liver surgeons, ideally those with expertise in liver transplantation, to ensure the best possible outcomes.

References

1. Schadde E, Ardiles V, Robles-Campos R, et al. Early survival and safety of ALPPS: first report of the International ALPPS Registry[J]. Ann Surg. 2014;260(5):829–36.
2. Linecker M, Björnsson B, Stavrou GA, et al. Risk adjustment in ALPPS is associated with a dramatic decrease in early mortality and morbidity[J]. Ann Surg. 2017;266(5):779–86.
3. Alvarez FA, Ardiles V, de Santibañes M, et al. Associating liver partition and portal vein ligation for staged hepatectomy offers high oncological feasibility with adequate patient safety: a prospective study at a single center[J]. Ann Surg. 2015;261(4):723–32.
4. Sandström P, Røsok BI, Sparrelid E, et al. ALPPS improves resectability compared with conventional two-stage hepatectomy in patients with advanced colorectal liver metastasis: results from a Scandinavian multicenter randomized controlled trial (LIGRO trial) [J]. Ann Surg. 2018;267(5):833–40.
5. Schnitzbauer AA, Lang SA, Goessmann H, et al. Right portal vein ligation combined with *in situ* splitting induces rapid left lateral liver lobe hypertrophy, enabling 2-staged extended right hepatic resection in small-for-size settings[J]. Ann Surg. 2012;255(3):405–14.
6. Balci D. Pushing the envelope in perihiler cholangiocellularcarcinoma surgery: TIPE-ALPPS[J]. Ann Surg. 2018;267(2):e21–2.
7. Liu CL, Fan ST, Cheung ST, et al. Anterior approach versus conventional approach right hepatic resection for large hepatocellular carcinoma: a prospective randomized controlled study[J]. Ann Surg. 2006;244(2):194–203.
8. Ribero D, Amisano M, Bertuzzo F, et al. Measured versus estimated total liver volume to preoperatively assess the adequacy of the future liver remnant: which method should we use? [J]. Ann Surg. 2013;258(5):801–6.
9. Belghiti J, Guevara OA, Noun R, et al. Liver hanging maneuver: a safe approach to right hepatectomy without liver mobilization[J]. J Am Coll Surg. 2001;193(1):109–11.
10. Chan A, Zhang WY, Chok K, et al. ALPPS versus portal vein embolization for hepatitis-related hepatocellular carcinoma: a changing paradigm in the modulation of future liver remnant before major hepatectomy[J]. Ann Surg. 2021;273(5):957–65.
11. Petrowsky H, Györi G, de Oliveira M, et al. Is partial-ALPPS safer than ALPPS? A single-center experience[J]. Ann Surg. 2015;261(4):e90–2.
12. Chan ACY, Chok K, Dai JWC, et al. Impact of split completeness on future liver remnant hypertrophy in associating liver partition and portal vein ligation for staged hepatectomy(ALPPS) in hepatocellular carcinoma: complete-ALPPS versus partial-ALPPS[J]. Surgery,2017,161(2):357–364.
13. Chia DKA, Yeo Z, Loh SEK, et al. ALPPS for hepatocellular carcinoma is associated with decreased liver remnant growth[J]. J Gastrointest Surg. 2018;22(6):973–80.
14. Hessheimer AJ, Fondevila C, Taurá P, et al. Decompression of the portal bed and twice-baseline portal inflow are necessary for the functional recovery of a "small-for-size" graft[J]. Ann Surg. 2011;253(6):1201–10.
15. Fondevila C, Hessheimer AJ, Taurá P, et al. Portal hyperperfusion: mechanism of injury and stimulus for regeneration in porcine small-for-size transplantation[J]. Liver Transpl. 2010;16(3):364–74.
16. Umeda Y, Yagi T, Sadamori H, et al. Effects of prophylactic splenic artery modulation on portal overperfusion and liver regeneration in small-for-size graft[J]. Transplantation. 2008;86(5):673–80.
17. Dahm F, Georgiev P, Clavien PA. Small-for-size syndrome after partial liver transplantation: definition, mechanisms of disease and clinical implications[J]. Am J Transplant. 2005;5(11):2605–10.
18. Pomposelli JJ, Goodrich NP, Emond JC, et al. Patterns of early allograft dysfunction in adult live donor liver transplantation: the A2ALL experience[J]. Transplantation. 2016;100(7):1490–9.
19. Schlegel A, Lesurtel M, Melloul E, et al. ALPPS: from human to mice highlighting accelerated and novel mechanisms of liver regeneration[J]. Ann Surg. 2014;260(5):839–46. discussion 846–7
20. Chan SC, Lo CM, Chok KS, et al. Modulation of graft vascular inflow guided by flowmetry and manometry in liver transplantation[J]. Hepatobiliary Pancreat Dis Int. 2011;10(6):649–56.
21. Troisi R, Cammu G, Militerno G, et al. Modulation of portal graft inflow: a necessity in adult living-donor liver transplantation? [J]. Ann Surg. 2003;237(3):429–36.
22. Matsuo K, Murakami T, Kawaguchi D, et al. Histologic features after surgery associating liver partition and portal vein ligation for staged hepatectomy versus those after hepatectomy with portal vein embolization[J]. Surgery. 2016;159(5):1289–98.
23. Budai A, Horváth G, Tretter L, et al. Mitochondrial function after associating liver partition and portal vein ligation for staged hepatectomy in an experimental model[J]. Br J Surg. 2019;106(1):120–31.
24. Biller-Andorno N, Jüni P. Abolishing mammography screening programs? A view from the Swiss medical board[J]. N Engl J Med. 2014;370(21):1965–7.
25. Tong YF, Meng N, Chen MQ, et al. Maturity of associating liver partition and portal vein ligation for staged hepatectomy-derived liver regeneration in a rat model[J]. World J Gastroenterol. 2018;24(10):1107–19.
26. Nadalin S, Capobianco I, Li J, et al. Indications and limits for associating liver partition and portal vein ligation for staged hepatectomy (ALPPS). Lessons learned from 15 cases at a single center [J]. Z Gastroenterol. 2014;52(1):35–42.
27. Cauchy F, Fuks D, Nomi T, et al. Incidence, risk factors and consequences of bile leakage following laparoscopic major hepatectomy[J]. Surg Endosc. 2016;30(9):3709–19.
28. Martin AN, Narayanan S, Turrentine FE, et al. Clinical factors and postoperative impact of bile leak after liver resection[J]. J Gastrointest Surg. 2018;22(4):661–7.
29. Chan ACY, Poon RTP, Lo CM. Modified anterior approach for the ALPPS procedure: how we do it[J]. World J Surg. 2015;39(11):2831–5.
30. Jakab F, Ráth Z, Schmal F, et al. Changes in hepatic hemodynamics due to primary liver tumors [J]. HPB Surg. 1996;9(4):245–8.

31. Săftoiu A, Ciurea T, Gorunescu F. Hepatic arterial blood flow in large hepatocellular carcinoma with or without portal vein thrombosis: assessment by transcutaneous duplex Doppler sonography[J]. Eur J Gastroenterol Hepatol. 2002;14(2):167–76.
32. Peng SY, Chen WJ, Lai PL, et al. High alpha-fetoprotein level correlates with high stage, early recurrence, and poor prognosis of hepatocellular carcinoma: significance of hepatitis virus infection, age, p53, and beta-catenin mutations[J]. Int J Cancer. 2004;112(1):44–50.
33. Jung HI, Jeong D, Ji S, et al. Overexpression of PD-L1 and PD-L2 is associated with poor prognosis in patients with hepatocellular carcinoma[J]. Cancer Res Treat. 2017;49(1):246–54.
34. Pang R, Poon RT. Angiogenesis and antiangiogenic therapy in hepatocellular carcinoma[J]. Cancer Lett. 2006;242(2):151–67.
35. Raskopf E, Vogt A, Sauerbruch T, et al. siRNA targeting VEGF inhibits hepatocellular carcinoma growth and tumor angiogenesis *in vivo*[J]. J Hepatol. 2008;49(6):977–84.
36. Di Stefano DR, de Baere T, Denys A, et al. Preoperative percutaneous portal vein embolization: evaluation of adverse events in 188 patients[J]. Radiology. 2005;234(2):625–30.
37. van Gulik TM, van den Esschert JW, de Graaf W, et al. Controversies in the use of portal vein embolization[J]. Dig Surg. 2008;25(6):436–44.

11 Laparoscopic ALPPS

Shuguo Zheng, Baolin Wang, and Kexi Liao

11.1 Introduction

As an innovative surgical method, associating liver partition and portal vein ligation for staged hepatectomy (ALPPS) represents a significant advancement in surgical techniques developed in recent years. It integrates the essence of portal vein ligation and traditional two-step hepatectomy, which is hailed as a milestone breakthrough in the field of hepatobiliary surgery [1]. By altering the hepatic blood flow distribution and inducing an inflammatory response, ALPPS prompts rapid hypertrophy of the remaining liver parenchyma within a short term. This enhances the liver's volume to increase tolerance to extreme hepatectomy effectively and reduces the incidence of postoperative liver failure. ALPPS provides a viable option for curative surgical intervention in cases of advanced or multifocal liver malignancies, whereas conventional resection approaches may be inadequate [2]. As a result, ALPPS shows favorable clinical efficacy and broad application prospects. Jian Zhou and colleagues first performed the ALPPS procedure in Asia in 2013 [3]. Since then, multiple hepatobiliary surgery centers have documented successful ALPPS cases and reported their experience. Some guiding suggestions for ALPPS in Chinese patients with liver cancer and/or liver cirrhosis were also put forward [4]. In recent years, with advancements in basic research and improvements in surgical approaches, the clinical application of ALPPS has been increasingly performed. Liver surgeons have widely recognized its safety, feasibility, and effectiveness. Remarkable achievements have been realized.

Stages 1 and 2 of classical ALPPS involve open abdominal surgery, subjecting patients to two separate liver surgeries in a short period of time. The liver parenchyma transection and right portal vein ligation during the first-stage procedure may lead to severe inflammatory reactions, bile leakage, infections, and postoperative adhesions, thereby increasing the difficulty and risks associated with the following procedure. This results in a higher incidence of postoperative complications and mortality, leading to doubts and limitations in its clinical application [5, 6]. Laparoscopic techniques offer advantages such as minimal invasiveness, rapid recovery, small incisions, lower complication rates, reduced abdominal adhesions, and a shorter interval between the two staged surgeries. Therefore, laparoscopic ALPPS becomes the key research direction to break through the dilemma of classical ALPPS.

Leveraging the high-definition magnified view by laparoscopy to achieve precise hilar plate anatomy and liver parenchymal transection, laparoscopic ALPPS represents a significant advancement in this surgical approach. Vascular structures could be visualized and clamped distinctly during liver parenchyma transection, facilitating safer manipulation of the portal vein and biliary tracts. This not only enhances surgical safety but also significantly reduces postoperative abdominal and transected surface adhesions after the first stage, thereby mitigating the difficulty and risks associated with the following stage. Moreover, it allows surgeons to choose the proper time to perform stage 2 surgery based on the patient's situation [7]. Additionally, performing liver transection and portal vein ligation laparoscopically minimizes tumor tissue compression compared to open surgery, thereby minimizing the risk of intraoperative cancer cell dissemination, which is in line with the principle of "tumor-free surgery." Therefore, the combination of laparoscopic techniques with classical ALPPS procedures fully embodies the advantages of minimal invasiveness, rapid rehabilitation, and precise liver resection [8].

The application of laparoscopic techniques in staged liver resection was first documented in 2008 by Chandrakanth Are et al. [9], which included nine patients (five with colorectal cancer metastases, three with bile duct cancer, and one with hepatocellular carcinoma), all of whom underwent laparoscopic ligation of the right branch of the portal vein without

S. Zheng (✉) · B. Wang · K. Liao
The First Hospital Affiliated to Army Medical University (Southwest Hospital), Chongqing, China
e-mail: shuguozh@163.com

J. Zhou (ed.), *Associating Liver Partition and Portal Vein Ligation for Staged Hepatectomy (ALPPS)*, https://doi.org/10.1007/978-981-96-7364-3_11

liver parenchymal transection. Five patients successfully completed two-stage liver resection procedures due to liver dysfunction and infection. In 2012, Marcel Autran C. Machado et al. [10] reported a successful case with colorectal cancer liver metastasis using pure laparoscopic ALPPS procedure, in addition to their previous success with laparoscopic two-stage liver resection. The smaller incision and fewer abdominal adhesions not only reduced the difficulty of the second-stage surgery but also improved surgical safety. In 2013, Cao Jun et al. [11] were the first in China to adopt laparoscopic-assisted ALPPS to perform the first-stage procedure, e.g., ligation of the right branch of the portal vein, liver parenchymal division, and cholecystectomy in a patient with a giant HCC of the right lobe. By postoperative day 7, the second-stage open right trisectionectomy was successfully performed since the patient's FLR reached the criteria for safe resection. In China, patients with liver cancer often have underlying chronic hepatitis and cirrhosis, leading to impaired liver regenerative capacity, which poses new challenges for ALPPS surgeons. To our knowledge, the authors' unit was the first to adopt purely laparoscopic ALPPS for hepatectomy for patients with hepatitis B-related cirrhosis. The results showed that patients with hepatocellular carcinoma and cirrhosis could properly extend the interval of the two-step operation under favorable preoperative planning, and the residual liver parenchyma could also grow to the standard of safe resection [12].

The first-stage ALPPS procedure is particularly crucial, as it is not only decisive for postoperative recovery, the extent of residual liver volume enlargement, and the incidence of postoperative complications, but also determines the interval between both stages of the procedure and the success of the entire procedure. With the progress of clinical research on ALPPS, the high incidence of perioperative bile leakage and infection, which might lead to higher mortality, has been a heated topic. The liver parenchymal transection in first-stage ALPPS surgery poses a potential risk for postoperative bile leakage. Enrico Gringeri et al. [13] and Tamara M.H. Gal et al. [14] used laparoscopic techniques to ligate the portal vein on the tumor side during the ALPPS first-stage procedure, opting against liver splitting and performed laparoscopic microwave coagulation and radiofrequency ablation under ultrasound guidance to create a coagulative necrotic zone between the resected tumor and the residual liver parenchyma. This approach resulted in satisfactory postoperative residual liver hypertrophy and a marked decrease in complications and mortality with no bile leakage or infection. During the subsequent second stage procedure, minimal adhesions were observed in the surgical field, facilitating a "bloodless" minimally invasive resection of the diseased liver parenchyma along the necrotic zone surface. Furthermore, Cai Xiujun et al. [15] reported laparoscopic liver hanging maneuvers and ligature at the pre-transection line to perform ligation of the left and right liver parenchyma instead of liver parenchymal transection, which is a reflection of integrating the advantages of laparoscopic techniques with traditional liver transection and liver hanging maneuvers. This strategy yielded significant short-term liver hypertrophy, thereby reducing the risks of postoperative bile leakage, bleeding, and abdominal infection following the first-stage procedure. The above reports represent notable advancements in laparoscopic ALPPS, which may effectively avoid the high incidence of complications related to liver parenchymal transection and the prolonged postoperative recovery period.

11.2 Indication

ALPPS reported abroad are primarily for liver metastasis of colorectal cancer, bile duct cancer, neuroendocrine tumors, etc. [16]. Based on the morbidity and treatment status of liver tumors in our country, surgeons in China have successfully performed ALPPS in the treatment of primary liver cancer with favorable therapeutic effects. They have also proposed the potential application of ALPPS in certain benign liver lesions, such as hepatic hydatid disease and giant hemangiomas with Kasabach-Merritt syndrome. With the advancement of laparoscopic techniques, laparoscopic ALPPS for liver tumors has been reported successively. Careful selection of indications for laparoscopic ALPPS remains one of the important methods to improve the success rate of surgery and reduce the incidence of complications and mortality.

Currently, from the authors' perspectives, the main indications for laparoscopic ALPPS are primary and metastatic liver cancer that cannot be resected by curative surgery, as well as other incurable benign and malignant liver lesions. These indications are generally subject to the following conditions: (a) The whole body was in good condition, there were no organic lesions in other vital organs, and CO_2 pneumoperitoneum was tolerated, which met the primary conditions of open and laparoscopic liver surgery; (b) Age $\leq$60 years, regardless of gender; (c) Curative resection with open approach could not be realized with no evidence of extrahepatic metastasis, bleeding due to tumor rupture, main trunk PVTT and common bile duct tumor thrombus, or invasion of the vena cava; (d) Presence of giant or multiple liver lesions, or tumors located in a complex area requiring extensive liver resection (e.g., hemihepatectomy or extended hemihepatectomy) to achieve R0 resection, with technical feasibility and preoperative evaluations showing a ratio of post-resection residual liver volume to standard liver volume of <25% (<35% in patients with cirrhosis or other underlying liver diseases); e. Liver function of Child-Pugh class B or above, ICG-R15 ≤20%, with absence of active hepatitis, decompensated liver cirrhosis, or severe portal hypertension; f. Treatment including surgery such as radiofrequency ablation, and transcatheter arterial embolization chemotherapy should not be performed within 6 weeks before surgery. Patients with liver metastases of colorectal cancer are completely or partially sensitive to systemic chemotherapy, and chemotherapy should be stopped for more than 4 weeks.

In addition to the indications above, the impact of tumor size and location on laparoscopic ALPPS should also be considered. The author believes that for patients with massive liver cancer or large liver benign tumors, due to the space-occupying effect of huge tumors, hyperplasia of the left liver, and possible splenomegaly, laparoscopy in stage 2 surgery leads to small abdominal space, difficulty in safe removal of free liver and specimens. We recommend laparoscopically assisted ALPPS (stage 1 surgery performed laparoscopically, stage 2 surgery performed laparoscopically). Conversely, for patients with centrally located liver malignancy of relatively more minor volume but situated at critical sites such as vascular bifurcation, or those with multifocal tumors necessitating an expanded liver resection to achieve a radical outcome (R0 resection), the use of totally laparoscopic ALPPS is advocated. During the second-stage surgery, specimen removal via a suprapubic incision above the pubic symphysis takes advantage of the minimally invasive nature of the laparoscopic approach.

11.3 Surgical Procedure

Two types of surgical approaches can be considered laparoscopic ALPPS: laparoscopic-assisted ALPPS and total laparoscopic ALPPS. The former, also known as semi-laparoscopic ALPPS, involves a laparoscopic first-stage surgery followed by an open second-stage surgery. In the latter approach, both stages are conducted entirely under laparoscopy. Although the initial surgical steps are similar for both approaches, the method differs for the second stage, while the core surgical techniques and principles remain largely consistent. The following outlines the operation process and steps for both stages of laparoscopic ALPPS with the example of a right hemihepatectomy.

11.3.1 Laparoscopic ALPPS: Stage 1 Procedure

11.3.1.1 Patient Positioning and Trocar Distribution

The patient is placed in a supine position with legs apart, followed by endotracheal intubation and general anesthesia via combined inhalation and intravenous approach. The surgical area is disinfected, and drapes are placed before CO_2 pneumoperitoneum initiation with a pressure of 12–14 mmHg. A 10 mm trocar port is placed 2 cm to the right of the umbilicus, and the patient is adjusted to reverse Trendelenburg position, with the head side raised by 15°–30°. The right side can be elevated by approximately 30° as required. A 12 mm operating port is established below the xiphoid process, and a 5 mm port is placed at the midpoint of the line between the xiphoid process and the umbilicus. Additionally, a 12 mm main operating port is established horizontally 2–3 cm above the umbilicus along the right midclavicular line, and a 5 mm auxiliary operating port is established slightly higher than the main operating port, between the anterior axillary line and the midaxillary line (Fig. 11.1).

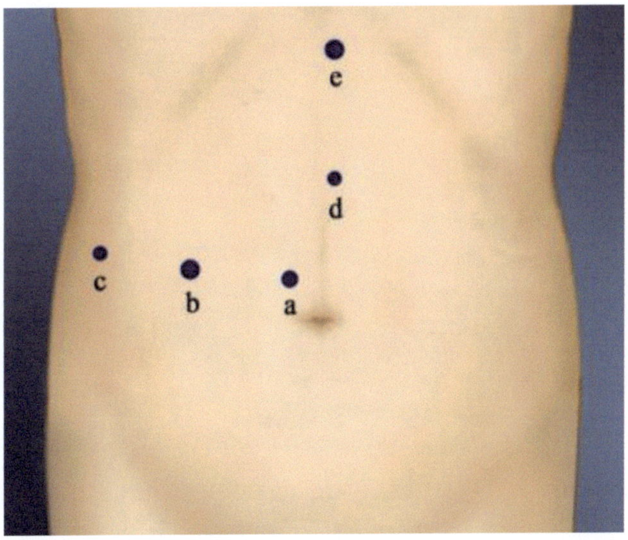

Fig. 11.1 Layout of trocar and operating ports. (**a**) 10 mm trocar port; (**b** and **e**) 12 mm operating ports; (**c** and **d**) 5 mm operating ports

11.3.1.2 Laparoscopy and Intraoperative Ultrasonography Exploration

Laparoscopic exploration is performed to assess the presence of ascites, liver size, texture, morphology, presence and degree of cirrhosis, tumor location, rupture, and bleeding. Additionally, it evaluates whether any previously undiscovered lesions in the hepatic hilum, enlargement of lymph nodes, metastases in the omentum, abdominal wall, or diaphragm are present. It assesses the surface of abdominal organs such as the stomach and intestines. Intraoperative ultrasound further determines the size and location of liver tumors, their relationship with surrounding major vascular structures, and the presence of cancer thrombus in major vessels. A comprehensive examination of the liver is warranted to identify any lesion in the pre-reserved liver parenchyma. Preoperative three-dimensional visualization and virtual surgical planning can help identify the correct plane for liver parenchymal transection.

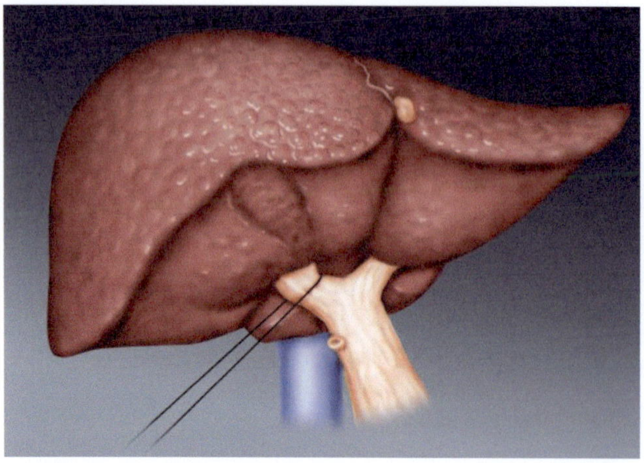

Fig. 11.2 Dissection of the right hepatic pedicle outside the glissonian sheath

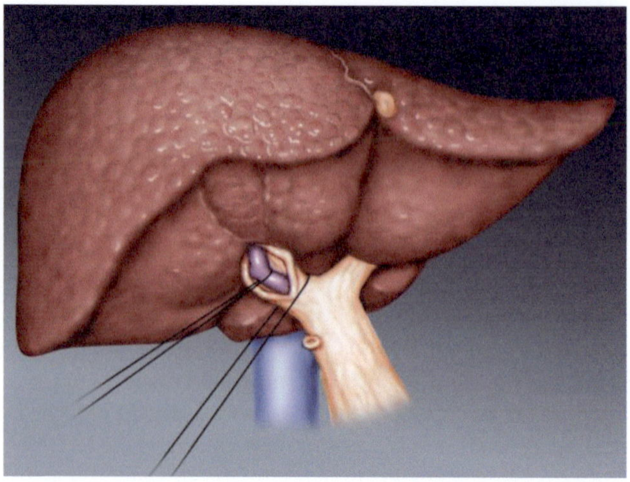

Fig. 11.3 Dissection and ligation of the right branch of the portal vein within the Glissonian sheath

11.3.1.3 Cholecystectomy

Calot's triangle is dissected using a harmonic scalpel or bipolar electrocoagulation. After careful ligation of the cystic artery and cystic duct, the gallbladder is dissected and removed with combined antegrade and retrograde approaches before thorough hemostasis of the gallbladder bed.

11.3.1.4 Dissection of the Glissonian Pedicle and Ligation of the Right Branch of the Portal Vein

The lesser omentum is opened anteriorly to the left lobe of the liver along the posterior aspect of the hepatic hilum through the Winslow hole. A laparoscopic liver blood flow occlusion device is pre-placed. Lowering the hepatic hilum to expose the bifurcation of the left and right hepatic pedicles. Dissect along the sheath of the Lannec's membrane and expose the right Glissonian pedicle, which is marked and suspended with a 7–0 silk suture (Fig. 11.2). The sheath of the right Glissonian pedicle is opened, and dissection within the sheath dissociates the right branch of the portal vein and the right hepatic artery. The right branch of the portal vein is ligated with a 4–0 silk suture (Fig. 11.3). The right hepatic artery is pre-placed with an absorbable suture for later use during the second-stage surgery. During the dissection of the Glissonian sheath, it is suggested to minimize the use of high-power energy devices to avoid damage to the arteries and bile ducts. Ligation of the portal vein must be thorough since incomplete ligation with residual blood flow perfusing the tumor side often leads to failure of the procedure. Anatomical variations of the portal vein branches may exist, and preoperative imaging and three-dimensional visualization can help surgeons identify these variations. During surgery, attention is given to ligating all tumor-feeding portal vein branches to prevent insufficient hypertrophy of the future liver remnant, in which case timely portal vein embolization (PVE) of the corresponding portal vein branches would be needed. The hepatocaval recess is exposed, followed by blunt dissection towards the foot side along the vena cava recess. The right liver is lifted to expose the anterior wall of the infrarenal vena cava and the retrohepatic space, typically using a Goldfinger dissector for blunt dissection towards the head direction with convergence from above and below to establish a retrohepatic tunnel. A tape is placed around the liver through the retrohepatic tunnel (Fig. 11.4) to guide the transection plane, expose the surgical field, and protect the vena cava during liver transection. Temporary occlusion of the right hepatic artery is performed using vascular clamps, and the ischemic demarcation line on the liver surface can be observed. After determining the ischemic plane, the planned incision line is marked on the liver surface using an electrocautery hook based on tumor location and surgical planning (Figs. 11.5 and 11.6).

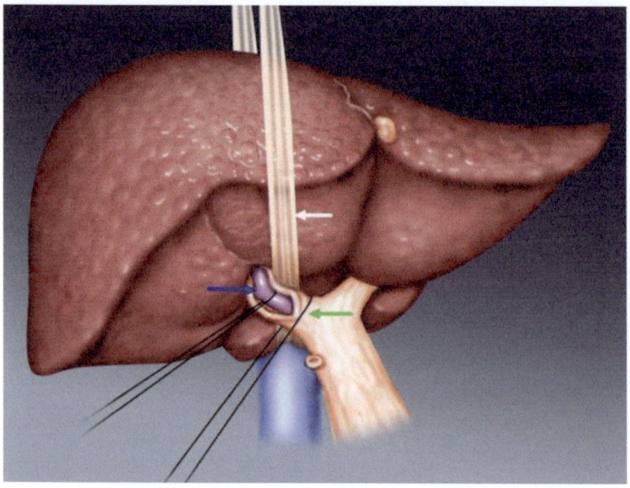

Fig. 11.4 Establishment of the hepatic tunnel and placement of the tape. White arrow: tape location; Green arrow: right hepatic pedicle; Blue arrow: right branch of the portal vein

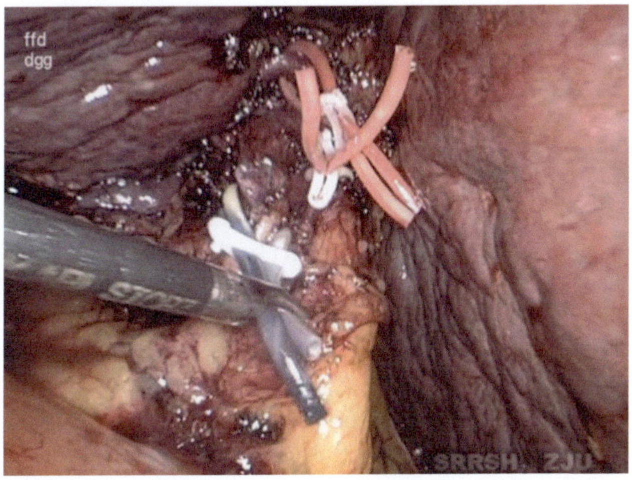

Fig. 11.5 Suspension of the common bile duct

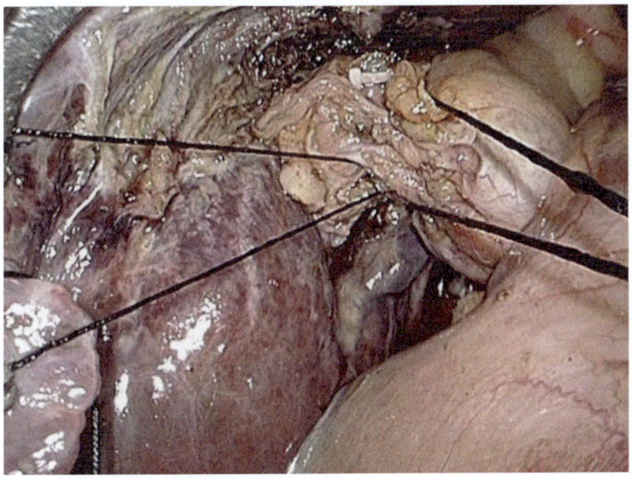

Fig. 11.6 Laparoscopic dissection of the right hepatic pedicle and right branch of the portal vein during stage 1 ALPPS

11.3.1.5 Laparoscopic Liver Parenchymal Transection

Liver parenchymal transection is performed using an ultrasonic scalpel/laparoscopic cavitron ultrasonic surgical aspirator (CUSA) along the ischemic demarcation line on the liver surface, directed towards the inferior vena cava from the ventral to dorsal and from caudal to cranial directions. The liver parenchyma is transected in a "book-opening" manner while maintaining optimal visualization and moderate tension. After complete exposure of the encountered ductal structures with 360° skeletonization, Hem-o-lok clips or LigaSure titanium clips are applied to both ends of the transected liver parenchyma, followed by transection in between. Bipolar electrocautery and Prolene sutures, as needed, are utilized for hemostasis. When transecting deeper into the liver parenchyma, the tissue anterior to IVC can be lifted by

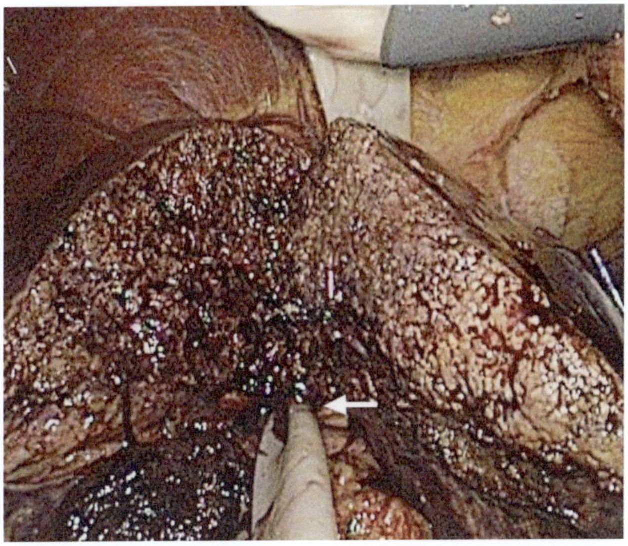

Fig. 11.7 Guiding the direction of liver parenchymal transection with retrohepatic tape

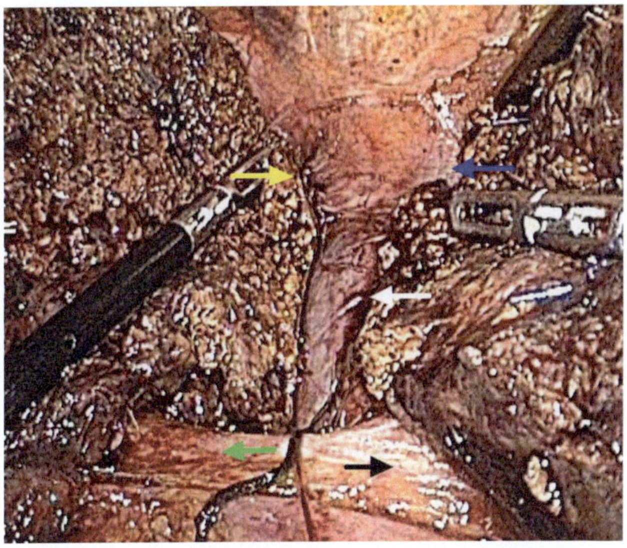

Fig. 11.8 Complete transection of liver parenchyma. Yellow arrow: right hepatic vein; Blue arrow: middle hepatic vein; White arrow: inferior vena cava; Green arrow: right hepatic pedicle; Black arrow: left hepatic pedicle

pulling the tape around the liver until complete transection is done (Figs. 11.7, 11.8 and 11.9). Controlled low central venous pressure techniques are performed during liver parenchymal transection to minimize bleeding. This involves close coordination with the anesthesiologist to restrict fluid input and use vasopressors to maintain central venous pressure within a predefined range if necessary. The Pringle maneuver may be adopted when necessary to temporarily occlude hepatic inflow.

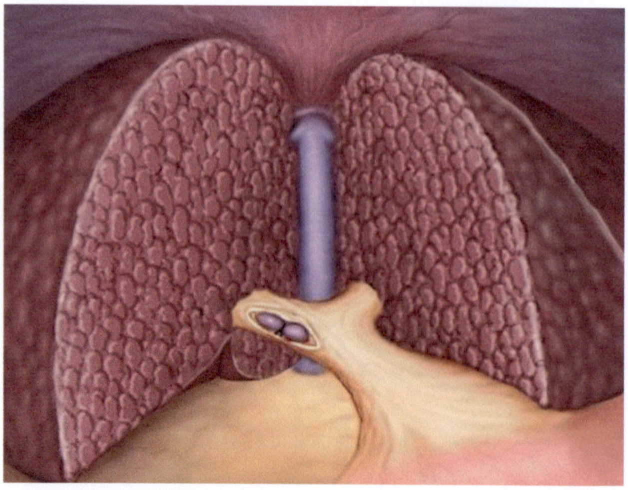

Fig. 11.9 Schematic diagram of complete liver parenchymal transection

11.3.1.6 Examination of the Transection Surface and Placement of Drainage

Following the completion of liver parenchymal transection, a routine examination is conducted to check for bleeding and bile leakage on both transection surfaces, particularly focusing on bile leakage. In cases of oozing from the transection surface, bipolar or monopolar electrocautery is typically used for hemostasis, while active bleeding may necessitate hemostasis with Prolene sutures. Some centers have reported using fat emulsion injection into the residual end of the cystic duct to detect bile leakage from the liver transection surface (bile leakage is indicated by the emergence of white fat emulsion). However, it is primarily applicable to traditional open ALPPS first-stage surgeries where laparoscopic access may be challenging. Laparoscopy's high-definition magnified view and angulation capability enable the detection of minor vascular oozing and bile leaks, thereby reducing the incidence of bleeding and bile leakage. The transection surface is typically irrigated with saline solution, followed by clean gauze coverage to detect bile staining and identify leakage points. Indocyanine green (ICG) staining under a fluorescence laparoscope can also be used if necessary to confirm bile leakage and guide precise suturing and management. The application of biological glue or hemostatic gauze to cover the transection surface can alleviate local adhesions and facilitate better separation of the left and right sides during the second-stage surgery. One negative pressure drain is left in place at the liver transection surface, with an additional latex drain placed under the right diaphragm. After deflating the pneumoperitoneum and closure of the trocar fascia, fascial closure devices and laparoscopic inverted suturing can be used to close the fascial defects and prevent postoperative abdominal fluid leakage.

11.3.2 Postoperative Management After Laparoscopic Stage 1 ALPPS

Patients receive anti-inflammatory, hepatoprotective, fluid replacement, antiviral, and symptomatic supportive therapy postoperatively, along with early initiation of oral intake and ambulation. Blood tests such as coagulation function, liver and kidney functions, and arterial blood gas analysis are routinely monitored. Abdominal drainage fluid should be observed, and intermittent compression of the drainage tube wall can facilitate drainage and maintain tube patency. The timing for removal of drainage tubes is determined based on drainage volume and content, typically within 3 to 5 days. In cases where encapsulated effusion develops on the liver transected surface postoperatively or when drainage fluid is inadequate, ultrasound-guided percutaneous liver puncture drainage may be performed. Thoracentesis drainage is conducted if pleural effusion restricts respiratory function or pulmonary infection occurs. Patients are instructed to consume a high-protein diet upon resumption of oral intake.

11.3.3 FLR Hypertrophy and Functional Assessment

Routine follow-up assessments for all patients include abdominal contrast-enhanced computed tomography angiography (CTA) and chest computed tomography (CT) scans on the seventh-day post-first-stage surgery to evaluate residual liver hypertrophy, tumor progression or metastasis, liver transection surface, abdominal drainage, and pulmonary function status. The ratio of residual liver volume to standard liver volume is calculated. Suppose FLR is 40% or higher of the total liver volume, meeting safety requirements for liver resection, with the patient's general condition improved, and hematological, coagulation, liver, and kidney function tests returning to normal. In that case, a decision regarding the indication for ALPPS stage 2 surgery is made through consultation with a hepatobiliary surgical expert panel. In the absence of surgical contraindications and with the consent of the patient and family, second-stage laparoscopic ALPPS is performed, with similar preoperative preparations to the first stage. Patients with underlying chronic liver diseases such as liver fibrosis, cirrhosis, or hepatic steatosis exhibit slower liver regeneration and typically require two weeks or longer. If hypertrophy is inadequate, weekly follow-up with abdominal CTA is conducted until FLR hypertrophy reaches the safety resection criteria, at which point a decision is made regarding a second-stage surgery or termination of the procedure. Postoperative CTA follow-up and re-measurement of liver volume should focus on the status of portal vein branch occlusion on the tumor side; incomplete ligation or overlooked variations of portal vein branches require timely salvage, such as portal vein embolization (PVE).

11.3.4 Total Laparoscopic Stage 2 ALPPS

Anesthesia and patient positioning for second-stage surgery are similar to the first stage. The operative field is routinely prepared and draped, and incisions are made at the previous Trocar sites from the first-stage procedure. The pneumoperitoneum is established at 12–14 mmHg, and entry into the abdominal cavity is made through the original laparoscopic ports. Adhesions in the abdominal cavity after first-stage laparoscopic ALPPS are generally mild, but patients with a longer interval after first-stage surgery or those who experience bile leakage or intra-abdominal infection may have more severe adhesions. Blunt dissection using an aspirator is helpful to manage adhesions between the abdominal wall and the liver, between the liver and the gastrointestinal tract or the omentum, and between the bilateral liver transection surfaces. Thus, the liver transection surface and Hilar structures can be exposed for the examination of the abdominal cavity and FLR hypertrophy (Fig. 11.10). Laparoscopic ultrasonography is used to confirm the absence of new lesions within the FLR, which is particularly important for patients undergoing ALPPS for colorectal cancer liver metastasis. The right hepatic pedicle marked and suspended during First-stage surgery is identified, and an endoscopic linear cutter is used for transection (Fig. 11.11). If bleeding occurs at the transection margin, reinforcement with 4–0 Prolene sutures is applied. The right liver is dissected from the anterior wall of IVC towards the cephalad direction, and any encountered short hepatic veins are double-clipped and divided using Hem-o-lok or LigaSure device to preserve the posterior aspect until the root of the right hepatic vein, which is then divided by an endoscopic linear cutter (Fig. 11.12). Ligaments around the right liver are dissected, tumors and the right liver specimen are completely removed, and a transverse incision of approximately 15 cm is made 5 cm above the pubic symphysis to retrieve the specimen (Fig. 11.13). The incision is closed layer by layer, and the pneumoperitoneum is reestablished. After confirming no bleeding or bile leakage, biological hemostatic materials can be applied to the liver transection surface. The liver round ligament and part of the falciform ligament are fixed to the anterior abdominal wall. An abdominal drainage tube is placed under the

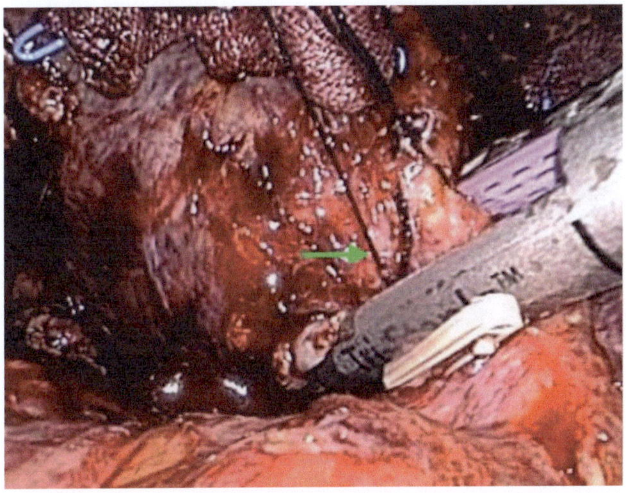

Fig. 11.11 Transection of the right hepatic pedicle with a cutting stapler

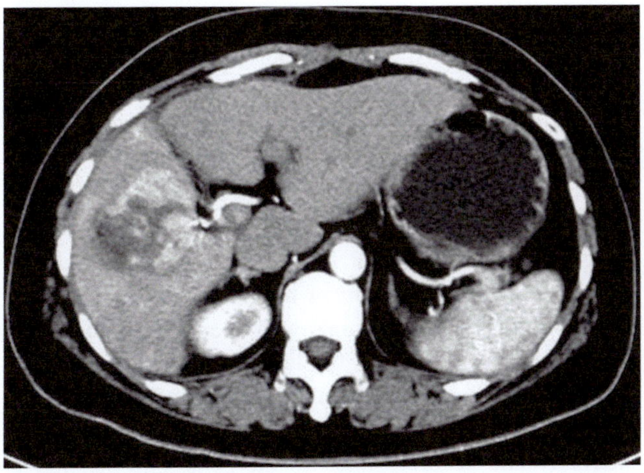

Fig. 11.10 Significant regeneration of the left liver after stage 1 ALPPS

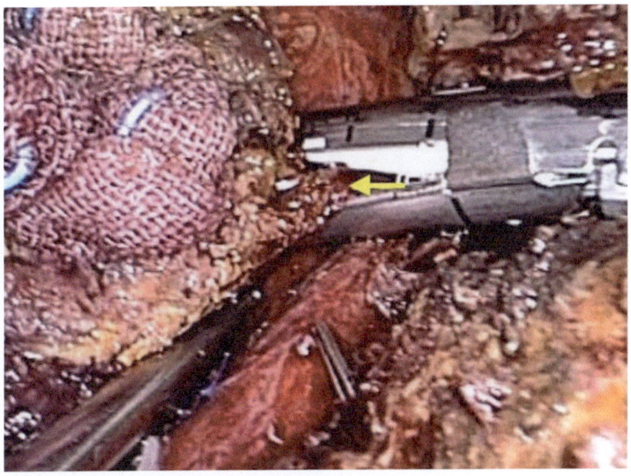

Fig. 11.12 Transection of the right hepatic vein with a cutting stapler

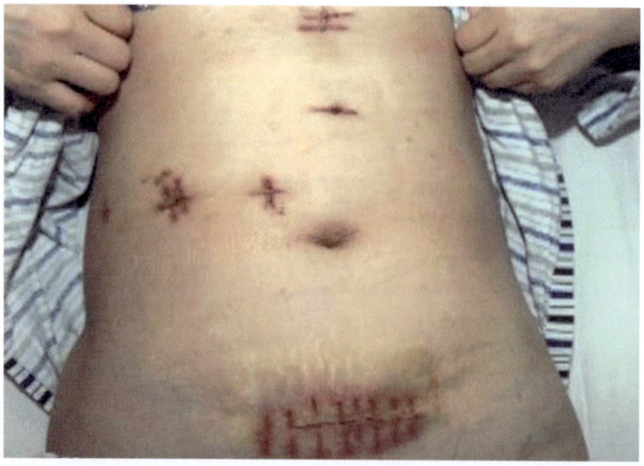

Fig. 11.13 Ports re-established for stage 2 ALPPS with same trocar locations, specimen retrieved through transverse incision above the pubic symphysis

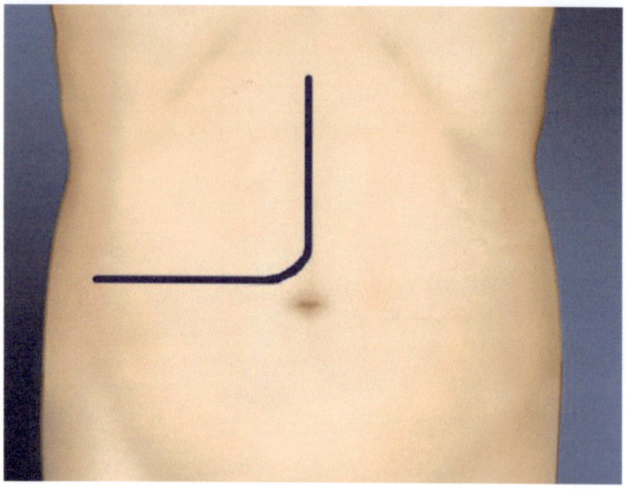

Fig. 11.14 Reverse "L"-shaped incision connecting the Trocar ports from first-stage surgery

right diaphragm, which is brought out through the main operating port, and securely fixed externally. The pneumoperitoneum is released before Trocar sites are sutured closed.

11.3.5 Laparoscopic-Assisted Stage 2 ALPPS (Open Surgery)

The patient is positioned supine, with anesthesia administered as previously introduced, and the Trocar distribution from first-stage surgery is connected to form a reverse "L"-shaped incision in the right upper abdomen (Fig. 11.14).

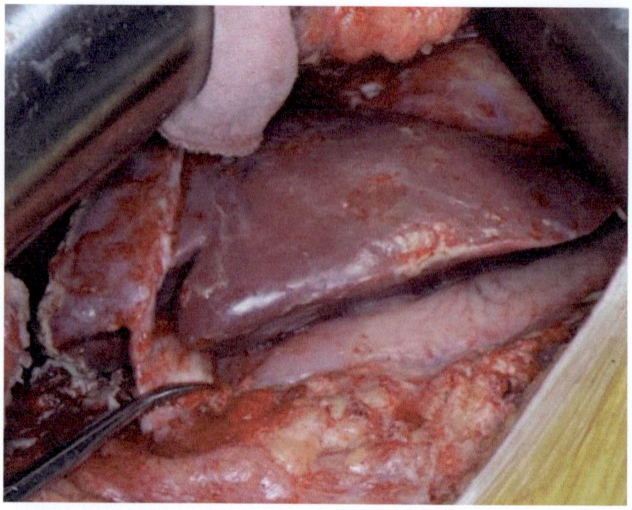

Fig. 11.15 Intraoperative finding—significant regeneration of the residual liver

Careful dissection of intra-abdominal adhesions is done while exploring the abdominal cavity and FLR (Fig. 11.15). Intraoperative ultrasound can help identify the presence of new lesions or metastases in the FLR or abdominal cavity. The hepatic hilum is dissected to locate the right hepatic pedicle marked during first-stage surgery, and the bilateral liver transection surfaces are separated, removing local adhesive tissue. Thorough debridement is needed if encapsulated effusion develops locally. After further dissection of the right hepatic pedicle for more operating space, an endoscopic linear cutter is used for transection, with reinforcement using 4–0 Prolene sutures if necessary. The liver is separated from the anterior wall of IVC towards the cephalad direction, and any short hepatic veins encountered are ligated or sutured before transection. An endoscopic linear cutter may be used for transection if large right posterior inferior or right posterior middle hepatic veins are encountered. The right hepatic vein is dissected and divided with an endoscopic linear cutter (Fig. 11.16). The liver is pulled downward and freed along the right side of the IVC, and the resected liver specimen is removed after dissecting the ligaments around the right liver (Fig. 11.17). After repeated inspection, it was confirmed that there was no bleeding or bile leakage from the liver transection surface, so biological hemostatic materials could be applied. The round and part of the falciform ligaments are fixed to the anterior abdominal wall at an appropriate position to prevent twisting of the left liver, which may affect blood reflux in the hepatic veins. A drainage tube is routinely placed under the right diaphragm, which is brought out externally and securely fixed to the skin. The incision is closed layer by layer, and the abdomen is closed.

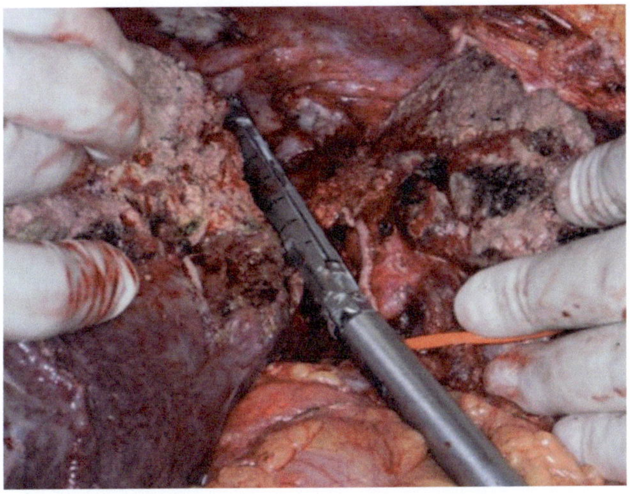

Fig. 11.16 Transection of the right hepatic pedicle followed by transection of the right hepatic vein using a cutting stapler

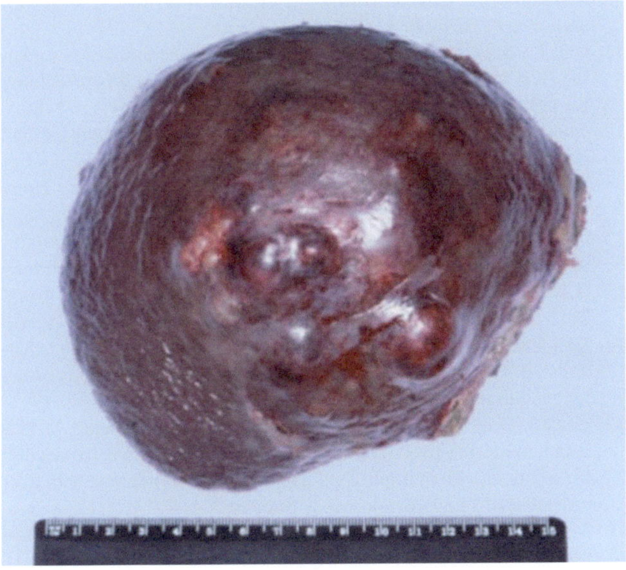

Fig. 11.17 Resected tumor and liver specimen

11.4 Key Points and Considerations for Laparoscopic ALPPS Surgery

The key points and considerations for laparoscopic ALPPS surgery are as follows:

Firstly, patients undergoing laparoscopic ALPPS surgery are often those with extensive or multiple hepatocellular carcinomas who have lost the opportunity for conventional surgical resection. Some patients may also have underlying liver cirrhosis, high tumor tension, significant mass effect, and a hard liver texture, posing challenges for intraoperative mobilization. Following the "no-touch" principle of tumor surgery, efforts should be made during first-stage surgery to minimize liver mobilization and aim for in situ liver transection to avoid flipping, squeezing, and preventing tumor rupture and bleeding. In second-stage surgery, liver mobilization and tumor removal should only be done after complete vascular occlusion.

Secondly, in first-stage surgery, an anterior approach is used to perform in situ liver transection to the level of the anterior wall of IVC, which completely separates the liver to be resected from the FLR. A retrohepatic tunnel is established from the retrocaval space to the anterior space between the liver and the posterior aspect of the IVC, allowing convergence from above and below. Pringle maneuver is applied, and the liver is transected only after complete vascular occlusion is confirmed.

Thirdly, during liver transection, both ends of encountered vascular structures should be carefully treated. Both sides of the liver transection surface should be thoroughly inspected to ensure no bleeding or bile leakage, with preoperative three-dimensional visualization and virtual surgical planning, if applicable, and intraoperative ultrasound to ensure the integrity of important vascular structures between the pre-resected liver and the residual liver. The use of ICG fluorescence fusion mode can help observe tumor staining and determine the liver transection plane in real-time intraoperatively in combination with anterograde and retrograde staining methods. Bile ducts in the hepatic hilum and bile leakage from the transection surface were also observed.

Fourthly, postoperative inflammation and adhesions after first-stage surgery are relatively milder compared to traditional open surgery but cannot be completely avoided. Particularly, adhesions at the hepatic hilum, between the liver transection surface and the abdominal wall, intra-abdominal organs, and between the deep aspect of the liver transection surface and the anterior wall of the retrohepatic IVC and hepatic vein root. Gentle maneuvers should be employed when dissociating adhesions. Blunt and sharp dissection should be combined, depending on the interval between surgeries and the degree of local tissue inflammation and edema, to protect important vascular structures. Due to tissue inflammation, edema, and fragility, the use of an endoscopic linear cutter to handle the hepatic pedicle and hepatic vein root may result in complications such as local tissue fragmentation, staple line dehiscence, and significant bleeding. Gentle maneuvers are required when using a cutting stapler to ensure a safe distance from the caval side of the transected end, and the direction of hepatic vein root transection should be as parallel as possible to the course of the IVC to reduce tension. If bleeding along the staple line occurs, prompt and decisive suturing should be performed. For patients with small stature, massive right liver tumors, or significant mass effect from a large spleen occupying the right and left subcostal spaces, resulting in insufficient abdominal space, laparoscopic techniques for second-stage surgery may pose challenges in liver mobilization and safe specimen removal. In such cases, an open approach may be more suitable, in the case patients can still benefit from the minimally invasive advantages of first-stage laparoscopic surgery.

Fifthly, in our center's practice, we found patients with liver cirrhosis can still have rapid regenerative capacity shortly after first-stage ALPPS surgery, although the speed of regeneration is slightly lower compared to normal liver tissue, with regeneration typically occurring over a period of approximately 2 weeks, followed by no significant further regeneration. For patients with massive tumors in the right hepatic lobe and a large spleen occupying the right and left subcostal areas, leading to inadequate abdominal space after first-stage ALPPS, left hepatic regeneration may be limited. However, after right hepatic resection in second-stage surgery, FLR can undergo rapid regeneration once again.

References

1. Schnitzbauer AA, Lang SA, Goessmann H, et al. Right portal vein ligation combined with *in situ* splitting induces rapid left lateral liver lobe hypertrophy enabling 2-staged extended right hepatic resection in small-for-size settings[J]. Ann Surg. 2012;255(3):405–14.
2. Lang H, Baumgart J, Mittler J. Associated liver partition and portal vein ligation for staged hepatectomy (ALPPS) registry: what have we learned?[J]. Gut Liver. 2020;14(6):699–706.
3. Torres OJ, de Souza Martins Fernandes E, Oliveira CV, et al. Associating liver partition and portal vein ligation for staged hepatectomy (ALPPS): the Brazilian experience[J]. Arq Bras Cir Dig. 2013;26(1):40–3.
4. Wang ZY, Yan YK, Zhang YC. The application status and research progress of laparoscopic-assisted associating liver partition and portal vein ligation[J]. Int J Dig Dis. 2017;37(4):217–20.
5. Maulat C, Philis A, Charriere B, et al. Rescue associating liver partition and portal vein ligation for staged hepatectomy after portal embolization: our experience and literature review[J]. World J Clin Oncol. 2017;8(4):351–9.
6. Linecker M, Björnsson B, Stavrou GA, et al. Risk adjustment in ALPPS is associated with a dramatic decrease in early mortality and morbidity[J]. Ann Surg. 2017;266(5):779–86.
7. Xiao Y, Gong LS, Li XL, et al. Experience of laparoscopic-assisted associating liver partition and portal vein ligation[J]. Chin J Mod Med. 2020;30(5):124–7.
8. Zheng SG. Value and evaluation of associating liver partition with portal vein ligation for staged hepatectomy (ALPPS) in the treatment of colorectal liver metastases[J]. Chin J Pract Surg. 2016;36:403–7.
9. Are C, Iacovitti S, Prete F, et al. Feasibility of laparoscopic portal vein ligation prior to major hepatectomy[J]. HPB (Oxford). 2008;10(4):229–33.
10. Machado MA, Makdissi FF, Surjan RC. Totally laparoscopic ALPPS is feasible and may be worthwhile[J]. Ann Surg. 2012;256(3):e13. author reply e16–e19
11. Cao J, Zhang HW, Zhang L, et al. Laparoscopic-assisted associating liver partition and portal vein ligation for staged hepatectomy for primary liver cancer[J]. Chin J Pract Surg. 2014;34(1):77–80.
12. Chan ACY, Chan CY. The role of associating liver partition and portal vein ligation for staged hepatectomy in the management of hepatocellular carcinoma[D]. Hong Kong: The University of Hong Kong Libraries, Master of Surgery; 2019.
13. Gringeri E, Boetto R, D'Amico FE, et al. Laparoscopic microwave ablation and portal vein ligation for staged hepatectomy (LAPS): a minimally invasive first-step approach[J]. Ann Surg. 2015;261(2):e42–3.
14. Gall TM, Sodergren MH, Frampton AE, et al. Radio-frequency-assisted liver partition with portal vein ligation (RALPP) for liver regeneration[J]. Ann Surg. 2015;261(2):e45–6.
15. Cai XJ, Peng SY, Duan L, et al. Completely laparoscopic ALPPS using round-the-liver ligation to replace parenchymal transection for a patient with multiple right liver cancers complicated with liver cirrhosis[J]. J Laparoendosc Adv Surg Tech A. 2014;24(12):883–6.
16. Machado MA, Makdissi FF, Surjan RC, et al. Two-stage laparoscopic liver resection for bilateral colorectal liver metastasis[J]. Surg Endosc. 2010;24(8):2044–7.

Robotic ALPPS

12

Xiaoying Wang

12.1 Introduction to Robotic ALPPS

In 2013, Solomonov et al. [1] accomplished the world's first robotic associating liver partition and portal vein ligation for staged hepatectomy (ALPPS) procedure for the management of hepatocellular carcinoma and subsequently presented this pioneering accomplishment at the Clinical Robotic Surgery Association (CRSA) Worldwide Congress. In 2014, Vicente et al. [2] reported the treatment of liver metastasis of colon cancer with a robotic ALPPS procedure at the CRSA Worldwide Congress. The first Chinese robotic ALPPS procedure was successfully completed at Zhongshan Hospital, Fudan University, in October 2014, which was reported at the 2015 CRSA Worldwide Congress. In 2021 and 2022, Benedetto et al. [3, 4] reported the treatment of intrahepatic cholangiocarcinoma and hilar cholangiocarcinoma with robotic ALPPS procedure, respectively.

12.2 Advantages and Limitations of Robotic ALPPS

12.2.1 Advantages of Robotic ALPPS

The robotic surgical system, which addresses the inherent constraints of conventional laparoscopy, offers the following technical advantages: (a) EndoWrist instruments provide seven degrees of freedom, enabling them to mimic the intricate movements of the human wrist with remarkable dexterity and precision. In addition, the instruments can effectively filter out hand tremors, achieving a level of flexibility and accuracy that meets or even surpasses the capabilities of the human hand; (b) The video imaging system provides surgeons with high-definition three-dimensional images magnified up to 10 times; (c) The robotic arm system offers a consistent and unwavering traction force; (d) The surgeon console prioritizes ergonomics. Therefore, the robotic surgical system is theoretically well-suited for complex liver surgeries and is particularly effective in enhancing the success rates of minimally invasive major hepatectomies, reducing the need for conversion to laparotomy, and reconstructing blood vessels and biliary tract.

The robotic ALPPS procedure confers the following potential advantages over conventional laparoscopy: (a) a more expeditious learning curve and more precise control; (b) safer and more precise dissection of the porta hepatis and the retrohepatic inferior vena cava; (c) superior hemostatic control because of straightforward suturing operations; (d) higher detectability of micrometastases, biliary variations, bile leakage, and hepatic lobar or segmental borders on the liver surface and resection margin, achieved with the aid of fluorescence imaging. As with laparoscopic ALPPS procedure, robotic ALPPS procedure induces less trauma and adhesion formation than open ALPPS procedure, facilitating stage 2 surgery, avoiding two major incisions, mitigating the risk of infections, and promoting rapid postoperative recovery.

12.2.2 Limitations of Robotic ALPPS

Given the substantial cost of disposable instruments for a robotic surgical system, coupled with the two-stage nature of the ALPPS procedure, the cost is remarkably higher for robotic ALPPS procedures as compared to laparoscopic or open ALPPS procedures. To prudently control surgical costs, our center implements a hybrid strategy, utilizing robotic surgery for stage 1 ALPPS procedure involving complex dissection while employing laparoscopic surgery for stage 2 ALPPS procedure entailing transecting the right hepatic pedicle, hepatic vein, and a small portion of the parenchyma.

X. Wang (✉)
Zhongshan Hospital, Fudan University, Shanghai, China
e-mail: wang.xiaoying1@zs-hospital.sh.cn

J. Zhou (ed.), *Associating Liver Partition and Portal Vein Ligation for Staged Hepatectomy (ALPPS)*,
https://doi.org/10.1007/978-981-96-7364-3_12

The operative time for the robotic approach may be longer than that for the laparoscopic approach. Docking needs extra time, particularly the divergent approaches necessary for liver and colorectal surgeries necessitate re-docking the robotic surgical system when the ALPPS procedure is indicated for patients who concurrently have colorectal cancer and hepatic metastases. Consequently, robotic surgery may require an extended duration than laparoscopic surgery. Furthermore, the successful execution of complex hepatectomies (e.g., robotic ALPPS procedure) relies heavily on the seamless collaboration between the primary surgeon and an experienced bedside assistant surgeon responsible for instrument exchanges and ancillary tasks.

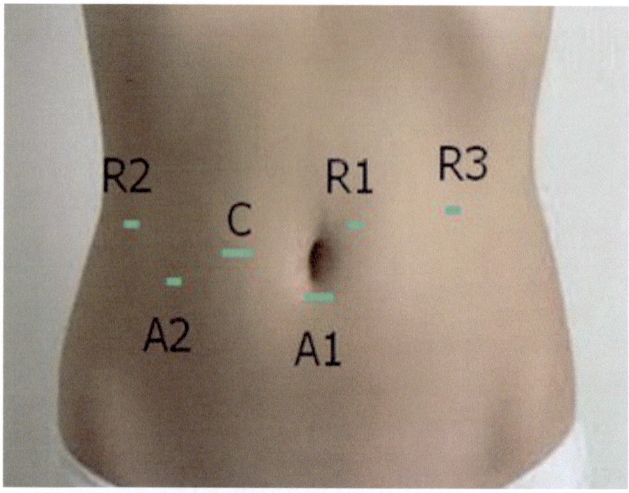

Fig. 12.1 Trocar placement for robotic ALPPS

12.3 Tips for Robotic ALPPS

12.3.1 Robotic ALPPS Procedure: Stage 1

12.3.1.1 Position

The patient is typically positioned in either a supine or 30°tilt to left and reverse Trendelenburg position.

12.3.1.2 Trocar Placement and Docking

The camera port is typically positioned 2 cm to the right of the umbilicus. The robotic arms R1 and R2 ports are distributed in an arc-shaped configuration on either side of the camera port, with the vertex of the arc aligned with the planned hepatic parenchymal transection line. The port for the traction arm R3 is placed beneath the left costal arch. The assistant port is positioned inferior to the midpoint of the line connecting the robotic arm port and the camera port (Fig. 12.1). The distance of the adjacent trocars is about 8 to 10 cm, which prevents collision between the robotic arms. The trocar positions may be adjusted based on tumor location, patient shape, and surgeon habits. The robotic surgical system is docked in a linear trajectory from the patient's cranial side (Fig. 12.2). The assistant surgeon stands on the patient's right side or between the patient's legs.

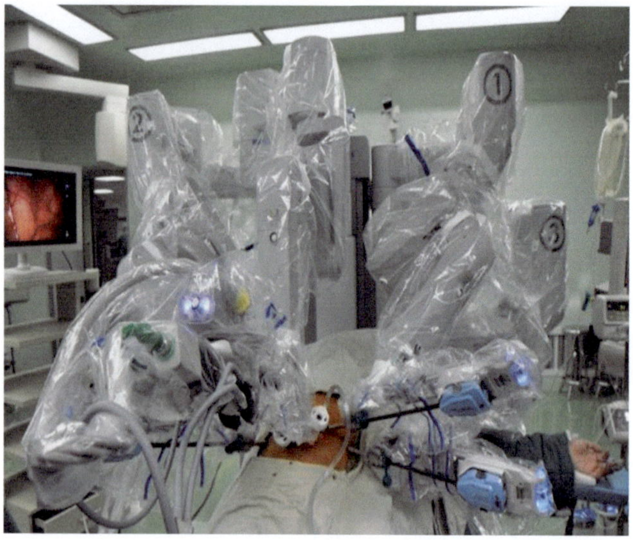

Fig. 12.2 Docking for robotic ALPPS

12.3.1.3 Exploration

Following the establishment of a pneumoperitoneum of 13 mmHg, the robotic camera is introduced to explore the abdominal cavity and the liver. The liver is scanned with intraoperative ultrasound (Fig. 12.3). Compared to preoperative percutaneous ultrasound, robotic or laparoscopic ultrasound enables the probe to be placed directly on the liver surface and provides clearer images of intrahepatic lesions. Intraoperative ultrasound utilizes multiple techniques (e.g., color Doppler, contrast-enhanced ultrasound, and real-time tissue elastography) to determine the location, size, number, nature, and extent of tumors. The Si and Xi surgical systems feature Firefly fluorescence imaging, achieving higher intraoperative detectability of small lesions situated within 1 cm from the liver surface or resection margin by intravenous injection of indocyanine green (ICG) 3 to 7 days preoperatively.

12.3.1.4 Dissection of the Porta Hepatis

Lifting the left medial section with the robotic arm R3 after transecting the round and falciform ligaments. The gallbladder is resected, and the cystic duct is retracted to the left. Next, the right portal vein and the right hepatic artery are dissected (Figs. 12.4 and 12.5), with particular attention devoted to safeguarding the artery. The hilar plate and bile duct should not be dissected to lessen the risk of bile leakage. Subsequently, the right hepatic artery and the right portal vein are marked with absorbable sutures, facilitating the

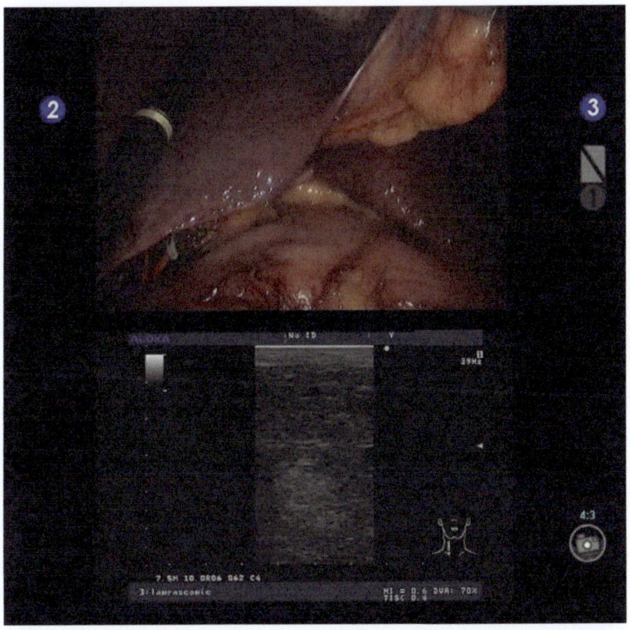

Fig. 12.3 Scanning the liver with laparoscopic ultrasound

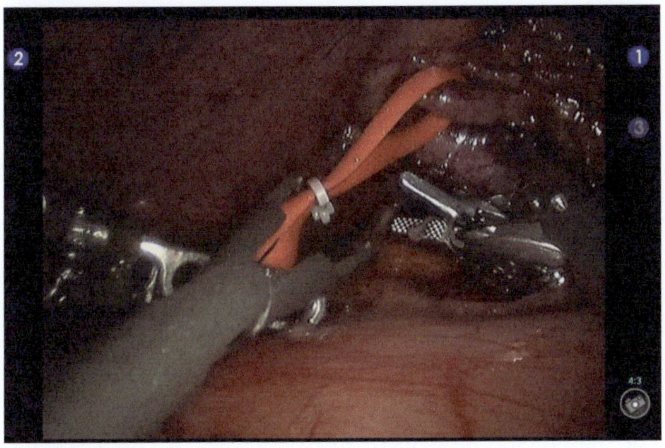

Fig. 12.4 Dissection of the right hepatic artery

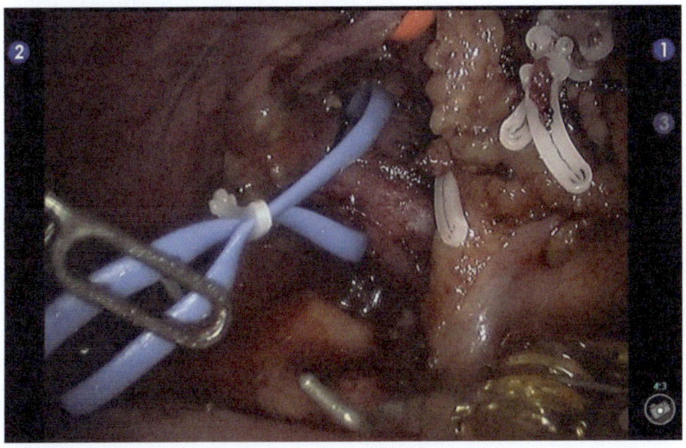

Fig. 12.5 Dissection of the right portal vein

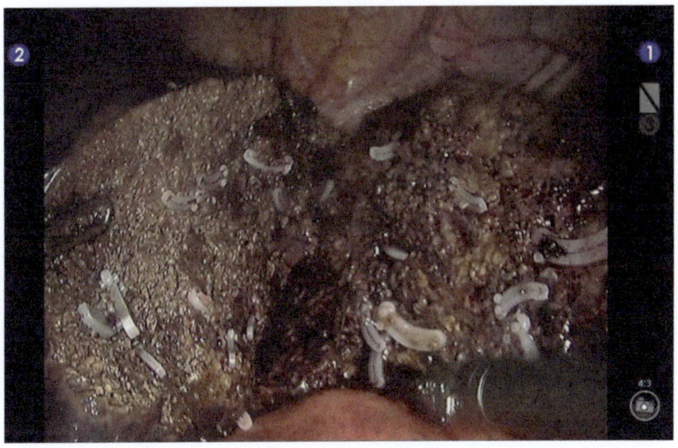

Fig. 12.6 Hepatic parenchymal transection

identification of the corresponding anatomical structures during stage 2 surgery. The hepatoduodenal ligament is encircled with an umbilical tape employed for Pringle maneuver.

12.3.1.5 Hepatic Parenchymal Transection

The anterior approach is recommended, as it does not necessitate mobilizing the right liver, mitigating the risk of abdominal adhesion formation and facilitating stage 2 surgery. This approach also alleviates compression on tumors, thereby diminishing the propensity for metastatic dissemination. Tumors residing within the preserved left lobe should be resected first. In the ALPPS procedure, the parenchymal transection line is contingent upon the tumor location and the volume of the preserved liver. Typically, right trisectionectomy entails the transection along the right border of the falciform ligament, while right hemihepatectomy necessitates the parenchymal transection along the Cantlie line. The hepatic parenchymal is transected by a robotic harmonic scalpel and Maryland bipolar electrocoagulation forceps (Fig. 12.6). Employing partial or complete hepatic parenchymal transection remains debated; however, either approach can induce rapid hypertrophy of the preserved liver. Partial parenchymal transection should go inferior to the plane of the middle hepatic vein, which encompasses the resection of the communicating branch in segment S4. Upon completion of the hepatic parenchymal transection, the transection plane should be meticulously examined for bile leakage. The Si and Xi surgical systems feature Firefly fluorescence imaging, enabling the utilization of ICG fluorescence cholangiography to detect bile leakage.

12.3.1.6 Right Portal Vein Ligation

Following the right portal vein ligation (Fig. 12.7), large Hem-o-lock clips are applied to clamp the right portal vein to ensure complete occlusion. This is followed by localized

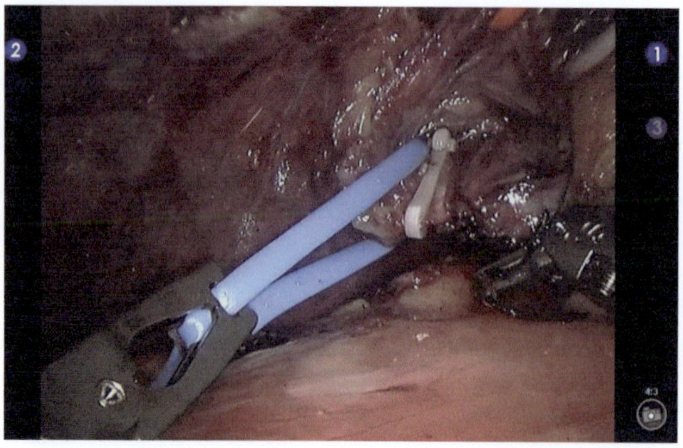

Fig. 12.7 Right portal vein ligation

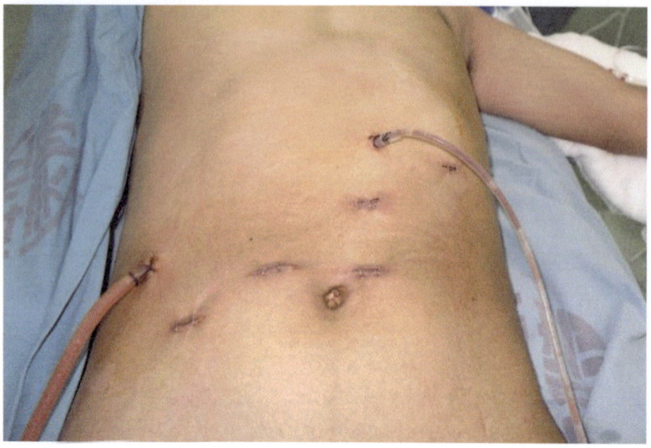

Fig. 12.8 Abdominal incisions during stage 1 robotic ALPPS procedure

application of chitosan in the hepatic portal area to prevent adhesion formation. Subsequently, the Surgicel Fibrillar hemostat is placed on the hepatic transection plane for hemostasis and isolation, facilitating the delineation of the hepatic transection plane during stage 2 surgery. Drainage tubes are positioned on the hepatic transection plane and inferior to the right diaphragm to allow for adequate drainage. The excised gallbladder or tumor specimen is retrieved (Fig. 12.8).

12.3.2 Stage 2 Robotic ALPPS Procedure

12.3.2.1 Exploration

The same trocar placement and docking as stage 1 surgery employed. Due to the meticulous execution using the robotic surgical system during stage 1 surgery, abdominal adhesions are minimized, allowing for straightforward delineation of the hepatic transection plane through a gentle blunt dissection approach. The right portal vein and the right hepatic artery are identified as guided by the markings placed during stage 1 surgery (Fig. 12.9).

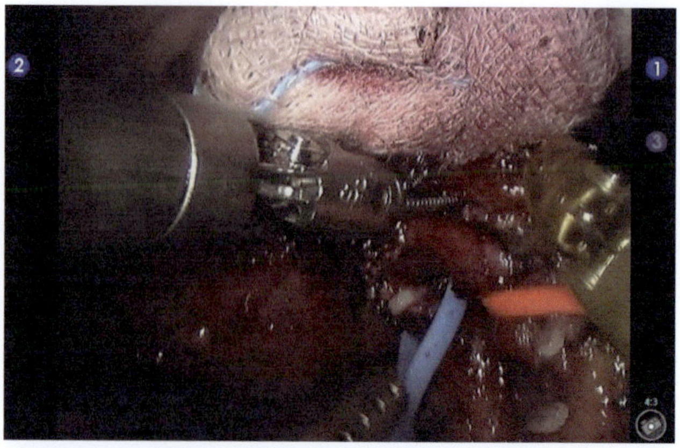

Fig. 12.9 Identification of the right hepatic artery and right portal vein during stage 2 surgery

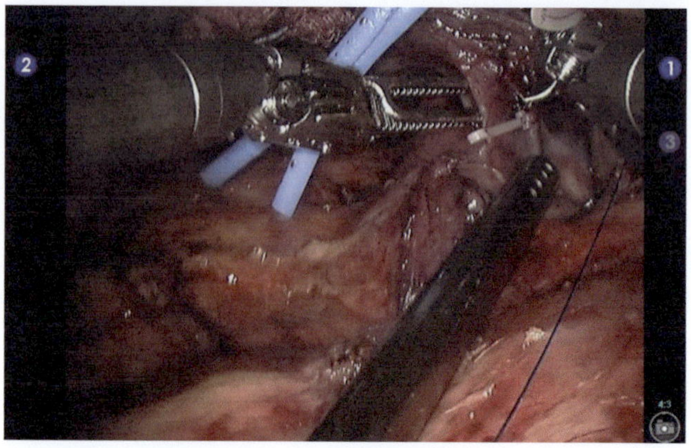

Fig. 12.10 Management of short hepatic veins

12.3.2.2 Mobilization of Retrohepatic Inferior Vena Cava

The right lobe is lifted using the robotic arm R3 to dissect the hepatorenal ligament, exposing the space between the inferior vena cava and the caudate lobe. The short hepatic veins are dissected, clamped, and transected by a harmonic scalpel. The thick, short hepatic veins, well sutured with the robotic surgical system, are resected (Fig. 12.10). The junction between the paracaval portion and the caudate process is dissected in a caudal-to-cephalic direction, progressively exposing the midline of the retrohepatic inferior vena cava. The dissection transgresses the dorsal aspect of the right hepatic pedicle.

12.3.2.3 Dissection of the Right Hepatic Pedicle

The right hepatic pedicle is dissected with an endoscopic linear cutter stapler (Fig. 12.11), with particular attention directed to avoiding any inadvertent injury to the bifurcation of the left and right hepatic ducts. If a tumor is adjacent to the right hepatic pedicle, the right hepatic duct, right hepatic artery, and right portal vein may be dissected separately.

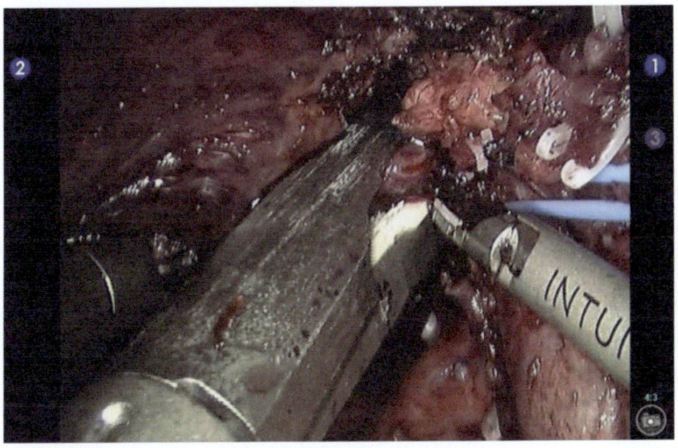

Fig. 12.11 Dissection of the right hepatic pedicle

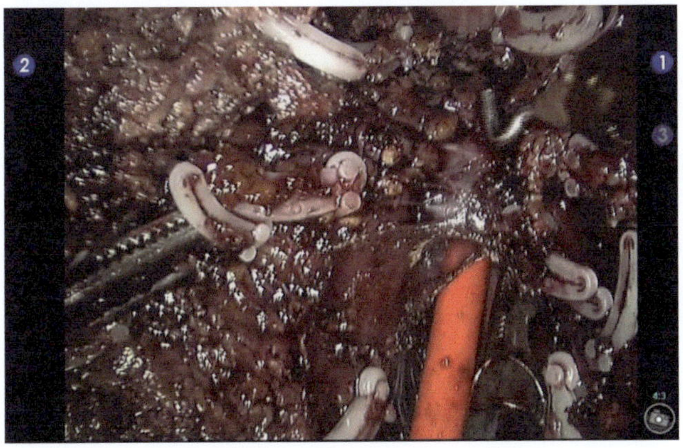

Fig. 12.12 Parenchymal transection of paracaval portion

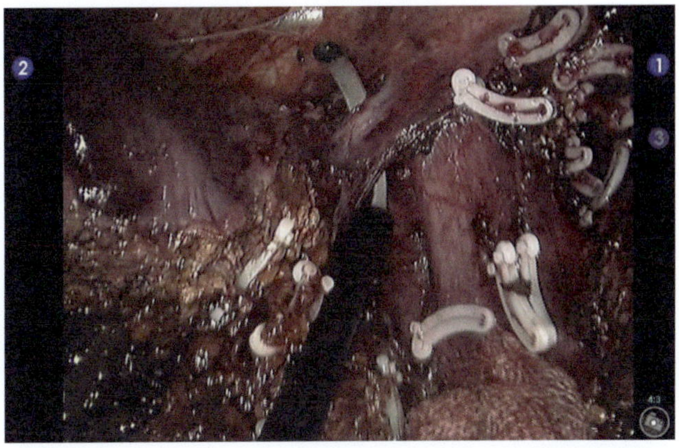

Fig. 12.13 Exposure of the right hepatic vein

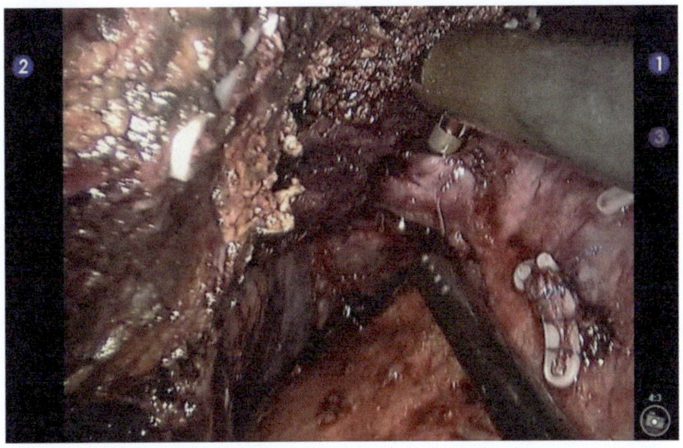

Fig. 12.14 Exposure of the inferior right hepatic vein

12.3.2.4 Parenchymal Transection in the FLR

Following the dissection of the right hepatic pedicle, a small portion of hepatic parenchyma remains in close proximity to the paracaval portion. To prevent any inadvertent injury to the inferior vena cava, a tunnel can be created between the avascular area anterior to the inferior vena cava and the liver, facilitating hepatic parenchymal transection achieved by hanging or lifting with grasping forceps (Fig. 12.12). Following the dissection of the hepatic parenchyma anterior to the inferior vena cava, the anterior wall of the inferior vena cava is exposed. If right trisectionectomy is performed, resecting the origin of the middle hepatic vein is necessary for exposing the anterior wall of the inferior vena cava. The right lobe is retracted to the right, and the right border of the inferior vena cava is dissected, thereby exposing the inferior right hepatic vein, venous ligament, and the origin of the right hepatic vein (Figs. 12.13 and 12.14). Subsequently, the right hepatic vein is transected with an endoscopic linear cutter stapler.

12.3.2.5 Mobilization of the Right Lobe

The right coronary ligament, right adrenal gland, bare area of the liver, and right triangular ligament are mobilized in a medial to lateral direction to completely mobilize the right lobe.

12.3.2.6 Specimen Retrieval and Drainage Tube Placement

The resected right lobe is placed into a specimen retrieval bag, and the specimen is retrieved through a Pfannenstiel's incision. Subsequently, the specimen retrieval incision is closed (Fig. 12.15). Following the re-establishment of the pneumoperitoneum, the abdominal cavity is cleaned. The hepatic transection plane is examined for any potential bile leakage or bleeding, and the falciform and round ligaments are secured with barbed sutures. Then, a drainage tube is positioned inferior to the right diaphragm and the hepatic transection plane, respectively.

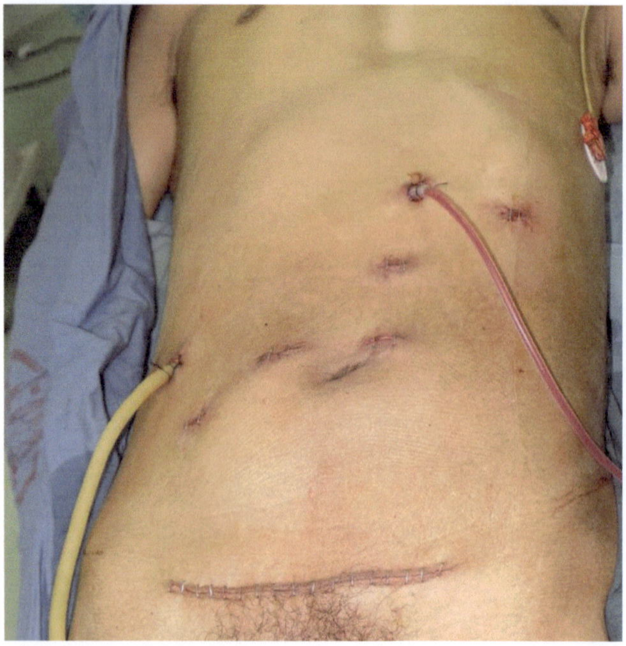

Fig. 12.15 An incision for stage 2 robotic ALPPS procedure

12.4 Prospects

The cumulative evidence from the existing literature and the extensive experience garnered at our center have unequivocally substantiated the safety and feasibility of the robotic ALPPS procedure. The judicious case selection criteria and precise surgical maneuvers are paramount to yielding favorable outcomes. The robotic ALPPS procedure confers the following distinct advantages over conventional laparoscopy: (a) shorter learning curve and enhanced precision in manipulation; (b) safer dissection of the porta hepatis and the retrohepatic inferior vena cava; (c) superior hemostatic control because of straightforward suturing operations; (d) convenient reconstruction of biliary and vascular anastomoses, achieved with the aid of micro-suturing techniques. Collectively, these advantages contribute to ameliorating the success rate of robotic ALPPS procedures.

Robotic ALPPS procedure circumvents the need for two major laparotomies, offering distinct advantages (e.g., small incisions and expedited postoperative recovery). Nonetheless, the current evidence supporting the robotic ALPPS procedure remains limited to individual case reports, and the laparoscopic or open ALPPS procedure and the robotic ALPPS procedure have yet to be comparatively investigated to date. Consequently, the safety profile and oncological efficacy of the robotic ALPPS procedure await a large-scale case evaluation. With the accumulation of cases and the continuous refinement and innovation of robotic surgical systems, the prospects for robotic ALPPS procedures hold considerable promise.

References

1. Solomonov E, Tzadok I, Stemmer S, et al. Case report: robotic ALPPS procedure for hepatocellular carcinoma in the right lobe of the liver[J]. Front Surg. 2021;8:655683.
2. Vicente E, Quijano Y, Ielpo B, et al. First ALPPS procedure using a total robotic approach[J]. Surg Oncol. 2016;25(4):457.
3. Di Benedetto F, Magistri P. First case of full robotic ALPPS for intrahepatic cholangiocarcinoma[J]. Ann Surg Oncol. 2021;28(2):865.
4. Di Benedetto F, Magistri P, Guerrini GP, et al. Robotic liver partition and portal vein embolization for staged hepatectomy for perihilar cholangiocarcinoma[J]. Updat Surg. 2022;74(2):773–7.

Hybrid ALPPS

13

Jun Li and I-Chin Lee

13.1 Introduction

In 2007, Professor Hans J. Schlitt from the University Hospital Regensburg in Germany performed the first associating liver partition and portal vein ligation for staged hepatectomy (ALPPS) on a patient with hilar cholangiocarcinoma. During exploratory laparotomy, the surgeon divided the liver along the falciform ligament and ligated the right branch of the portal vein to promote the enlargement of the future liver remnant (FLR). CT on the 8th postoperative day showed that the FLR volume increased by 94%, and the second-stage hepatectomy was completed the next day [1, 2]. In 2012, Professor Schnitzbauer et al. reported and reviewed 25 cases of two-staged liver resection performed in five medical centers in Germany from September 2007 to January 2011. On average, CT scans on the 9th postoperative day after the first stage revealed an increase of FLR by a mean value of 74% (21%–192%) without irreversible post-hepatectomy liver failure (PHLF). The in-hospital mortality rate was 12%, and the median 6-month survival rate was 86% [1]. Then, the ALPPS procedure immediately gained the attention of the hepatobiliary surgery community. In the same year, Professor Santibanes E. and Professor Clavien P. A. published a paper in the *Annals of Surgery*, using the "associating liver partition and portal vein ligation for staged hepatectomy" with "ALPPS" as the acronym to name this novel procedure [3], that is, classical ALPPS that we know today.

ALPPS has been rapidly executed worldwide thanks to its rapid postoperative FLR growth, high reproducibility, and the fact that it does not require interventional radiologists to perform precise embolization of multiple portal veins in the fourth segment of the liver. Professor Jian Zhou et al. from Zhongshan Hospital, Fudan University, first reported in 2013 that a patient with giant hepatocellular carcinoma (HCC) successfully treated by ALPPS [4], attracting many Chinese scholars for joint exploration, most of which were applications in the surgical treatment of HCC [5, 6].

With a large number of ALPPS implementations and case reports, concerns and discussions continue to arise, which can be majorly divided into two categories: (a) Rates of severe complications after ALPPS surgery (including mortality) are relatively high [7]. (b) Some tumors are located close to the right porta hepatis. In the first stage of ALPPS, the surgical procedure needs to be performed there without tumor resection, which goes against the principle of "no touch" [8].

To reduce the incidence of postoperative complications, scholars from many countries have modified and progressed in various aspects, especially for the first-stage surgical step. Varies procedures have been proposed [9–13] to reduce complications (such as bleeding, bile leakage, liver ischemia, and infection) and associated mortality. Professor Jun Li from the University of Hamburg in Germany reported two cases of hybrid ALPPS that he performed in 2012 in the *Annals of Surgery*, reconciliating the "no-touch" principle of oncology surgery and ALPPS [14]. Hybrid ALPPS divides the operation into two stages. The first one is to determine the resectability intraoperatively, split the liver along the pre-cut line, and divide the portal vein of the fourth liver segment. The second one is to embolize the right branch of the portal vein via interventional techniques. In this way, the first stage of ALPPS not only achieves considerable simplification and reduces the occurrence of postoperative complications but keeps the tumor-invaded right portal hepatitis intact, adhering to the "no-touch" principle. Applying interventional techniques to embolize the right branch of the portal vein is technically simpler than additional embolization of liver segment 4. Moreover, in case of abnormal vessel structures, the right anterior branch from the left branch of the portal vein can be embolized more accurately, thereby increasing the growth rate of FLR after surgery. At the same time, hybrid

J. Li (✉) · I.-C. Lee
Jiahui International Hospital Shanghai, Jiahui Health, Shanghai, China
e-mail: j.li@uke.de

J. Zhou (ed.), *Associating Liver Partition and Portal Vein Ligation for Staged Hepatectomy (ALPPS)*,
https://doi.org/10.1007/978-981-96-7364-3_13

ALPPS enabled an expand of indications, especially in cases where the tumor directly invades the right branch of the portal vein.

Since the concept of "Hybrid ALPPS" was proposed, surgeons were no longer in thrall to specific surgical methods but followed the two basic concepts of ALPPS to divide the portal vein and split the liver on both sides and carried out different combinations of techniques to achieve better results, reduce postoperative complications, and improve patient survival. Thus, a series of procedures have emerged and been developed, including Mini ALPPS and ATLPS [10, 15, 16].

In 2017, Italian professor Lai Q. et al. reported two successful cases of hybrid ALPPS, one in a patient with a giant intrahepatic cholangiocarcinoma (a diameter of 18 cm) that invaded the right portal vein and the other in a patient with multiple colorectal liver metastases (CRLM) that involved the right portal vein, the hepatic vein, and the inferior vena cava. Results confirmed the feasibility and safety of this surgical procedure in resecting huge tumors [17, 18]. In 2020, Professor Oldhafer K. J. et al. from Germany reported the combination of laparoscopic hybrid ALPPS and extracorporeal circulation for a patient with giant HCC accompanied by superior vena cava and right atrium invasion and pulmonary embolism, further expanding the application scope of hybrid ALPPS [19, 20].

13.2 Indications

ALPPS was first used in patients with biliary malignant tumors who are expected to undergo extensive liver resection, including the tumor, with no extrahepatic metastasis but insufficient FLR. After more than a decade of popularization and exploration, according to the current statistics of the ALPPS Registry, the most common indications for ALPPS per application frequency are as follows: CRLM, HCC, intrahepatic cholangiocarcinoma (ICC), perihilar cholangiocarcinoma (PHC), neuroendocrine liver metastases (NETLM), and other liver occupancies [9, 21–23].

The core of hybrid ALPPS is combining the basics of classical ALPPS and the "no contact" principle in surgical oncology. R0 radical resection is the treatment goal of surgery where two essential concepts need to be abided by the no-touch and the en bloc resection proposed by German Professor Peter Neuhaus in the surgical treatment of PHC [24, 25] to improve long-term surgical outcomes. In the classical ALPPS, it is necessary to mobilize the right hemi-liver, dissect the porta hepatis, separate the portal vessels, skeletonize the hepatoduodenal ligament, dissect regional lymph nodes, and divide liver parenchyma at the first stage. In contrast, the tumor is removed only till the second stage. This is considered to be contrary to the "no-touch" but being "all-touch" that can lead to tumor dissemination [14, 17, 18].

Compared with classical ALPPS, there are many differences in the first stage of hybrid ALPPS: An anterior approach for exploration and in situ liver parenchymal transection is performed. Mobilization of the right liver is not carried out. Dissection of the porta hepatis is not performed without touching the right side of the hepatoduodenal ligament. The blood flow of the right portal vein is blocked by PVE, which is usually carried out after the parenchyma split. The approach for PVE can be chosen according to the tumor size and the location. The right portal vein could be accessed by puncturing the sagittal part of the left portal vein or the right portal vein branch directly. The embolization can also be executed intraoperatively via the ileocolic vein, avoiding puncture-related complications. In the second stage, the left and right portal vein bifurcations should be removed, if possible, to ensure an R0 resection and end-to-end anastomosis of the left portal vein and the main portal vein trunk then be performed [14, 17, 18, 20].

Hybrid ALPPS, like classic ALPPS, is a highly invasive two-stage extensive liver resection. A comprehensive preoperative assessment should be conducted, including basic health status, primary lesions, resectability of metastases, anatomic variations of liver vessels and bile ducts, liver function, liver volume, and functions of other organs. Currently, FLR/SLV ratio, FLR/BWR ratio, Child-Pugh score, ICG-R15, and model for end-stage liver disease (MELD) are used to evaluate FLR and liver functional reserve [26] comprehensively. Recently, Mebrofenin has been applied to measure left-side and right-side liver function for a more accurate assessment of effective liver function, reducing the risk of PHLF [27]. In China, there is an expert consensus on precision liver resection regarding this, which should be adapted to the individual situation in each center [28].

Based on the abovementioned information, indications for hybrid ALPPS can be summarized as the following:

(a) CRLM, HCC, or ICC with suspicion of the right branch of the portal vein invasion, as well as gallbladder cancer and PHC requiring right trisectionectomy.
(b) Having the general indication of ALPPS, but the ligation of the right portal vein is technically difficult due to the anatomic variation, such as the right anterior branch of the portal vein coming from the left branch of the portal vein (Fig. 13.1). Such patients, especially when the tumor is close to the right hepatic pedicle, need to use a special retractor to lift the right bile duct (Fig. 13.2). Sometimes, the location of the right anterior branch is rather concealed and is easy to miss during surgery. The radiology intervention is easier and more accurate in this case.
(c) Combining with laparoscopic liver parenchymal transection, the first stage would be carried out more minimally invasively by hybrid ALPPS [14, 17–20, 23].

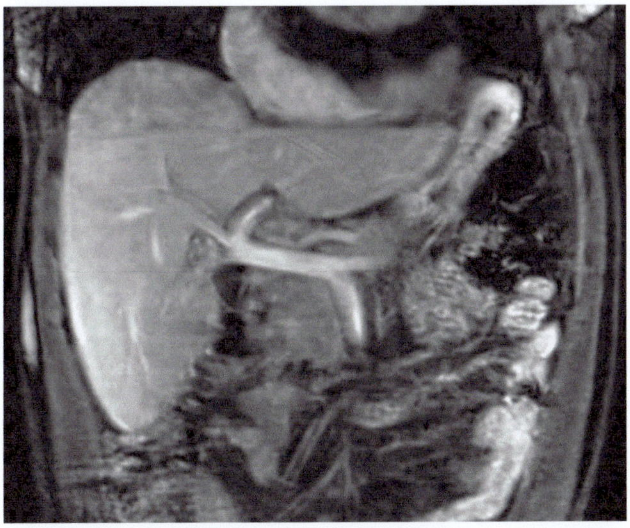

Fig. 13.1 HCC patient. The right anterior branch of the portal vein comes from the left branch of the portal vein, and the tumor has invaded the right posterior branch of the portal vein

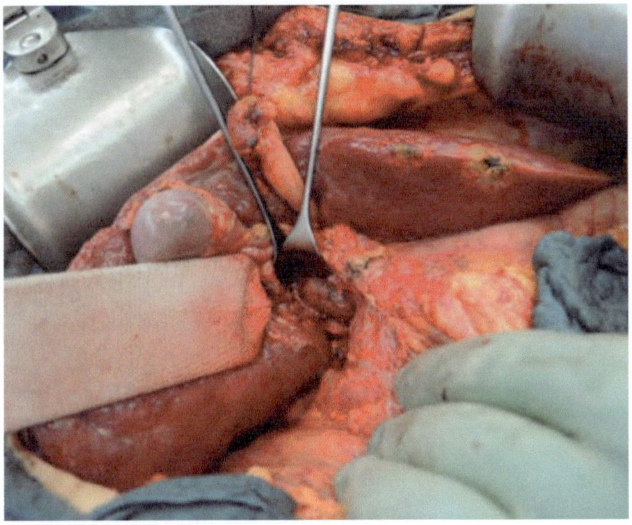

Fig. 13.2 HCC patient. A vascular retractor is used during the operation to lift the right bile duct and the base of segment 4 to fully expose the right anterior branch from the left portal vein

13.3 Surgical Procedures

Hybrid ALPPS was initially performed by open surgery [14]. Successful cases of laparoscopically assisted or laparoscopic surgery have been reported [19, 20, 29]. In the foreseeable future, hybrid ALPPS will be performed using all kinds of surgical techniques, sharing the same basic concepts and oncological principles.

Two cases are selected to explain the surgical procedures of hybrid ALPPS with different indications.

13.3.1 Case 1: PHC or Gallbladder Cancer Requiring Right Trisectionectomy

The patient was a 52-year-old female with suspected Bismuth type IIIa PHC. She underwent exploratory laparotomy at the referral hospital 9 months ago and subsequently received bile duct metal stenting and systemic chemotherapy (gemcitabine plus cisplatin). No extrahepatic metastasis was found in the preoperative evaluation, and another laparotomy was planned to evaluate the feasibility of ALPPS intraoperatively for a right trisectionectomy, including segment 1. The preoperative estimated FLR was 329 mL (only 15.3% of the total liver volume and 0.37% of the body weight).

13.3.1.1 Surgical Procedures for Stage 1 Hybrid ALPPS

1. Exploration: The patient was placed in a supine position, and a reverse "L" shape surgical incision was made. An appropriate retractor was then used to expose the field of view, exploring the whole abdominal cavity, including the main body of the tumor, liver, porta hepatis, hepatoduodenal ligament, hepatogastric ligament, greater omentum, and lesser omentum for extrahepatic lesions to rule out surgical contraindications. Intraoperative ultrasound was performed to examine the structural relationships between the tumor and the hepatic veins, the portal vein (especially the bifurcation), the biliary system, and the FLR. Combining preoperative imaging data, the predetermined transection plane of the liver was delineated. Then, the suitability and feasibility of two-stage liver resection were reassessed. Since Bismuth type IIIa PHC or malignant tumor from the cystic duct were highly suspected, hybrid ALPPS was determined without dissecting the right part of the hepatoduodenal ligament.
2. Porta hepatis dissection and liver parenchyma transection: The ligamentum teres was lifted, and the peritoneum of the round ligament at the sagittal part of the portal vein was then opened up. The portal vein branches of segment 4 were then carefully separated. Division and ligation were done at the starting point of the portal vein branch (Pay attention to preserving the dorsal branch of segment 4a to avoid damaging the bile duct of this segment) to the base of the left portal vein branch. The portal vein branches to the caudate lobe were exposed on the left side and divided. The left part of the hepatoduodenal ligament was opened, and the LHA was isolated and marked with a vascular sling for easy identification during the second stage (Fig. 13.3). The rest part of the hepatoduodenal ligament was not touched. Liver parenchyma transection was performed using the anterior approach without mobilizing the right hemiliver. Combining CUSA with bipolar electrocoagulation, the liver was then precisely transected

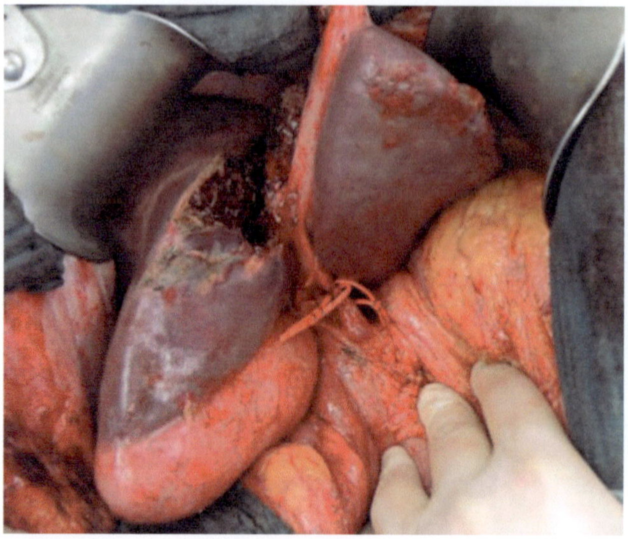

Fig. 13.3 Liver parenchyma transection in hybrid ALPPS. The liver parenchyma and the portal vein branches of segment 4 were gradually separated along the right side of the falciform ligament and ligamentum teres while protecting the confluence of the bile ducts of this segment. The left hepatic artery was dissected out and marked with a sling

along the predetermined plane. The intermittent inflow occlusion can be performed during the transection. When dissecting the liver tissue, care should be taken to preserve tissues near the porta hepatis and the confluence of the hepatic vein and inferior vena cava to avoid injuring the left hepatic vein and the segment 4 bile duct. After transection, the presence of bile leakage should be checked, especially at the site near the porta hepatis. Then, two tube drains could be introduced between the transected surfaces to separate the tumor-side liver from the remaining liver. Another drain should be placed at the porta hepatis and led out through the right abdominal wall. Avoid using silicone films or plastic bags to isolate the liver from the adjacent tissues to prevent infection of the collection.

13.3.1.2 Portal Vein Embolization (PVE)

Portal vein embolization can be performed during the operation or within a few days postoperatively, according to the situation in each center. The intervention approach could be chosen per tumor size and location obtained via exploration, including:

(a) Puncture the sagittal part of the left portal vein and then perform PVE of the contralateral right portal vein.
(b) Puncture the right portal vein branch and perform ipsilateral PVE.
(c) Intraoperative PVE that is performed through ileocolic vein catheterization, which can avoid puncture-related complications.

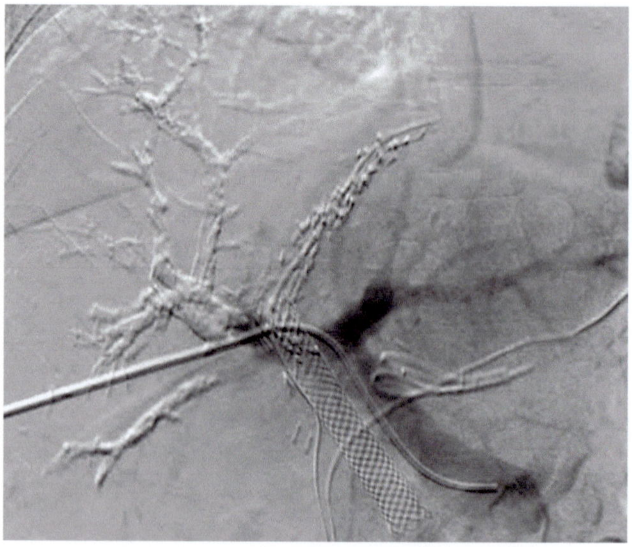

Fig. 13.4 Portal vein embolism in hybrid ALPPS

In this case, the ipsilateral PVE method was used with needle insertion on the right side (Fig. 13.4) [14].

13.3.1.3 Volumetric Study After the First Stage of Hybrid ALPPS

The patient was discharged on the 7th day after surgery. On the 14th day, she returned to the hospital for an abdominal CT to measure FLR. The volume of the left lateral lobe was found to be 544 mL (accounting for 25.4% of the total liver volume and 0.60% of the body weight), and the second stage of surgery was thus feasible. For patients with chronic liver disease, liver fibrosis, or cirrhosis, the waiting time till the volumetric reassessment and the second stage surgery is generally longer because of the reduced hypertrophic potential of the liver.

13.3.1.4 Surgical Procedures for Stage 2 Hybrid ALPPS

A laparotomy was performed layer by layer along the original incision. Compared with conventional or classical ALPPS, inflammatory changes around the liver after the first stage were milder in hybrid ALPPS. The hepatoduodenal ligament was dissected, and lymph nodes were resected up to the celiac axis. The right hepatic artery and distal bile duct were severed, and the left branch and the main trunk of the portal vein were isolated. The caudate lobe and right liver lobe were divided, the remaining liver tissues were dissociated at the confluence of the hepatic vein and inferior vena cava, and the middle hepatic vein and right hepatic vein were cut off. The remaining liver tissues at the porta hepatis were divided, along with the left branch and the main trunk of the portal vein. Finally, the left hepatic duct was cut off on the left side of the sagittal part of the portal vein, and the speci-

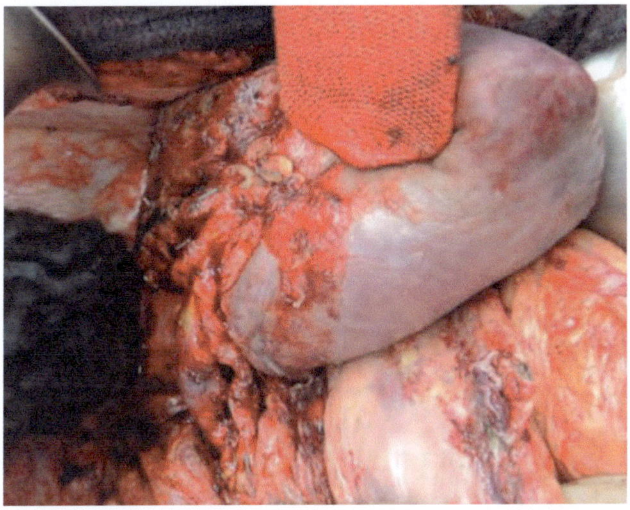

Fig. 13.5 After the right trisectionectomy of the liver, the left lateral lobe grew significantly. End-to-end anastomosis of the main trunk and the left branch of the portal vein was performed

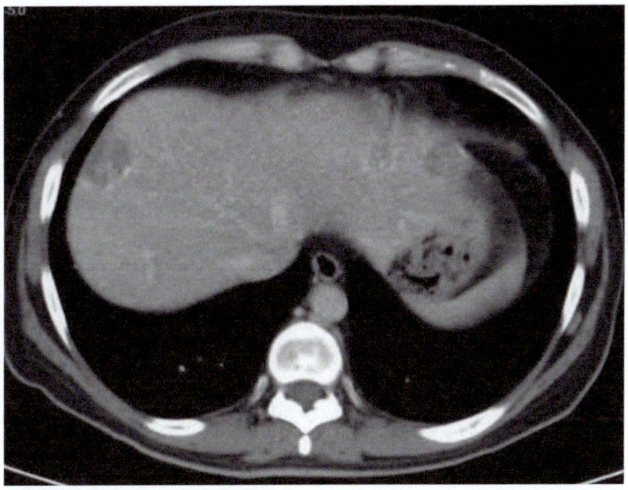

Fig. 13.6 Preoperative CT showed that the tumor metastases were distributed in both lobes of the liver

men was sent for pathological examination. An end-to-end anastomosis between the main trunk and the left branch of the portal vein was performed with a 5-0 Prolene (Fig. 13.5). The liver transection surface was checked, and hemostasis was conducted when necessary. Bile leakage at the transection site was checked meticulously. In case of bile leakage, 5-0 Prolene sutures were needed for closure, and Roux-en-Y hepatobiliary-jejunal reconstruction was performed. Drains were placed in the liver transection region, and the porta hepatis and the abdominal cavity were closed layer by layer.

This case showed the ipsilateral PVE method with needle insertion on the right side. Post-embolization angiography of the portal vein visualized the right portal vein but not the liver parenchyma of segments 4 to 8. Visible in the background were the metal biliary stent, the marker band of the left hepatic artery, and the drains located along the liver transection line and below the left lateral lobe.

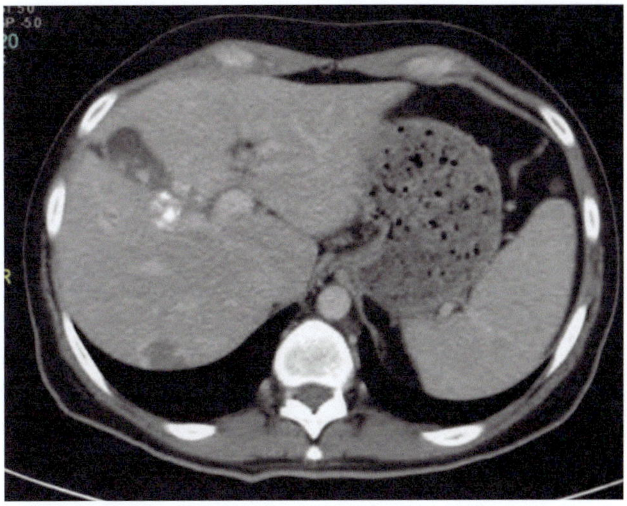

Fig. 13.7 Preoperative CT showed that the tumor metastases were distributed in both lobes of the liver

13.3.2 Case 2: Multiple Liver Metastases of Colon Cancer

The patient was a 44-year-old male. Due to extensive liver metastases of colorectal cancer and intestinal obstruction, he underwent palliative transverse colostomy and chemotherapy. The tumor shrank significantly, and he came for further treatment. After a multidisciplinary discussion, resection of the primary tumor after liver metastases removal was planned. In his CT scans, two tumors were located in the right anterior and posterior branches of the portal vein. There were also several metastases in segments 2 and 4. Because the left lobe was relatively large (338 mL, accounting for 21.3% of the total liver volume and 0.5% of the body weight), it was expected that after tumor enucleation in the left lateral lobe, hybrid ALPPS could be performed for the final right trisectionectomy (Figs. 13.6 and 13.7). Since the patient had a transverse colon stoma, which interfered with the conventional reverse "L"-shaped incision (Fig. 13.8). Thus, a laparoscopic resection of the metastases in segment 2 was determined, dividing the liver parenchyma of the left lateral lobe and segment 4. The right branch of the portal vein was closed by interventional embolization.

13.3.2.1 Surgical Procedures for Stage 1 of Hybrid ALPPS

1. Exploration: The patient was placed in a supine position with legs straddled. Four laparoscopic portals were inserted in sequence after marking the future incisions for

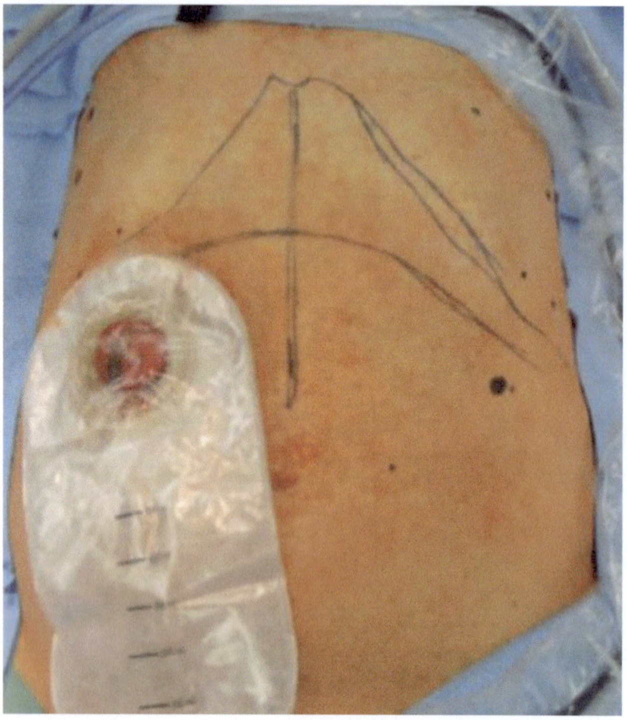

Fig. 13.8 Selection of intraoperative incisions: the patient had a transverse colon stoma, which was located close to the conventional reverse "L"-shaped incision

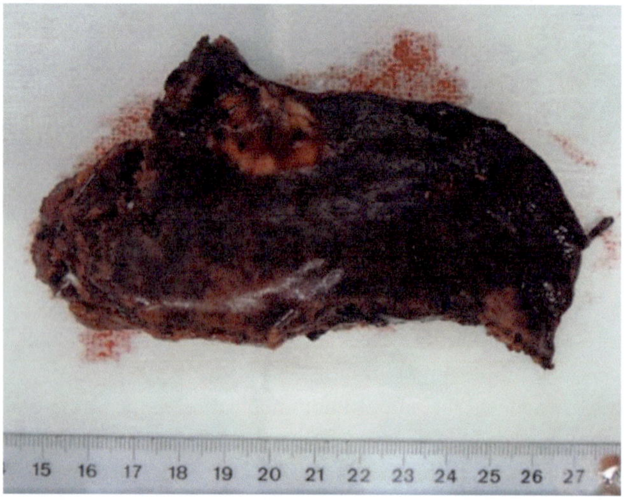

Fig. 13.9 Specimen of segment 2

the second-stage surgery. Adhesions were separated, and the ligamentum teres and falciform ligament were divided. The coronary ligament and left triangular ligament were opened to reveal the left and right hepatic lobes. Laparoscopic ultrasound was performed to locate metastases.

2. Resection of segment 2 and liver parenchyma transection: Under intermittent liver inflow occlusion, resection of segment 2 was conducted (Fig. 13.9). Then, along the right side of the falciform ligament, CUSA was applied to open the liver parenchyma of segment 4. The liver on the caudal side was divided to about 5 mm from the porta hepatis to avoid bile duct injury. The liver parenchyma on the cranial side was dissected until the left hepatic vein was exposed. A drain was placed at the section site. The specimen was retrieved via the supraumbilical incision (Fig. 13.10).

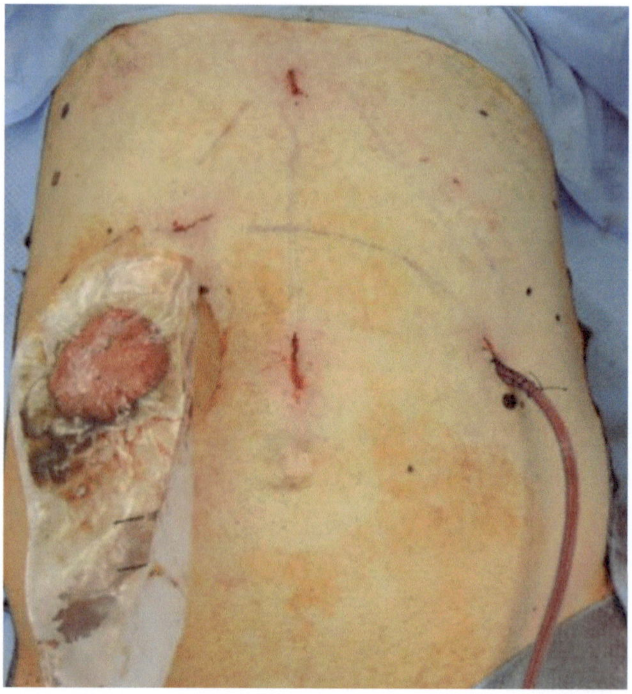

Fig. 13.10 Laparoscopic incision selection. Specimen removed via the supraumbilical incision

The ipsilateral PVE method was adopted with needle insertion on the right side. Post-embolization angiography of the portal vein trunk showed that segment 4 remained partially visualized, indicating incomplete liver splitting.

13.3.2.2 PVE

On the 2nd day after surgery, the ipsilateral PVE method was adopted with needle insertion on the right side. The right anterior and posterior branches of the portal vein were embolized, respectively (Fig. 13.11).

13.3.2.3 Volume Measurement After the First Stage of Hybrid ALPPS

The patient was discharged on the 10th day after the operation. On the 21st day, he returned to the hospital for an abdominal CT to measure future liver remnant volume. The volume of the left lateral lobe was 542 mL (accounting for 32.9% of the total liver volume and 0.73% of the body weight), and thus, the second-stage surgery could be performed.

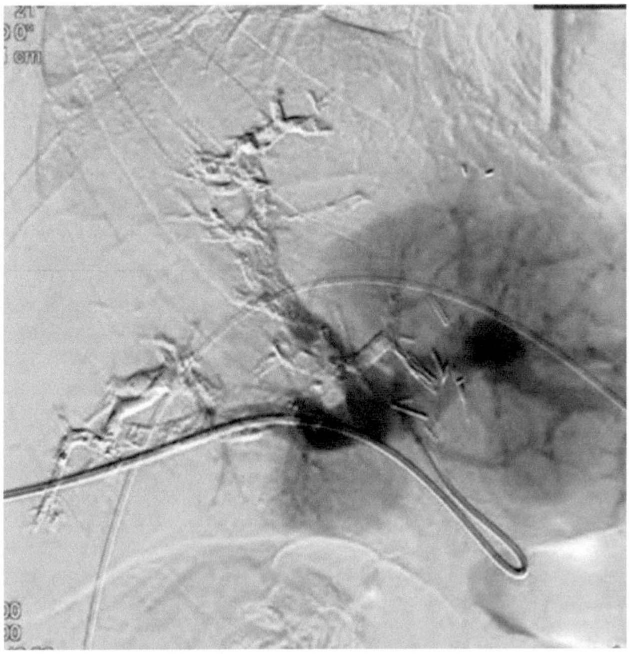

Fig. 13.11 PVE in hybrid ALPPS

13.3.2.4 Surgical Procedures for Stage 2 of Hybrid ALPPS

The patient was placed in the left lateral recumbent position. The hepatorenal ligament and the right triangular ligament were opened laparoscopically, and the right liver was dissociated to the vena cava. Because the right liver had not been divided before, mild adhesions occurred. After removing the laparoscope, the patient was then put in a supine position. A laparotomy was conducted along the midline incision to expose the liver. The adhesions were separated, the porta hepatis dissected, and the right hepatic artery divided. After lowering the portal plate, transect the remaining parenchyma in segment 4, cut off the right hepatic duct and the right branch of the portal vein, gradually transected the liver parenchyma caudally to cranially along the right side of the vena cava, and severed the middle hepatic vein and the right hepatic vein respectively. Specimens were sent for pathological tests. The liver transection site was checked, and hemostasis was conducted when necessary. Bile leakage at this site was checked meticulously. Drains were placed in the liver transection region, and the porta hepatis, and the abdominal cavity was closed layer by layer.

13.4 Pearls and Pitfalls of the Surgery

The core concept of hybrid ALPPS is the application of the "no-touch" principle in the first stage of ALPPS, mainly aiming at increasing the FLR rapidly to avoid postoperative liver failure. Technical-wise, different liver transection and PVE techniques can be combined. For example, when partial liver parenchymal transection is performed, the whole procedure should be called "hybrid partial ALPPS" [17, 18]. In 2013, the Zurich group found in an experimental study that partial (75%–80%) and complete liver parenchymal transection had similar outcomes regarding FLR growth. On average, 7 days after the first stage, a median growth rate of 60% was observed in the partial ALPPS group and 61% in the classical ALPPS group (complete liver parenchyma transection). In 2015, Petrowsky H. et al. proposed the standard definition of "partial ALPPS" as "ALPPS procedures that do not perform complete liver parenchymal transection in the first stage" [11]. Linecker M. et al. demonstrated that dividing the liver by more than 50% of the total transection surface brought about the same FLR growth as that of complete division. To reduce the risk of bile leakage after the first-stage surgery, hybrid ALPPS draws upon techniques of partial ALPPS and improves the liver parenchyma transection step in the first stage:

(a) Preserve the segment 4a branch of the portal vein to avoid bile duct injury in the same segment.
(b) Preserve the middle hepatic vein.

The above procedures can reduce the risk of bile leakage after the first stage of surgery.

The "anterior approach" can be adopted in liver parenchyma transection. (**a**) The right liver lobe is not mobilized. (**b**) The porta hepatis is not routinely dissected. When the porta hepatis has to be dissected, the right porta hepatis should remain untouched. (**c**) The gallbladder is generally not removed, especially for intrahepatic and extrahepatic malignant bile duct tumors or gallbladder cancer that invade the right hilus and biliary tract. (**d**) Do not dissect and ligate the right branch of the portal vein [14, 17–20, 29]. These four aspects need to be followed during the first stage of ALPPS in a "no-touch" manner. Performing "en bloc resection" in the second stage, achieving R0 resection would improve long-term oncological efficacy [23].

To follow the "no-touch" principle, hybrid ALPPS uses radiological intervention such as PVE instead of portal vein ligation in the first stage of classical ALPPS, reducing the risk of tumor dissemination during dissection of the right hepatic hilus and right portal vein. PVE can be performed during or after the first stage of surgery. The approach for the portal vein puncture shall be determined based on the preoperative imaging data and intraoperative exploration. Depending on the anatomy and variations of the portal vein, the location and size of the tumor, and the invasion of the right hepatic portal vein, PVE can be performed via the ileocolic vein during surgery or via the ipsilateral or contralateral portal vein branch after surgery. During interventional procedures, care should be taken to avoid damaging the main trunk and the left branch of the portal vein to reduce PVE complications and tumor dissemination [14, 17–19, 29, 30].

In conclusion, hybrid ALPPS is a modified ALPPS procedure carrying the "no-touch" principle of surgical oncology [14, 31]. Combined with partial liver parenchymal transection, the surgical complication rate and mortality rate would be reduced [18]. Hybrid ALPPS is specifically suitable for malignant tumors that invade the right hepatic portal, right portal vein, or the confluence of the left and right bile ducts [14, 17–20, 29, 30]. The surgery can be performed in open, laparoscopically assisted, or complete laparoscopic manners.

References

1. Schnitzbauer AA, Lang SA, Goessmann H, et al. Right portal vein ligation combined with *in situ* splitting induces rapid left lateral liver lobe hypertrophy enabling 2-staged extended right hepatic resection in small-for-size settings[J]. Ann Surg. 2012;255(3):405–14.
2. Schlitt HJ, Hackl C, Lang SA. 'In-situ split' liver resection/ ALPPS – historical development and current practice[J]. Visc Med. 2017;33(6):408–12.
3. de Santibañes E, Clavien PA. Playing Play-Doh to prevent postoperative liver failure: the "ALPPS" approach[J]. Ann Surg. 2012;255(3):415–7.
4. Zhou J, Wang Z, Sun J, et al. Associating liver partition and portal vein ligation for staged hepatectomy[J]. Chin J Dig Surg. 2013;12(7):485–9.
5. Hong DF, Peng SY, Wanyee YY. Ten-year retrospect of ALPPS in the treatment of hepatocellular carcinoma: an eternal concept with cautious technologic choice[J]. Zhonghua Wai Ke Za Zhi. 2022;60(2):113–6.
6. Xin HY, Wang Z, Zhou J. Research progress of associating liver partition and portal vein ligation for staged hepatectomy[J]. Chin J Dig Surg. 2019;18(2):194–8.
7. Eshmuminov D, Raptis DA, Linecker M, et al. Meta-analysis of associating liver partition with portal vein ligation and portal vein occlusion for two-stage hepatectomy[J]. Br J Surg. 2016;103(13):1768–82.
8. Aloia TA, Vauthey JN. Associating liver partition and portal vein ligation for staged hepatectomy (ALPPS): what is gained and what is lost?[J]. Ann Surg. 2012;256(3):e9.
9. Lang H, Baumgart J, Mittler J. Associated liver partition and portal vein ligation for staged hepatectomy (ALPPS) registry: what have we learned?[J]. Gut Liver. 2020;14(6):699–706.
10. Campos RR, Brusadin R, Conesa AL, et al. Staged liver resection for perihilar liver tumors using a tourniquet in the umbilical fissure and sequential portal vein embolization on the fourth postoperative day (a modified ALTPS)[J]. Cir Esp. 2014;92(10):682–6.
11. Petrowsky H, Györi G, de Oliveira M, et al. Is partial-ALPPS safer than ALPPS? A single-center experience[J]. Ann Surg. 2015;261(4):e90–2.
12. Michal K, Sau M, Tamara GMH, et al. A better route to ALPPS: minimally invasive vs open ALPPS[J]. Surg Endosc. 2020;34(6):2379–89.
13. López-López V, Robles-Campos R, Brusadin R, et al. Tourniquet-ALPPS is a promising treatment for very large hepatocellular carcinoma and intrahepatic cholangiocarcinoma[J]. Oncotarget. 2018;9(46):28267–80.
14. Li J, Kantas A, Ittrich H, et al. Avoid "all-touch" by hybrid ALPPS to achieve oncological efficacy[J]. Ann Surg. 2016;263(1):e6–7.
15. Balci D. Pushing the envelope in perihiler cholangiocellularcarcinoma surgery: TIPE-ALPPS[J]. Ann Surg. 2018;267(2):e21–2.
16. de Santibañes E, Alvarez FA, Ardiles V, et al. Inverting the ALPPS paradigm by minimizing first stage impact: the mini-ALPPS technique[J]. Langenbeck's Arch Surg. 2016;401(4):557–63.
17. Lai Q, Melandro F, Rossi M. Hybrid partial ALPPS: a feasible approach in case of right trisegmentectomy and macrovascular invasion[J]. Ann Surg. 2018;267(4):e80–2.
18. Li J, Nashan B. Reply to: "minimize the surgical damage at the stage-1 operation by combining hybrid ALPPS and nontotal parenchymal transection"[J]. Ann Surg. 2018;267(4):e82–3.
19. Oldhafer KJ, Wagner KC, Kantas A, et al. Hybrid-ALPPS followed by ante situm with cardiopulmonary bypass: rapid liver augmentation and complex surgery[J]. Ann Surg Oncol. 2020;27(9):3341.
20. Fard-Aghaie MH, Oldhafer KJ. ASO author reflections: hybrid-ALPPS followed by ante situm with cardiopulmonary bypass: pushing the boundaries for resectability by combining two controversial methods[J]. Ann Surg Oncol. 2020;27(9):3342–3.
21. Lang H, de Santibañes E, Schlitt HJ, et al. 10th anniversary of ALPPS-lessons learned and quo vadis[J]. Ann Surg. 2019;269(1):114–9.
22. Petrowsky H, Linecker M, Raptis DA, et al. First long-term oncologic results of the ALPPS procedure in a large cohort of patients with colorectal liver metastases[J]. Ann Surg. 2020;272(5):793–800.
23. Li J, Moustafa M, Linecker M, et al. ALPPS for locally advanced intrahepatic cholangiocarcinoma: did aggressive surgery lead to the oncological benefit? An international multi-center study[J]. Ann Surg Oncol. 2020;27(5):1372–84.
24. Neuhaus P, Blumhardt G. Extended bile duct resection – a new oncological approach to the treatment of central bile duct carcinomas? Description of method and early results[J]. Langenbecks Arch Chir. 1994;379(2):123–8.
25. Neuhaus P, Thelen A, Jonas S, et al. Oncological superiority of hilar en bloc resection for the treatment of hilar cholangiocarcinoma[J]. Ann Surg Oncol. 2012;19(5):1602–8.
26. Linecker M, Stavrou GA, Oldhafer KJ, et al. The ALPPS risk score: avoiding futile use of ALPPS[J]. Ann Surg. 2016;264(5):763–71.
27. Serenari M, Collaud C, Alvarez FA, et al. Interstage assessment of remnant liver function in ALPPS using hepatobiliary scintigraphy: prediction of posthepatectomy liver failure and introduction of the HIBA index[J]. Ann Surg. 2018;267(6):1141–7.
28. Chinese Research Hospital Association, Society for Hepatopancreatobiliary Surgery. Expert consensus on precision liver resection[J]. Chin J Dig Surg. 2017;16(9):883–93.
29. Schmelzle M, Öllinger R, Gebauer B, et al. Stage 1-laparoscopy partial PVE-ALPPS followed by step 2-hand-assisted laparoscopic extended right hepatectomy in a patient with gallbladder cancer[J]. Zentralbl Chir. 2019;144(1):21–3.
30. Hybrid ALPPS[EB/OL]. [2022-10-10]. http://www.alpps.net/?q=Forum_Hybrid_ALPPS
31. Li J, Girotti P, Königsrainer I, et al. ALPPS in right trisectionectomy: a safe procedure to avoid postoperative liver failure?[J]. J Gastrointest Surg. 2013;17(5):956–61.

Reversal ALPPS

14

Jian Zhou and Yuanfei Peng

14.1 Introduction

In 2007, Professor Hans J. Schlitt et al. established the associating liver partition and portal vein ligation for staged hepatectomy (ALPPS). Following its formal report and naming in 2012 [1–3], ALPPS has garnered widespread attention and has been rapidly adopted [4–14]. ALPPS has been demonstrated to induce rapid and extensive future liver remnant (FLR) hypertrophy and achieve a high tumor resection rate, providing curative surgery opportunities for many liver tumor patients who were previously inoperable. In recent years, with the publication of numerous clinical controlled studies, including prospective randomized controlled trials (RCTs), and the accumulation of long-term follow-up data, ALPPS has been proven to benefit patients. Compared to traditional treatment methods, it significantly improves patients' medium and long-term survival rates [15–19].

The application of ALPPS is flexible and diverse, with no restrictions on the tumor location, future liver remnant (FLR) location, number of liver segments, or extent of resection. Initially, ALPPS was used for right trisectionectomy (classical right trisectionectomy ALPPS) and was quickly adapted for extended right hepatectomy and right hemihepatectomy ALPPS. The extensive practice with ALPPS has enabled surgeons to apply it more flexibly. ALPPS has been utilized for left trisectionectomy (reversal ALPPS), middle segmentectomy, and single-segment ALPPS (monosegment ALPPS). FLR is no longer limited to the left lateral segment or left hemiliver; any liver lobe or segment, or even any liver region with independent and complete vascular structure and function, can serve as FLR for inducing regeneration and then performing tumor resection [20, 21]. Procedures that meet the two core elements (separation of the tumor-side liver from FLR and ligation of the portal vein on the tumor side) can induce hypertrophy in the corresponding FLR, allowing for the resection of areas outside the FLR.

Reversal ALPPS refers to left trisectionectomy ALPPS, where FLR is the right posterior lobe of the liver [21, 22]. It was applied as early as 2012 [23]. Obed et al. formally reported a reversal of ALPPS in 2016 [22]. A 36-year-old female patient with sigmoid colon cancer liver metastasis involving segments V and VII of the left liver required a left trisectionectomy. Preoperatively, the FLR to total liver volume (TLV) ratio was only 22%. In first-stage ALPPS, the liver parenchyma between the right anterior and right posterior lobes was transected, and the right anterior branch of the portal vein was divided (without ligating the left portal vein, only dissecting the left hepatic artery and portal vein). Postoperatively, the right posterior lobe (FLR) of the liver increased by 100%. Seven days later, the patient underwent left trisectionectomy and left hemicolectomy, achieving an R0 resection. Reversal ALPPS variants have also been reported using modification techniques, including minimally invasive approaches, partial partition, and transileocolic portal vein embolization (TIPE) as an alternative to portal vein ligation [21, 24, 25]. Reversal ALPPS has been applied for colorectal liver metastasis (CRLM), hepatocellular carcinoma (HCC), and perihilar cholangiocarcinoma (PHCC). In 2016, Professor Machado [21] reported fully laparoscopic reversal ALPPS. In stage 1 ALPPS, three superficial metastatic lesions in the right posterior lobe were resected, followed by transection of the liver parenchyma between the right anterior and posterior lobes, division of the right anterior Glisson branch, and ligation of the left portal vein. The postoperative FLR increase was 70%, and 3 weeks later, stage 2 ALPPS (left trisectionectomy) was performed with uneventful recovery. An 18-month follow-up showed no recurrence. In China, in 2017, we completed the first case of reversal ALPPS, successfully excising a huge HCC involving the left and medial lobes.

The initial definition of reversal ALPPS refers to the left trisectionectomy ALPPS, with the FLR being the right

J. Zhou (✉) · Y. Peng
Zhongshan Hospital, Fudan University, Shanghai, China
e-mail: zhou.jian@zs-hospital.sh.cn

J. Zhou (ed.), *Associating Liver Partition and Portal Vein Ligation for Staged Hepatectomy (ALPPS)*,
https://doi.org/10.1007/978-981-96-7364-3_14

Table 14.1 Literature reports of the reversal ALPPS

Author	Year	Age	Tumor	FLR increase	Extent of resection	Complications	Survival follow-up
Sala S. et al. [23]	2012	50	CRLM	108%	Left trisectionectomy	None	NA
Gauzolino et al. [26]	2012	NA	CRLM	10.6%	Left trisectionectomy	Atrial fibrillation, biloma	NA
Petrowsky H. et al. [24]	2015	61	CRLM	NA	Left trisectionectomy	NA	NA
Obed A. et al. [22]	2016	36	CRLM	100%	Left trisectionectomy	Sepsis, renal failure	NA
Zattar-Ramos L. C. et al. [27]	2016	58	CRLM	15%	Left trisectionectomy	None	NA
Machado M. A. et al. [21]	2016	42	CRLM	70%	Left trisectionectomy	None	Tumor-free survival 18 months
Ji R. et al. [28]	2018	37	PNETM	58%	Left trisectionectomy + pancreaticoduodenectomy ileum	None	Tumor-free survival 4 years
Voskanyan et al. [29]	2018	44	HCC	78.8%	Left trisectionectomy	None	Tumor-free survival 12 months
Sakamoto et al. [25]	2018	39	PHCC	NA	Left trisectionectomy	NA	NA

Note: *CRLM* colorectal liver metastases, *PNET* pancreatic neuroendocrine tumor liver metastases, *HCC* hepatocellular carcinoma, *PHCC* perihilar cholangiocarcinoma, *NA* not available data reported

posterior lobe of the liver [21, 22]. From the perspective of ALPPS development, similar to the evolution of classical ALPPS, reversal ALPPS is merely a relative definition. The definition should be expanded to include instances where the FLR is on the right side of the liver, not limited to the right posterior lobe. Due to the variability of liver anatomy, some patients have a hypertrophic left lobe and a smaller right lobe, and the portal vein distribution in the right lobe is more complex and variable than in the left lobe. Reversal ALPPS is significantly more complex than classical ALPPS, making it more challenging to perform and consequently few cases (Table 14.1). According to existing reports, reversal ALPPS demonstrates the same FLR induction efficiency as conventional ALPPS, with FLR hypertrophy reaching 70% to 124.3%. However, as most reports are case studies, data on complications, mortality, long-term oncological benefits, and other outcomes remain largely unknown. Final conclusions await further research results. Regardless, reversal ALPPS provides a surgical opportunity for patients requiring extensive left-sided liver resection but who have insufficient FLR.

14.2 Indications

The following criteria are indications for reversal ALPPS: primary or secondary malignant liver tumors or perihilar cholangiocarcinoma that are potentially resectable; no extrahepatic metastases or extrahepatic lesions can be simultaneously radically resected and no expected residual extrahepatic lesions after surgery; lesions locate on the left side of the liver and involve the right anterior lobe, requiring left trisectionectomy, extended left hepatectomy, or left hemihepatectomy; insufficient FLR on the right side [normal liver parenchyma, FLR to standard liver volume (SLV) ratio < (25%–30%); liver parenchyma with damage or chronic liver disease, including chemotherapy-related liver injury, liver fibrosis/cirrhosis, cholestasis and severe steatosis, FLR/SLV ratio < (30%–40%)] [3, 30, 31]; FLR without lesions or lesions that can be simultaneously radically resected, with no expected residual lesions after surgery; normal liver function, Child-Pugh A, or mild reversible damage with an indocyanine green retention rate at 15 min (ICG-R15) < 15%; and good performance status, able to tolerate major surgery.

14.3 Surgical Steps

Reversal ALPPS (Fig. 14.1) involves surgical elements that are fundamentally the same as those in conventional ALPPS, including liver separation and tumor-side portal vein occlusion. Both the classic liver parenchymal transection combined with portal vein ligation and modified procedures can be applied [21, 22, 24, 25]. Reversal ALPPS surgery can be performed via open surgery or laparoscopic surgery, with the basic operational elements remaining consistent. The following describes the classical open reversal ALPPS (left trisectionectomy ALPPS).

14.3.1 Positioning

The patient is usually in a left lateral position of 30° to 45°, depending on the degree of the transection plane to right side.

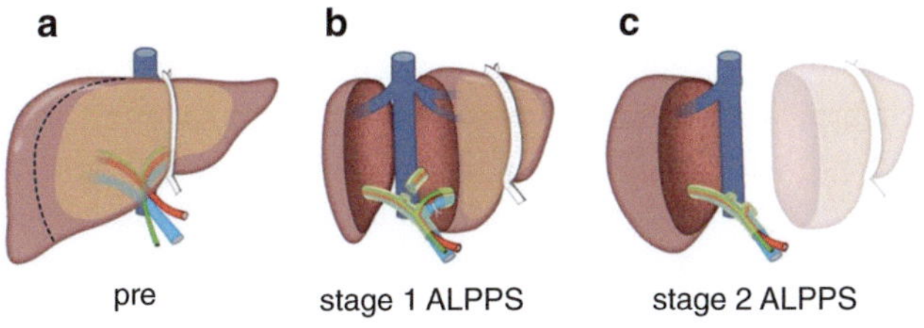

Fig. 14.1 Schematic diagram of reversal ALPPS. (**a**) Preoperative pre-cutting plane. (**b**) Stage 1 ALPPS: the liver parenchyma between the right anterior lobe and the right posterior lobe is partitioned, the right anterior Glisson pedicle is divided, and the left portal vein is ligated. (**c**) Stage 2 ALPPS: left trisectionectomy

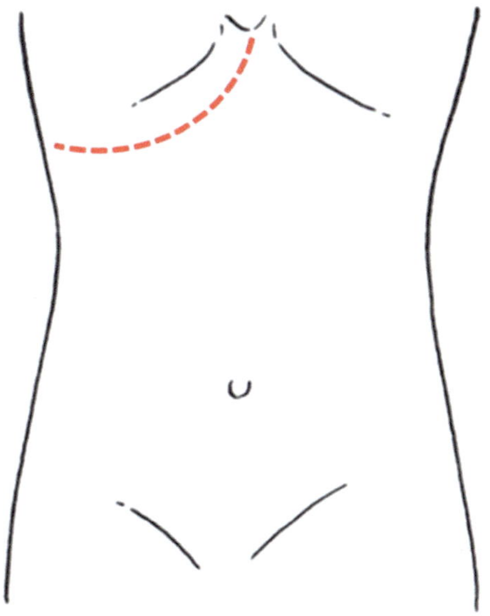

Fig. 14.2 Incisions for open reversal ALPPS: right subcostal incision

14.3.2 Stage 1 ALPPS

14.3.2.1 Surgical Incision

The right subcostal incision is usually used (Fig. 14.2).

14.3.2.2 Abdominal Exploration

After access into the abdomen, the abdominal cavity is exposed by placing a liver retractor. Full exploration is performed to exclude any extrahepatic lesions not detected by preoperative imaging and other surgical contraindications.

14.3.2.3 Mobilization of the Right Liver

The right liver is fully mobilized by dividing the round ligament (ligament teres), falciform ligament, right triangular ligament, coronary ligament, and hepatorenal ligament. If the left side allows mobilization, the ligaments on the left side are dissociated to facilitate rotating the liver and exposure of the right posterior lobe. Due to the deep position of the right posterior lobe, the transection plane is often horizontal or even has a posterior tilt. Complete mobilization of the right liver facilitates the exposure of the transection plane, reducing the difficulty of liver parenchyma partition. Meanwhile, rotating the liver to the left shifts the right hepatic vein vertically, reducing pressure in the distal right hepatic vein and minimizing bleeding. The common trunk of the left and middle hepatic veins, the root of the right hepatic vein, is dissected, and the hepatic vein fossa is exposed and marked with electrocautery. The liver is then flipped to the left, and the right side of the inferior vena cava (IVC) is dissected. Taking care not to divide the short hepatic veins on the right side of the IVC, preserving the outflow of the right posterior lobe and caudate lobes into the IVC.

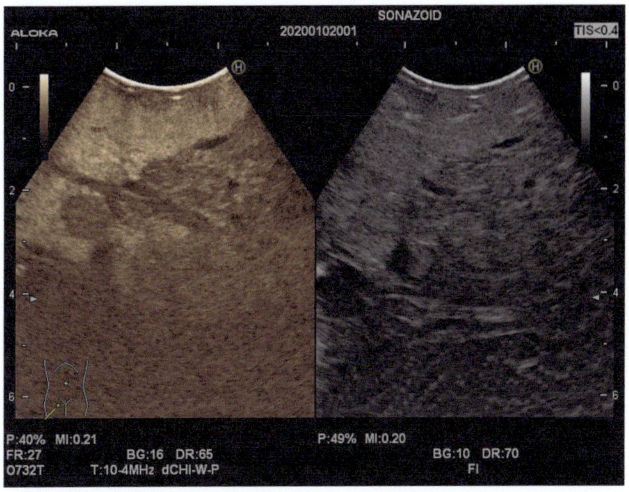

Fig. 14.3 Ultrasound examination with Sonazoid contrast agent is used to exclude tumors in FLR

14.3.2.4 Intraoperative Ultrasound

The liver is comprehensively examined using intraoperative ultrasound to confirm preoperative diagnosed lesions and check for any other lesions, especially whether there are preoperatively undetected lesions in the FLR. For CRLM, it is recommended to use a Sonazoid contrast agent for contrast-enhanced imaging (Fig. 14.3) to fully screen for potential small metastatic lesions. The right hepatic vein is located using ultrasound and marks on the liver surface (Fig. 14.4). The adjacent relationship between the tumor, FLR, and major vascular structures is explored and clarified. In combination with preoperative virtual surgical planning, the pre-cut line is delineated on the liver surface and determines the liver parenchymal transection plane.

14.3.2.5 Cholecystectomy

Calot's triangle is dissected; the cystic duct and the cystic artery are exposed, ligated, and divided; and then the gallbladder is removed. The cystic duct is divided close to the gallbladder side, and a certain length is reserved at the stump. After the parenchymal partition, a bile leakage check will be

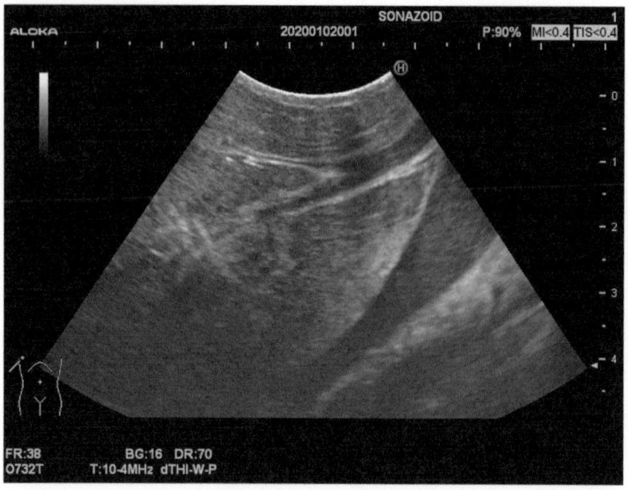

Fig. 14.4 Intraoperative ultrasound location of the right hepatic vein and inferior vena cava are common. If bile duct variation is suspected before surgery but is not clearly shown by MRI or other examinations, contrast agents can be injected through the cystic duct for cholangiography. ICG can also be injected through the cystic duct to clarify the variations using fluorescence technology

performed via the stump of the cyst duct by injecting a contrast agent or a color-developing agent such as fat emulsion. Anatomical variations in the bile duct.

14.3.2.6 Liver Parenchymal Partition, Division of the Left Portal Vein and the Right Anterior Glisson Pedicle

Liver parenchymal partition involves separating the right anterior lobe and right posterior lobe, ligating the left portal vein, and transecting the right anterior branch of the hepatic artery. Unlike conventional ALPPS (right trisectionectomy ALPPS), the right anterior Glisson pedicle is directly divided rather than dissecting and ligating the right anterior branch of the portal vein. Isolation of the right anterior branch of the portal vein is relatively difficult, as the right posterior branch of the bile duct usually runs above and behind the right anterior branch of the portal vein (Fig. 14.5), increasing the risk of damaging the right posterior branch of the bile duct. Furthermore, the right anterior lobe occupies a smaller area, so Glissonean pedicle transection is used to directly divide the right anterior pedicle. The division of the right anterior pedicle also facilitates liver parenchyma transection. The method and sequence of steps of the procedure may vary based on the tumor location, anatomical variations, and the surgeon's preferences. If the tumor is close to the hilum or compresses the Glisson pedicle, it is inadvisable to perform Glissonean dissection due to the potential risk of tumor rupture. In such cases, an intrahepatic approach may be more appropriate. The intrahepatic approach involves initially dissecting the hepatoduodenal ligament, isolating the portal vein's left and right branches, and subsequently exposing the right posterior branch of the portal vein through careful dissection. The right posterior branch of the portal vein is clamped with a nontraumatic Bulldog clamp, and the ischemia line is identified to delineate the transection plane, as previously mapped with ultrasound. The parenchyma is then transected using either a Cavitron ultrasonic surgical aspirator (CUSA), bipolar coagulation, or an ultrasonic scalpel to separate the right anterior hepatic pedicle from the tumor site in the left/medial liver. The right anterior Glisson pedicle is then clamped and divided. Because of the specific course of the right posterior bile duct, a certain distance should be maintained when transecting the right anterior Glisson pedicle to avoid injury or suturing the right posterior bile duct (Fig. 14.5). A nontraumatic Satinsky clamp can be used to occlude the right anterior Glisson pedicle, with proximal suture ligation using polypropylene suture. Next, the left portal vein is ligated. Suppose the tumor is sufficiently distant from the hilum and the surgeon is skilled in Glissonean transection. In that case, the Laennec capsule can be opened to separate and ligate the right anterior, left, and right posterior Glisson pedicles. The right posterior lobe (FLR) can then be confirmed based on the ischemia line, and the right anterior Glisson pedicle is ligated. Following the right anterior pedicle ligation, the ischemic demarcation of the right anterior lobe is clearly visible, providing a clear boundary for further parenchyma transection between the right posterior and right anterior lobes. Finally, the hepatoduodenal ligament is dissected to isolate and ligate the left portal vein. It is crucial to note that due to common anatomical variations of the hepatic inflow and outflow tracts and the relatively complex blood supply to the right posterior lobe, both preoperative and intraoperative assessments should carefully consider these variations' impacts on the surgical procedure. The following sections will describe the surgical steps in three parts, focusing on the most commonly used intrahepatic method, while also addressing other surgical techniques.

14.3.2.7 Dissection of the Porta Hepatis

Adjusting the liver hook traction, pulling the liver upward to fully expose the hilum (Fig. 14.6); if the tumor is close to the hepatic hilum, dissect the hepatic hilum first, separating the proper hepatic artery and the left (middle) and right branches of hepatic arteries, left and right branches of portal vein, and the bile duct; marking the portal vein, bile duct, and hepatic artery with blue, yellow, and red color ribbons, respectively (Figs. 14.7, 14.8 and 14.9). If the tumor is intrahepatic cholangiocarcinoma or hilar cholangiocarcinoma, the hepatoduodenal ligament should be skeletonized, and regional lymphadenectomy including No.12 lymph nodes should be performed; the separation of the right anterior branch is very important, relying on it to determine the ischemic right anterior lobe, but the right anterior branch is relatively difficult to

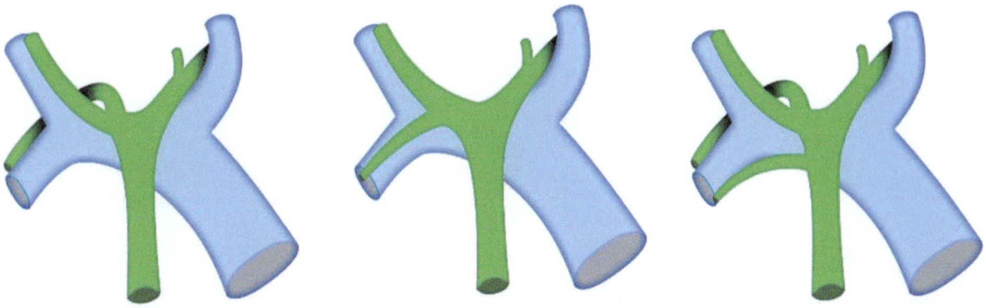

Fig. 14.5 Common variations of the right posterior bile duct

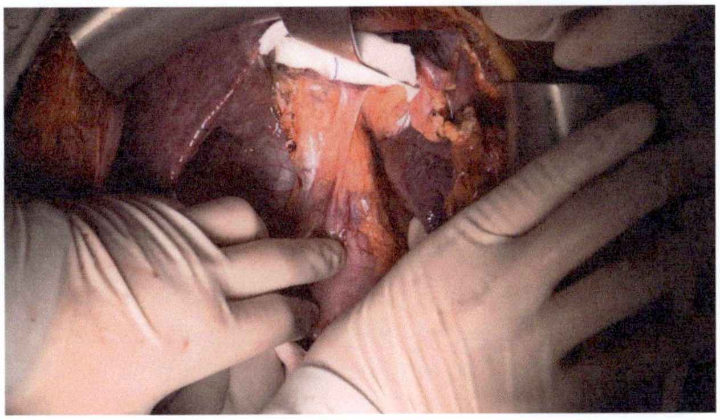

Fig. 14.6 Using a retractor to pull the liver upwards to fully expose the porta hepatis

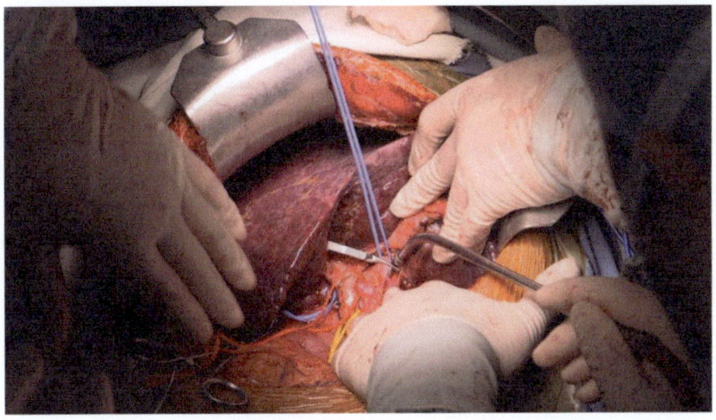

Fig. 14.9 Dissecting the portal vein trunk and left branch of the portal vein (blue ribbon), and clamping with Bulldog clamp for ischemia confirmation

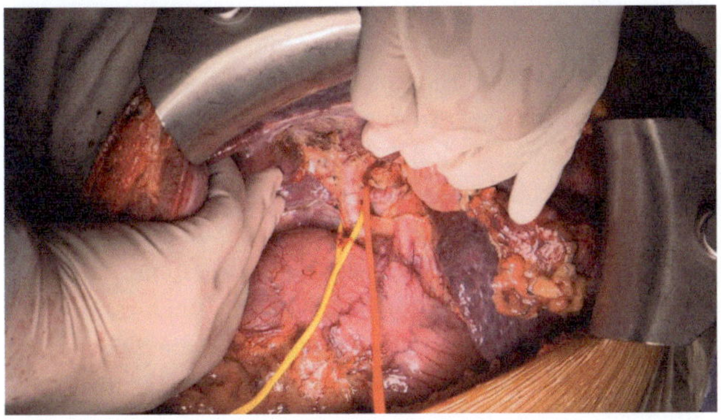

Fig. 14.7 Dissecting the porta hepatis and exposing the artery and bile duct

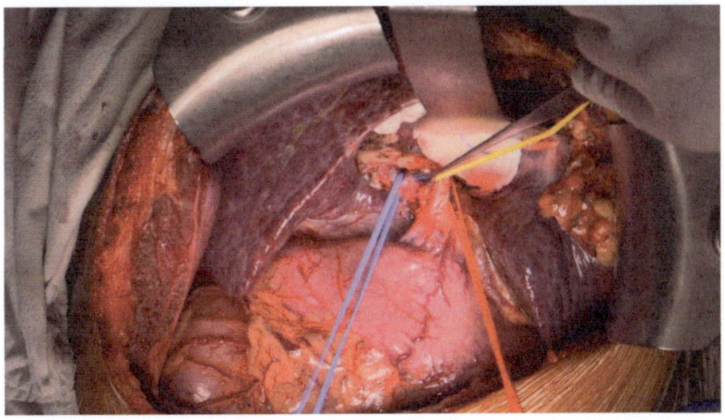

Fig. 14.8 Dissecting the porta hepatis and exposing the portal vein trunk and right branch of the portal vein

separate. In contrast, the right posterior branch is easy to determine and separate from the right branch of the portal vein, which is easy to separate from below. The right anterior branch is relatively difficult to separate, and because the right posterior bile duct mostly takes a northward course, separation is prone to damage the bile duct. Therefore, in practice, the boundary of the right posterior lobe (FLR) can be determined by confirming the right posterior branch, without the need to forcibly separate the right anterior branch. Using a Bulldog clamp to occlude the right posterior portal vein to expose the ischemic right posterior lobe, in combination with intraoperative ultrasound location of the right hepatic vein and other liver markers, the liver partition line is determined (Fig. 14.10). If there is a fluorescence laparoscopy, positive staining can be used to visualize the right posterior lobe to better determine the right posterior lobe (FLR). Suppose the tumor is a certain distance from the hilum. In that case, Laennec's capsule can be directly opened to separate the right anterior, left, and right posterior Glisson pedicles and occlude them to confirm the right posterior lobe, making the operation more convenient.

14.3.2.8 Liver Parenchymal Transection

The liver parenchyma is transected along the pre-marked line toward the anterior wall of the IVC. The specific method for liver transection can vary according to individual preference. Typically, the Cavitron ultrasonic surgical aspirator (CUSA) is used in combination with bipolar/unipolar electrocautery

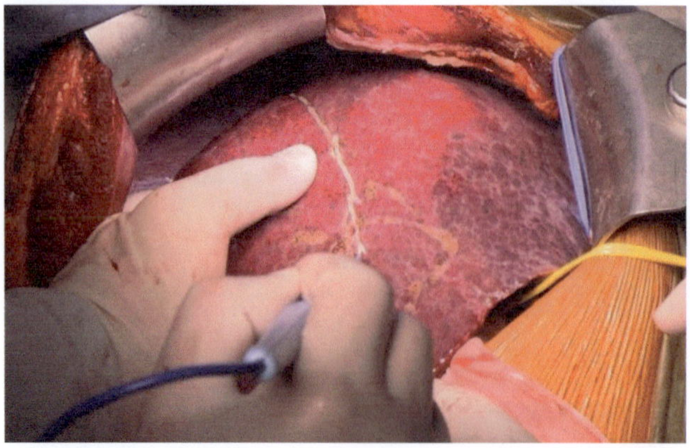

Fig. 14.10 Marking the pre-cutting line after intraoperative ultrasound examination

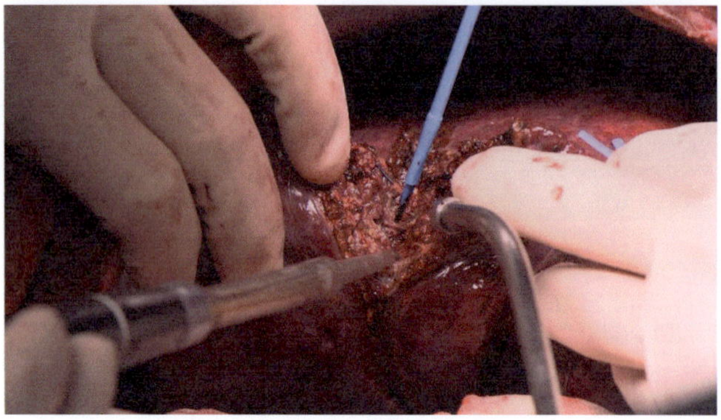

Fig. 14.11 Liver parenchymal partition: liver parenchymal partition is performed using CUSA combined with bipolar/unipolar electrocoagulation

for precise transection of the liver parenchyma (Fig. 14.11). During the transection, branches of the Glisson, hepatic veins, and other encountered ducts are coagulated, ligated with silk sutures, or clipped with titanium clips as needed. Hemostasis must be meticulously maintained throughout the procedure. Other devices such as the Harmonic scalpel can also be used for liver parenchymal transection. Intraoperative low central venous pressure (CVP) techniques are commonly employed to reduce bleeding during liver parenchymal transection. This involves close coordination with the anesthesiologist to restrict fluid intake, deepen anesthesia, and minimize tidal volume, while restricting positive end-expiratory pressure (PEEP). The patient's position can be adjusted to a reverse Trendelenburg position, and vasoactive drugs (e.g., dobutamine, nitroglycerin) may be used to control CVP as necessary. If there is significant bleeding, hepatic inflow occlusion may be utilized. The intermittent Pringle maneuver (clamping for 15 min, releasing for 5 min, repeated as necessary) is generally used. Selective blood flow occlusion can also be employed. Similar to the routine use of the

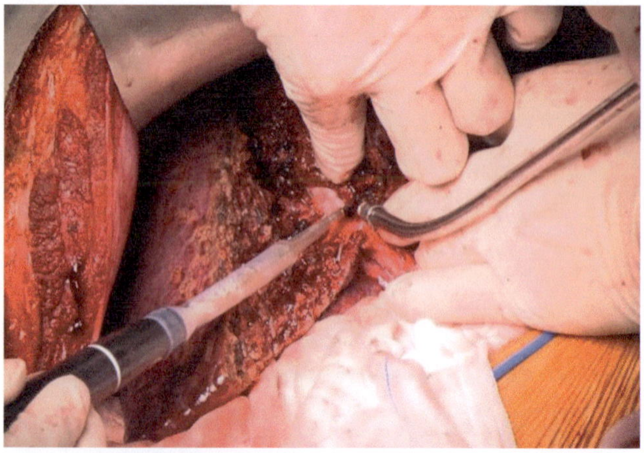

Fig. 14.12 Dissecting the right anterior Glisson pedicle

Pringle maneuver in live donor liver transplantation [32], its use for ALPPS is safe. Techniques such as the Belghiti suspension can assist in liver parenchyma transection. The liver parenchyma is transected up to the anterior wall of the IVC, completely separating the tumor-bearing liver from the FLR.

14.3.2.9 Division of the Right Anterior Glisson Pedicle

The right anterior Glisson pedicle is usually divided using the intrahepatic approach, but the Glissonean transection method can also be employed. For the intrahepatic approach, the liver parenchyma is divided using the CUSA until the hilum is reached, exposing the right anterior Glisson pedicle. At the same time, ensure adequate exposure of the right posterior Glisson pedicle and the junctional area of the left pedicle, taking special care to protect the right posterior Glisson pedicle. The right anterior pedicle is clamped at its root with a Satinsky clamp, then transected, and the stump is closed with a continuous polypropylene suture. When transecting the right anterior branch, it is important to maintain a certain distance from the root, as the right posterior bile duct typically loops around the right branch of the portal vein and the posterior aspect of the right anterior branch (Figs. 14.5 and 14.12). Suturing too close to the root risks inadvertently including the right posterior bile duct in the suture, leading to catastrophic consequences. It is recommended to use an atraumatic arterial clamp (Fig. 14.13) to clamp the right anterior pedicle at a safe distance from the root, then continuously suture the stump above the clamp site (Figs. 14.13 and 14.14). If using the Glissonean transection method, this is performed before dissecting the hepatoduodenal ligament. The Pringle maneuver is applied to occlude the hepatic pedicle, the Laennec's capsule is opened, and the right anterior Glisson pedicle is isolated and suspended in preparation for subsequent transection.

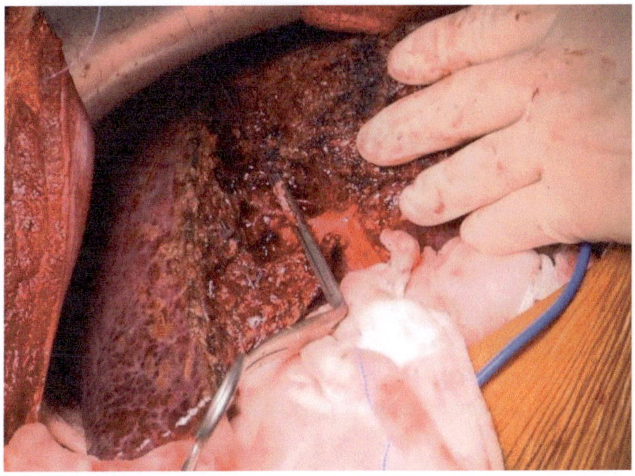

Fig. 14.13 Dividing the right anterior Glisson pedicle and suturing the stump

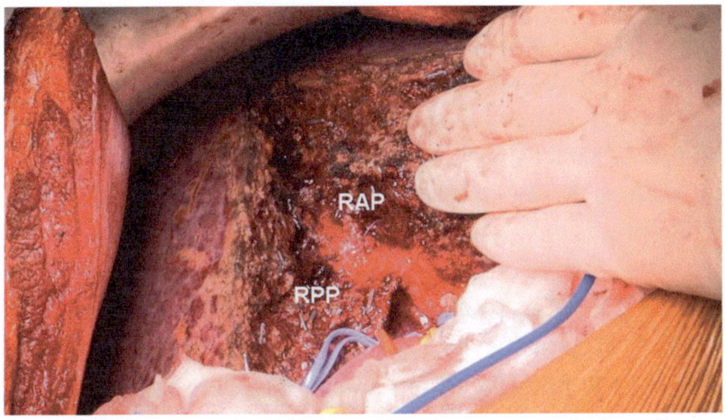

Fig. 14.14 The right anterior Glisson pedicle (RAP) is divided, and the right posterior Glisson pedicle (RPP) is exposed

14.3.2.10 Ligation of the Left Portal Vein

After the liver parenchyma has been transected and the right anterior Glisson pedicle has been divided, the left portal vein is ligated using 4-0 polypropylene suture or silk sutures, leaving a long tag for easier identification during the second stage of the surgery (Fig. 14.15). The ligation of the portal vein must be reliable. It is recommended to use a double ligation technique. During laparoscopic surgery, titanium clips should not be used; instead, Hem-o-lok clips should be applied, ensuring they pass the opposite wall of the portal vein for a complete and secure closure. Alternatively, sutures can be used under direct laparoscopic visualization. The portal vein has a certain degree of variability (commonly classified using the Cheng Y. F. classification [33] or Nakamura classification [34]). TypesI, II, andIII portal vein left branches are easy to manage. For type IV variants, where the right anterior branch of the portal vein cannot be isolated from outside the liver, the right anterior branch and the left branch

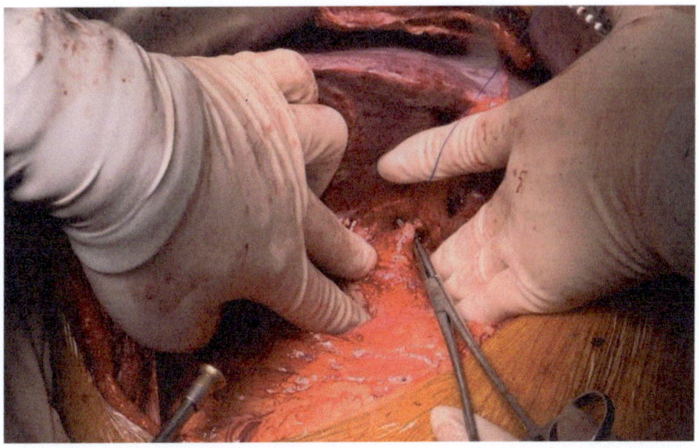

Fig. 14.15 Ligation of the left portal vein

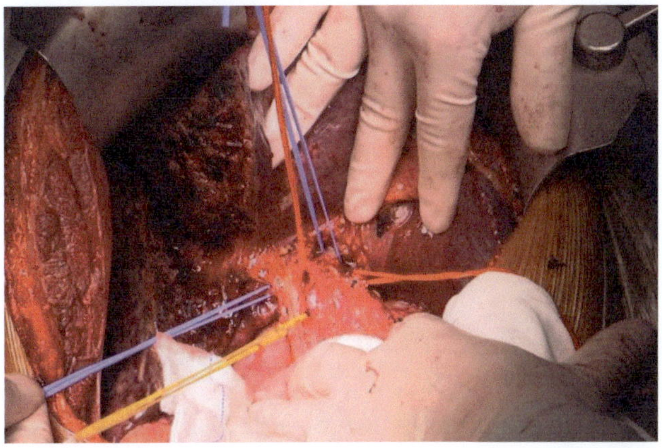

Fig. 14.16 Hepatic tracts display after the dissection of the porta hepatis (from right to left) the right portal vein, common bile duct, right hepatic artery, left portal vein, and left hepatic artery

of the portal vein are ligated together. For other challenging types, the principle is to ensure that the portal vein branches supplying the FLR are preserved while all other branches are ligated. After ligation, an ultrasound examination is performed to check blood inflow. Additionally, interventional procedures can be combined, such as ultrasound-guided portal vein embolization, to embolize the portal vein branches on the tumor side completely. The caudate lobe is managed based on the situation. If simultaneous resection is necessary, the left caudate lobe is also resected.

14.3.2.11 Color Ribbon Marking

Marking the hepatic portal ducts with color ribbons (Fig. 14.16) and hemostasis of transection surface (Figs. 14.17 and 14.18).

14.3.2.12 Bile Leakage Check

A Strict bile leakage check is performed after liver parenchymal partition. If the handling of the duct during the liver parenchymal partition is precise and reliable and bile leakage

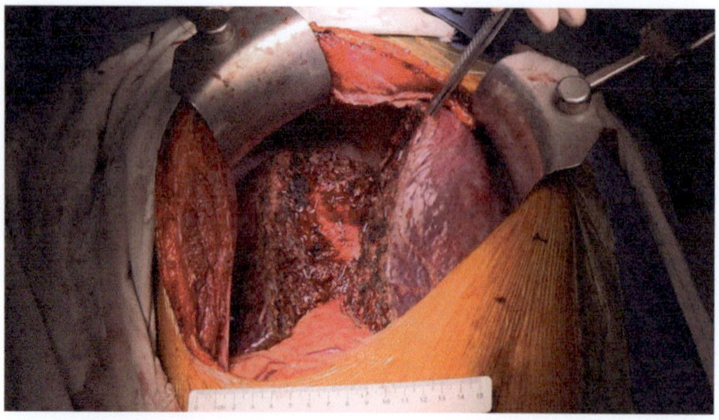

Fig. 14.17 Transection surface of the right posterior lobe (right lobe has been padded up)

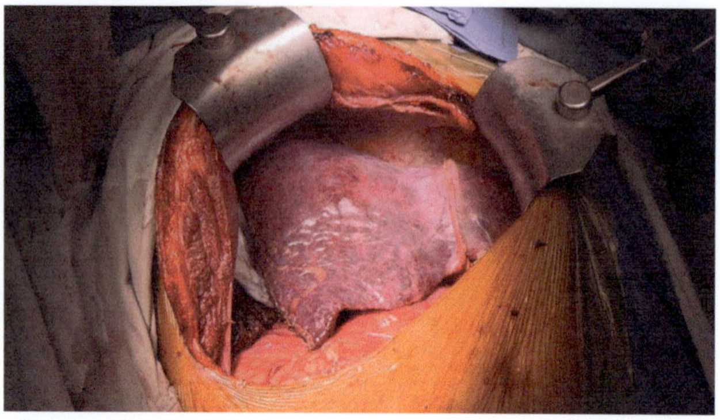

Fig. 14.18 The left lobe and the right anterior lobe (in situ positioning)

is not expected to occur, this step can be skipped. In our center, we often use the diluted fat emulsion injection method to check for bile leakage; the procedure is as follows: open the gallbladder duct, clamp the common bile duct below the gallbladder duct stump, insert a needle catheter from the gallbladder duct stump to inject diluted fat emulsion, and observe for bile leakage on the transection surface (if there is bile leakage, white fat emulsion will flow out from the leakage point, making it easy to be detected). After confirming no bile leakage, suture the gallbladder duct stump.

14.3.2.13 Management of the Transection Surface

The practice of using plastic bags to wrap the tumor side liver during the early years of ALPPS has now been abandoned, as it is prone to causing abdominal fluid accumulation that can lead to serious abdominal infections if combined with infection. The abdominal infections are also difficult to drain. Moreover, if the FLR cannot reach the requirements for the stage 2 ALPPS, the plastic bag will become a foreign object left in the body, requiring another surgery for removal. Currently, most cases use fibrin and absorbable hemostatic gauze to cover the transection surface (Fig. 14.19), which

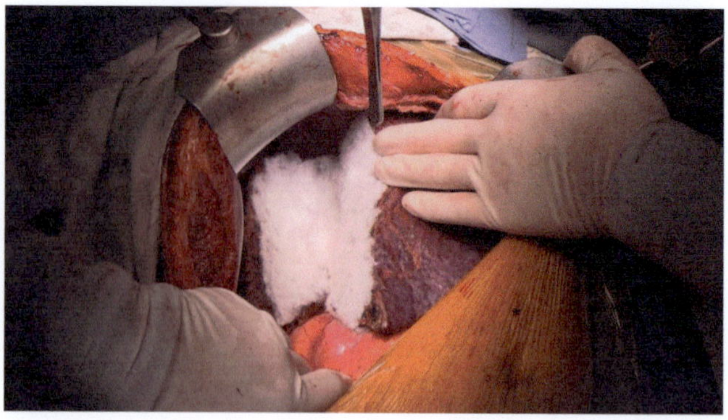

Fig. 14.19 Covering the transection surface with absorbable hemostatic gauze

usually provides good separation. Adhesions are not severe during the second stage of surgery, and it is not difficult to separate the left and right sides.

14.3.2.14 Drainages

A drain tube (usually Jackson-Pratt drain) is placed on the transection surface. If necessary, another drainage tube can be placed under the right diaphragm. Foley catheters can be introduced to the transected surface for further drainage while preventing adhesions on both sides [35].

14.3.2.15 Coating with Anti-adhesion Materials

Coating around the liver with anti-adhesion materials can reduce abdominal adhesions and facilitate the stage 2 ALPPS surgery. The author's center usually applies chitosan to reduce abdominal adhesions after the first stage of surgery.

14.3.2.16 Close the Abdomen

Use absorbable sutures to close the abdomen layer by layer. In particular, the peritoneal layer must be well-closed to ensure the smoothness of the inferior lining and reduce postoperative adhesions. For laparoscopic ALPPS, closure of the fascia at the trocar sites is needed, which can be done using fascial closure devices or laparoscopic inverted suturing techniques. Some patients may have a large amount of ascites after stage 1 ALPPS, closing the trocar sites can prevent leakage of ascites from the trocar sites when abdominal drainage is not smooth.

14.3.3 Postoperative FLR Volume Remeasurement After Stage 1 ALPPS

After the first stage of ALPPS surgery, the liver volume is remeasured after a certain interval, usually remeasured at 1 week, and the specific interval can be determined by the operating surgeon based on the actual situation. Patients with a history of drug treatment, liver fibrosis, cirrhosis, and other chronic

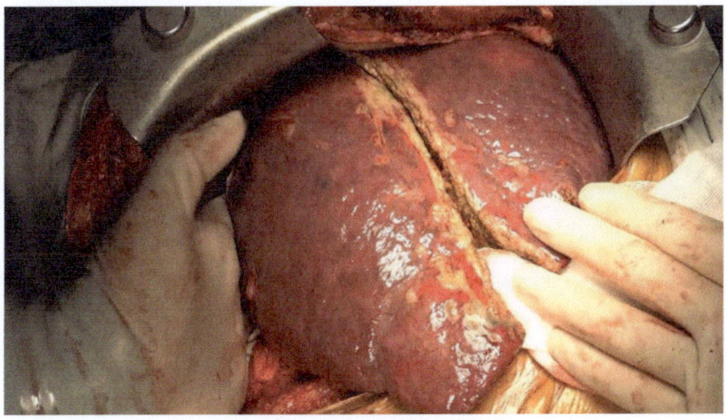

Fig. 14.20 Significant hypertrophy of the right posterior lobe

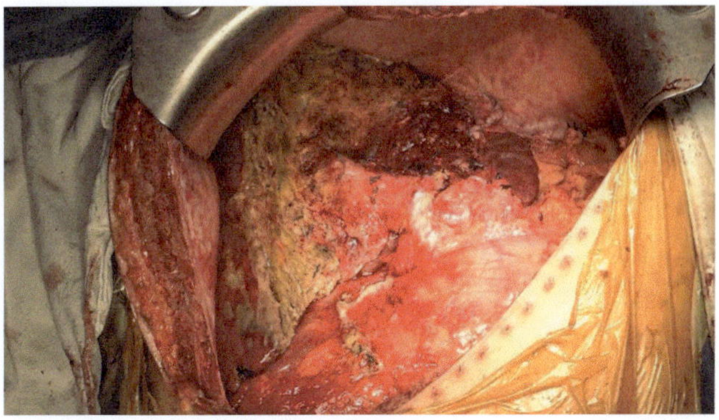

Fig. 14.21 Operative view after tumor removal

liver diseases often require a longer time. After reaching the FLR volume required, the stage 2 ALPPS is performed. During the postoperative CT angiography (CTA) examination, attention should be paid to the portal vein flow simultaneously.

14.3.4 Stage 2 ALPPS

14.3.4.1 Reentering the Abdomen Through the Previous Incision

Following the stage 1 ALPPS surgery, the abdominal cavity typically exhibits some degree of adhesions, local congestion, and edema. Care must be taken to avoid damaging the gastrointestinal tract located beneath the incision. After entering the abdomen, the hypertrophic condition of the right posterior lobe is examined (Fig. 14.20).

14.3.4.2 Adhesions Lysis

Most adhesions within the abdominal cavity are not difficult to separate. However, if the waiting period has been prolonged or if an intra-abdominal infection occurred after the first stage of surgery, adhesions can be severe. After the adhesions are lysed, the FLR is further inspected to expose the liver transection surface and the hepatic hilum.

14.3.4.3 Intraoperative Ultrasound Examination of the FLR

This is particularly important for patients undergoing ALPPS for colorectal liver metastases (CRLM). To detect potential lesions, it is recommended to use a Sonazoid contrast agent for contrast-enhanced ultrasound. If necessary, these lesions should be treated promptly with radiofrequency ablation or resection.

14.3.4.4 Transection of the Hepatic Artery, Portal Vein, and Bile Duct on the Tumor Side

Given the numerous variations in bile duct anatomy, the bile duct is usually transected as the final step. Following transection, a bile duct probe is used to ensure the smooth flow of bile fluid in the FLR. In the case where the liver parenchyma was incompletely transected during the stage 1 ALPPS surgery, any remaining parenchyma should be further divided, especially the parenchyma connecting the FLR and the right side of the IVC. The stage 2 ALPPS surgery presents challenges such as inflammation, congestion, and edema from the first stage of surgery, making the liver parenchyma more susceptible to bleeding. This often results in a significant increase in blood loss compared to the first stage of surgery. To address this, the Pringle maneuver can be employed to control bleeding, or a Bulldog clamp can be used to clamp the portal vein trunk. It is essential to expose the hepatic veins, transect the middle and left hepatic veins or their common trunk, and close the stumps with a 4-0 polypropylene suture. Alternatively, a stapler can be utilized for quicker transection of the hepatic veins.

14.3.4.5 Removal of the Tumor

The residual ligaments surrounding the tumor side of the liver are divided, and the tumor is removed (Figs. 14.21 and 14.22).

14.3.4.6 Hemostasis and Bile Leakage Check

At the center where the authors work, an emulsion injection method is often used to check for bile leaks. A Bulldog or Satinsky clamp is used to clamp the common bile duct, and a diluted emulsion is injected through a catheter inserted into the stump of the left bile duct. The liver transection surface is then observed for any bile leaks. If no bile leaks are detected, the left bile duct is sutured and closed (Fig. 14.23). The liver transection surface is sprayed with fibrin and covered with absorbable hemostatic gauze.

14.3.4.7 Close the Abdomen

A drain tube (usually Jackson-Pratt drain) is placed on the transection surface. Close the abdomen layer by layer.

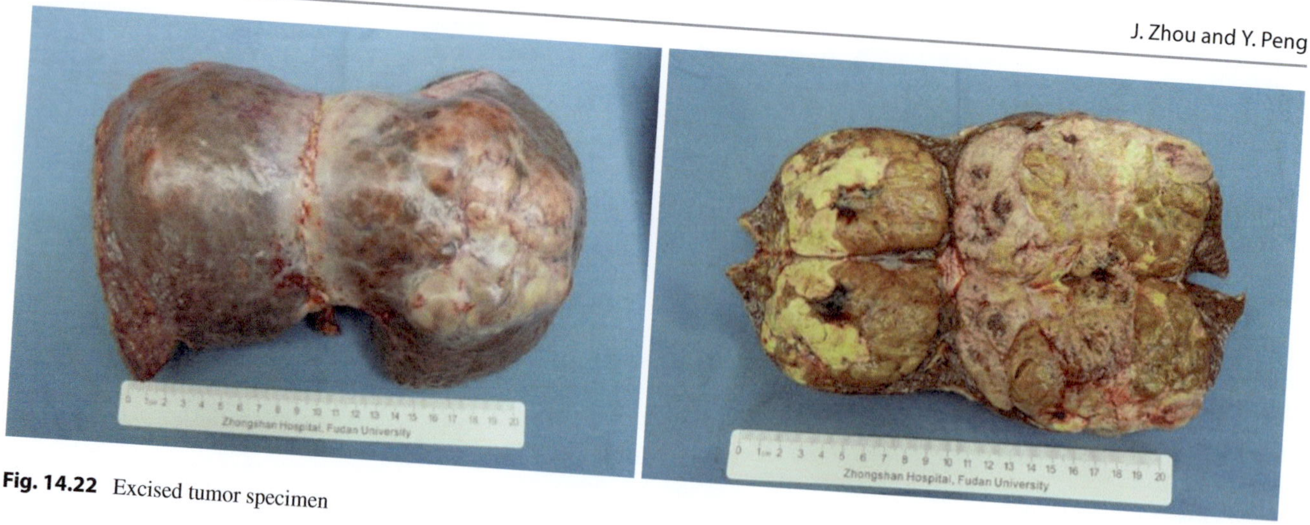

Fig. 14.22 Excised tumor specimen

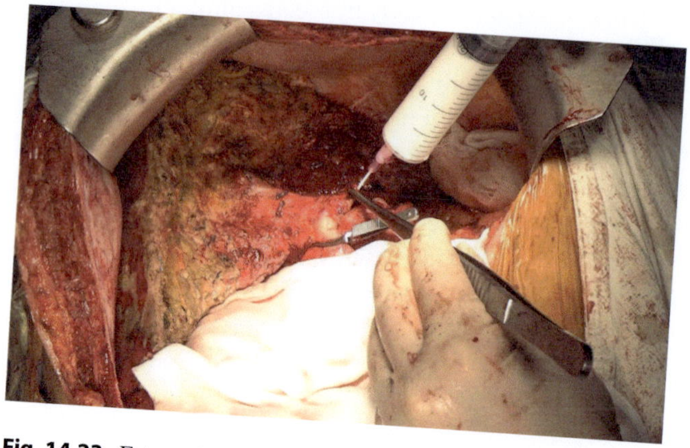

Fig. 14.23 Fat emulsion injection method for bile leakage check: the diluted fat emulsion is injected into the left bile duct to investigate bile leakage on the transection surface

14.4 Key Points and Notes of the Surgery

The key points and notes of the reversal ALPPS surgery are as follows.

14.4.1 Management of the Transection Surface

Reversal ALPPS is more complex than conventional ALPPS due to the curved plane of the right posterior lobe. This requires careful operation to determine the cut surface, including precise preoperative planning, virtual cutting, and thorough planning. During the operation, it is essential to comprehensively consider the tumor location, margins, and the requirements for a safe cutting edge, particularly adjacent to blood vessels like the right hepatic vein, to ensure the structural and functional integrity of the right posterior lobe.

If fluorescence equipment (such as fluorescence laparoscopy) is available, positive staining of the right posterior lobe can be utilized. Additionally, combining the Glissonean transection technique with reversal fluorescence staining techniques can fully expose the FLR. Conducting liver parenchymal transection under fluorescence guidance can enhance precision and reduce the difficulty of the surgical operation.

14.4.2 Position and Exposure

The transection plane of the right posterior lobe is usually horizontal and located posteriorly, necessitating a sufficient left lateral decubitus position and adequate mobilization of the right liver for optimal exposure. With this, achieving leftward liver rotation and proper FLR exposure becomes easier. In reversal ALPPS cases, where the tumor burden on the left side is often substantial, it can be challenging to rotate the liver to the left and secure enough right-sided operating space if a large liver tumor occupies the left side. This situation complicates the exposure of the right posterior lobe transection plane. In such scenarios, complete mobilization of the liver and the use of strong retractors to open the right subcostal area can provide better exposure.

14.4.3 Management of the Right Anterior Glisson Pedicle

The management of the right anterior pedicle is crucial. If the situation allows (i.e., if the tumor is far from the hepatic hilum), an external Glissonean transection can be directly performed by opening the Laennec capsule to ligate the right anterior hepatic pedicle. If the situation is not suitable, the liver parenchyma should be adequately dissected to expose the right anterior hepatic pedicle from within the liver. The surgeon must be familiar with the bile duct anatomy, particularly the course of the right posterior branch of the bile duct. The right anterior hepatic pedicle must be ligated at a sufficient distance from the confluence of the right anterior and right posterior hepatic pedicles to avoid damaging the right posterior bile duct, which could lead to bile duct stricture or biliary obstruction. Currently, in reversal ALPPS procedures, the right anterior hepatic pedicle is mainly transected directly. This approach is preferred because separating the right anterior branch of the portal vein is relatively difficult and carries a risk of injuring the right posterior branch of the bile duct. Embolization of the right anterior branch of the portal vein (portal vein embolization (PVE) can be performed intraoperatively through the colonic vein or mesenteric vein, or postoperatively via percutaneous transhepatic PVE) may achieve the same FLR induction while simultaneously reducing the risk of right anterior lobe necrosis and other potential adverse effects. However, further studies are needed to clarify the efficacy and safety of this approach.

14.4.4 Hepatic Duct Variations

Variations of the hepatic ducts can significantly affect surgical procedures. Although portal vein variations have a lesser impact on reversal ALPPS than conventional ALPPS, they still require careful attention, especially Type IV and other less common variations. The Glissonean transection technique is challenging to implement in these cases and necessitates a different approach than handling Types I–III variations. Bile duct variations are more complex. Only some patients with bile duct variations also exhibit portal vein variations, and these variations are often challenging to fully ascertain preoperatively. During surgery, it is crucial to thoroughly investigate the bile duct variation. If necessary, during the stage 1 ALPPS surgery, a fine 2 mm biliary probe can be inserted through the cystic duct to trace the bile duct. Alternatively, indocyanine green (ICG) can be injected through the cystic duct and visualized using fluorescence equipment. Otherwise, the iodinated contrast agents can be used for cholangiography to delineate the bile duct course. Variations in hepatic veins are less common but still notable. An inferior right hepatic vein (IRHV) drain Segment IV is common and should be identified during preoperative planning and intraoperative exploration to prevent injury, especially when mobilizing the liver or dissecting around the right side of the IVC. Additionally, care must be taken to avoid damaging the short hepatic veins on the right side during mobilization and ensure they are preserved intact.

References

1. Schlitt HJ, Hackl C, Lang SA. "In-situ split" liver resection/ALPPS – historical development and current practice[J]. Visc Med. 2017;33(6):408–12.
2. Baumgart J, Lang SA, Lang H. A new method for induction of liver hypertrophy prior to right trisectionectomy: a report of three cases[J]. HPB (Oxford). 2011;13(supple 2):71–2.
3. Schnitzbauer AA, Lang SA, Goessmann H, et al. Right portal vein ligation combined with *in situ* splitting induces rapid left lateral liver lobe hypertrophy enabling 2-staged extended right hepatic resection in small-for-size settings[J]. Ann Surg. 2012;255(3):405–14.
4. D'Haese JG, Neumann J, Weniger M, et al. Should ALPPS be used for liver resection in intermediate-stage HCC?[J]. Ann Surg Oncol. 2016;23(4):1335–43.
5. Enne M, Schadde E, Björnsson B, et al. ALPPS as a salvage procedure after insufficient future liver remnant hypertrophy following portal vein occlusion[J]. HPB. 2017;19(12):1126–9.
6. Eshmuminov D, Raptis DA, Linecker M, et al. Meta-analysis of associating liver partition with portal vein ligation and portal vein occlusion for two-stage hepatectomy[J]. Br J Surg. 2016;103(13):1768–82.
7. Linecker M, Kron P, Lang H, et al. Too many languages in the ALPPS: preventing another tower of babel?[J]. Ann Surg. 2016;263(5):837–8.
8. Linecker M, Stavrou GA, Oldhafer KJ, et al. The ALPPS risk score: avoiding futile use of ALPPS[J]. Ann Surg. 2016;264(5):763–71.
9. Olthof PB, Coelen RJS, Wiggers JK, et al. High mortality after ALPPS for perihilar cholangiocarcinoma: case-control analysis including the first series from the international ALPPS registry[J]. HPB. 2017;19(5):381–7.
10. Olthof PB, Huiskens J, Wicherts DA, et al. Survival after associating liver partition and portal vein ligation for staged hepatectomy (ALPPS) for advanced colorectal liver metastases: a case-matched comparison with palliative systemic therapy[J]. Surgery. 2017;161(4):909–19.
11. Schadde E, Ardiles V, Robles-Campos R, et al. Early survival and safety of ALPPS: first report of the International ALPPS Registry[J]. Ann Surg. 2014;260(5):829–83.
12. Schadde E, Raptis DA, Schnitzbauer AA, et al. Prediction of mortality after ALPPS stage 1: an analysis of 320 patients from the international ALPPS registry[J]. Ann Surg. 2015;262(5):780–5.
13. Viganò L, Cimino MM, Adam R, et al. Improving the safety of ALPPS procedure: the optimal compromise between dropout and mortality risk. Comment on schadde E et al prediction of mortality after ALPPS stage 1: an analysis of 320 patients from the international ALPPS registry[J]. Ann Surg, 2015(262): 780–786. Ann Surg. 2017;266(6):e101–2.
14. Wanis KN, Buac S, Linecker M, et al. Patient survival after simultaneous ALPPS and colorectal resection[J]. World J Surg. 2017;41(4):1119–25.
15. Wang Z, Peng YF, Hu JW, et al. Associating liver partition and portal vein ligation for staged hepatectomy for unresectable hepatitis B virus-related hepatocellular carcinoma: a single center study of 45 patients[J]. Ann Surg. 2020;271(3):534–41.
16. Hasselgren K, Røsok BI, Larsen PN, et al. ALPPS improves survival compared with TSH in patients affected of CRLM: survival analysis from the randomized controlled trial LIGRO[J]. Ann Surg. 2021;273(3):442–8.
17. Sandström P, Røsok BI, Sparrelid E, et al. ALPPS improves resectability compared with conventional two-stage hepatectomy in patients with advanced colorectal liver metastasis: results from a Scandinavian multicenter randomized controlled trial (LIGRO trial)[J]. Ann Surg. 2018;267(5):833–40.

18. Li PP, Huang G, Jia NY, et al. Associating liver partition and portal vein ligation for staged hepatectomy versus sequential transarterial chemoembolization and portal vein embolization in staged hepatectomy for HBV-related hepatocellular carcinoma: a randomized comparative study[J]. Hepatobiliary Surg Nutr. 2022;11(1):38–51.
19. Chan A, Zhang WY, Chok K, et al. ALPPS versus portal vein embolization for hepatitis-related hepatocellular carcinoma: a changing paradigm in modulation of future liver remnant before major hepatectomy[J]. Ann Surg. 2021;273(5):957–65.
20. Schadde E, Malagó M, Hernandez-Alejandro R, et al. Monosegment ALPPS hepatectomy: extending resectability by rapid hypertrophy[J]. Surgery. 2015;157(4):676–89.
21. Machado MA, Surjan R, Basseres T, et al. Total laparoscopic reversal ALPPS[J]. Ann Surg Oncol. 2017;24(4):1048–9.
22. Obed A, Jarrad A, Bashir A. First left hepatic trisectionectomy including segment one with new associated liver partition and portal vein ligation with staged hepatectomy (ALPPS) modification: how to do it?[J]. Am J Case Rep. 2016;17:759–65.
23. Sala S, Ardiles V, Ulla M, et al. Our initial experience with ALPPS technique: encouraging results[J]. Updat Surg. 2012;64(3):167–72.
24. Petrowsky H, Györi G, de Oliveira M, et al. Is partial-ALPPS safer than ALPPS? A single-center experience[J]. Ann Surg. 2015;261(4):e90–2.
25. Sakamoto Y, Matsumura M, Yamashita S, et al. Partial TIPE ALPPS for perihilar cancer[J]. Ann Surg. 2018;267(2):e18–20.
26. Gauzolino R, Castagnet M, Blanleuil ML, et al. The ALPPS technique for bilateral colorectal metastases: three "variations on a theme"[J]. Updat Surg. 2013;65(2):141–8.
27. Zattar-Ramos LC, Bezerra RO, Siqueira LT, et al. Associating liver partition and portal vein ligation for staged hepatectomy (ALPPS) in colorectal liver metastasis: the radiologist's perspective[J]. Abdom Radiol. 2016;41(11):2150–60.
28. Ji R, Zuo S, Qiu SY, et al. Combined associating liver partition and portal vein ligation for staged hepatectomy (ALPPS) followed by left trisectionectomy and Whipple operation for PNET[J]. Gland Surg. 2018;7(1):47–53.
29. Voskanyan SE, Rudakov VS, Shabalin MV, et al. "Reversal" ALPPS in patient with hepatocellular carcinoma and liver cirrhosis. First clinical case in Russia[J]. Ann HPB Surg. 2021;26(3):142–8.
30. Nadalin S, Capobianco I, Li J, et al. Indications and limits for associating liver partition and portal vein ligation for staged hepatectomy (ALPPS). Lessons Learned from 15 cases at a single centre[J]. Z Gastroenterol. 2014;52(1):35–42.
31. Alvarez FA, Ardiles V, Sanchez Claria R, et al. Associating liver partition and portal vein ligation for staged hepatectomy (ALPPS): tips and tricks[J]. J Gastrointest Surg. 2013;17(4):814–21.
32. Imamura H, Takayama T, Sugawara Y, et al. Pringle's manoeuvre in living donors[J]. Lancet. 2002;360(9350):2049–50.
33. Cheng YF, Huang TL, Lee TY, et al. Variation of the intrahepatic portal vein; angiographic demonstration and application in living-related hepatic transplantation[J]. Transplant Proc. 1996;28(3):1667–8.
34. Nakamura T, Tanaka K, Kiuchi T, et al. Anatomical variations and surgical strategies in right lobe living donor liver transplantation: lessons from 120 cases[J]. Transplantation. 2002;73(12):1896–903.
35. Alexandrescu S, Stoica L, Grigorie R, et al. Primary hepatic lymphoma resected by ALPPS procedure (associating liver partition and portal vein ligation for staged hepatectomy)[J]. J Transl Med Res. 2016;21(2):153.

TAE-Salvaged ALPPS (Zhou's ALPPS)

15

Jian Zhou and Yuanfei Peng

15.1 Introduction

Associating liver partition and portal vein ligation for staged hepatectomy (ALPPS) is a great innovation in hepatic surgery, providing short-term curative resection opportunities for patients with previously unresectable liver tumors [1, 2]. Despite existing controversy, ALPPS has been increasingly applied in hepatic surgery in recent years, extending to hepatocellular carcinoma (HCC) with chronic liver disease [3–8]. In China, HCC is a major indication, and the experience of ALPPS in this patient population mainly comes from China's contribution [4, 9–14]. In recent years, with reports from large Chinese liver cancer centers and evidence generated by clinical studies, including randomized controlled trials (RCT), the effectiveness of ALPPS for HCC has been elucidated [4, 10–14]. According to China's practical experience, in highly selective patients, ALPPS enables optimal clinical outcomes. The overall safety profile has been significantly improved compared to early years, with satisfactory tumor resection and R0 resection rates. Mid/long-term survival benefits are reassuring, better than nonsurgical treatments such as transarterial chemoembolization (TACE), equivalent to the postoperative survival of those undergoing one-stage hepatectomy, and superior or non-inferior to traditional two-stage hepatectomy (TSH), including portal vein embolization (PVE)-TSH and TACE-PVE-TSH [4, 10–14]. For HCC patients with no or mild chronic liver disease, ALPPS can effectively induce future liver remnant (FLR) hypertrophy, and its effectiveness and safety are comparable to those of colorectal cancer liver metastasis (CRLM) and other tumors. However, the application of ALPPS for severe liver fibrosis or cirrhosis remains challenging. Studies have shown that FLR growth is negatively correlated with the severity of liver fibrosis/cirrhosis [3, 4, 10, 11]. The more severe the fibrosis/cirrhosis, the less potent the FLR induction. These patient populations often have limited FLR regeneration, predisposing them to ALPPS failure. Data reported by the International ALPPS Registry (35 HCC cases) showcased that the FLR kinetic growth ratios (KGR) in patients with cirrhosis and METAVIR grade 3 liver fibrosis were only (1.52 ± 0.40) mL/d and (2.98 ± 0.65) mL/d, respectively. In contrast, those in patients without fibrosis/cirrhosis and those with METAVIR grade 1 liver fibrosis were (30.94 ± 10.95) mL/d and (12.34 ± 4.38) mL/d, respectively [3]. Report from Zhongshan Hospital, Fudan University (45 HCC cases) also revealed that the median FLR KGR of patients with cirrhosis (METAVIR grade 4) and METAVIR grade 3 liver fibrosis were 9.6 mL/d and 19.8 mL/d, respectively. In comparison, patients with normal liver parenchyma (METAVIR grade 0) had a KGR of 50.1 mL/d [4]. Furthermore, it was found that the KGR of these patients in the second week after stage 1 ALPPS was usually significantly lower than that in the first week postoperatively. Due to limited FLR hypertrophy, the time required for liver regeneration in these patients was significantly longer than that in cases with normal livers (14 days vs. 7 days) [4]. A longer interstage interval is associated with tumor progression. Furthermore, the change of portal vein-arterial blood supply led by portal vein ligation (PVL) also exerts oncological effects. There is a compensatory increase in hepatic artery perfusion after PVL, and the tumor may grow with the increase in arterial blood supply [15–17]. This is more common when ALPPS is used to treat HCC (mostly large HCC). These factors often lead to a higher incidence of surgical failure or post-hepatectomy liver failure (PHLF) when ALPPS is used in this population. In the authors' center, before the emergence of the new transarterial embolization salvaged ALPPS (TAE-salvaged ALPPS), two HCC patients failed to achieve sufficient FLR hypertrophy 3–4 weeks after stage 1 ALPPS and were unable to undergo the stage 2 surgery, thus being converted to other treatments; another HCC patient directly developed PHLF after stage 1 ALPPS [4]. In China, HCC patients are often

J. Zhou (✉) · Y. Peng
Zhongshan Hospital, Fudan University, Shanghai, China
e-mail: zhou.jian@zs-hospital.sh.cn

J. Zhou (ed.), *Associating Liver Partition and Portal Vein Ligation for Staged Hepatectomy (ALPPS)*,
https://doi.org/10.1007/978-981-96-7364-3_15

complicated by chronic liver diseases such as liver fibrosis and cirrhosis. The implementation of ALPPS in patients with cirrhosis or severe fibrosis remains challenging, and appropriate solutions are urgently needed.

The TAE-salvaged ALPPS (Zhou's ALPPS, Fig. 15.1) created by the authors' team is expected to address the above problems [18, 19]. In 2017, a patient with huge HCC and severe liver fibrosis underwent ALPPS. Insufficient FLR growth occurred after the first-stage surgery, and the tumor progressed during the interstage interval. Imaging examination revealed FLR arterial steal (mainstream inflow of arterial blood into the huge tumor on the right side), which was confirmed by digital subtraction angiography (DSA). The patient immediately underwent TAE, embolizing the feeding vessels to control tumor progression and improve the arterial blood supply of the FLR [18]. One week after TAE, it was unexpectedly observed that in addition to effective control over tumor progression, FLR hypertrophy was reactivated and rapidly grew to the volume required for stage 2 surgery. The ALPPS was salvaged from failure, and the tumor was successfully resected [18]. After the success of the first case, this new ALPPS procedure was applied to nine other patients with similar conditions, and all triumphed. Based on this, the authors established a novel ALPPS variant that can efficiently induce FLR growth in patients with chronic liver disease: TAE-salvaged ALPPS [18]. In 2022, the authors reviewed and reported their successful experiences of these ten cases [19]. The median age of the patients was 56 years (43–66 years). Among them, nine had a single tumor (median diameter 14.0 cm), and one had multiple tumors (one major lesion with a diameter of 14.0 cm and two satellite foci of 2.0 cm and 3.0 cm in diameter, respectively). Six patients were pathologically diagnosed with cirrhosis (METAVIR grade 4), one with METAVIR grade 3 fibrosis, and three with METAVIR grade 2 fibrosis. Preoperative liver stiffness measurement by transient elastography was 13.2 (5.1–16.4) kpa. All patients (100%) achieved R0 resection. The preoperative FLR/standard liver volume (SLV) of these 10 patients was 24.5% (19.7%–36.3%), with an FLR volume of 306.9 mL (236.6–467.0 mL). A rapid FLR increase was observed during the first postoperative week after stage 1 ALPPS. Nonetheless, in the second week, the FLR hypertrophy was significantly attenuated (KGR at week 1 and 2 after stage 1 ALPPS were 15.7 mL/d and 2.6 mL/d, respectively) (Fig. 15.2). None of these patients had adequate FLR hypertrophy at postoperative week 2 (POW2) after the first stage. Meanwhile, an increase in tumor size was observed in eight patients (80%) from 800.5 mL preoperatively to 832.6 mL at POW2. Six of the eight alpha-fetoprotein (AFP)-positive patients had complete postoperative AFP follow-up data. All of them showed an increase after the stage 1 ALPPS at a median of postoperative day 10 (8–13 days). Elevated levels of AFP and increasing tumor size indicate tumor progression that could be detected within approximately 2 weeks after stage 1 ALPPS. After TAE of feeding arteries, the FLR volume increased significantly (absolute and relative KGR after TAE were 19.5 mL/d and 4.1%, respectively). The FLR rapidly increased to the desired volume required for stage 2 surgery, and all these patients subsequently underwent the stage 2 operation successfully. Besides, AFP levels were significantly reduced after TAE. The interstage interval was 21 days (18–24 days), and the increase in FLR was 69.7% (34.4%–143.9%). The absolute and relative KGR were 9.9 mL/d (7.1–17.3 mL/d) and 3.4% (1.9%–7.2%), respectively. TAE

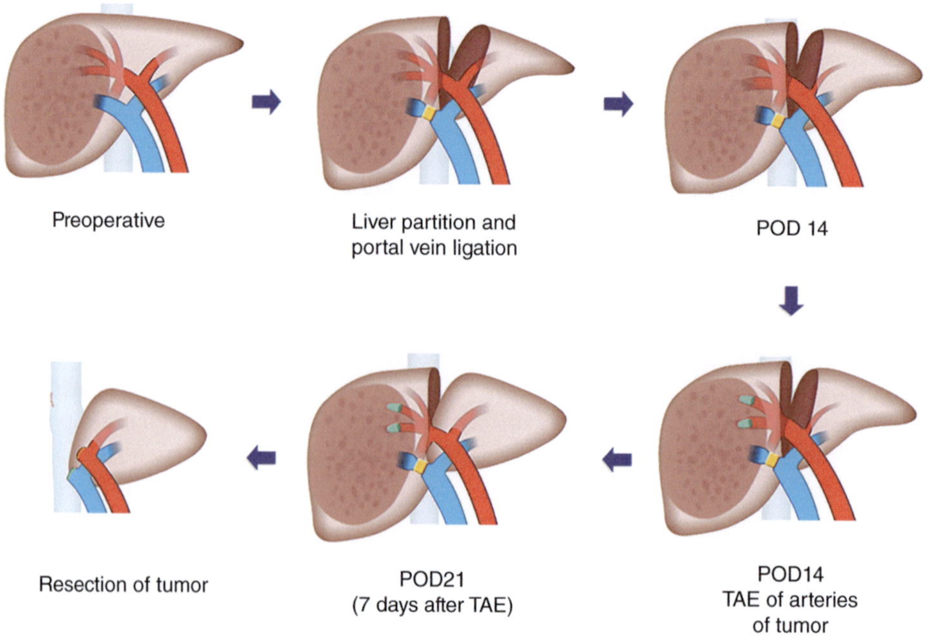

Fig. 15.1 Schematic diagram of TAE-salvaged ALPPS [19]. The TAE-salvaged ALPPS procedure comprises the conventional stage 1 ALPPS (liver partition and portal vein ligation), transcatheter arterial embolization (TAE) of arteries supplying the tumor at 2 weeks after stage 1 ALPPS, and conventional stage 2 ALPPS (resection of tumor)

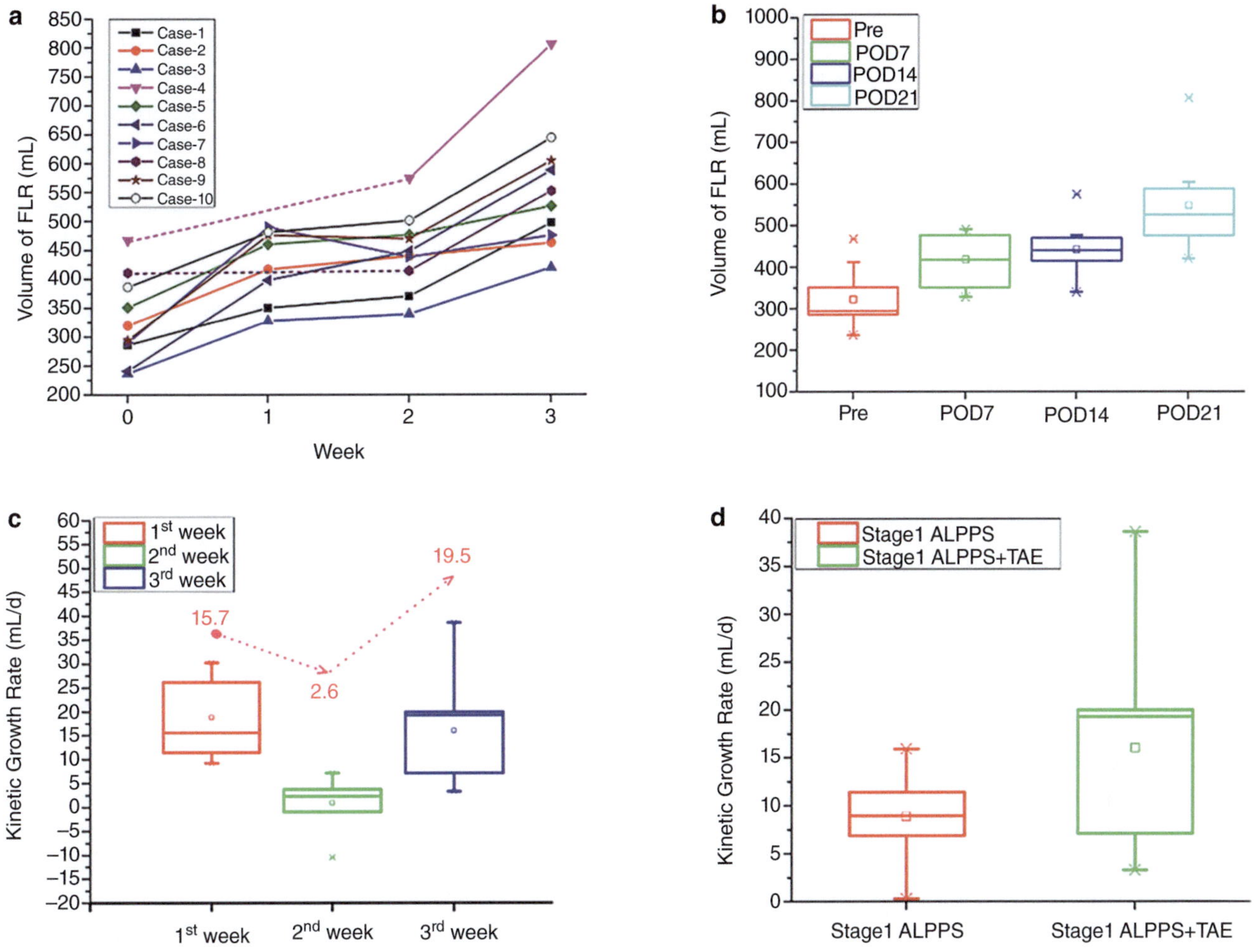

Fig. 15.2 FLR increase after TAE-salvaged ALPPS (This figure is reprinted with permission from the source of [19]). (**a**) Individual FLR hypertrophy in the ten patients who received TAE-salvaged ALPPS; (**b**) The median FLR volumes before operation and on postoperative days 7, 14, and 21 after the stage 1 ALPPS were 306.9 mL, 438.5 mL, 443.7 mL, and 539.1 mL, respectively; (**c**) The median KGR of FLR was 15.7 mL/d, 2.6 mL/d, and 19.5 mL/d at postoperative weeks 1, 2, and 3 after the first stage, respectively. The FLR growth weakened in the second week after stage 1 ALPPS but was revoked after TAE; (**d**) The median KGR after ALPPS stage 1 (1st + 2nd week) and ALPPS stage 1 + TAE (3rd week) were 8.9 and 19.5 mL/d, respectively

prominently accelerated FLR regeneration: the absolute and relative KGR after TAE were 19.5 mL/d and 3.2%, while those before TAE were 8.9 mL/d and 1.9%, respectively (Fig. 15.2). The safety of TAE-salvaged ALPPS is equivalent to that of conventional ALPPS. After stage 1 operation, TAE, and stage 2 operation, the overall complication rates were 50% (5/10), 20% (2/10), and 70% (7/10), respectively, with a 90-day mortality of 10% (1/10). Most patients recovered uneventfully. There were 26 postoperative complication (POC) events (7, 4, and 15 events after stage 1, TAE, and stage 2, respectively), of which one patient claimed 8 POC events. Among them, Clavien-Dindo grade I and II POCs were common, while severe ones (>grade IIIa) were uncommon (none occurred after stage 1 ALPPS and TAE, and only 1 event after the second stage). PHLF did not require special treatment in most patients. According to the definition and grading system of the International Study Group of Liver Surgery (ISGLS), two patients (20%) developed grade A PHLF after stage 1 ALPPS, and another one (10%) after TAE. This complication was more common after stage 2 ALPPS, where five patients (50%) were complicated with grade A and 2 (20%) with grade B PHLF. All these patients recovered well with conservative treatment and did not require special medications. One patient (10%) suffered from severe oncolytic syndrome and renal function insufficiency after the first stage, progressing into multiorgan dysfunction, and unfortunately died after the second stage. Oncolysis was not observed in the rest of the cohort. Relative to classical ALPPS, especially when performed in patients with HCC and liver fibrosis/cirrhosis, TAE-salvaged ALPPS exemplified similar or lower morbidity and mortality [3, 4, 11, 13, 20] and encouraging survival benefits. The median overall survival (OS) reached 40 months (median follow-up 24.1 months), comparable to large tumors treated by one-stage resection [21, 22]. The authors' research demonstrated that TAE-salvaged ALPPS achieved a 100% R0 resection rate in HCC patients with severe fibrosis/cirrhosis. Before this novel modification, 16 patients with cirrhosis underwent ALPPS in the authors' center, four of whom failed to complete the stage 2 ALPPS, and the tumor resection rate was only 75% (12/16). New TAE-salvaged ALPPS enables a perfect R0 resection rate.

TAE-salvaged ALPPS is indicated for HCC patients with severe fibrosis or cirrhosis who are scheduled to undergo ALPPS but fail to induce sufficient FLR hypertrophy after conventional stage 1 ALPPS. The hepatic surgery team of Zhongshan Hospital, Fudan University, has developed an algorithm for ALPPS in this patient population (Fig. 15.3). TAE-salvaged ALPPS can not only induce satisfactory FLR growth but also control tumor progression. The underlying mechanism of action remains unclear, possibly related to the improvement of arterial blood supply to FLR, which is critical for liver regeneration. Studies on patients with small liver syndrome after liver transplantation have shown that poor hepatic artery flow can lead to functional de-arterialization and liver parenchymal infarction, and ligation of the FLR artery during partial hepatectomy can also cause the failure of FLR hypertrophy [23, 24]. The hepatic arterial buffer response (HABR) played an important role in regulating FLR hepatic artery blood flow, and ligation of the right portal vein was correlated with HABR-induced dilation of the right hepatic artery [24]. Studies have showcased that the compensatory increase in arterial flow after PVE or PVL facilitated disease progression [25, 26]. Nagino et al. [27] reported an increase in the arterial blood flow of the embolized liver segment immediately after PVE. Multiple studies validated that in living donor liver transplantation, when all portal blood flows through the "small liver graft," the pressure accumulated in the portal vein may block the hepatic arterial flow, causing liver "de-arterialization" [23, 24]. Therefore, the HABR effect caused by tumor "arterial blood steal" and right PVL may engender a reduction in the arterial blood supply to the FLR, ultimately hindering its growth. Analysis of the FLR arteries showed that the cross-sectional area ratios (left vs right hepatic arteries) before the operation, 2 weeks after ALPPS stage 1, and 2 week after TAE were 27.16% (12.81%–172.98%), 13.37% (7.44%–55.15%), and 22.41% (13.22%–50.36%), respectively. These findings indicate that TAE significantly improves the arterial blood supply to the FLR, eliminates tumor blood "steal," and reduces the negative impact of HABR.

In summary, TAE-salvaged ALPPS permits rapid FLR hypertrophy and controls tumor progression to a certain extent. It did not significantly increase operative morbidity and mortality rates compared to classical ALPPS. It can be used as a new strategy to enhance the resectability of HCC patients with cirrhosis or severe liver fibrosis, since these populations are prone to inadequate FLR growth after the conventional stage 1 ALPPS.

First, conventional stage 1 ALPPS (liver partition and PVL) is performed to induce FLR hypertrophy. Two weeks later, if FLR growth is insufficient, TAE of arteries supplying the tumor is performed to further induce FLR growth and finally followed by tumor resection, and the procedure is called TAE-salvaged ALPPS; if the FLR increases sufficiently, the conventional stage 2 ALPPS is directly performed to remove the tumor.

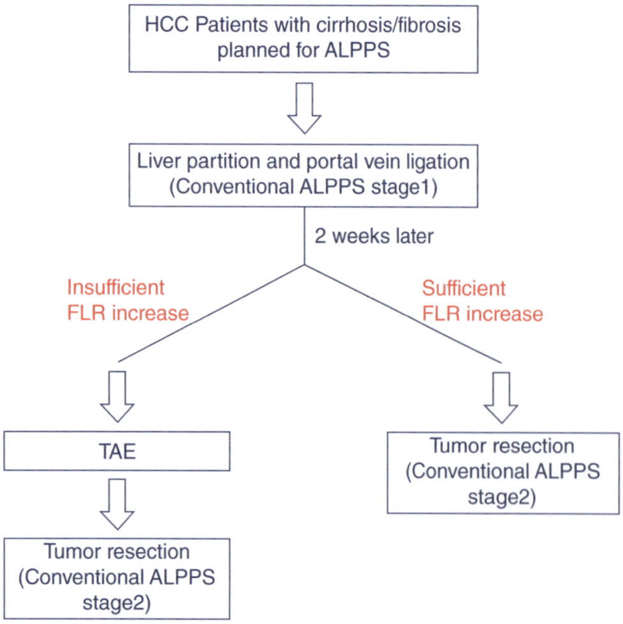

Fig. 15.3 Algorithm of ALPPS for HCC patients with severe liver fibrosis or cirrhosis. (This figure is reprinted with permission from the source of [19])

15.2 Indications

TAE-salvaged ALPPS can be performed in HCC patients with insufficient FLR hypertrophy two weeks after conventional stage 1 ALPPS (Fig. 15.3). Its indications are the same as conventional ALPPS in HCC cases with chronic liver disease: age < 67 years [28], potentially resectable but with inadequate FLR (FLR/SLV < 40%), no extrahepatic metastasis, normal or mildly injured but reversible liver function, Child-Pugh class A, indocyanine green retention rate at 15 min (ICG-R15) <20%, and patients in sound general condition with normal functions in the heart, brain, lungs, kidneys, and other organs, capable of tolerating major operations. Those who have received interventional therapy and/or medication management (such as targeted therapy combined with immunotherapy) before surgery are still applicable and are not contraindicated. Severe cirrhotic cases whose FLR/SLV is too low should undergo surgery with caution [13, 20]. Patients with severe portal hypertension are ineligible.

15.3 Surgical Procedures

TAE-salvaged ALPPS consists of three steps (Fig. 15.1): stage 1 ALPPS (liver parenchyma partition + PVL), TAE (tumor-feeding artery embolization), and stage 2 ALPPS (tumor resection). The surgical approaches of stage 1 and stage 2 operations are the same as those of conventional ALPPS. It can be completed through laparotomy, laparoscopy, or robot-assisted surgery, which is decided by the surgeon in a personalized manner. The following surgical procedures are the operating steps of TAE-salvaged ALPPS based on its classical counterpart.

15.3.1 Body Position

The patient is usually in a supine position. If the transection plane is to the right, the patient can also lie on the left side at 30°.

15.3.2 Stage 1 ALPPS

15.3.2.1 Surgical Incision

The right subcostal incision is usually used (Fig. 15.4a). In cases with massive tumors, or the porta hepatis is involved by a tumor, or when regional lymphadenectomy is required simultaneously, a reverse "L"-shaped incision may be used (Fig. 15.4b).

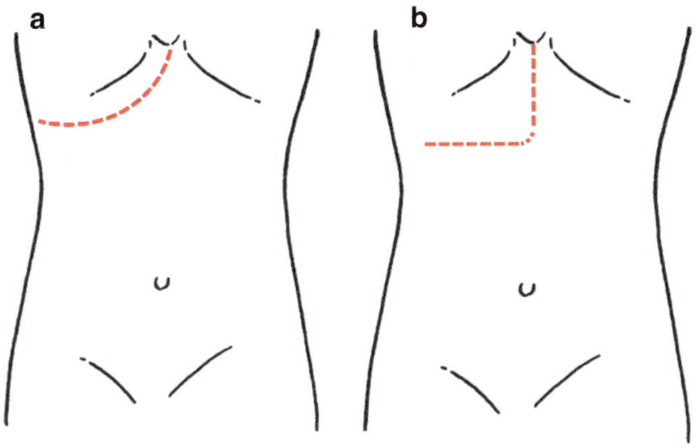

Fig. 15.4 Surgical incisions. (**a**) A right subcostal incision is commonly used. (**b**) A reverse "L"-shaped incision (also called "J"-shaped incision) can also be used when necessary

15.3.2.2 Abdominal Exploration and Liver Biopsy

After access into the abdomen, the abdominal cavity is exposed by placing a liver retractor. Full exploration is performed to exclude any extrahepatic lesions not detected by preoperative imaging and eliminate other surgical contraindications. Liver parenchyma in FLR is sampled for pathological examination to determine the degree of liver fibrosis, cirrhosis, and other parenchymal damage.

15.3.2.3 Right Liver Mobilization

The round ligament (ligament teres) and falciform ligament are divided. The hepatic vein fossa is exposed and marked. The right triangular ligament, the right coronary ligament, and the hepatorenal ligament are divided. Then, the right liver is rotated to the left, the bare area and the right adrenal gland are dissociated, and the right IVC ligament and the short hepatic vein are divided. The right liver is fully mobilized. For giant tumors where liver mobilization is not feasible or inappropriate, the anterior approach ALPPS can also be performed.

15.3.2.4 Intraoperative Ultrasound (IOUS)

The liver is comprehensively examined using intraoperative ultrasound to confirm preoperatively diagnosed lesions and check for any other lesions, especially whether there are preoperatively undetected lesions in the FLR. The adjacent relationship among the tumor, FLR, and major vessels is explored and clarified. In combination with preoperative virtual surgical planning, the pre-cut line is delineated on the liver surface, and the liver parenchymal transection plane is determined.

15.3.2.5 Cholecystectomy

The Calot's triangle is dissected; the cystic duct and the cystic artery are exposed, ligated, and divided; and then the gallbladder is removed. If antegrade cholecystectomy is not feasible, the gallbladder can also be resected retrogradely. The cystic duct is divided close to the gallbladder side, and a certain length is reserved at the stump. After parenchymal partition, the cutting surface is strictly checked to exclude bile leakage by injecting a contrast agent or a color-developing agent, such as diluted fat emulsion or methylene blue, through the cystic duct. Anatomical variation of the bile duct is common. If variation of the bile duct is suspected before surgery but is not clearly shown by MRI and/or other examinations, a contrast agent can be injected from the cystic duct for cholangiography. The ICG-based fluorescence technique can serve as another option for observing the variation.

15.3.2.6 Porta Hepatis Dissection

Dividing the arteries first and then the portal vein should be executed rigorously. The proper hepatic artery and the branches of the left (middle) and right hepatic arteries, the

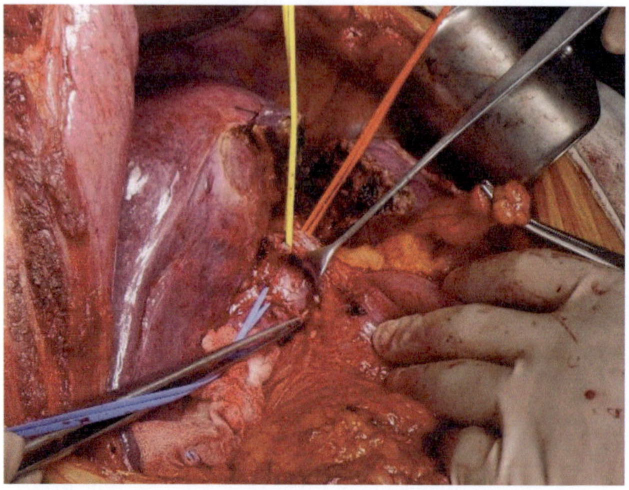

Fig. 15.5 Dissect the porta hepatis, separate the proper hepatic artery and its left and right branches, the left and right branches of the portal vein, and the common bile duct

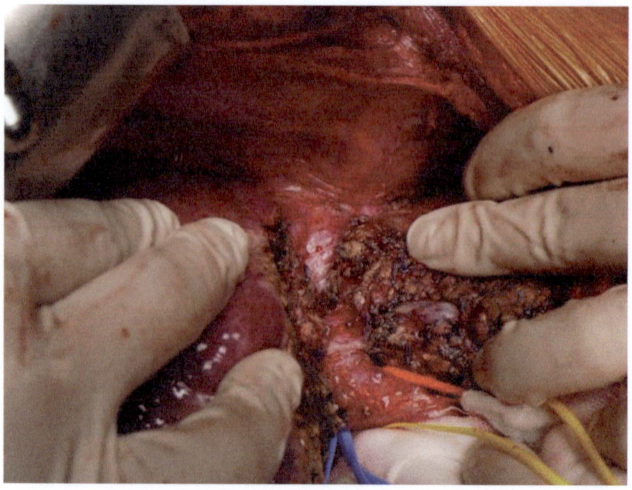

Fig. 15.6 The liver parenchyma is partitioned completely to the anterior wall of the IVC

left and right branches of the portal vein, and the common bile duct are separated, respectively. The right branch of the portal vein, the common bile duct, and the right hepatic artery are marked with blue, yellow, and red ribbons, respectively (Fig. 15.5). Arteries must be strictly protected regardless of the FLR side or the tumor side. High-power energy equipment should be avoided to prevent arterial damage when isolating these vessels. During division, special attention should be paid to the anatomic variations of the hepatic artery, and the diameter of the left and right hepatic arteries should be compared and observed. If the left hepatic artery is thin and the liver tumor is huge, it is necessary to be prepared for TAE-salvaged ALPPS.

15.3.2.7 Parenchymal Partition

A complete, rather than partial, parenchymal partition is needed. Studies have demonstrated that classical ALPPS with a complete partition (complete ALPPS) yields better FLR growth than ALPPS with a partial partition (partial ALPPS) for patients with chronic liver disease. Albert Chan et al. [29] compared ALPPS with complete and partial partition. Results showcased that for HCC patients with chronic liver disease, compared with the partial partition group, FLR grew faster and more significant in the complete partition group (64.1%/7 days vs. 43.1%/10.5 days), with lower incidence of severe complication (7.7% vs. 25%) and 90-day mortality (0% vs. 16.7%). The authors concluded that complete partition ALPPS induced FLR hypertrophy more significantly than its partial partition counterpart, with a shorter interstage interval, faster liver function recovery after stage 2, and lower complications and mortality. For HCC with chronic liver disease, it should be the first choice to achieve optimal results [29]. Consistent results were shown by our center. For all HCC cases complicated with chronic liver diseases, classical ALPPS with complete partition was performed, generating satisfactory FLR hypertrophy, high tumor resection rates, and low incidence of severe complication and mortality after surgery. Hence, intraoperative complete division to the anterior wall of the IVC is essential. If the tumor is adjacent to the IVC, rendering the complete partition not feasible, at least 80% shall be divided (Fig. 15.6). Methods of parenchyma partition may vary per personal habits. Usually, Cavitron ultrasonic surgical aspirator (CUSA) and bipolar electrocoagulation devices are used for finely parenchymal division. The Glisson branches, hepatic vein branches, and other vessels encountered during the transection are coagulated, ligated, or clamped with titanium clip. Strict hemostasis is required during this process. Ultrasonic dissector can also be applied for the parenchymal transection. During the operation, the central vein pressure (CVP) shall be controlled at a low level to reduce bleeding. If the CVP is not well controlled by fluid restriction and medication, adjusting the body to a reverse Trendelenburg position and/or clamping the lower IVC can be applied to further reduce its level. In case of severe bleeding, block the inflow to the liver. Generally, the Pringle maneuver is used for intermittent hepatic occlusion (clamp for 15 min, release for 5 min, and repeat this). This maneuver can be safely and routinely performed in ALPPS as used in living donor liver transplantation [30]. Selective inflow occlusion is an alternative. Belghiti's hanging maneuver and other techniques can assist the partition, generating a better safety profile.

15.3.2.8 Ligation of the Tumor-Bearing Side Portal Veins

After liver partition, the portal vein branches on the tumor side are ligated with 4-0 polypropylene suture or double silk sutures. The suture is kept with a long end as mark to facilitate the identification during stage 2 ALPPS operation. An alternative is dividing the portal vein and suturing the stump with polypropylene suture during stage 1 ALPPS surgery. The PVL should be reliable and thorough since an incomplete ligation causes residual perfusion into the tumor side, leading to failure of FLR induction. It is recommended to use double ligation. During laparoscopy, a Hem-o-lok clip rather than titanium clip is used, with the tip crossing the contralateral wall of the portal vein to ensure complete and reliable clamping. Ligation or stitching with suture under the laparoscopic view is another option. Pay attention to the anatomic variations of the portal vein. In case of portal vein variation, all of the branches on the tumor side must be ligated. An accidental omission often engenders inadequate FLR growth, where timely PVE of the omitted portal vein is required. After PVL, mark portal tracts with colored strings (the right branch of the portal vein, the common bile duct, and the right hepatic artery) to facilitate identification in the stage 2 operation.

15.3.2.9 Bile Leakage Check

After liver parenchymal partition, the transection surface is checked for bile leakage. The transection of segment IV due to complete partition is potentially correlated with a relatively high incidence of postoperative bile leakage. Therefore, it is recommended that bile leakage checking is strictly performed. If, judged by the surgeon, the vessels are handled accurately and reliably during liver partition and bile leakage is not expected to occur, this step can be skipped. In our center, we use fat emulsion injection to check for bile leakage. The steps are as follows: open the cystic duct, clamp the common bile duct below it, use an indwelling needle to inject normal saline diluted fat emulsion from the cystic duct orifice into the bile duct, and check the existence of bile leakage on the transection surface. In case of bile leakage, the white fat emulsion, gushing out from the leakage point, could be easily spotted. After the testing, the cystic duct is sutured.

15.3.2.10 Management of the Transection Surface

The transection surface is covered with fibrin and absorbable hemostatic gauze to guarantee satisfactory hemostasis and separation. In spite of a 3-week interstage interval, the adhesion is often not serious during stage 2 operation, and it is easy to separate the FLR side from the tumor side.

15.3.2.11 Drainage Insertion

A drain tube (usually Jackson-Pratt drain) is placed on the transection surface. If necessary, another drainage tube can be placed under the right diaphragm.

15.3.2.12 Coating with Anti-adhesion Materials

Coating with anti-adhesion materials is recommended to routinely use to relieve abdominal adhesions and facilitate the stage 2 surgery. The authors' center usually applies chitosan around the liver.

15.3.2.13 Close the Abdomen

The abdomen is closed using absorbable sutures layer by layer. In particular, the peritoneal layer must be well closed to ensure the smoothness of the inferior lining and reduce postoperative adhesions. If laparoscopic ALPPS is performed, the fascia of port site needs to be closed with reliable methods such as fascial closure devices and laparoscopic inversion sutures. Some patients produce a large amount of ascites after the first stage of ALPPS. Closing the port site can prevent ascites from leaking via these sites when abdominal drainage is poor.

15.3.3 FLR Volume Remeasurement and Tumor Progression Monitoring After Stage 1 Surgery

The FLR volume is measured once a week after the stage 1 ALPPS and changes in tumor markers are monitored. CT angiography (CTA) with 3D reconstruction is recommended for better reassessment and comparison of the left and right hepatic arteries. If the FLR fails to achieve the desired volume 2 weeks after stage 1 ALPPS, TAE is required to embolize tumor-feeding arteries. If the FLR hypertrophy is significantly attenuated, unable to obtain sufficient growth at the established time, or/and tumor progression is observed at the same time, TAE shall be applied at an appropriate time, not necessarily at POW2. The principle is to control tumor progression and promote FLR growth.

15.3.4 TAE

TAE is performed to embolize arteries supplying the tumor. A 4F RH catheter is inserted into the femoral artery using the Seldinger technique and accesses the hepatic artery superselectively. Hepatic arteriography is performed before pushing the tip of the guiding catheter to the tumor-feeding artery

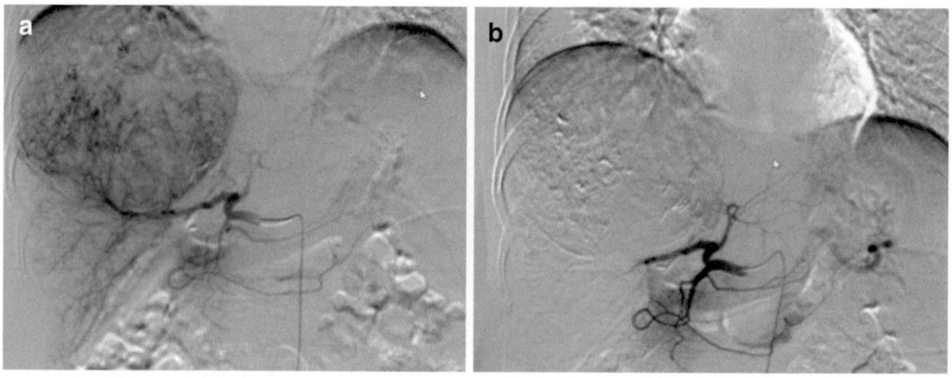

Fig. 15.7 Insufficient FLR growth 2 weeks after stage 1 ALPPS and TAE was performed to embolize tumor-feeding arteries. (**a**) Before TAE. (**b**) After TAE

for selective embolization (Fig. 15.7). Guided by angiography, appropriate amounts of lipiodol, microsphere, and gelatin sponge are injected for thorough embolization of the feeding arteries.

15.3.5 FLR Volume Remeasurement after TAE

The FLR volume is reassessed 1 week after TAE with 3D reconstruction to enable accurate volume calculation (Fig. 15.8). The stage 2 ALPPS proceed when an adequate FLR hypertrophy is achieved.

15.3.6 Stage 2 ALPPS

15.3.6.1 Access the Abdomen Via the Original Incision

There is usually a certain degree of adhesions and local congestion and edema in the abdominal cavity after the first stage surgery. When entering the abdomen, care must be taken to avoid damage to the gastrointestinal tract under the incision.

15.3.6.2 Adhesions Lysis

Stage 1 ALPPS (liver parenchymal partition + PVL) plus TAE and tumor necrosis render the intra-abdominal inflammatory reaction more severe than a conventional stage 1 ALPPS alone, resulting in more serious abdominal adhesions. However, when anti-adhesion measures are in place, adhesion lysis is not difficult in most cases. After adhesion lysis, the FLR is explored, and the transection surface and portal tracts are exposed. Due to inflammatory reactions after TAE, the arteries should be dissected cautiously.

15.3.6.3 IOUS Reassessment of FLR

Since the interstage interval is longer than that of conventional ALPPS (3 weeks vs. 1–2 weeks), tumor progression may occur during this period. Examination is required to completely rule out possible lesions in the FLR.

15.3.6.4 Division of the Right Hepatic Artery, the Right Portal Vein, and the Right Bile Duct

Be careful when ligating arteries. The intima may be damaged, sometimes inflamed, and swollen after TAE. When ligating, protect the intima to prevent laceration-induced entrapment of the artery. The authors adopt the double ligation method, where the proximal end is ligated with appropriate strength (only closing the inner lumen of the arteries), and the distal end is routinely ligated. There are many anatomic variations in the biliary tract, and its dissection is usually performed at the end, after which a biliary tract probe is introduced in to confirm that the biliary tract of the FLR is intact and unobstructed. If the parenchyma is not completely transected during the first stage of surgery, continue to separate the residual FLR parenchyma and the right junction between the parenchyma and the IVC. During stage 2 ALPPS, due to the inflammation, congestion, and edema caused by the first stage, the liver parenchyma becomes brittle and prone to bleeding. The blood loss is often significantly greater than that during the first stage of surgery. If necessary, the Pringle maneuver or clamping the portal vein trunk with Bulldog can be used to control bleeding. The hepatic vein is exposed and divided. The stumps are sutured continuously with a 4–0 polypropylene suture. Alternatively, a linear cutting stapler can be applied directly, making the procedure faster.

15.3.6.5 Tumor Removal

If the stage 1 ALPPS is performed via an anterior approach, perihepatic ligaments on the tumor side need to be mobilized, and finally, the tumor is removed.

15.3.6.6 Hemostasis and Bile Leakage Check

The authors' center applies fat emulsion injection for bile leakage check as follows: clamp the common bile duct, use an indwelling needle to inject diluted fat emulsion from the stump orifice of the right hepatic duct into the FLR bile duct and check the existence of bile leakage in the transection surface. After confirming that there is no leakage, the right bile duct is closed with suturing (Fig. 15.9).

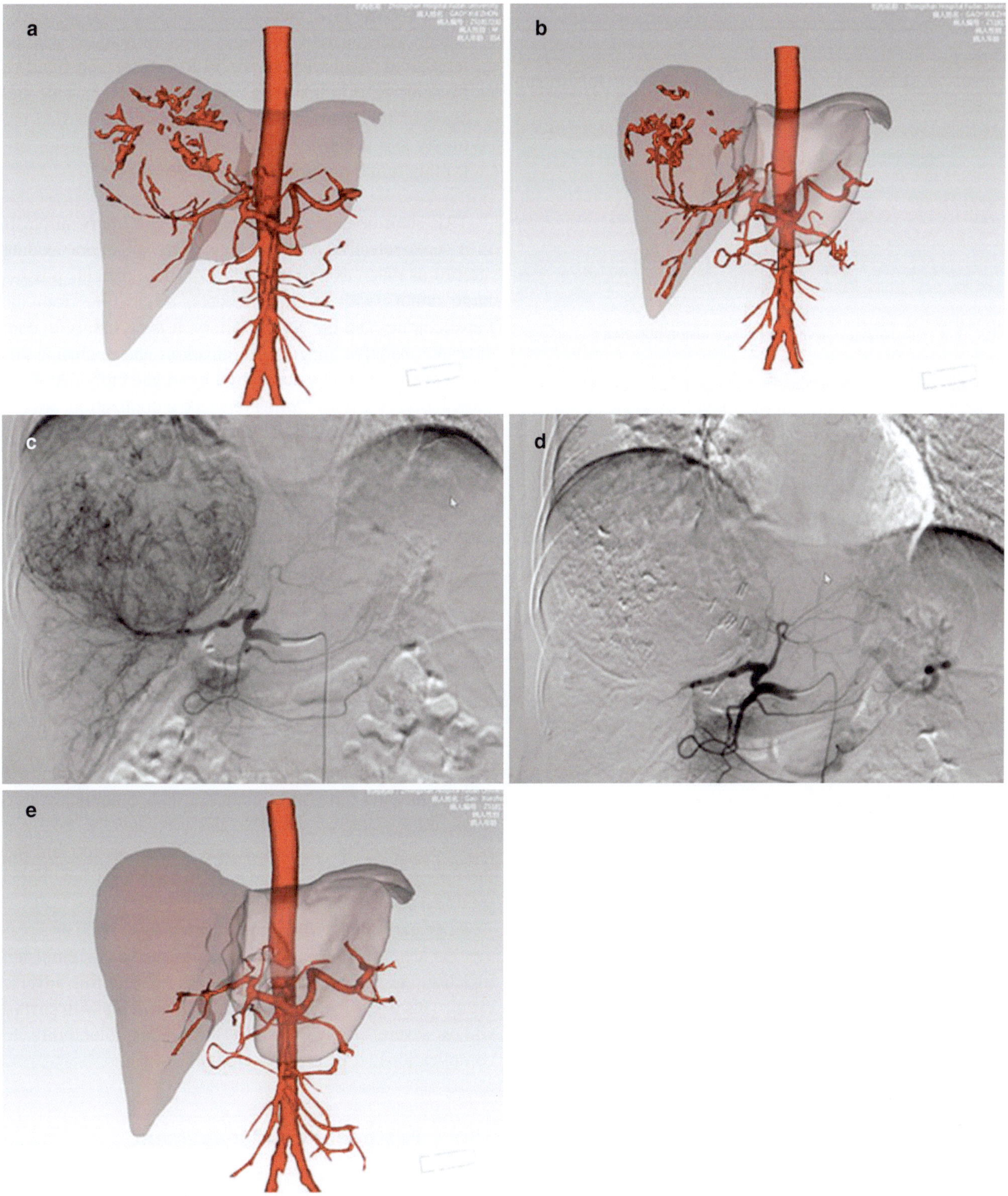

Fig. 15.8 FLR volume remeasurement after stage 1 ALPPS. (**a**) Before stage 1 ALPPS. (**b**) One week after stage 1 ALPPS. (**c**) TAE is performed 2 weeks after stage 1 ALPPS. (**d**) Tumor-feeding arteries are embolized after TAE; (**e**) One week after TAE

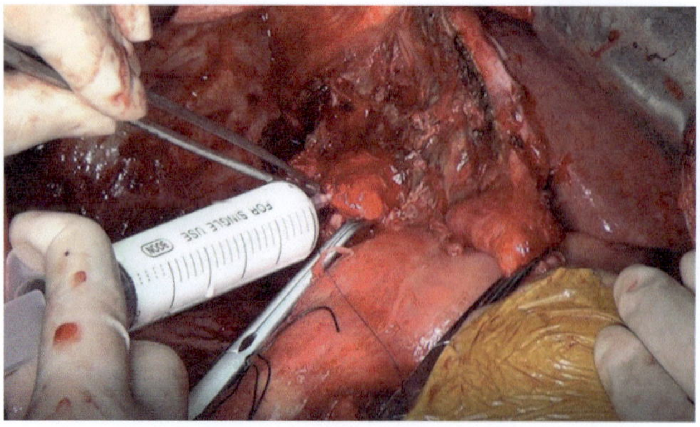

Fig. 15.9 Bile leakage check using fat emulsion injection

Clamp the common bile duct using a Satinsky clamp, and inject fat emulsion from the right bile duct to check for bile leakage in the transection surface.

15.3.6.7 Treatment of the Transection Surface

The liver transection surface is sprayed with fibrin and covered with absorbable hemostatic gauze.

15.3.6.8 Drainage

A drain tube (usually Jackson-Pratt drain) is placed on the transection surface.

15.3.6.9 Closing the Falciform Ligament

The falciform ligament is sutured, and the left FLR is fixed to prevent it from twisting around the left hepatic vein.

15.3.6.10 Closing the Abdomen

The abdominal cavity is closed layer by layer using continuous absorbable sutures.

15.4 Pearls and Pitfalls

The pearls and pitfalls of TAE-salvaged ALPPS are similar to those in conventional ALPPS, but it has its own characteristics, which are described below.

Stage 1 ALPPS: During this stage, complete partition needs to be done in patients with severe liver fibrosis or cirrhosis. Unlike patients with a healthy liver, patients with chronic hepatitis, liver fibrosis, and cirrhosis are not suitable for partial ALPPS (see Chap. 9, Partial ALPPS), which may lead to insufficient FLR hypertrophy. For this population, complete partition can maximize FLR growth and reduce morbidity and mortality [29]. Therefore, during the first stage, parenchyma between the FLR and the tumor needs to be thoroughly partitioned to the anterior wall of the IVC, as long as the conditions are allowed.

Timing of TAE: FLR volume shall be measured regularly, whereas postoperative changes in tumor markers shall be monitored. According to the FLR volume and trend of FLR increase (whether it is limited or attenuated) and signs of tumor progression, TAE should be carried out timely and decisively to revoke FLR growth while controlling tumor progression.

TAE shall be performed by experienced interventionists in a super-selective manner to embolize all tumor-feeding arteries as much as possible. Most of these patients possess large tumors with multiple feeders, originating from the hepatic artery and the phrenic artery. It is necessary to consider preoperative imaging examinations and to change different angles in the angiography to find and embolize all of these blood suppliers. During repeated embolization, arterial damage shall be prevented. Should it occur after TAE, the function of the auxiliary liver would be compromised, bringing about serious adverse events such as liver failure.

In principle, the stage 2 ALPPS shall be performed as soon as possible since the combination of PVL and TAE produces severe or even complete ischemia of the tumor. Necrosis is usually severe in large tumors (more so when complicated with infection). The FLR volume is remeasured 1 week after TAE. If desirable, resection could proceed. In case of severe necrosis and oncolysis or with an almost sufficient FLR before TAE, volume reassessment and tumor resection can be performed in advance after integrated evaluation.

Pay special attention to hepatic artery status, including the ratio of left and right hepatic arteries and anatomical variations, during stage 1 ALPPS, and prejudge the potential adverse effect. If the arteries on the FLR side are too thin and the tumor is huge, it is mandatory to watch out for "blood steal" associated with insufficient FLR hypertrophy [18].

After parenchymal partition, bile leakage check and prevention are essential. Reliable methods such as fat emulsion injection are recommended to strictly rule out this adverse event. This is particularly vital for HCC patients with cirrhosis or severe fibrosis due to their poor tolerability to complications.

15.5 Postoperative Management

Postoperative management is generally the same as conventional ALPPS, with special attention to liver protection and supportive care. Because patients undergoing this procedure are often complicated with cirrhosis or severe fibrosis, whose liver compensation function is compromised. They are prone to liver dysfunction after surgery. Postoperative changes in liver function shall be monitored and liver protection treatment administered to facilitate function recovery. Abdominal effusion after surgery is common. Special care shall be given to fluid, electrolyte, and acid-base imbalance monitoring, albumin supplement, and hypoproteinemia prevention. Antibiotics are given routinely after surgery to prevent abdominal infection and secondary PHLF. Kidney function needs special attention as well. Since this technique is most commonly used in huge HCC patients, the application of classical ALPPS in this population per se often leads to renal insufficiency. Once it occurs, disastrous results ensue if appropriate treatment is not initiated in time. Huang et al. [31] reported two cases of acute kidney injury (AKI) after ALPPS. One patient, treated with delayed renal replacement therapy (RRT), died of multi-organ dysfunction syndrome. The other, receiving early RRT, recovered the renal function gradually after the stage 2 ALPPS. These findings indicated that HCC patients with cirrhosis are prone to AKI after ALPPS, highlighting the value of early RRT [31]. Pooled analysis of the ALPPS registry [32] showed that patients with interstage renal dysfunction suffered from more major complications, higher mortality (1% vs. 8%), and more frequent and severe complications after stage 2 ALPPS. The mortality rates of patients with and without interstage renal dysfunction were 38% and 8%, respectively. In the former subgroup, renal function in 41% recovered before the second stage. However, their post-stage 2 mortality remained high, standing at 28%. AKI after stage 1 ALPPS is a predictive factor for interstage and post-stage 2 complications and perioperative deaths. For TAE-salvaged ALPPS, the combination of stage 1 ALPPS and TAE theoretically engenders significant tumor necrosis, which leads to AKI. The only one death among the 10 patients undergoing TAE-salvaged ALPPS reported by the authors was related to an oncolytic syndrome that caused renal dysfunction and secondary multi-organ failure. It is recommended to ensure sufficient hydration and appropriate amounts of diuretics after surgery, monitor renal function and electrolytes (creatinine, urea nitrogen, uric acid, blood phosphorus, and blood calcium), and prevent oncolytic syndrome (hyperuricemia, hypertension, and hypocalcemia). In the case of oncolysis and AKI, aggressive treatment should be initiated, starting with medication (hydration and diuretics). RRT could be given when necessary. Postoperative pleural effusion needs to be dealt with in time. In case of severe effusion, a drainage tube should be introduced percutaneously. Intraoperative drainage via the diaphragm is another option during stage 2 ALPPS. Suppose patients with liver failure who are not responding to medication and artificial liver support system (ALSS), liver transplantation, and other rescue regimens could be considered. Postoperative follow-up is the same as that of HCC patients subjected to conventional ALPPS. Prophylactic TACE could be routinely performed for the eligible 1 month after surgery. Since this procedure is mostly used for patients with giant HCC and large tumor burden, the overall waiting time before tumor resection is longer than that in conventional ALPPS. It is necessary to pay attention to postoperative follow-up results and adopt active strategies accordingly to prevent and treat relapse and metastasis.

References

1. Sandström P, Røsok BI, Sparrelid E, et al. ALPPS improves resectability compared with conventional two-stage hepatectomy in patients with advanced colorectal liver metastasis: results from a Scandinavian multicenter randomized controlled trial (LIGRO trial)[J]. Ann Surg. 2018;267(5):833–40.
2. Lang H, de Santibañes E, Schlitt HJ, et al. 10th anniversary of ALPPS-lessons learned and quo vadis[J]. Ann Surg. 2019;269(1):114–9.
3. D'Haese JG, Neumann J, Weniger M, et al. Should ALPPS be used for liver resection in intermediate-stage HCC?[J]. Ann Surg Oncol. 2016;23(4):1335–43.
4. Wang Z, Peng YF, Hu JW, et al. Associating liver partition and portal vein ligation for staged hepatectomy for unresectable hepatitis B virus-related hepatocellular carcinoma: a single center study of 45 patients[J]. Ann Surg. 2020;271(3):534–41.
5. van Lienden KP, van den Esschert JW, de Graaf W, et al. Portal vein embolization before liver resection: a systematic review[J]. Cardiovasc Intervent Radiol. 2013;36(1):25–34.
6. Chan AC, Poon RT, Chan C, et al. Safety of ALPPS procedure by the anterior approach for hepatocellular carcinoma[J]. Ann Surg. 2016;263(2):e14–6.
7. Vennarecci G, Grazi GL, Sperduti I, et al. ALPPS for primary and secondary liver tumors[J]. Int J Surg. 2016;30:38–44.
8. Vennarecci G, Laurenzi A, Levi Sandri GB, et al. The ALPPS procedure for hepatocellular carcinoma[J]. Eur J Surg Oncol. 2014;40(8):982–8.
9. Zhou J, Wang Z, Sun J, et al. Associating liver partition and portal vein ligation for staged hepatectomy[J]. Chin J Dig Surg. 2013;12(7):485–9.
10. Chan A, Zhang WY, Chok K, et al. ALPPS versus portal vein embolization for hepatitis-related hepatocellular carcinoma: a changing paradigm in modulation of future liver remnant before major hepatectomy[J]. Ann Surg. 2021;273(5):957–65.
11. Li PP, Huang G, Jia NY, et al. Associating liver partition and portal vein ligation for staged hepatectomy versus sequential transarterial chemoembolization and portal vein embolization in staged hepatectomy for HBV-related hepatocellular carcinoma: a randomized comparative study[J]. Hepatobiliary Surg Nutr. 2022;11(1):38–51.
12. Deng ZF, Jin ZR, Qin YH, et al. Efficacy of the association liver partition and portal vein ligation for staged hepatectomy for the treatment of solitary huge hepatocellular carcinoma: a retrospective single-center study[J]. World J Surg Oncol. 2021;19(1):95.
13. Zhang JW, Xu YY, Yang HY, et al. Application of associating liver partition and portal vein ligation for staged hepatectomy for hepatocellular carcinoma related to hepatitis B virus: comparison with traditional one-stage right hepatectomy[J]. Transl Cancer Res. 2020;9(9):5371–9.
14. Peng CH, Li C, Liu C, et al. The outcome of the HCC patients underwent ALPPS: retrospective study[J]. Medicine (Baltimore). 2019;98(38):e17182.

15. Imamura H, Seyama Y, Makuuchi M, et al. Sequential transcatheter arterial chemoembolization and portal vein embolization for hepatocellular carcinoma: the university of Tokyo experience[J]. Semin Intervent Radiol. 2008;25(2):146–54.
16. Aoki T, Imamura H, Hasegawa K, et al. Sequential preoperative arterial and portal venous embolizations in patients with hepatocellular carcinoma[J]. Arch Surg. 2004;139(7):766–74.
17. De Carlis L, Sguinzi R, De Carlis R, et al. Residual right portal branch flow after first-step ALPPS: artifact or homeostatic response?[J]. Hepato-Gastroenterology. 2014;61(134):1712–6.
18. Wang Z, Peng YF, Sun QM, et al. Salvage transhepatic arterial embolization after failed stage I ALPPS in a patient with a huge HCC with chronic liver disease: a case report[J]. Int J Surg Case Rep. 2017;39:131–5.
19. Peng YF, Wang Z, Qu XD, et al. Transcatheter arterial embolization-salvaged ALPPS, a novel ALPPS procedure especially for patients with hepatocellular carcinoma and severe fibrosis/cirrhosis[J]. Hepatobiliary Surg Nutr. 2022;11(4):504–14.
20. Cai XJ, Tong YF, Yu H, et al. The ALPPS in the treatment of hepatitis B-related hepatocellular carcinoma with cirrhosis: a single-center study and literature review[J]. Surg Innov. 2017;24(4):358–64.
21. Shrager B, Jibara GA, Tabrizian P, et al. Resection of large hepatocellular carcinoma (≥10 cm): a unique western perspective[J]. J Surg Oncol. 2013;107(2):111–7.
22. Yang LY, Fang F, Ou DP, et al. Solitary large hepatocellular carcinoma: a specific subtype of hepatocellular carcinoma with good outcome after hepatic resection[J]. Ann Surg. 2009;249(1):118–23.
23. Michalopoulos GK. Liver regeneration after partial hepatectomy: critical analysis of mechanistic dilemmas[J]. Am J Pathol. 2010;176(1):2–13.
24. Eipel C, Abshagen K, Vollmar B. Regulation of hepatic blood flow: the hepatic arterial buffer response revisited[J]. World J Gastroenterol. 2010;16(48):6046–57.
25. Ribero D, Curley SA, Imamura H, et al. Selection for resection of hepatocellular carcinoma and surgical strategy: indications for resection, evaluation of liver function, portal vein embolization, and resection[J]. Ann Surg Oncol. 2008;15(4):986–92.
26. Shindoh J, Tzeng CWD, Vauthey JN. Portal vein embolization for hepatocellular carcinoma[J]. Liver Cancer. 2012;1(3–4):159–67.
27. Nagino M, Nimura Y, Kamiya J, et al. Immediate increase in arterial blood flow in embolized hepatic segments after portal vein embolization: CT demonstration[J]. AJR Am J Roentgenol. 1998;171(4):1037–9.
28. Raptis DA, Linecker M, Kambakamba P, et al. Defining benchmark outcomes for ALPPS[J]. Ann Surg. 2019;270(5):835–41.
29. Chan ACY, Chok K, Dai JWC, et al. Impact of split completeness on future liver remnant hypertrophy in associating liver partition and portal vein ligation for staged hepatectomy (ALPPS) in hepatocellular carcinoma: complete-ALPPS versus partial-ALPPS[J]. Surgery. 2017;161(2):357–64.
30. Imamura H, Takayama T, Sugawara Y, et al. Pringle's manoeuvre in living donors[J]. Lancet. 2002;360(9350):2049–50.
31. Huang HC, Lu X, Yang HY, et al. Acute kidney injury after associating liver partition and portal vein ligation for staged hepatectomy for hepatocellular carcinoma: two case reports and a literature review[J]. Ann Transl Med. 2019;7(23):795.
32. Reese T, Fard-Aghaie MH, Makridis G, et al. Renal impairment is associated with reduced outcome after associating liver partition and portal vein ligation for staged hepatectomy[J]. J Gastrointest Surg. 2020;24(11):2500–7.

16 ALPPS vs Traditional Two-Stage Hepatectomy

Weiping Zhou and Pengpeng Li

16.1 Conventional Two-Stage Hepatectomy: Portal Vein Embolization

Liver resection has become an effective treatment for primary and secondary liver malignancies. Clinical practices validate that patients eligible for liver resection can often achieve the best radical treatment results. For patients without underlying liver diseases, the mortality rate after major liver resection is 3.2–7%. In contrast, for those with fibrotic livers, the postoperative mortality rate can be as high as 32% [1–3], mostly due to postoperative liver failure caused by insufficient future liver remnant (FLR) [4]. Safe liver resection depends on preserving sufficient FLR and ensuring adequate inflow, outflow, and bile drainage of the FLR parenchyma. Preoperative portal vein embolization (PVE) is a traditional and safe interventional procedure, embolizing the portal vein on the tumor-bearing side to redistribute intrahepatic blood flow, thereby promoting FLR hypertrophy. PVE improves the safety of extensive liver resection and reduces its mortality rate to 3.3% [5]. This technique induces FLR growth, providing 70–80% of patients with the opportunity for extensive hepatectomy [6, 7].

16.1.1 Mechanism of PVE

Following liver injury, partial hepatectomy, and hepatic vascular obstruction, changes in hemodynamics and metabolic pathways stimulate normal liver regeneration. In this process, the portal vein plays a central role in transporting growth-stimulating substances. After PVE on the affected side, portal vein blood flow is redistributed to the non-embolized side, increasing blood flow on the unaffected side until it gradually returns to baseline levels 11 days after the procedure [8–11]. Liver regeneration largely involves an increase in hepatocyte quantity rather than cell volume enlargement [9]. At the cellular level, this process initiates a few hours after stimulating factors begin to act. For most patients, it usually takes a few weeks to reach growth requirements, with an average of approximately 4 weeks (using traditional gelatin sponge + spring coils as embolic agents). The liver grows to 40–62% of pre-PVE FLR [12], and the effect lasts 1 year after embolization [13]. Only about 25% of the total volume growth occurs in the first month, 50% in the first 3 months, and 75% in the first 8 months [13]. The FLR regeneration rate peaks about 2 weeks post-PVE, at around 12–21 cm^3/d, plateaus at 3 weeks, and maintains at 6–11 cm^3/d 1 month after the intervention [14]. The rate of regeneration after PVE is influenced by multiple factors, such as the scope of embolism, underlying liver diseases (viral hepatitis cirrhosis, alcoholic cirrhosis, and fatty liver), and systemic diseases (diabetes).

16.1.2 Liver Volume and Functional Volume Assessment

To assess the necessity of preoperative PVE, we first need to determine the FLR. It is essential to understand and appropriately estimate FLR and functional liver volume. Regardless of the method used for such measurements, there will always be a discrepancy between the estimated and the actual volumes.

The FLR is usually measured by tomographic imaging systems, including enhanced triple-phase liver CT or MRI. A more advanced clinical approach is three-dimensional (3D) visualization reconstruction using thin-section CT or MRI of the liver (slice thickness is required to be at most 5 mm, preferably 1.25 mm), and the volume is calculated by a 3D reconstruction voxel-based algorithm [15]. This method allows surgeons to self-determine the liver resection plane

W. Zhou (✉) · P. Li
The Third Affiliated Hospital of Naval Medical University (Eastern Hepatobiliary Surgery Hospital), Shanghai, China
e-mail: ehphwp3@126.com

J. Zhou (ed.), *Associating Liver Partition and Portal Vein Ligation for Staged Hepatectomy (ALPPS)*,
https://doi.org/10.1007/978-981-96-7364-3_16

based on the preoperative resection plan and calculate the FLR more intuitively and individually. Since liver volume is directly correlated to body size, patients with greater statures require larger remaining parenchyma to support physiological hepatic function requirements [16]. Therefore, standardized future liver remnant (sFLR) is often used clinically to evaluate the remaining liver volume, sFLR = fFLR/TLV (total liver volume). This assessment methodology has been widely verified in clinical practices [17, 18]. The following formula is applied to estimate the TLV: TLV = −794.41 + 126.28 × BSA, where BSA stands for the body surface area [17, 18].

The FLR volume required for safe liver resection varies among patients with underlying liver diseases. For those without these conditions, hepatectomy can be safely performed when their sFLR >20% [14, 18–20], whereas, for those with potential liver damage (including chemotherapy, fatty liver disease, viral infection, or other iatrogenic injuries), sFLR is required to be >30% [3, 21–23]. For patients with liver diseases (including cirrhosis), the sFLR needs to be greater than 40% [21, 22]. FLR/BW (body weight) is another way to evaluate. In patients free from liver diseases, FLR/BW should be >0.8% [24], while for fibrotic patients, the ratio should be greater than 1.4% [25].

Liver parenchymal functional tests usually include indocyanine green (ICG) clearance [26] and asialoglycoprotein receptor scintigraphy using ^{99m}Tc-galactosyl-human serum albumin (^{99m}Tc-GSA) as the imaging agent [27].

ICG clearance is a widely applied analytical method in clinical practices to quantify liver function, especially in cirrhotic patients. Combining with FLR, it helps predict functional FLR [28]. ICG is a nontoxic dye that binds to albumin and is eliminated through biliary excretion. Its excretion rate can be measured using serum samples or a fingertip optical sensor. Generally, serum ICG retention 15 minutes after injection (ICG-R15) should be less than 10% [26, 29, 30]. Hence, ICG-R15 can be used clinically to evaluate liver function reserve and roughly estimate the extent of liver resection that can be tolerated. Patients with an ICG-R15 <14% can withstand extensive hepatectomy (≥3 liver segments), while those with an ICG-R15 between 14% and 22% can tolerate small liver resection (≤2 liver segments). In clinical practices, FLR and ICG-R15 are often combined to assess the risk of post-hepatectomy liver failure (PHLF). For patients with a liver function classification of Child-Pugh class A [31], ICG-R15 <10% + FLR/TLV >40% or 10% ≤ ICG-R15 <20% + FLR/TLV >50% is considered eligible for liver resection [32].

16.1.3 Indications of PVE

In patients who are expected to have insufficient FLR, PVE on the affected side may be considered before hepatectomy. As the required FLR gradually increases, the probability of successful liver regeneration to the target FLR after PVE decreases. With the worsening of underlying liver diseases, the likelihood of actual liver growth after PVE also drops [33]. Therefore, the indications for PVE are classified as follows based on liver condition:

(a) Normal livers: sFLR <20% or FLR/BW <0.5 (Truant standard) [34]
(b) Livers with significant steatosis, cholestasis, chemotherapy-related steatohepatitis, and chronic hepatitis: sFLR <30% or FLR/BW <0.8
(c) Cirrhotic livers (liver function classification of Child-Pugh A); sFLR <40% or FLR/BW <1.4%

16.1.4 Contraindications of PVE

Specific contraindications are as follows:

(a) Patients who are unable to undergo extensive liver resection, including those with severe cardiopulmonary comorbidities, poor performance status (PS score >3 points) [35], cirrhosis of Child-Pugh grade C, and severe portal hypertension
(b) Patients who are not suitable for interventional therapy, including those with uncorrectable coagulation disorders and renal failure requiring dialysis
(c) Patients who are technically unable to undergo PVE, including those with anatomic variations of the portal vein and intraportal vein tumor thrombus
(d) Patients whose tumors are too large to receive radical treatment, including those with extrahepatic metastases or intrahepatic tumor dissemination, where R0 resection is unachievable
(e) Patients whose baseline FLR volume is too small and who are not expected to achieve adequate FLR growth through PVE
(f) Patients with biliary tract obstruction.

16.1.5 Preoperative Preparation for PVE

Before PVE, the patient must undergo a comprehensive assessment, the proposed liver resection plan must be determined, and the FLR volume must be measured. The rationale for PVE is determined by the sFLR criteria. Simultaneously, the location and scope of the embolization are decided based on the tumor site and the proposed surgical plan. If the FLR is lesion-bearing, these neoplasms must be treated before performing PVE. Pre-PVE transarterial chemoembolization (TACE) may benefit patients by cutting off the arterial blood supply and nutrients to the tumor, preventing disease progression during the liver regeneration period after PVE. Additionally, the inflammatory response induced by

TACE may help promote FLR hypertrophy [36]. Many studies have demonstrated that TACE followed by PVE not only increases FLR more and faster but also facilitates tumor necrosis and improves the prognosis of hepatocellular carcinoma (HCC) [37–42]. If the segment IV hepatic artery or inferior phrenic artery supplies the tumor, these vessels need to be embolized during TACE. PVE can usually be performed 1–2 weeks after TACE, when liver function has basically recovered [38].

(a) Assessment of underlying diseases and important organ function: medical history collection (hypertension, diabetes and their control status, recent history of stroke and myocardial infarction, renal insufficiency, viral hepatitis, alcohol intake, and medication); blood routine, liver and kidney function, coagulation function, HBV panel, HCV antibody, HBV DNA and HCV RNA (further examination if the relevant virus screening is positive), echocardiography (age ≥60 years old), and electrocardiogram; pulmonary function; chest X-ray; and gastroscopy.
(b) Tumor assessment: tumor markers (AFP, CEA, and CA199); liver thin-section contrast-enhanced CT or MRI; for cholangiocarcinoma and metastatic liver cancer (such as colorectal cancer and neuroendocrine tumors) where there is a higher risk of metastasis to other organs, PET-CT examination should be considered.
(c) Liver-related assessment: ICG-R15; FibroScan for liver stiffness; 3D visualization liver reconstruction based on thin-section CT or MRI to identify any anatomical variations and intrahepatic portal vein tortuosity; using three-dimensional visualization technology to calculate the volumes of the liver to be resected and the FLR based on the liver resection plan proposed by the surgeon following the evaluation of the tumor conditions.

CT scan standards and requirements: All patients undergoing preoperative CT scans must receive triple-phase contrast-enhanced CT scans. The scanning range should encompass all liver sections with a slice thickness of 1.25 mm. The original scan data is saved in a digital imaging and communications in medicine (DICOM) format on the server for subsequent 3D visualization processing.

MRI scan standards and requirements: All patients undergoing preoperative MRI scans must receive triple-phase enhanced scans. The scanning range should encompass all liver sections with a slice thickness of 3 mm. The raw scan data should be stored in DICOM (Digital Imaging and Communications in Medicine) format on the server for subsequent 3D visualization processing.

16.1.6 PVE Techniques and Embolization Materials

PVE is usually performed under local anesthesia using a percutaneous transhepatic approach under B-ultrasound guidance in an interventional radiology suite or an intraoperative transileocolic venous approach. Studies have shown that the compensatory FLR growth is more significant with the percutaneous transhepatic approach [43], which can be classified into ipsilateral and contralateral percutaneous transhepatic PVE according to the relationships between the puncture site and the liver to be resected [44]. The advantage of the ipsilateral approach is the avoidance of accidental damage to the remaining liver during PVE, and it facilitates easier catheter access to segment IV of the portal vein when an extended right hepatectomy is planned [45]. However, the placement of embolic material is against the direction of blood flow, requiring special care to prevent the embolic material from dislodging and causing unintended segmental embolization. Conversely, the contralateral approach offers easier puncture and catheter placement, and the embolic material is placed in the direction of blood flow. Nevertheless, it carries a risk of damaging the FLR and poses challenges in embolizing segment IV of the portal vein. Studies have shown no significant differences in post-embolization complications between the ipsilateral and contralateral approaches [20, 46].

It is essential to embolize the whole target portal vein tree, including terminal branches, so as to refrain from portal vein shunting and optimize the embolization effect. In addition, it is also crucial to treat all diseased liver segments during portal vein embolization to promote compensatory hypertrophy of the future liver remnant (FLR) and avoid hypertrophy of the liver segments planned for resection.

Many embolization materials are currently available for clinical use, including gelatin sponges, micro coils, n-butyl cyanoacrylate (NBCA), fibrin glue, and polyvinyl alcohol (PVA), among others [43]. To date, there have been no randomized controlled trials (RCTs) comparing the pros and cons of these materials.

From our own experience, the embolization effect of gelatin sponge needs to be sufficiently reliable. As the material dissolves, portal vein recanalization is prone to occur after PVE. Besides, it cannot effectively block either peripheral branches or potential communicating vessels between the left and right sides. Therefore, its stimulatory effect on liver hypertrophy is relatively weak. Patients often require a longer time to achieve sufficient FLR regeneration, and nearly one-third of patients fail to gain surgical opportunities through PVE.

NBCA, on the other hand, has demonstrated excellent embolization effects in our clinical applications, showing rapid and reliable performance in promoting FLR growth. Studies have indicated that NBCA-based PVE produced a stable embolization effect that lasted for 4 weeks, while using a gelatin sponge and thrombin only yielded a temporary effect, where portal vein recanalization was prone to occur. The former method induced a 90% FLR growth from baseline within 30 days, while the latter generated only 35% within 43 days [44]. Nonetheless, NBCA also caused significant inflammatory reactions, including fibrosis around the biliary tract and sclerotic casts within the portal vein, rendering the subsequent surgery more difficult [47].

16.1.7 Postoperative Patient Management of PVE

The follow-up evaluation interval of patients after PVE varies per embolization material. In general, patients who receive NBCA-based embolization experience faster FLR regeneration, which can be evaluated every 2 weeks. For those who accept gelatin sponge + spring coil, due to inadequate embolization and slower FLR hypertrophy, the remnant is usually evaluated every 4 weeks. Typically, liver resection is performed 3–6 weeks after PVE.

If patients with colorectal liver metastases receive neoadjuvant chemotherapy prior to PVE, it can be continued after PVE to avoid tumor progression during the waiting period [48]. Many studies have shown that continuing chemotherapy does not significantly impact liver volume hypertrophy following PVE [49–51].

Each assessment should include a liver function test, hepatitis viral levels (if the patient is complicated by viral hepatitis infection), contrast-enhanced CT or MRI of the liver, and 3D visualization reconstruction to calculate liver volume, tumor size, and number.

If liver regeneration meets the sFLR criteria, the planned hepatectomy may proceed. However, preoperative imaging examinations, such as chest CT or imaging of other metastasis-prone sites, are still required to rule out extrahepatic tumor metastasis following PVE.

16.1.8 Complications of PVE

PVE is generally well tolerated by patients, and severe complications are uncommon (2–3%), including portal vein thrombosis, non-targeted vascular embolism, infection, bile leakage, biliary tract hemorrhage, pseudoaneurysm, arteriovenous fistula, arterial-portal shunt, liver hematoma, pneumothorax, and esophageal-gastric variceal bleeding (EGVB) caused by increased portal venous pressure after PVE [5, 46, 52, 53]. Minor complications such as fever and abdominal discomfort occur in 20–30% of patients and are usually self-limiting. Aminotransferase levels typically peak on the third day after PVE, generally less than three times the normal value, and return to baseline by the tenth day. Bilirubin levels may increase slightly, while albumin levels and prothrombin time are usually unaffected [14].

16.1.9 Benefits and Risks of PVE

Preoperative PVE can reduce the incidence of post-hepatectomy and pulmonary complications, minimize the impact of post-PVE hepatectomy on liver function, and shorten both ICU length-of-stay (LoS) and the overall LoS [3]. This intervention grants patients who are ineligible for radical resection due to insufficient FLR the opportunity for curative surgery. According to a study on extensive resection of liver metastases from colorectal cancer, the curative resection rate increased from 46% to 79% after PVE [54]. Sequential TACE and PVE induced complete tumor necrosis [42]. Therefore, combining TACE and PVE can serve as a tumor treatment strategy for some patients, rather than solely to stimulate FLR hypertrophy. Subclinical or rapidly progressive tumors can be screened out through repeated imaging examinations during the surgery-pending follow-up period after PVE, thereby avoiding unnecessary resections. A suboptimal FLR hypertrophy after embolization indicates the ineligibility of extensive hepatectomy.

In addition to the abovementioned postoperative complications, PVE poses potential risks of promoting tumor proliferation. Approximately 1/6–1/3 of patients suffered from post-embolization disease progression, being deprived of surgical opportunities [48], partially led by PVE per se. One study showed that the tumor growth rate after this procedure was higher than that in the control group (0.36 mL/d vs 0.05 mL/d) [55]. However, this phenomenon varies among different tumor types. For colorectal cancer liver metastasis, tumor growth was similar between embolized and non-embolized liver lobes [48, 56, 57]. The speed of tumor growth increased by 2.65-fold after PVE for HCC, and by 1.16-fold for cholangiocarcinoma [58].

16.1.10 Outlook of PVE

PVE combined with hematopoietic stem cells injection into the portal vein can facilitate liver regeneration [59, 60]. Current studies have illustrated that early infusion of bone marrow-derived progenitor cells into the FLR after PVE may induce greater and faster FLR hypertrophy without increasing the incidence of complications [61, 62]. A small sample-size RCT indicated that PVE combined with branched-chain amino acid supplementation significantly ameliorated the function of FLR after liver resection and partially enhanced the FLR function after PVE [63].

In recent years, a strategy called liver venous deprivation (LVD) that integrates PVE and hepatic vein embolization (HVE) has emerged, further advancing FLR growth. It promotes the formation of collateral branches of the hepatic vein in the FLR. When PVE alone fails to induce sufficient FLR hypertrophy, sequential HVE can be applied as a remedial measure [64]. Some centers have adopted this simultaneous PVE and HVE strategy and achieved promising results [65].

16.2 Comparison Between ALPPS and PVE

ALPPS is a two-stage hepatectomy combined with liver partition and portal vein ligation [66]. Through the first operation, the parenchyma of the affected and the unaffected sides are separated, and the portal vein on the affected side is ligated at the same time. Then, FLR growth on the unaffected side is rapidly promoted in a short time frame. The second operation is performed after liver function requirements are met, completely resecting the diseased liver. Compared with PVE, ALPPS is significantly more effective in facilitating FLR growth, shortening interstage intervals (usually 1–2 weeks), and increasing the proportion of patients undergoing radical liver resection. Although ALPPS patients face greater surgical risks and a higher incidence of postoperative complications [67–70], the higher resection rate and OS drive the broad application of ALPPS. It is also an effective salvage procedure after PVE failure [12].

16.2.1 Liver Hypertrophy and Increase in Liver Function Reserve

The degree of hypertrophy (DH) and kinetic growth rate (KGR) are accurate metrics for comparing liver volume and growth rate between ALPPS and PVE and other comparisons. Studies have reported that ALPPS induced greater FLR hypertrophy than PVE [(84.3 ± 7.8)% vs (36.0 ± 27.2)%, $P < 0.001$] [71]. This finding was also supported by a systematic review and meta-analysis conducted in 2019. Compared with PVE, ALPPS enabled greater DH (RR = 6.30, 95%CI: 3.97–8.64) [68], revealing that the interval to the second stage of hepatectomy in ALPPS was significantly shortened, thereby reducing the incidence of tumor progression and increasing the rate of radical resection.

Kenichi Matsuo et al. shared their experience on the histological characteristics of the liver after ALPPS and PVE, concluding that the estimated KGR of ALPPS was better than that of PVE [(14.4 ± 4.8) mL/d vs (3.6 ± 2.2) mL/d, $P < 0.001$] [72]. In 2021, Albert Chan et al. compared the FLR growth rate between these two strategies. The results suggested that patients treated with ALPPS had faster FLR volume growth (7.4%/d vs 1.6%/d), shorter median waiting time for stage 2 resection (7 days vs 48 days), and higher tumor resection rate (97.8% vs 67.7%) [73]. Similarly, another study validated that the KGR of patients receiving ALPPS was higher than that of patients undergoing PVE [(10.8 ± 4.5)%/d vs (0.98 ± 0.75)%/d, $P < 0.001$] [71]. This evidence clearly manifests that patients treated with ALPPS have better DH and KGR than those treated with PVE.

In the process of ALPPS or PVE to promote FLR regeneration, measuring liver function before and after surgery can prevent patients from undergoing inappropriate resection due to insufficient FLR function, which may lead to PHLF. Many studies measured FLR function by liver scintigraphy imaging, and the results showed that the function increased by 28–29% at 6–7 days after ALPPS [74, 75], while at 4–8 weeks after PVE, the average improvement in FLR function was 16% and 9% in patients with normal livers and in those with underlying liver diseases, respectively [3]. These findings also illustrate the superiority of ALPPS over PVE in promoting liver functional growth in the short term.

16.2.2 Complication and Mortality Rates

Postoperative complications of ALPPS and PVE were classified using the Clavien-Dindo classification (grades I–V) [76]. In a systematic review and meta-analysis conducted in 2019, Yanmo Liu et al. compared the advantages and disadvantages of the two methods and reported their overall safety. Their results showed that the complication rate of ALPPS was higher than that of PVE (25% vs 21%, RR = 1.37, 95%CI: 0.84–2.21) [68]. Junichi Shindoh et al. also reported that the incidence of total postoperative complications and the incidence of major complications in the ALPPS group were higher than those in the PVE group (64% and 40% vs 57.7% and 32.7%). The authors also pointed out that the occurrence of postoperative bile leakage, sepsis, and unplanned reoperation in the ALPPS group was higher compared to the PVE group (24.0%, 20.0%, and 28.0% vs 5.8%, 0.0%, and 2.9%) [12].

In contrast, in a study conducted in Hong Kong, China, Albert Chan et al. revealed similar postoperative complication rates between ALPPS and PVE (20.7% vs 30.4%, $P = 0.159$) [73]. Jan Bednarsch et al., defining postoperative grade II–IV complications as major events, proposed that although the incidence of major postoperative complications in ALPPS was higher than that in PVE (64% vs 38%), the difference between the two groups was not statistically significant [77]. Hence, there remains considerable controversy regarding the differences in postoperative complication rates between ALPPS and PVE, highlighting the need for further large-sample studies to provide fair and objective evaluations of both procedures.

Compared with PVE, the stage 2 resection rate of ALPPS is significantly higher, but the comparison of mortality between the two strategies remains disputed. According to Albert Chan et al., the postoperative mortality rates of ALPPS and PVE were similar (6.5% vs 5.8%, $P = 1.000$) [73]. Yanmo Liu et al. pointed out that in three studies, the adjusted mortality rate of ALPPS was higher than that of PVE (10% vs 5%, RR = 2.26, 95%CI: 0.88–5.80) [68].

The limitation of the above studies is the need for a randomized controlled comparison of the two treatments, rendering it difficult for the authors to make a fair and objective comparison. More high-quality studies are therefore necessary. In recent years, the strict selection of indications for ALPPS and the application of minimally invasive surgical techniques have significantly reduced the postoperative complication and mortality rates associated with ALPPS.

16.2.3 Oncological Outcomes

Disease-free survival (DFS) or recurrence-free survival (RFS) and overall survival (OS) are essential indicators for evaluating the oncological outcomes of PVE and ALPPS. A study published by Albert Chan et al. [73] in 2021 illustrated no significant differences in the 1-, 3-, and 5-year DFS between ALPPS (63.2%, 34.9%, 25.5%) and PVE (61.4%, 41.8%, 40.7%, $P = 0.267$). Jan Bednarsch et al. reported in a 2020 study that the median RFS of the ALPPS group was 19 months, better than that of the PVE group (10 months). Nevertheless, the authors found no significant differences in oncological outcomes between the two groups [77]. The above studies suggest a comparable DFS between these two strategies.

Some studies showcased that the OS rates between the two were also comparable. According to Albert Chan et al., there were no significant differences in the 1-, 3-, and 5-year OS between the ALPPS and PVE groups (84.7%, 60.2%, and 46.8% vs 88.2%, 73.5%, and 64.1%, $P = 0.234$). Further stratified analysis based on tumor stage was conducted on both groups, finding similar OS results [73]. These were consistent with Jan Bednarsch et al., who reported that the median OS of the ALPPS and PVE groups was 28 months and 34 months, respectively. In addition, no significant differences were found in 3- and 5-year OS between the ALPPS and the PVE groups (37% and 37% vs 44% and 33%, $P = 0.297$). The above studies all compared the survival outcomes of patients who have completed tumor resection in both arms.

16.3 Comparison of ALPPS and PVE in Patients with Hepatitis B-Related HCC

In a randomized controlled study conducted by the Third Affiliated Hospital of Naval Medical University (Eastern Hepatobiliary Surgery Hospital), Professor Weiping Zhou compared the use of ALPPS and TACE + PVE for treating hepatitis B virus (HBV)-related hepatocellular carcinoma (HCC) patients who were ineligible for one-stage resection due to insufficient FLR [70]. Patients were randomly assigned to the ALPPS or TACE + PVE groups in a 1:1 ratio. Inclusion criteria included the following: age 18–75 years, tumor treatment-naive patients with hepatitis B-related HCC ineligible for liver resection due to insufficient FLR volume, BCLC stage 0, A, B, Child-Pugh Grade A, serum alanine aminotransferase (ALT) <2 times the upper limit of normal. Patients with intra- or extra-hepatic metastases, portal hypertension, and American Society of Anesthesiologists (ASA) operative risk ≥III were excluded.

In the ALPPS group, patients underwent weekly contrast-enhanced CT scans and three-dimensional visualization imaging to assess FLR volume after the first-stage surgery. If the FLR volume increased sufficiently, the stage 2 hepatectomy was proceeded; otherwise, the assessment was repeated weekly until adequate FLR hypertrophy was achieved or the treatment was deemed a failure. Due to the slower FLR hypertrophy rate after PVE, and to avoid tumor progression during the waiting period, patients in the TACE + PVE group first received TACE. After 2 weeks, when the liver function returned to baseline levels, PVE was performed [38]. The same method was applied to evaluate the FLR hypertrophy every 4 weeks until adequate FLR hypertrophy was achieved or the treatment was deemed a failure. For patients with insufficient liver hypertrophy in the TACE + PVE group, salvage ALPPS was recommended. Treatment failure was defined as intrahepatic or extrahepatic tumor metastasis, KGR below 2% per week at any time, and complications that hampered stage 2 hepatectomy. In such cases, patients were switched to TACE, targeted drugs, or supportive care.

All patients underwent preoperative upper abdominal contrast-enhanced CT for 3D reconstruction and liver volume calculation, ICG-R15, FibroTouch (to assess the degree of liver fibrosis), gastroscopy, and ultrasound. Antiviral treatment with entecavir (0.5 mg/d) or tenofovir (300 mg/d) was administered to all before surgery, covering the whole treatment process unless unacceptable toxicity occurred [78, 79].

The KGR was calculated either by the mean volume increase per day from the baseline to the final volume before stage 2 liver resection or by the following formula: KGR = degree of FLR increase (%)/time elapsed (weeks) from the baseline to the final volume before stage 2 liver resection [80].

All surgeries were performed by a single surgical team following previously reported techniques for hepatectomy [81, 82]. For the first stage of ALPPS, the portal vein on the tumor-containing side was ligated. Both partial and complete parenchymal transections were carried out. The middle hepatic vein was preserved during the first-stage surgery. In the second stage, the portal vein, hepatic artery, bile duct, and hepatic veins of the affected side were divided, and the tumor was resected. The middle hepatic vein was resected during left or right hemihepatectomy.

All TACE and PVE procedures were performed by one team of interventional radiologists using previously reported techniques [38]. Superselective catheterization of the tumor artery was performed by injecting 40 mg of doxorubicin, 15 mg of hydroxy camptothecin, 16 mL of lipiodol, 1/3 of gelatin sponge particles (diameter 560–710 μm), and 1/4 of microspheres (diameter 1000–1400 μm). After liver function returned to normal 2 weeks later, a contralateral portal vein puncture was performed under ultrasound guidance for PVE under mild sedation. Embolization was then carried out using gelatin sponges and steel coils.

The primary endpoints were the tumor resection and 3-year survival rates. Secondary endpoints included:

(a) The rate of FLR volume increase
(b) The time to reach the predefined FLR volume for the stage 2 resection
(c) Intraoperative data
(d) Postoperative mortality and morbidity rates

Portal hypertension was defined as the presence of thrombocytopenia (PLT <100 × 10^9/L), splenomegaly (a spleen length >12 cm) [83], or gastroesophageal varices on preoperative gastroscopy. Severe liver fibrosis was defined as liver stiffness ≥12.5 kPa [84]. The incidence of complications was categorized according to the Clavien-Dindo classification [76], with major complications defined as grade ≥IIIa and severe complications as grade ≥IIIb. PHLF was defined and graded using the "ISGLS" criteria [85]. The degree of liver fibrosis is assessed using the METAVIR scoring system [86]. The surgical margin was defined as the shortest macroscopic distance from the tumor edge to the resection plane. R0 resection was defined as the nonexistence of tumor cells at the plane of transection on microscopic examination.

After treatment, follow-up visits were scheduled once a month. Contrast-enhanced CT or MRI, liver function test, AFP, HBV-DNA, and chest radiography were performed once every 3 months. For patients diagnosed with HCC recurrence or metastasis, active treatment was given depending on the location and number of recurrences, liver functional status, and the patient's general condition.

Previous studies have shown that more than 90% of patients receiving ALPPS completed two-stage hepatectomy, while approximately 60% of patients did so using PVE [69, 82, 87]. Using an alpha risk of 0.05 and a power of 80%, a sample size of 30 cases in each group was required. Considering possible dropouts and loss to follow-up, the final enrollment for each group was 38 patients.

A multidisciplinary tumor board, consisting of radiologists, oncologists, and liver surgeons, assessed patients for eligibility for ALPPS and TACE + PVE and randomized the patients. Eligible patients were randomly assigned to two the groups in a 1:1 ratio using a computer-generated random number list. A research nurse who was not involved in the study assigned the treatments according to consecutive numbers, which were kept in sealed envelopes. Since the two procedures differed, masking was not applied for group assignment.

Continuous variables were expressed as medians (ranges), and categorical variables as counts or ratios. The Mann-Whitney U test was used as the nonparametric test for two independent samples. Categorical variables were analyzed using Pearson's chi-square or Fisher exact test. Correlation analyses were carried out using the Pearson test. Multiple linear regression analyses were performed to identify significant factors influencing FLR increase rate. OS was estimated using the Kaplan-Meier method, which is defined as the time from first treatment to death (all causes). A log-rank test was used to compare the survival outcomes of the two groups. Cox regressions examined the association between OS and demographic features and other covariates. All calculations were performed using standard software (SPSS Statistics version 24.0). A two-sided $P < 0.05$ was considered as statistically significant. All data were analyzed on an intention-to-treat (ITT) basis.

From November 2014 to June 2016, 1146 HCC patients were treated at our center, of whom 921 underwent direct liver resection; 139 were suitable for staged hepatectomy, of whom 63 received TACE + sorafenib. Finally, 76 patients enrolled in this study.

The two patient groups had no statistically significant differences in the general and preoperative clinical data (Table 16.1). All 38 patients in the ALPPS group completed the first-stage surgery, and 37 patients (97.4%) completed the second-stage surgery. Only one patient with portal hypertension failed to achieve adequate FLR hypertrophy and, therefore, did not undergo tumor resection.

All 38 patients in the TACE + PVE group underwent the initial TACE treatment and PVE. Tumor resection was completed in 25 patients (65.8%). The difference in the completion rate of stage 2 surgery between the ALPPS group and the TACE + PVE group was statistically significant (HR = 1.48, 95%CI: 1.17–1.87, $P < 0.001$). All six patients who failed to undergo stage 2 surgery due to insufficient

Table 16.1 Baseline characteristics of two patients

Characteristics	Results	
	ALPPS group ($n = 38$)	TACE + PVE group ($n = 38$)
Age (years)	48.5 (27–68)	51 (32–72)
Sex, male, *n* (%)	34 (89.5)	32 (84.2)
BMI	23.7 (19.7–31.1)	23.0 (20.6–28.6)
ASA operative risk, *n* (%)		
I	5 (13.2)	7 (18.4)
II	33 (86.8)	31 (81.6)
III	0	0
ECOG score, *n* (%)		
0	30 (78.9)	28 (73.7)
1	8 (21.1)	10 (26.3)
2	0	0
HBV-DNA >50 IU/mL, *n* (%)	18 (47.4)	21 (55.3)
HCV+, *n* (%)	0	1 (2.6)
TB (μmol/L)	13.3 (6.7–28.0)	13.2 (5.4–31.0)
ALT (U/L)	33 (11–123)	34 (14–96)
ALB (g/L)	41.5 (35.1–51.3)	40.1 (33.6–48.7)
Portal hypertension+, *n* (%)	14 (36.8)	12 (31.6)
Gastroesophageal varices, *n* (%)	2 (5.3)	2 (5.3)
Platelet count ($\times 10^9$/L)	152 (70–369)	162 (65–365)
Spleen diameter (mm)	101 (77–140)	103 (79–136)
AFP >20 μg/L, *n* (%)	23 (60.5)	27 (71.1)
FibroTouch (kPa)	8.4 (4–21.2)	10.4 (5.1–20.3)
Single tumor, *n* (%)	19 (50)	17 (44.7)
Tumor diameter (cm)	8 (3–13)	8(4–13)
Multiple tumors, *n* (%)	19 (50)	21 (55.3)
Sum of tumor diameters (cm)	12 (7–17)	11 (5–15)
Sum of tumor volume (mL)	451 (18–2493)	397 (9–1677)
FLR1/BW (%)	0.72 (0.39–0.79)	0.65 (0.39–0.79)
Child-Pugh classification (%)		
A	100	100
BCLC stage (%)		
A	50	44.7
B	50	55.3
C	0	0
D	0	0

This table is reprinted with permission from the source of Ref. [70]
Note: *BMI* body mass index, *TB* total bilirubin, *ALT* alanine aminotransferase, *ALB* albumin, *ASA* American Society of Anesthesiologists, *ECOG* Eastern Cooperative Oncology Group, *FLR/BW* future liver remnant volume/body weight, *BCLC stage* Barcelona Clinic Liver Cancer classification. FibroTouch is a noninvasive detection system for liver fibrosis and has been approved by FDA

FLR growth refused to switch to the ALPPS group for salvage ALPPS and were finally treated with TACE + sorafenib. One patient refused hepatectomy after PVE due to tumor necrosis and did not receive further treatment beyond the 3-month follow-up. When the TACE + PVE group was further subdivided into the portal hypertension ($n = 12$) and the non-portal hypertension ($n = 26$) subgroups, the completion rate of two-stage hepatectomy was higher in the non-portal hypertension subgroup than in the portal hypertension subgroup, the completion rate of two-stage hepatectomy in the non-portal hypertension subgroup was higher, though insignificantly, than that in the portal hypertension subgroup (41.7% vs 76.9%, $P = 0.078$), which may be related to the small sample size (Table 16.2).

The daily FLR hypertrophy rate ($P < 0.001$) and the waiting time for the second-stage surgery were significantly better in the ALPPS group compared to the TACE + PVE group ($P < 0.001$). There were no statistically significant differences in the final volume of FLR and tumor volume changes (ALPPS, $P = 0.408$; TACE + PVE, $P = 0.433$) (Table 16.3) between the two groups.

Analysis of significant factors influencing the FLR growth rate showed that only the ALPPS staged liver resection strategy ($\beta = 13.03$, 95%CI: 10.03–16.02, $P < 0.001$) and low

Table 16.2 Intraoperative and postoperative clinical data of the two patient groups

Index	Findings		*P* value
	ALPPS group	TACE + PVE group	
Data on first operation			
First operation/procedure	ALPPS stage 1 ($n = 38$, 100%) Rt PVL ($n = 32$, 84.2%) Lt PVL ($n = 6$, 15.8%)	TACE ($n = 38$, 100%) PVE ($n = 38$, 100%) Rt PVE ($n = 28$, 73.7%) Rt + Segment 4 PVE ($n = 8$, 21.1%) Lt + Segment 5, 8 PVE ($n = 2$, 5.3%)	
Intraoperative findings (median, range)			
Operating time (min)	147.5 (55–255)	140 (100–175)	$P = 0.274$
Pringle's maneuver (min)	15 (0–22)	0	
Intraoperative blood loss (mL)	200 (100–800)	0	
Intraoperative blood transfusion (units)	0 (0–4)	0	
Postoperative complications (Clavien Dindo)			
≥Grade IIIa	($n = 6$, 15.8%)	($n = 1$, 2.6%)	$P = 0.108$
Grade III	Ascites ($n = 1$, 2.6%)		
	Pleural effusion ($n = 1$, 2.6%) Bile duct obstruction ($n = 1$, 2.6%) Bile leakage ($n = 1$, 2.6%) Abdominal infection ($n = 2$, 5.3%)	$P = 0.108$	
Grade IV	($n = 0$)	Liver failure ($n = 1$, 2.6%)	$P = 1.000$
Data on second operation			
Second operation	ALPPS stage 2 ($n = 37$, 97.4%)	Stage 2 hepatectomy ($n = 25$, 65.8%)	$P < 0.001$
Reasons for not proceeding to stage 2 hepatectomy	Total: $n = 1$ (2.6%) Insufficient FLR hypertrophy ($n = 1$, 2.6%)	Total: $n = 13$ (34.2%) Tumor progression ($n = 5$, 13.2%) Insufficient FLR hypertrophy ($n = 6$, 15.8%) Liver decompensation ($n = 1$, 2.6%) Refuse surgery due to tumor necrosis ($n = 1$, 2.6%)	
Second operation time (min)	145 (105–380)	210 (140–270)	$P < 0.001$
Intraoperative data			
Pringle maneuver duration (min)	12 (0–22)	21 (0–47)	$P < 0.001$
Number of blood transfusion, *n* (%)	18/37 (48.6)	14/25 (56.0)	$P = 0.570$
Intraoperative blood loss (mL)	400 (100–4700)	800 (150–4400)	$P = 0.280$
Type of hepatectomy, *n* (%)			
Right hemihepatectomy	22 (59.5)	17 (68.0)	
Left hemihepatectomy	2 (5.4)	0	
Right trisectionectomy	9 (24.3)	6 (24.0)	
Left trisectionectomy	4 (10.8)	2 (8.0)	
Clinical data after stage 2 surgery			
Complications, *n* (%)	35/37 (94.6)	22/25 (88)	$P = 0.385$
Major complications (≥IIIa)	20/37 (54.1)	5/25 (20)	$P = 0.007$
Grade III	($n = 18$, 48.6)	($n = 4$, 16.0)	
Bile leak ± ascites ± pleural effusion	11 (29.7)	1 (4.0)	
Atelectasis + intra-abdominal infection	1 (2.7)	0	
Pleural effusion + hemorrhage	2 (5.4)	0	
Pleural effusion + disruption of wound	1 (2.7)	0	
Pleural effusion	1 (2.7)	2 (8.0)	
Hemorrhage	0	1 (4.0)	
Ascites	1 (2.7)	0	
Bile leakage	1 (2.7)	0	
Grade IV	($n = 2$, 5.4)	($n = 1$, 4.0)	
Liver failure	2 (5.4)	1 (4.0)	

(continued)

Table 16.2 (continued)

Index	Findings		P value
	ALPPS group	TACE + PVE group	
Resection margin (cm)	1 (0.5–2.0)	1 (0.5–2.2)	$P = 0.602$
Postoperative liver failure, *n* (%)	13/37 (35.1)	6/25 (24.0)	$P = 0.351$
Grade A	5	3	
Grade B	5	2	
Grade C	3	1	
Death in 90 days, *n* (%)	2/38 (5.3)	2/38 (5.3)	$P = 1.000$
Cause of death: liver failure	2	2	
HCC recurrence on follow-up	19/37 (51.4)	13/25 (52.0)	
Treatment of recurrence			
Rehepatectomy	1 (2.7)	1 (4.0)	
TACE	2 (5.4)	5 (20.0)	
TACE + sorafenib	5 (13.5)	0	
Percutaneous microwave coagulation therapy (PMCT)	2 (5.4)	1 (4.0)	
PMCT + TACE	0	1 (4.0)	
PMCT + radiofrequency ablation (RFA)	2 (5.4)	0	
External radiation	2 (5.4)	0	
Sorafenib	3 (8.1)	3 (12.0)	
Supportive treatment	2 (5.4)	2 (8.0)	

Note: *PVL* portal vein ligation, *Lt* left portal vein trunk, *Rt* right portal vein trunk

Table 16.3 FLR growth in the groups

Index	Result				P value
	ALPPS group		TACE + PVE group		
	$n = 38$	P value	$n = 38$	P value	
Liver hypertrophy time/d	12 (8.0–30)		42(28.0–131)		<0.001
FLR before 1st operation	462.5 (299.0–666)		440 (249.0–635)		0.114
ΔFLR, median (range)/mL	172 (97.0–457)		158.5 (3.0–460)		0.169
$\Delta FLR/FLR_1$, median (range)/%	38 (18.0–104)		39 (1.0–163)		0.618
ΔFLR/d (mL/d)	15.4 (4.843.4)		3.8(0.1–8.0)		<0.001
Tumor volume before the 1st operation/mL	451(18.0–2493)	0.408	397(9.0–1677)	0.433	0.728
Tumor volume before the 2nd operation or the last examination/mL	489 (23.0–2503)		480 (7.0–2965)		0.685

Note: Liver hypertrophy time, the waiting time between the two operations or the time span from the first stage operation to treatment failure. ΔFLR, the increase in future liver remnant volume between the two operations. ΔFLR/FLR1, the increase of future liver remnant volume between the two operations divided by the volume of future liver remnant before the first operation

FibroTouch elastography value ($\beta = -0.58$, 95%CI: −0.92–0.23, $P = 0.001$) significantly associated with FLR growth rate.

The METAVIR score of 37 patients undergoing second-stage hepatectomy in the ALPPS group showed that KGR was negatively correlated with the severity of liver fibrosis and cirrhosis ($P = 0.007$). ALPPS group was divided into the portal hypertension subgroup ($n = 14$) and the non-portal hypertension subgroup ($n = 24$). There was a significant difference in KGR between the two subgroups ($P = 0.022$) but no statistically significant difference in FLR increase ($P = 0.126$).

When the TACE + PVE group was further divided into the portal hypertension subgroup (n = 12) and the non-portal hypertension subgroup (n = 26), the latter showed a significantly faster KGR ($P < 0.001$) and greater FLR hypertrophy ($P = 0.001$).

Most patients in both groups underwent right hemihepatectomy or right trisectionectomy, except for two patients in the ALPPS group whose left liver was larger than the right liver and underwent left hemihepatectomy. In the TACE + PVE group, the second-stage operation time and Pringle's maneuver time were significantly longer than those in the ALPPS group. Patients in this group had more intraoperative blood loss than the other group, but the difference was not statistically significant.

There was a statistically significant difference in major complications (≥IIIa) between the two groups of patients after stage 2 hepatectomy (Table 16.2). In the ALPPS group, 20 out of 37 patients (54.1%) experienced major complications, whereas in the TACE + PVE group, five out of 25 patients (20.0%) developed major complications (HR = 2.70, 95%CI: 1.17–6.25, $P = 0.007$). Postoperative complications were all resolved successfully with active treatment. Two patients in each group died of liver failure within 90 days after surgery. Except for one patient with persistently low serum prealbumin and cholinesterase level, liver functions in all other liver failure patients fully recovered. There were no R1/R2 resections and no viral reactivation during the follow-up period.

Median follow-up time was 42 months (IQR: 38–45). The 3-year OS rate in the ALPPS group was 65.8% (95%CI: 50.7–80.9), significantly better than that in the TACE + PVE group (42.1%, 95%CI: 26.4–57.8) (HR = 0.50, 95%CI: 0.26–0.98, two-sided $P = 0.036$). This significant difference is primarily attributed to the higher tumor resection rate with ALPPS compared to PVE. Cox regression analysis showed that ALPPS treatment (HR = 0.34, 95%CI: 0.16–0.74, $P = 0.006$), smaller tumor size (HR = 1.00, 95%CI: 1.00–1.00, $P = 0.0028$), solitary tumor (HR = 11.83, 95%CI: 3.98–35.15, $P < 0.001$), and the absence of severe fibrosis (HR = 2.49, 95%CI: 1.22–5.10, $P = 0.012$) were significant risk factors affecting OS. No significant difference was observed in OS after tumor resection between the two groups (HR = 0.80, 95%CI: 0.35–1.83, two-sided $P = 0.595$). Nonetheless, a significant difference was shown in OS between patients who did and did not undergo liver resection in the TACE + PVE group (HR = 4.45, 95%CI: 1.85–10.68, two-sided $P < 0.001$). There was no statistically significant difference in DFS after tumor resection between the two groups (HR = 0.94, 95%CI: 0.47–1.91, two-sided $P = 0.869$). The 3-year DFS of 37 patients in the ALPPS group and 25 patients in the TACE + PVE group were 48.6% (95%CI: 32.5–64.8) and 48% (95%CI: 28.4–67.6), respectively, with no significant difference between the two groups (Fig. 16.1).

Surgeons who support ALPPS believe that it significantly improves the success rate of liver resection [69, 73, 88]. Conversely, those who oppose this procedure argue that its morbidity and mortality rates are excessively high [89]. Over more than a decade of development, improvements in technique and stringent patient selection have led to a reduction in the morbidity and mortality rates associated with ALPPS [90, 91]. However, the majority of reports on ALPPS pertain to colorectal liver metastasis, with relatively few studies addressing its application in HCC [92, 93]. The former usually involves multiple secondary tumors in a normal liver, whereas the latter features larger primary tumors arising in a liver complicated by viral hepatitis. Recent reports indicate that cirrhosis affects the rate of FLR hypertrophy and the recovery of liver function after ALPPS. It remains unclear whether ALPPS can be used for patients with primary or metastatic liver cancer and whether it can replace PVE.

Based on our results, ALPPS facilitated a sufficient increase in FLR even in HCC patients with HBV-related

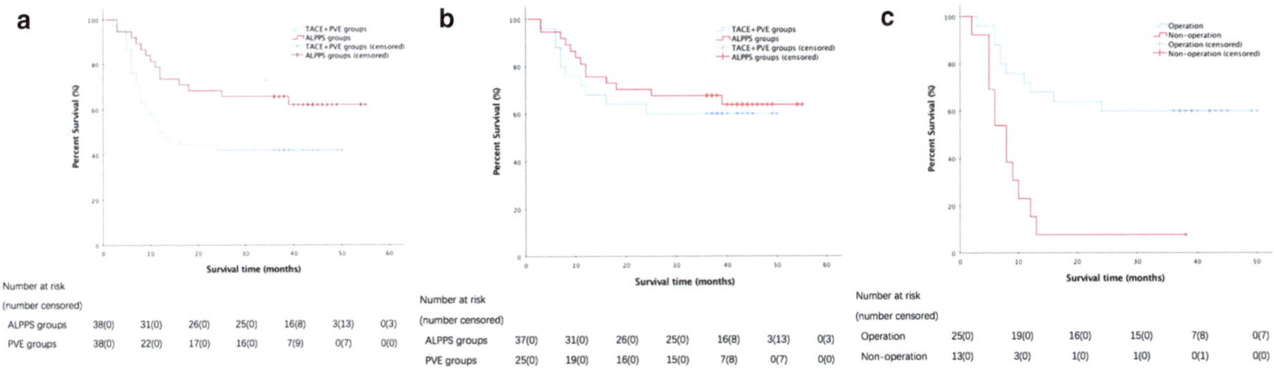

Fig. 16.1 Overall survivals between different groups. (**a**) Comparison of overall survivals between all the patients (including the patients with or without tumor resection) in 2 groups. (**b**) Comparison of overall survivals between the patients who had undergone stage-2 tumor resection in 2 groups. (**c**) Comparison of overall survivals between the patients with and without tumor resection in PVE groups. (This figure is reprinted with permission from the source of Ref. [70])

liver fibrosis. Nonetheless, for those with more severe cirrhosis, the growth rate and volume of FLR were limited and could not meet the criteria for stage 2 resection in one patient. Results also showed superiority of ALPPS over TACE + PVE in the following aspects.

(a) The interval between the first- and second-stage surgeries was significantly shortened.
(b) The tumor resection rate was significantly higher.
(c) The waiting time for the second stage was significantly reduced.

These significantly increased the surgical resection rate and prolonged the OS of patients in the ALPPS group. Nevertheless, among those who successfully underwent the stage 2 resection, there was no significant difference in OS between the two groups. In the PVE group, the OS rate was significantly better in those patients who were able to undergo stage 2 hepatectomy, suggesting that improving the tumor resection rate after PVE shall be a focus of future research. Similar to other reported studies, the incidence of major complications (≥IIIa) in the ALPPS group in this study was significantly higher than that in the PVE group, but there was no significant difference in the 90-day mortality rate between the two groups. Stringent patient selection and the adoption of minimally invasive surgical techniques can significantly reduce postoperative complications and mortality rates. Techniques such as three-dimensional visualization can preoperatively display the three-dimensional anatomy and anatomical variations of major intrahepatic vessels, and the application of laparoscopic techniques and microwave ablation can make ALPPS minimally invasive.

Latest studies have shown that PVE with small spherical particles results in improved liver hypertrophy and resection rates compared with larger, nonspherical particles [45]. In addition, as n-butyl cyanoacrylate (NBCA) can completely embolize the terminal branches of the portal vein and the portal venous communicating branches, the increase in FLR volume has been reported to be rapid enough to allow a significant proportion of patients to undergo stage 2 hepatectomy before tumor progression [94].

The study showed that portal hypertension reduced the rate of increase in FLR volume and the rate of stage 2 liver resection. The KGR was negatively correlated with the severity of liver fibrosis and cirrhosis. These findings indicated that ALPPS or PVE should be carried out with great caution in patients with severe cirrhosis and portal hypertension.

This study also found that the increase in liver volume after ALPPS or PVE did not necessarily correlate with synchronous recovery of liver function. One patient in the study had persistently low levels of prealbumin and cholinesterase, suggesting a suboptimal recovery of synthetic function [72]. The decision on the second-stage surgery should be made based on a comprehensive assessment of FLR, ICR-R15, prealbumin and cholinesterase levels, and 99mTc-GSA scintigram [95, 96].

The results of this study demonstrated that the OS of patients undergoing ALPPS was significantly higher than that of patients undergoing PVE, with no significant difference in the postoperative mortality rate between the two groups (Table 16.4).

In summary, ALPPS is a breakthrough in hepatic surgery over the past decade. Whether it can replace PVE requires validation through large-sample, multicenter, randomized controlled trials.

Table 16.4 Comparison between ALPPS and PVE

Authors, year of publication	Title	Study type, population, sample size	Complication and mortality rates	Oncological outcomes
Bednarsch et al. [77], 2020, Germany	ALPPS versus two-stage hepatectomy for colorectal liver metastases—a comparative retrospective cohort study	Retrospective controlled cohort study Colorectal cancer liver metastasis patients who received ALPPS or PVE from 2011 to 2017 Total sample size $n = 58$ (ALPPS = 21, PVE = 37)	There were no significant differences in the incidence of complications and mortality between the two groups after the first and the second stages	[a]The median survival of the ALPPS group and the PVE group were 28 months and 34 months, respectively ($P = 0.297$); the 3- and 5-year disease-free survival rates of the ALPPS group and the PVE group were 43% and 43% versus 8% and 8%, respectively; the 3- and 5-year OS of the ALPPS group and the PVE group were 37% and 37% versus 44% and 33%, respectively

(continued)

Table 16.4 (continued)

Authors, year of publication	Title	Study type, population, sample size	Complication and mortality rates	Oncological outcomes
Chan et al. [73], 2021, China	ALPPS versus portal vein embolization for hepatitis-related hepatocellular carcinoma: a changing paradigm in modulation of future liver remnant before major hepatectomy	Retrospective controlled cohort study Hepatocellular carcinoma patients who underwent FLR hyperplasia due to insufficient FLR from 2002 to 2018 Total sample size $n = 148$ (ALPPS = 46, PVE = 102)	There were no significant differences in the incidence of complications (20.7% vs 30.4%, $P = 0.159$) and mortality (6.5% vs 5.8%, $P = 1.000$) between the ALPPS group and the PVE group	[a]The 1, 3, and 5-year DFS of the ALPPS group and the PVE group were 63.2%, 34.9%, 25.0% versus 61.4%, 41.8%, 40.7%, respectively ($P = 0.267$); the 1-, 3-, and 5-year OS of the ALPPS group and the PVE group were 84.7%, 60.2%, 46.8% versus 88.2%, 73.5%, 64.1%, respectively ($P = 0.234$)
Liu et al. [68], 2019, China	A systematic review and meta-analysis of associating liver partition and portal vein ligation for staged hepatectomy (ALPPS) versus traditional staged hepatectomy	Meta-analysis Included nine studies comparing ALPPS and PVE Total sample size $n = 557$	Compared with conventional staged liver resection, ALPPS had a higher postoperative complication rate after the second stage (RR = 1.19, 95%CI: 0.96–1.47) and a higher mortality (RR = 2.11, 95%CI: 1.02–4.33)	NA
Shindoh et al. [12], 2013, United States	Analysis of the efficacy of portal vein embolization for patients with extensive liver malignancy and very low future liver remnant volume, including a comparison with the associating liver partition with portal vein ligation for staged hepatectomy approach	Retrospective study The post-PVE results were compared with the ALPPS results reported in the literature The sample size in the PVE group was $n = 144$, and that in the ALPPS group was $n = 25$	There were differences in the incidence of complications and mortality between the two groups of patients. The incidence of bile leakage (Grade B or C), sepsis, and unplanned reoperation among patients in the ALPPS group was higher than those in the PVE group (24%, 20%, 28% versus 5.8%, 0%, 2.9%)	NA
Li et al. [70], 2021, China	Associating liver partition and portal vein ligation for staged hepatectomy versus sequential transarterial chemoembolization and portal vein embolization in staged hepatectomy for HBV-related hepatocellular carcinoma: a randomized comparative study	Prospective randomized controlled study Patients with hepatitis B-related liver cancer who received ALPPS or PVE from 2014 to 2016 Total sample size $n = 76$ (ALPPS = 38, PVE = 38)	There was a difference in the incidence of major complications between the ALPPS group and the PVE group after the second stage (54.1% vs 20.0%, $P = 0.007$)	[b]There was no statistically significant difference in DFS between the ALPPS group and the PVE group (HR = 0.94, 95%CI: 0.47–1.91, $P = 0.869$). The 3-year DFS of patients in the ALPPS group and PVE group were 48.6% and 48%, respectively; The 3-year OS of the ALPPS group (65.8%) was significantly better than that of the PVE group (42.1%) (HR = 0.50, 95%CI: 0.26–0.98, $P = 0.036$)

Note: [a]The above analysis is based on patients who have completed tumor resection in both the ALPPS and PVE groups
[b]The above analysis is based on all patients in the ALPPS and PVE groups, including those who have not completed tumor resection

References

1. Broering DC, Hillert C, Krupski G, et al. Portal vein embolization *vs.* portal vein ligation for induction of hypertrophy of the future liver remnant [J]. J Gastrointest Surg. 2002;6(6):905–13.
2. Hemming AW, Reed AI, Howard RJ, et al. Preoperative portal vein embolization for extended hepatectomy [J]. Ann Surg. 2003;237(5):686–91.
3. Farges O, Belghiti J, Kianmanesh R, et al. Portal vein embolization before right hepatectomy: prospective clinical trial [J]. Ann Surg. 2003;237(2):208–17.
4. Yamanaka N, Okamoto E, Kuwata K, et al. A multiple regression equation for prediction of posthepatectomy liver failure [J]. Ann Surg. 1984;200(5):658–63.
5. van Lienden KP, van den Esschert JW, de Graaf W, et al. Portal vein embolization before liver resection: a systematic review [J]. Cardiovasc Intervent Radiol. 2013;36(1):25–34.
6. Yamashita S, Sakamoto Y, Yamamoto S, et al. Efficacy of preoperative portal vein embolization among patients with hepatocellular carcinoma, biliary tract cancer, and colorectal liver metastases: a comparative study based on single-center experience of 319 cases [J]. Ann Surg Oncol. 2017;24(6):1557–68.
7. Shindoh J, Tzeng CW, Aloia TA, et al. Safety and efficacy of portal vein embolization before planned major or extended hepatectomy: an institutional experience of 358 patients [J]. J Gastrointest Surg. 2014;18(1):45–51.
8. Schweizer W, Duda P, Tanner S, et al. Experimental atrophy/hypertrophy complex (AHC) of the liver: portal vein, but not bile duct obstruction, is the main driving force for the development of AHC in the rat [J]. J Hepatol. 1995;23(1):71–8.
9. Fausto N, Campbell JS, Riehle KJ. Liver regeneration [J]. Hepatology. 2006;43(2 Suppl 1):S45–53.
10. Goto Y, Nagino M, Nimura Y. Doppler estimation of portal blood flow after percutaneous transhepatic portal vein embolization [J]. Ann Surg. 1998;228(2):209–13.
11. Taub R. Liver regeneration: from myth to mechanism [J]. Nat Rev Mol Cell Biol. 2004;5(10):836–47.
12. Shindoh J, Vauthey JN, Zimmitti G, et al. Analysis of the efficacy of portal vein embolization for patients with extensive liver malignancy and very low future liver remnant volume, including a comparison with the associating liver partition with portal vein ligation for staged hepatectomy approach [J]. J Am Coll Surg. 2013;217(1):126–33.
13. Corrêa D, Schwartz L, Jarnagin WR, et al. Kinetics of liver volume changes in the first year after portal vein embolization [J]. Arch Surg. 2010;145(4):351–4.
14. Abdalla EK, Hicks ME, Vauthey JN. Portal vein embolization: rationale, technique and future prospects [J]. Br J Surg. 2001;88(2):165–75.
15. Bégin A, Martel G, Lapointe R, et al. Accuracy of preoperative automatic measurement of the liver volume by CT-scan combined to a 3D virtual surgical planning software (3DVSP) [J]. Surg Endosc. 2014;28(12):3408–12.
16. Johnson TN, Tucker GT, Tanner MS, et al. Changes in liver volume from birth to adulthood: a meta-analysis [J]. Liver Transpl. 2005;11(12):1481–93.
17. Ribero D, Chun YS, Vauthey JN. Standardized liver volumetry for portal vein embolization [J]. Semin Intervent Radiol. 2008;25(2):104–9.
18. Vauthey JN, Abdalla EK, Doherty DA, et al. Body surface area and body weight predict total liver volume in Western adults [J]. Liver Transpl. 2002;8(3):233–40.
19. Kishi Y, Abdalla EK, Chun YS, et al. Three hundred and one consecutive extended right hepatectomies: evaluation of outcome based on systematic liver volumetry [J]. Ann Surg. 2009;250(4):540–8.
20. Ribero D, Abdalla EK, Madoff DC, et al. Portal vein embolization before major hepatectomy and its effects on regeneration, resectability and outcome [J]. Br J Surg. 2007;94(11):1386–94.
21. Azoulay D, Castaing D, Krissat J, et al. Percutaneous portal vein embolization increases the feasibility and safety of major liver resection for hepatocellular carcinoma in injured liver [J]. Ann Surg. 2000;232(5):665–72.
22. Adam R, Pascal G, Castaing D, et al. Tumor progression while on chemotherapy: a contraindication to liver resection for multiple colorectal metastases? [J]. Ann Surg. 2004;240(6):1052–61.
23. Shindoh J, Tzeng CW, Aloia TA, et al. Optimal future liver remnant in patients treated with extensive preoperative chemotherapy for colorectal liver metastases [J]. Ann Surg Oncol. 2013;20(8):2493–500.
24. Kiuchi T, Kasahara M, Uryuhara K, et al. Impact of graft size mismatching on graft prognosis in liver transplantation from living donors [J]. Transplantation. 1999;67(2):321–7.
25. Lin XJ, Yang J, Chen XB, et al. The critical value of remnant liver volume-to-body weight ratio to estimate posthepatectomy liver failure in cirrhotic patients [J]. J Surg Res. 2014;188(2):489–95.
26. Imamura H, Sano K, Sugawara Y, et al. Assessment of hepatic reserve for indication of hepatic resection: decision tree incorporating indocyanine green test [J]. J Hepato-Biliary-Pancreat Surg. 2005;12(1):16–22.
27. Hirai I, Kimura W, Fuse A, et al. Evaluation of preoperative portal embolization for safe hepatectomy, with special reference to assessment of nonembolized lobe function with ^{99m}Tc-GSA SPECT scintigraphy [J]. Surgery. 2003;133(5):495–506.
28. Lee SG, Hwang S. How I do it: assessment of hepatic functional reserve for indication of hepatic resection [J]. J Hepato-Biliary-Pancreat Surg. 2005;12(1):38–43.
29. Makuuchi M, Kosuge T, Takayama T, et al. Surgery for small liver cancers [J]. Semin Surg Oncol. 1993;9(4):298–304.
30. Fan ST. Liver functional reserve estimation: state of the art and relevance for local treatments: the Eastern perspective [J]. J Hepatobiliary Pancreat Sci. 2010;17(4):380–4.
31. Pugh RN, Murray-Lyon IM, Dawson JL, et al. Transection of the oesophagus for bleeding oesophageal varices [J]. Br J Surg. 1973;60(8):646–9.
32. Shindoh J, Tzeng CW, Vauthey JN. Portal vein embolization for hepatocellular carcinoma [J]. Liver Cancer. 2012;1(3–4):159–67.
33. Kuo SC, Azimi-Tabrizi A, Briggs G, et al. Portal vein embolization prior to major liver resection [J]. ANZ J Surg. 2014;84(5):341–5.
34. Truant S, Oberlin O, Sergent G, et al. Remnant liver volume to body weight ratio > or =0.5%: a new cut-off to estimate postoperative risks after extended resection in noncirrhotic liver [J]. J Am Coll Surg. 2007;204(1):22–33.
35. Oken MM, Creech RH, Tormey DC, et al. Toxicity and response criteria of the Eastern Cooperative Oncology Group [J]. Am J Clin Oncol. 1982;5(6):649–55.
36. Michalopoulos GK. Liver regeneration [J]. J Cell Physiol. 2007;213(2):286–300.
37. Ronot M, Cauchy F, Gregoli B, et al. Sequential transarterial chemoembolization and portal vein embolization before resection is a valid oncological strategy for unilobar hepatocellular carcinoma regardless of the tumor burden [J]. HPB. 2016;18(8):684–90.
38. Aoki T, Imamura H, Hasegawa K, et al. Sequential preoperative arterial and portal venous embolizations in patients with hepatocellular carcinoma [J]. Arch Surg. 2004;139(7):766–74.
39. Sugawara Y, Yamamoto J, Higashi H, et al. Preoperative portal embolization in patients with hepatocellular carcinoma [J]. World J Surg. 2002;26(1):105–10.
40. Terasawa M, Allard MA, Golse N, et al. Sequential transcatheter arterial chemoembolization and portal vein embolization versus portal vein embolization alone before major hepatectomy for

patients with large hepatocellular carcinoma: an intent-to-treat analysis [J]. Surgery. 2020;167(2):425–31.
41. Yoo H, Kim JH, Ko GY, et al. Sequential transcatheter arterial chemoembolization and portal vein embolization versus portal vein embolization only before major hepatectomy for patients with hepatocellular carcinoma [J]. Ann Surg Oncol. 2011;18(5):1251–7.
42. Ogata S, Belghiti J, Farges O, et al. Sequential arterial and portal vein embolizations before right hepatectomy in patients with cirrhosis and hepatocellular carcinoma [J]. Br J Surg. 2006;93(9):1091–8.
43. Abulkhir A, Limongelli P, Healey AJ, et al. Preoperative portal vein embolization for major liver resection: a meta-analysis [J]. Ann Surg. 2008;247(1):49–57.
44. de Baere T, Roche A, Elias D, et al. Preoperative portal vein embolization for extension of hepatectomy indications [J]. Hepatology. 1996;24(6):1386–91.
45. Madoff DC, Abdalla EK, Gupta S, et al. Transhepatic ipsilateral right portal vein embolization extended to segment IV: improving hypertrophy and resection outcomes with spherical particles and coils [J]. J Vasc Interv Radiol. 2005;16(2 Pt 1):215–25.
46. Di Stefano DR, de Baere T, Denys A, et al. Preoperative percutaneous portal vein embolization: evaluation of adverse events in 188 patients [J]. Radiology. 2005;234(2):625–30.
47. Imamura H, Shimada R, Kubota M, et al. Preoperative portal vein embolization: an audit of 84 patients [J]. Hepatology. 1999;29(4):1099–105.
48. Fischer C, Melstrom LG, Arnaoutakis D, et al. Chemotherapy after portal vein embolization to protect against tumor growth during liver hypertrophy before hepatectomy [J]. JAMA Surg. 2013;148(12):1103–8.
49. Goéré D, Farges O, Leporrier J, et al. Chemotherapy does not impair hypertrophy of the left liver after right portal vein obstruction [J]. J Gastrointest Surg. 2006;10(3):365–70.
50. Covey AM, Brown KT, Jarnagin WR, et al. Combined portal vein embolization and neoadjuvant chemotherapy as a treatment strategy for resectable hepatic colorectal metastases [J]. Ann Surg. 2008;247(3):451–5.
51. Zorzi D, Chun YS, Madoff DC, et al. Chemotherapy with bevacizumab does not affect liver regeneration after portal vein embolization in the treatment of colorectal liver metastases [J]. Ann Surg Oncol. 2008;15(10):2765–72.
52. Kodama Y, Shimizu T, Endo H, et al. Complications of percutaneous transhepatic portal vein embolization [J]. J Vasc Interv Radiol. 2002;13(12):1233–7.
53. Nagino M, Kamiya J, Nishio H, et al. Two hundred forty consecutive portal vein embolizations before extended hepatectomy for biliary cancer: surgical outcome and long-term follow-up [J]. Ann Surg. 2006;243(3):364–72.
54. Shindoh J, Tzeng CW, Aloia TA, et al. Portal vein embolization improves rate of resection of extensive colorectal liver metastases without worsening survival [J]. Br J Surg. 2013;100(13):1777–83.
55. Pamecha V, Levene A, Grillo F, et al. Effect of portal vein embolisation on the growth rate of colorectal liver metastases [J]. Br J Cancer. 2009;100(4):617–22.
56. Spelt L, Sparrelid E, Isaksson B, et al. Tumour growth after portal vein embolization with pre-procedural chemotherapy for colorectal liver metastases [J]. HPB. 2015;17(6):529–35.
57. Pommier R, Ronot M, Cauchy F, et al. Colorectal liver metastases growth in the embolized and non-embolized liver after portal vein embolization: influence of initial response to induction chemotherapy [J]. Ann Surg Oncol. 2014;21(9):3077–83.
58. Hayashi S, Baba Y, Ueno K, et al. Acceleration of primary liver tumor growth rate in embolized hepatic lobe after portal vein embolization [J]. Acta Radiol. 2007;48(7):721–7.
59. Li TJ, Zhu J, Ma KS, et al. Autologous bone marrow-derived mesenchymal stem cell transplantation promotes liver regeneration after portal vein embolization in cirrhotic rats [J]. J Surg Res. 2013;184(2):1161–73.
60. Kaibori M, Adachi Y, Shimo T, et al. Stimulation of liver regeneration after hepatectomy in mice by injection of bone marrow mesenchymal stem cells via the portal vein [J]. Transplant Proc. 2012;44(4):1107–9.
61. Fürst G, Schulte am Esch J, Poll LW, et al. Portal vein embolization and autologous $CD133^+$ bone marrow stem cells for liver regeneration: initial experience [J]. Radiology. 2007;243(1):171–9.
62. am Esch JS, Schmelzle M, Fürst G, et al. Infusion of $CD133^+$ bone marrow-derived stem cells after selective portal vein embolization enhances functional hepatic reserves after extended right hepatectomy: a retrospective single-center study [J]. Ann Surg. 2012;255(1):79–85.
63. Beppu T, Nitta H, Hayashi H, et al. Effect of branched-chain amino acid supplementation on functional liver regeneration in patients undergoing portal vein embolization and sequential hepatectomy: a randomized controlled trial [J]. J Gastroenterol. 2015;50(12):1197–205.
64. Hwang S, Lee SG, Ko GY, et al. Sequential preoperative ipsilateral hepatic vein embolization after portal vein embolization to induce further liver regeneration in patients with hepatobiliary malignancy [J]. Ann Surg. 2009;249(4):608–16.
65. Guiu B, Chevallier P, Denys A, et al. Simultaneous trans-hepatic portal and hepatic vein embolization before major hepatectomy: the liver venous deprivation technique [J]. Eur Radiol. 2016;26(12):4259–67.
66. de Santibañes E, Clavien PA. Playing Play-Doh to prevent postoperative liver failure: the "ALPPS" approach [J]. Ann Surg. 2012;255(3):415–7.
67. Eshmuminov D, Raptis DA, Linecker M, et al. Meta-analysis of associating liver partition with portal vein ligation and portal vein occlusion for two-stage hepatectomy [J]. Br J Surg. 2016;103(13):1768–82.
68. Liu YM, Yang YX, Gu SL, et al. A systematic review and meta-analysis of associating liver partition and portal vein ligation for staged hepatectomy (ALPPS) versus traditional staged hepatectomy [J]. Medicine (Baltimore). 2019;98(15):e15229.
69. Schadde E, Ardiles V, Slankamenac K, et al. ALPPS offers a better chance of complete resection in patients with primarily unresectable liver tumors compared with conventional-staged hepatectomies: results of a multicenter analysis [J]. World J Surg. 2014;38(6):1510–9.
70. Li PP, Huang G, Jia NY, et al. Associating liver partition and portal vein ligation for staged hepatectomy versus sequential transarterial chemoembolization and portal vein embolization in staged hepatectomy for HBV-related hepatocellular carcinoma: a randomized comparative study [J]. Hepatobiliary Surg Nutr. 2022;11(1):38–51.
71. Croome KP, Hernandez-Alejandro R, Parker M, et al. Is the liver kinetic growth rate in ALPPS unprecedented when compared with PVE and living donor liver transplant? A multicentre analysis [J]. HPB. 2015;17(6):477–84.
72. Matsuo K, Murakami T, Kawaguchi D, et al. Histologic features after surgery associating liver partition and portal vein ligation for staged hepatectomy versus those after hepatectomy with portal vein embolization [J]. Surgery. 2016;159(5):1289–98.
73. Chan A, Zhang WY, Chok K, et al. ALPPS versus portal vein embolization for hepatitis-related hepatocellular carcinoma: a changing paradigm in modulation of future liver remnant before major hepatectomy [J]. Ann Surg. 2021;273(5):957–65.
74. Olthof PB, Tomassini F, Huespe PE, et al. Hepatobiliary scintigraphy to evaluate liver function in associating liver partition and portal vein ligation for staged hepatectomy: liver volume overestimates liver function [J]. Surgery. 2017;162(4):775–83.
75. Sparrelid E, Jonas E, Tzortzakakis A, et al. Dynamic evaluation of liver volume and function in associating liver partition and por-

tal vein ligation for staged hepatectomy [J]. J Gastrointest Surg. 2017;21(6):967–74.
76. Dindo D, Demartines N, Clavien PA. Classification of surgical complications: a new proposal with evaluation in a cohort of 6336 patients and results of a survey [J]. Ann Surg. 2004;240(2):205–13.
77. Bednarsch J, Czigany Z, Sharmeen S, et al. ALPPS versus two-stage hepatectomy for colorectal liver metastases—a comparative retrospective cohort study [J]. World J Surg Oncol. 2020;18(1):140.
78. Sarin SK, Kumar M, Lau GK, et al. Asian-Pacific clinical practice guidelines on the management of hepatitis B: a 2015 update [J]. Hepatol Int. 2016;10(1):1–98.
79. Huang G, Li PP, Lau WY, et al. Antiviral therapy reduces hepatocellular carcinoma recurrence in patients with low HBV-DNA levels: a randomized controlled trial [J]. Ann Surg. 2018;268(6):943–54.
80. Shindoh J, Truty MJ, Aloia TA, et al. Kinetic growth rate after portal vein embolization predicts posthepatectomy outcomes: toward zero liver-related mortality in patients with colorectal liver metastases and small future liver remnant [J]. J Am Coll Surg. 2013;216(2):201–9.
81. Schnitzbauer AA, Lang SA, Goessmann H, et al. Right portal vein ligation combined with in situ splitting induces rapid left lateral liver lobe hypertrophy enabling 2-staged extended right hepatic resection in small-for-size settings [J]. Ann Surg. 2012;255(3):405–14.
82. Sandström P, Røsok BI, Sparrelid E, et al. ALPPS improves resectability compared with conventional two-stage hepatectomy in patients with advanced colorectal liver metastasis: results from a Scandinavian multicenter randomized controlled trial (LIGRO trial) [J]. Ann Surg. 2018;267(5):833–40.
83. Augustin S, Millán L, González A, et al. Detection of early portal hypertension with routine data and liver stiffness in patients with asymptomatic liver disease: a prospective study [J]. J Hepatol. 2014;60(3):561–9.
84. Foucher J, Chanteloup E, Vergniol J, et al. Diagnosis of cirrhosis by transient elastography (FibroScan): a prospective study [J]. Gut. 2006;55(3):403–8.
85. Rahbari NN, Garden OJ, Padbury R, et al. Posthepatectomy liver failure: a definition and grading by the International Study Group of Liver Surgery (ISGLS) [J]. Surgery. 2011;149(5):713–24.
86. Bedossa P, Poynard T. An algorithm for the grading of activity in chronic hepatitis C. The METAVIR Cooperative Study Group [J]. Hepatology. 1996;24(2):289–93.
87. Zhang GQ, Zhang ZW, Lau WY, et al. Associating liver partition and portal vein ligation for staged hepatectomy (ALPPS): a new strategy to increase resectability in liver surgery [J]. Int J Surg. 2014;12(5):437–41.
88. Jiao LR, Fajardo Puerta AB, Gall TMH, et al. Rapid induction of liver regeneration for major hepatectomy (REBIRTH): a randomized controlled trial of portal vein embolisation versus ALPPS assisted with radiofrequency [J]. Cancers. 2019;11(3):302.
89. Ratti F, Schadde E, Masetti M, et al. Strategies to increase the resectability of patients with colorectal liver metastases: a multi-center case-match analysis of ALPPS and conventional two-stage hepatectomy [J]. Ann Surg Oncol. 2015;22(6):1933–42.
90. Li J, Ewald F, Gulati A, et al. Associating liver partition and portal vein ligation for staged hepatectomy: from technical evolution to oncological benefit [J]. World J Gastrointest Surg. 2016;8(2):124–33.
91. Linecker M, Björnsson B, Stavrou GA, et al. Risk adjustment in ALPPS is associated with a dramatic decrease in early mortality and morbidity [J]. Ann Surg. 2017;266(5):779–86.
92. Chan ACY, Chok K, Dai JWC, et al. Impact of split completeness on future liver remnant hypertrophy in associating liver partition and portal vein ligation for staged hepatectomy (ALPPS) in hepatocellular carcinoma: complete-ALPPS versus partial-ALPPS [J]. Surgery. 2017;161(2):357–64.
93. Wang Z, Peng YF, Hu JW, et al. Associating liver partition and portal vein ligation for staged hepatectomy for unresectable hepatitis B virus-related hepatocellular carcinoma: a single center study of 45 patients [J]. Ann Surg. 2020;271(3):534–41.
94. Luz JHM, Luz PM, Bilhim T, et al. Portal vein embolization with n-butyl-cyanoacrylate through an ipsilateral approach before major hepatectomy: single center analysis of 50 consecutive patients [J]. Cancer Imaging. 2017;17(1):25.
95. Truant S, Baillet C, Deshorgue AC, et al. Drop of total liver function in the interstages of the new associating liver partition and portal vein ligation for staged hepatectomy technique: analysis of the "auxiliary liver" by HIDA scintigraphy [J]. Ann Surg. 2016;263(3):e33–4.
96. Kwon AH, Matsui Y, Ha-Kawa SK, et al. Functional hepatic volume measured by technetium-99m-galactosyl-human serum albumin liver scintigraphy: comparison between hepatocyte volume and liver volume by computed tomography [J]. Am J Gastroenterol. 2001;96(2):541–6.

17 Liver Surgery in the Era of ALPPS

Albert Chan

ALPPS is considered one of the most monumental advancements in liver surgery over the past decade. This technique has undoubtedly revolutionized the management of patients undergoing extensive hepatic resection with an inadequate future liver remnant (FLR). In the initial development phase of ALPPS, the rapid augmentation of the FLR induced prior to liver resection sparked some debate concerning the safety of this procedure and whether it would enhance the safety margin of subsequent extensive hepatectomies. In the early series of cases documented by Andreas A. Schnitzbauer et al., the surgical mortality rate was 12% [1]. A global registry documented a 40% rate of significant complications (Clavien-Dindo IIIa or above) and a 9% surgical mortality rate [2]. Recognizing the risk factors associated with postoperative complications and death can enhance patient selection processes and improve overall results.

17.1 Posthepatectomy Liver Failure

Posthepatectomy liver failure (PHLF) accounts for 75% of ALPPS-related fatalities [2, 3]. According to the 5050 criteria [4], the ALPPS registry reported a 9% incidence of this complication. Although the median FLR volume escalates rapidly by 80% before the Stage 2 procedure, 80% of PHLF patients possess an FLR that surpasses 30% of total hepatic volume before this stage. Critics have contended that the swift FLR growth in ALPPS results from tissue edema rather than mere hypertrophy [5]. Others have voiced concerns regarding whether the volumetric increase is accompanied by a corresponding enhancement in function [6, 7]. Functional volume assessment employing hepatobiliary scintigraphy (HBS) has exhibited a discordance between FLR volume augmentation and functional improvement, with ^{99}mTc mebrofenin HBS testing revealing that the functional increase is merely half of the volumetric expansion [8]. This could partly explain why PHLF continues to be notably more common following Stage 2 ALPPS, even with adequate FLR volume increase.

A study of 320 patients from the ALPPS registry showed that the leading risk factor for 90-day mortality was being over 60 years old (OR = 14.3, P = 0.001) [3]. Additionally, biochemical markers measured between the two ALPPS stages can help predict postoperative mortality. A Model for End-Stage Liver Disease (MELD) score exceeding 10 prior to the second phase of ALPPS (odds ratio [OR] = 4.9, P = 0.006) and post-hepatectomy liver failure (PHLF) after the initial stage, indicated by a sustained increase in international normalized ratio (INR) and elevated serum bilirubin levels on day 5 post-operation as defined by the International Study Group for Liver Surgery (ISGLS) (OR = 3.9, P = 0.011), are independent predictors of PHLF following ALPPS [9]. These laboratory indicators are straightforward, objective, and reproducible, enabling clinicians to evaluate the risk of conducting Stage 2.

Another study based on the data from the ALPPS registry developed a postoperative mortality risk prediction model for the staged procedure. Risk factors for Stage 1 include older age (>67 years, odds ratio [OR] = 5.7) and biliary malignancy (OR = 3.8). For Stage 2, predictive factors include the cumulative risk score from Stage 1 (OR = 1.9), severe complications from Stage 1 (greater than grade IIIb, OR = 3.4), and increased levels of serum bilirubin (OR = 4.4) and creatinine (OR = 5.4). The findings underscore the importance of patient selection prior to Stage 1. The risk score for advanced age is 3, while those for biliary tumors and non-colorectal liver metastases/non-biliary tumors are 2 and 1, respectively. The surgery-related mortality rates for total scores of 0, 1, 2, 3, 4, and 5 are 3%, 5%, 9%, 15%, 24%, and 37%, respectively [10]. This risk model provides an objective assessment of mortality risk. Its scoring system

A. Chan (✉)
Queen Mary Hospital, University of Hong Kong, Hong Kong, China
e-mail: acchan@hku.hk

J. Zhou (ed.), *Associating Liver Partition and Portal Vein Ligation for Staged Hepatectomy (ALPPS)*,
https://doi.org/10.1007/978-981-96-7364-3_17

helps determine whether to delay or cancel the second stage of the procedure. The incorporation of serum bilirubin and creatinine levels suggests that Stage 2 surgery should be postponed until liver and kidney function return to normal, consistent with Erik Schadde et al.'s finding that mortality increased when surgery was conducted in patients with a high preoperative MELD score (>10, odds ratio [OR] = 4.9) in Stage 2 (P = 0.006) [3]. However, it's important to note that the inclusion of the Stage 1 cumulative score (reflecting factors like age and indication) and Stage 1 complications indicate that these unfavorable risk factors will continue to impact Stage 2 outcomes, even if liver and kidney function normalize.

Experience with portal vein embolization (PVE) has illustrated that the growth rate of FLR is correlated with hepatic regeneration potential [11, 12]. Patients with a kinetic growth rate (KGR) >2% per week exhibit fewer instances of PHLF following liver resection. Patryk Kambakamba et al. investigated its relevance in ALPPS. A retrospective analysis of 38 ALPPS patients revealed that KGR was more reliable in predicting PHLF than FLR volume alone [13]. A KGR ≥6% per day and an FLR >30% 1 week after Stage 1 ALPPS were correlated with the absence of postoperative PHLF. This closely aligns with the median KGR cutoff of 7% per day in the ALPPS registry [2]. Conversely, Matteo Serenari et al. [14] employed ^{99m}Tc methylbrompheniramine HBS to evaluate FLR function during the between-stage period and formulated a model known as the "HIBA index" to predict PHLF. In a cohort of 20 ALPPS patients, a critical value below 15% demonstrated a sensitivity of 100% and a specificity of 94% for such prediction. These results indicate that hepatic scintigraphy (HBS) can serve as an additional tool, complementing biochemical tests and liver volume assessments, to evaluate the function of the FLR. They demonstrate that patients with compromised FLR function may need more time for additional tissue hypertrophy to achieve sufficient liver growth, ensuring a safer tumor resection.

17.2 Bile Leakage

In the early stages of ALPPS, bile leakage was one of the most common surgical complications. Data from the ALPPS registry indicate that this adverse event occurred in 17% of ALPPS procedures [2]. The most common site of leakage was the tumor-side liver transection plane, attributed to segment IV ischemia caused by portal vein ligation (PVL) and the separation of liver parenchyma between the left internal lobe and the left lateral lobe. The risk associated with right trisegmentectomy in ALPPS is particularly high [15], as cutting off the perfusion of the segment IV portal vein and artery can lead to necrosis, bile leakage, and sepsis, which are major problems in this approach.

Cholangiocarcinoma is an additional risk factor for bile leakage [16]. Tumor infiltration makes hilar anatomical dissection technically difficult, while portal lymph node dissection further disrupts the blood supply to the transection plane [17]. Complications in ALPPS are strongly tied to the complexity of the surgery. Data from the ALPPS registry highlight that independent risk factors for severe complications (Clavien-Dindo grade IIIb or higher) include a prolonged Stage 1 operation time (over 300 minutes, odds ratio [OR] = 4.42, P = 0.004), the need for blood transfusion (OR = 5.26, P = 0.001), and liver metastases from non-colorectal origins (OR = 2.73, P = 0.049) [2]. In cases of hilar cholangiocarcinoma, ALPPS is associated with a higher incidence of posthepatectomy liver failure (PHLF) and surgical mortality [16, 18].

17.3 Strategies to Improve Outcomes

Many new surgical techniques initially yield suboptimal results. However, with accumulating experience, improved outcomes are possible through careful patient selection and technical refinements. Establishing an international registry could systematically collect data on ALPPS cases [2]. As knowledge and understanding of the procedure grow, hepatobiliary surgeons can better identify appropriate candidates and enhance their methods to optimize results.

Elderly patients are generally not ideal candidates for ALPPS. Data from the ALPPS registry indicate that those over 60 face a higher risk of severe complications (Clavien-Dindo grade IIIb or higher, odds ratio [OR] = 3.76, P = 0.007) and elevated mortality rates (OR = 14.3, P = 0.001) [2, 3]. Colorectal cancer liver metastasis (CRLM) and hepatocellular carcinoma (HCC) in the elderly also exhibit poor survival rates [2, 19]. ALPPS is a physiologically demanding procedure. While chronological cutoff values may be impractical, it is prudent to avoid this procedure in patients with advanced physiological age whose life expectancy is limited in the event of major complications, which are not uncommon. From an oncological perspective, complete involvement of the right portal vein and a small contralateral FLR constitute another relative contraindication for ALPPS. Given that the tumor-bearing liver segment has already been embolized, adding in situ liver resection will hardly induce further liver hypertrophy. In such cases, alternative treatments for tumor downstage to ameliorate respectability would be a more sensible approach.

For extensive hepatectomy, the ratio of FLR to estimated standard liver volume (ESLV) must reach 25% to ensure adequate hepatic function post-surgery in patients with liver tumors without underlying liver disease [20–22]. For patients with underlying hepatic conditions (such as cirrhosis and cholestasis), a ratio exceeding 30% is required [21]. When the FLR is considered insufficient, two-stage hepatectomy (TSH) with portal vein embolization (PVE) or portal vein ligation (PVL) is a well-recognized approach that can increase FLR volume by 10–30% throughout 4–6 weeks [23]. Despite this, 10–40% of patients are ineligible for TSH due to suboptimal FLR hypertrophy and tumor progression [24–29].

ALPPS can swiftly induce significant FLR hypertrophy—growth of 40–80% within 7–10 days [24–29]—but at the expense of higher morbidity and mortality. In theory, when the FLR is critically small, or there's a significant risk of tumor progression between stages—such as increased invasiveness and widespread metastasis—and PVE/PVL is unlikely to succeed, ALPPS may offer the greatest advantage. In the prospective LIGRO trial, ALPPS was directly compared to PVE/PVL, with the FLR standardized to an estimated standard liver volume (FLR/ESLV) of less than 30% as part of the study design [30]. In general, ALPPS can accommodate a lower FLR/ESLV ratio. Francesca Ratti et al. [31] suggested this approach for patients with an FLR below 20% who could not attain sufficient FLR volume through traditional two-stage hepatectomy (TSH). However, there is still no agreement on the optimal FLR for ALPPS. Accepting elevated surgical risks might be justifiable when conventional TSH is unlikely to yield sufficient FLR growth. Based on data from the International ALPPS registry, the median FLR/ESLV prior to Stage 1 is 21% (interquartile range [IQR] 17–27%), and with an 80% FLR increase within 7 days, the FLR/ESLV rises to 40% (IQR 31–47%) [2]. ALPPS is expected to increase surgical complications and mortality in high-risk patients with critically low FLR and should be reserved for experienced centers.

17.4 Is ALPPS Superior to TSH?

The principle of hepatectomy is to completely remove the tumor while retaining sufficient FLR. Large bilobar tumors and insufficient FLR are frequent barriers to radical resection. Before ALPPS was introduced, PVE and PVL were used to enhance FLR prior to major hepatectomy. PVE increases FLR by 12–62% in 3–8 weeks [24, 26, 32–34]. For patients with tumors involving both lobes, complete resection can be accomplished by TSH. In the first stage, the tumor in the FLR is removed, and during the interval before the second stage to excise all remaining tumors, the FLR grows while systemic treatment is administered to control disease progression. Second-stage liver resection can be combined with PVL to facilitate FLR augmentation. Some recent studies have compared ALPPS with TSH (PVL or PVE) in terms of surgical and oncological results.

17.4.1 Surgical Outcomes

A case-control comparison of ALPPS and TSH demonstrated that ALPPS induced more prominent FLR hypertrophy (50–80% vs. 10–40%) in a shorter time interval (7–11 days vs. 20–103 days) and a higher tumor resection rate (80–100% vs. 60–90%) [24, 26, 32–35]. In terms of major complications (Clavien-Dindo grade IIIa or higher), the results were less consistent, but the incidence for both approaches generally ranged from 20% to 40% [24, 26, 28, 33–35]. Common complications included bile leak, peritoneal effusion, and pleural effusion [34]. According to a pooled-data meta-analysis, no statistically significant difference in the overall complication rate was detected, but the major complication rate has not yet been compared [36]. The rates of PHLF (10% vs. 14%, OR = 0.86) and 90-day mortality (9% vs. 5%, OR = 1.44) were comparable between the two groups [36].

In a prospective randomized trial [30], all participants (100 CRLM patients with FLR/ESLV <30%) received preoperative chemotherapy and obtained oncological remission or at least stable disease. The average FLR/ESLV values were 22% in the ALPPS group and 21% in the TSH group. In the ALPPS group, which included 48 patients, 44 (92%) achieved sufficient FLR/ESLV growth (≥30%) and successfully completed Stage 2 hepatectomy within 14 days. Conversely, in the TSH group (n = 49), 13 patients (27%) failed to achieve adequate FLR expansion, and eight patients (16%) could not proceed to Stage 2 due to tumor progression. Notably, 12 of them (24% in the TSH group) successfully received rescue ALPPS. Prospective trials have shown that ALPPS is correlated with a higher resection rate (92% vs. 57%, $P < 0.001$). Nevertheless, the two strategies shared similar major complication rates (43% vs. 43%, $P = 0.99$) and 90-day mortality rates (8% vs. 6%, $P = 0.68$).

17.4.2 Oncological Results

From an oncological point of view, ALPPS is considered a viable surgical option thanks to its remarkable FLR augmentation effect, which facilitates tumor resection in patients with borderline FLR. Rapid induction of FLR growth shortens the between-stage interval and reduces treatment failure due to disease progression. However, leaving a high-burden tumor in the body within an immunosuppressive and stressful environment remains a concern, as stimulating FLR hypertrophy may also cause residual tumor progression [37, 38]. When performing TSH for CRLM patients, imaging and pathological examinations (including Ki67 index), verified tumor progression [39–42]. Nonetheless, these findings were not replicated in ALPPS patients. K. Tanaka et al. [33] examined Ki67 expression in both approaches and found a notable increase in this marker with PVE, but not in ALPPS cases. Similarly, Katharina Joechle et al. [43] reported that markers of tumor proliferation and angiogenesis were comparable between patients undergoing ALPPS and those receiving standard liver resection.

Data from the ALPPS registry illustrated that the 1- and 2-year overall survival (OS) rates for CRLM were 76% and 62%, respectively [2], which are comparable to the results of large-scale studies of TSH [44]. The indications of most case-control studies are mixed and heterogeneous, and comparative studies of CRLM patients alone are limited to two small retrospective series. Francesca Ratti et al. [26] compared 12 patients who received ALPPS with 36 patients who received TSH, matching them according to local staging and liver tumor status. With the lowest dropout rate in the TSH group (6%), the one-year OS (92% vs. 94%) and disease-free survival (DFS) (67% vs. 80%) of the two groups were comparable, and the R0 resection rate of patients who completed tumor resection in both groups was 100%.

According to Rene Adam et al. [34], in spite of a higher tumor resection rate (100% vs. 63%, $P < 0.001$), the 2-year median OS rate of patients in the ALPPS group was lower (42% vs. 77%, $P = 0.006$). This result differs significantly from the data of the ALPPS registry (2-year OS of 62%) and must be interpreted with caution. The R0 resection rate was low in both groups (17.6% vs. 19.5%, $P = 0.67$). Most patients in this study experienced early recurrence (1-year DFS: 0 vs. 10%, $P = 0.21$). The advanced tumor stage before surgery may be the primary reason. Six patients (35%) in the ALPPS group and 12 (29%) in the TSH group had extrahepatic metastases, with a median number of 10 extrahepatic metastases (five cases in the study of Francesca Ratti et al. [26]). The inferior oncological outcomes could be the result of aggressive tumor biology rather than the choice of surgical approach.

Recently, the results of a prospective randomized controlled trial reported by Per Sandstrom et al. [30] demonstrated that the R0 resection rates of ALPPS and TSH were analogous (77% vs. 57%, $P = 0.11$), but long-term survival data have not yet been obtained. Given that ALPPS has only been implemented for a relatively brief period, long-term oncological data are scarce. It remains uncertain whether the theoretical benefits of ALPPS will ultimately result in tangible improvements compared to TSH.

17.5 ALPPS and "Super" ALPPS: RAPID

The enhanced comprehension of ALPPS and its associated clinical physiological alterations has spurred the development of innovative methodologies and their integration into liver transplantation practices. In 2015, surgeons from Norway described a new procedure called "resection and partial segment 2/3 transplantation followed by delayed total hepatectomy" (RAPID) for the treatment of unresectable bilobar CRLM [45]. During the operation, segments II and III of the liver are initially resected, and then the graft (left lateral lobe) is implanted, followed by ligation of the right branch of the portal vein. After 2–3 weeks, the graft achieves sufficient growth, making the complete resection of the tumor-bearing liver possible. RAPID combines auxiliary liver transplantation and ALPPS (PVL combined with liver partition). Further modifications have been reported, including the use of partial living donor liver grafts [46] and expanded applications to cirrhotic patients [47]. Nevertheless, the procedure remains largely experimental, especially for cirrhosis, and more data is warranted before it can become standard treatment.

In summary, ALPPS challenges the concept of unresectable hepatectomy. It offers patients with insufficient FLR a chance of cure. This innovative technique pushes the boundaries of liver surgery but is controversial due to high morbidity and mortality. The surgical mortality rate is typically due to PHLF, which can be reduced by carefully choosing suitable patients. Older patients have reduced capacity to handle major surgery, while those with CRLM possess healthy livers, making them strong candidates for ALPPS. Nonetheless, performing ALPPS for cholangiocarcinoma is technically difficult and often leads to unfavorable results after surgery. Increased serum bilirubin and creatinine levels between the two stages and surgical complications can predict mortality after the second stage. KGR and HBS testing of FLR can guide the decision to proceed with Stage 2 or to postpone/cancel it. Compared with traditional PVE or PVL TSH, ALPPS offers a higher resection rate for CRLM without increasing complications or mortality. In terms of oncological benefit, ALPPS enables a higher tumor resection rate and possesses a clear theoretical advantage over TSH. Nonetheless, further prospective studies are required to determine the long-term outcomes.

References

1. Schnitzbauer AA, Lang SA, Goessmann H, et al. Right portal vein ligation combined with *in situ* splitting induces rapid left lateral liver lobe hypertrophy enabling 2-staged extended right hepatic resection in small-for-size settings [J]. Ann Surg. 2012;255(3):405–14.
2. Schadde E, Ardiles V, Robles-Campos R, et al. Early survival and safety of ALPPS: first report of the International ALPPS Registry [J]. Ann Surg. 2014;260(5):829–83.
3. Schadde E, Raptis DA, Schnitzbauer AA, et al. Prediction of mortality after ALPPS stage-1: an analysis of 320 patients from the international ALPPS registry [J]. Ann Surg. 2015;262(5):780–5.
4. Balzan S, Belghiti J, Farges O, et al. The "50-50 criteria" on postoperative day 5: an accurate predictor of liver failure and death after hepatectomy [J]. Ann Surg. 2005;242(6):824–8.

5. Aloia TA. Insights into alpps [J]. Eur J Surg Oncol. 2015;41(5):610–1.
6. Cieslak KP, Olthof PB, van Lienden KP, et al. Assessment of liver function using ^{99m}Tc-mebrofenin hepatobiliary scintigraphy in ALPPS (associating liver partition and portal vein ligation for staged hepatectomy) [J]. Case Rep Gastroenterol. 2015;9(3):353–60.
7. Truant S, Baillet C, Deshorgue AC, et al. Drop of total liver function in the interstages of the new associating liver partition and portal vein ligation for staged hepatectomy technique: analysis of the "auxiliary liver" by HIDA scintigraphy [J]. Ann Surg. 2016;263(3):e33–4.
8. Sparrelid E, Jonas E, Tzortzakakis A, et al. Dynamic evaluation of liver volume and function in associating liver partition and portal vein ligation for staged hepatectomy [J]. J Gastrointest Surg. 2017;21(6):967–74.
9. Rahbari NN, Garden OJ, Padbury R, et al. Posthepatectomy liver failure: a definition and grading by the International Study Group of Liver Surgery (ISGLS) [J]. Surgery. 2011;149(5):713–24.
10. Linecker M, Stavrou GA, Oldhafer KJ, et al. The ALPPS risk score: avoiding futile use of ALPPS [J]. Ann Surg. 2016;264(5):763–71.
11. Shindoh J, Truty MJ, Aloia TA, et al. Kinetic growth rate after portal vein embolization predicts posthepatectomy outcomes: toward zero liver-related mortality in patients with colorectal liver metastases and small future liver remnant [J]. J Am Coll Surg. 2013;216(2):201–9.
12. Leung U, Simpson AL, Araujo RLC, et al. Remnant growth rate after portal vein embolization is a good early predictor of post-hepatectomy liver failure [J]. J Am Coll Surg. 2014;219(4):620–30.
13. Kambakamba P, Stocker D, Reiner CS, et al. Liver kinetic growth rate predicts postoperative liver failure after ALPPS [J]. HPB (Oxford). 2016;18(10):800–5.
14. Serenari M, Collaud C, Alvarez FA, et al. Interstage assessment of remnant liver function in ALPPS using hepatobiliary scintigraphy: prediction of posthepatectomy liver failure and introduction of the HIBA index [J]. Ann Surg. 2018;267(6):1141–7.
15. Alghamdi T, Viebahn C, Justinger C, et al. Arterial blood supply of liver segment IV and its possible surgical consequences [J]. Am J Transplant. 2017;17(4):1064–70.
16. Li J, Girotti P, Königsrainer I, et al. ALPPS in right trisectionectomy: a safe procedure to avoid postoperative liver failure? [J]. J Gastrointest Surg. 2013;17(5):956–61.
17. Hernandez-Alejandro R, Bertens KA, Pineda-Solis K, et al. Can we improve the morbidity and mortality associated with the associating liver partition with portal vein ligation for staged hepatectomy (ALPPS) procedure in the management of colorectal liver metastases? [J]. Surgery. 2015;157(2):194–201.
18. Olthof PB, Coelen RJS, Wiggers JK, et al. High mortality after ALPPS for perihilar cholangiocarcinoma: case-control analysis including the first series from the international ALPPS registry [J]. HPB (Oxford). 2017;19(5):381–7.
19. D'Haese JG, Neumann J, Weniger M, et al. Should ALPPS be used for liver resection in intermediate-stage HCC? [J]. Ann Surg Oncol. 2016;23(4):1335–43.
20. Shoup M, Gonen M, D'Angelica M, et al. Volumetric analysis predicts hepatic dysfunction in patients undergoing major liver resection [J]. J Gastrointest Surg. 2003;7(3):325–30.
21. Ferrero A, Viganò L, Polastri R, et al. Postoperative liver dysfunction and future remnant liver: where is the limit? Results of a prospective study [J]. World J Surg. 2007;31(8):1643–51.
22. Guglielmi A, Ruzzenente A, Conci S, et al. How much remnant is enough in liver resection? [J]. Dig Surg. 2012;29(1):6–17.
23. Abulkhir A, Limongelli P, Healey AJ, et al. Preoperative portal vein embolization for major liver resection: a meta-analysis [J]. Ann Surg. 2008;247(1):49–57.
24. Shindoh J, Vauthey JN, Zimmitti G, et al. Analysis of the efficacy of portal vein embolization for patients with extensive liver malignancy and very low future liver remnant volume, including a comparison with the associating liver partition with portal vein ligation for staged hepatectomy approach [J]. J Am Coll Surg. 2013;217(1):126–33.
25. Croome KP, Hernandez-Alejandro R, Parker M, et al. Is the liver kinetic growth rate in ALPPS unprecedented when compared with PVE and living donor liver transplant? A multicentre analysis [J]. HPB. 2015;17(6):477–84.
26. Ratti F, Schadde E, Masetti M, et al. Strategies to increase the resectability of patients with colorectal liver metastases: a multicenter case-match analysis of ALPPS and conventional two-stage hepatectomy [J]. Ann Surg Oncol. 2015;22(6):1933–42.
27. Chia DKA, Yeo Z, Loh SEK, et al. Greater hypertrophy can be achieved with associating liver partition with portal vein ligation for staged hepatectomy compared to conventional staged hepatectomy, but with a higher price to pay? [J]. Am J Surg. 2018;215(1):131–7.
28. Matsuo K, Murakami T, Kawaguchi D, et al. Histologic features after surgery associating liver partition and portal vein ligation for staged hepatectomy versus those after hepatectomy with portal vein embolization [J]. Surgery. 2016;159(5):1289–98.
29. Røsok BI, Björnsson B, Sparrelid E, et al. Scandinavian multicenter study on the safety and feasibility of the associating liver partition and portal vein ligation for staged hepatectomy procedure [J]. Surgery. 2016;159(5):1279–86.
30. Sandström P, Røsok BI, Sparrelid E, et al. ALPPS improves resectability compared with conventional two-stage hepatectomy in patients with advanced colorectal liver metastasis: results from a Scandinavian multicenter randomized controlled trial (LIGRO trial) [J]. Ann Surg. 2018;267(5):833–40.
31. Ratti F, Cipriani F, Gagliano A, et al. Defining indications to ALPPS procedure: technical aspects and open issues [J]. Updates Surg. 2014;66(1):41–9.
32. Chia DKA, Yeo Z, Loh SEK, et al. ALPPS for hepatocellular carcinoma is associated with decreased liver remnant growth [J]. J Gastrointest Surg. 2018;22(6):973–80.
33. Tanaka K, Matsuo K, Murakami T, et al. Associating liver partition and portal vein ligation for staged hepatectomy (ALPPS): short-term outcome, functional changes in the future liver remnant, and tumor growth activity [J]. Eur J Surg Oncol. 2015;41(4):506–12.
34. Adam R, Imai K, Castro Benitez C, et al. Outcome after associating liver partition and portal vein ligation for staged hepatectomy and conventional two-stage hepatectomy for colorectal liver metastases [J]. Br J Surg. 2016;103(11):1521–9.
35. Schadde E, Ardiles V, Slankamenac K, et al. ALPPS offers a better chance of complete resection in patients with primarily unresectable liver tumors compared with conventional-staged hepatectomies: results of a multicenter analysis [J]. World J Surg. 2014;38(6):1510–9.
36. Zhou Z, Xu MX, Lin N, et al. Associating liver partition and portal vein ligation for staged hepatectomy versus conventional two-stage hepatectomy: a systematic review and meta-analysis [J]. World J Surg Oncol. 2017;15(1):227.
37. Alvarez FA, Ardiles V, de Santibañes E. The ALPPS approach for the management of colorectal carcinoma liver metastases [J]. Curr Colorectal Cancer Rep. 2013;9(2):168–77.
38. Aloia TA, Vauthey JN. Associating liver partition and portal vein ligation for staged hepatectomy (ALPPS): what is gained and what is lost? [J]. Ann Surg. 2012;256(3):e9.
39. de Graaf W, van den Esschert JW, van Lienden KP, et al. Induction of tumor growth after preoperative portal vein embolization: is it a real problem? [J]. Ann Surg Oncol. 2009;16(2):423–30.

40. Kokudo N, Tada K, Seki M, et al. Proliferative activity of intrahepatic colorectal metastases after preoperative hemihepatic portal vein embolization [J]. Hepatology. 2001;34(2):267–72.
41. Hoekstra LT, van Lienden KP, Doets A, et al. Tumor progression after preoperative portal vein embolization [J]. Ann Surg. 2012;256(5):812–7.
42. Pamecha V, Levene A, Grillo F, et al. Effect of portal vein embolisation on the growth rate of colorectal liver metastases [J]. Br J Cancer. 2009;100(4):617–22.
43. Joechle K, Moser C, Ruemmele P, et al. ALPPS (associating liver partition and portal vein ligation for staged hepatectomy) does not affect proliferation, apoptosis, or angiogenesis as compared to standard liver resection for colorectal liver metastases [J]. World J Surg Oncol. 2017;15(1):57.
44. Brouquet A, Abdalla EK, Kopetz S, et al. High survival rate after two-stage resection of advanced colorectal liver metastases: response-based selection and complete resection define outcome [J]. J Clin Oncol. 2011;29(8):1083–90.
45. Lim C, Turco C, Balci D, et al. Auxiliary liver transplantation for cirrhosis: from APOLT to RAPID: a scoping review [J]. Ann Surg. 2022;275(3):551–9.
46. Königsrainer A, Templin S, Capobianco I, et al. Paradigm shift in the management of irresectable colorectal liver metastases: living donor auxiliary partial orthotopic liver transplantation in combination with two-stage hepatectomy (LD-RAPID) [J]. Ann Surg. 2019;270(2):327–32.
47. Balci D, Kirimker EO, Bingol Kologlu M, et al. A new approach for increasing availability of liver grafts and donor safety in living donor liver transplantation: LD-RAPID procedure in the cirrhotic setting with hepatocellular carcinoma [J]. Liver Transpl. 2021;27(4):590–4.

18 ALPPS-Based Dual Conversion Therapy

Yajin Chen, Changzhen Shang, and Zhiqin Xie

Comprehensive treatment based on surgery remains the major pillar for hepatocellular carcinoma (HCC) management. Nevertheless, due to the poor early diagnosis rate, most HCC patients are diagnosed with intermediate-to-advance-stage diseases, losing the opportunity for radical resection. Evidence from the literature showed that only 20–30% of this patient population are candidates for radical resection when initially diagnosed. The first cause of unresectable HCC is the advanced stage of the tumor, where surgical resection generates no benefit or is less effective than other comprehensive treatments. Insufficient future liver remnant (FLR) and decompensated liver function are the second and third causes. Current guidelines recommend that the FLR/SLV (standard liver volume) ratio among patients without underlying liver disease should be greater than 20–30%. In contrast, those with underlying hepatic conditions should be greater than 30–40% [1, 2]. To address the concern of unresectability caused by insufficient FLR in HCC, portal vein embolization (PVE) on the affected side is usually applied to increase the volume of FLR in the earlier years. However, it takes a long time for liver growth with suboptimal increments. In 2007, Hans J. Schlitt et al. took the lead in performing staged hepatectomy combined with liver partition and portal vein ligation (PVL). In 2012, the procedure was named ALPPS (associating liver partition and portal vein ligation for staged hepatectomy) [3]. ALPPS integrates PVL of the affected side and liver parenchyma partition, rapidly promoting FLR growth and improving the resection rate. According to a systematic review [4], for HCC patients undergoing ALPPS, the growth rate of FLR reached 54.9% on the 11th-day average, 98% of patients completed the second stage of liver resection with a total complication rate of approximately 38%, and 3-year and 5-year overall survival (OS) rates standing at 60.2% [5] and 46.8% [6], respectively.

Although ALPPS has enhanced the resection and survival rates of some intermediate and advanced HCC patients, the tumor burden during the second stage of surgery remains heavy, and its postoperative recurrence rate is still high. A combination with a multi-measure strategy needs to be taken to further reduce relapses and elongate survival. Therefore, we designed a liver partition technique based on stage 1 of ALPPS, combining targeted therapy, immunotherapy, and local interventional therapy (such as transarterial chemoembolization, TACE/hepatic arterial infusion chemotherapy, HAIC) after PVL and liver parenchyma partition to reduce tumor burden. An elective stage 2 resection will be performed when the increased FLR volume is sufficient with improved function. Preliminary data showed that elective ALPPS integrated with systemic and local therapies after stage 1 of surgery achieved the "dual conversion" goal of reducing tumor burden and enabling sufficient FLR growth, obtaining safer perioperative results, higher resection rates, and more prolonged survival.

18.1 The Philosophy of Dual Conversion

The conventional ALPPS/PVE that improves the resection rate by increasing FLR volume and the conversion/downstaging treatment of HCC that has evolved with the advancement of systemic therapies in recent years is not without certain limitations. On the one hand, conventional ALPPS requires two stages of surgery in a short period of time, which is highly invasive. Despite the improvement in resection rate, it results in a high recurrence rate for patients with a heavy tumor burden, especially those with macroscopic tumor thrombus. However, the average resection rate after HCC conversion therapy, which is mainly based on targeted therapy and immunotherapy, is only 15–30%. The *Chinese Expert Consensus on Conversion Therapy for Liver Cancer*

Y. Chen (✉) · C. Shang · Z. Xie
Sun Yat-Sen Memorial Hospital, Sun Yat-Sen University, Guangdong, China
e-mail: cyj0509@126.com

J. Zhou (ed.), *Associating Liver Partition and Portal Vein Ligation for Staged Hepatectomy (ALPPS)*,
https://doi.org/10.1007/978-981-96-7364-3_18

(2021 Edition) [7] clearly states that conversion therapy for initially unresectable liver cancer requires both surgical and oncological conversion. In particular, for patients with China liver cancer staging (CNLC) stage IIb and IIIa whose FLR remains insufficient, the dual-conversion treatment model that increases FLR volume and reduces tumor burden is expected to improve resection rate and mid- and long-term survival.

18.2 Techniques of Dual Conversion

Based on its philosophy, dual-conversion techniques involve two components: one aims at increasing FLR volume (with liver partitioning in stage 1 of ALPPS as the bedrock), and the other focuses on tumor downstaging and conversion (largely hinges upon a comprehensive treatment model that combines targeted therapy and immunotherapy with TACE/HAIC). During implementation, it is necessary to organically integrate these two techniques to minimize tumor burden, optimize functional liver volume, guarantee perioperative safety, and obtain mid- and long-term benefits.

18.2.1 Portal Vein Ligation and Liver Parenchyma Partition Techniques Based on Stage 1 of ALPPS

Liver partition in the conventional ALPPS boasts two essential advantages. First, after portal vein branch ligation and liver parenchyma division, the unaffected side rapidly grows in a short period. Compared with PVE, it renders higher liver growth efficiency and a better resection rate. Second, ligating portal vein branches and dissociating parenchyma theoretically block the spread of tumor cells from the affected side to the healthy side along the portal vein, ensuring the tumor-free status of the unaffected part. According to our practical experience, after such procedures, the unaffected component remains relatively tumor-free for a long time (maximum 7 years after stage 1 of ALPPS) even if the tumor progresses on the affected side (Fig. 18.1).

In conventional ALPPS, the second stage is generally performed 2–3 weeks after the first stage, leading to two major risks. One is surgical, that is, the trauma caused by two surgeries in a short time frame [3]. In addition, some cirrhotic patients fail to achieve ideal FLR promptly due to limited liver growth capability in the healthy part. Even if a sufficient FLR is obtained rapidly, the function may not be desirable. This deprives some patients of the opportunity to complete the second stage after the first surgery. The second risk is oncological. Compromised immunity, led by the trauma of two operations, may facilitate tumor dissemination and metastasis. At the same time, even if the second stage is completed, patients' postoperative recurrence rate remains high due to the vast tumor burden and the presence of vascular tumor thrombus, which affects long-term survival.

Thus, the key to dual conversion is leveraging ALPPS's advantages while avoiding risks.

18.2.2 Tumor Downstaging and Conversion Therapy Combining Targeted Therapy and Immunotherapy with TACE/HAIC

In recent years, both concepts and new drugs for the comprehensive treatment of HCC have made great strides. In par-

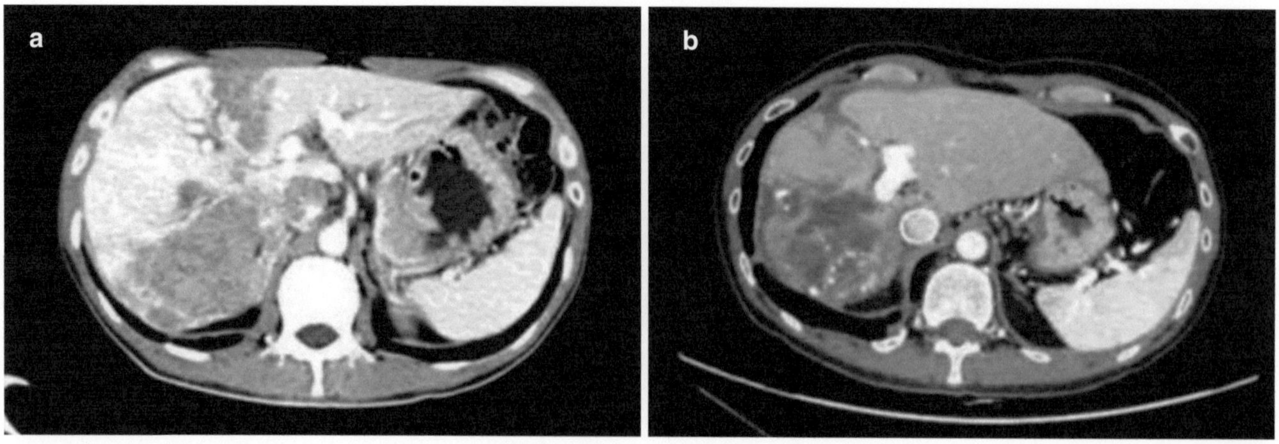

Fig. 18.1 The healthy component remains tumor-free for a long time after stage 1 ALPPS. (**a**) Multiple HCC in the left and right liver with tumor thrombi in the inferior vena cava (IVC) and the right branch of the portal vein (at initial diagnosis in 2014). (**b**) Seven years after ligating the right branch of the portal vein + parenchymal partition of the left lateral lobe + IVC stenting (2021), the left lateral lobe grew and remained tumor-free

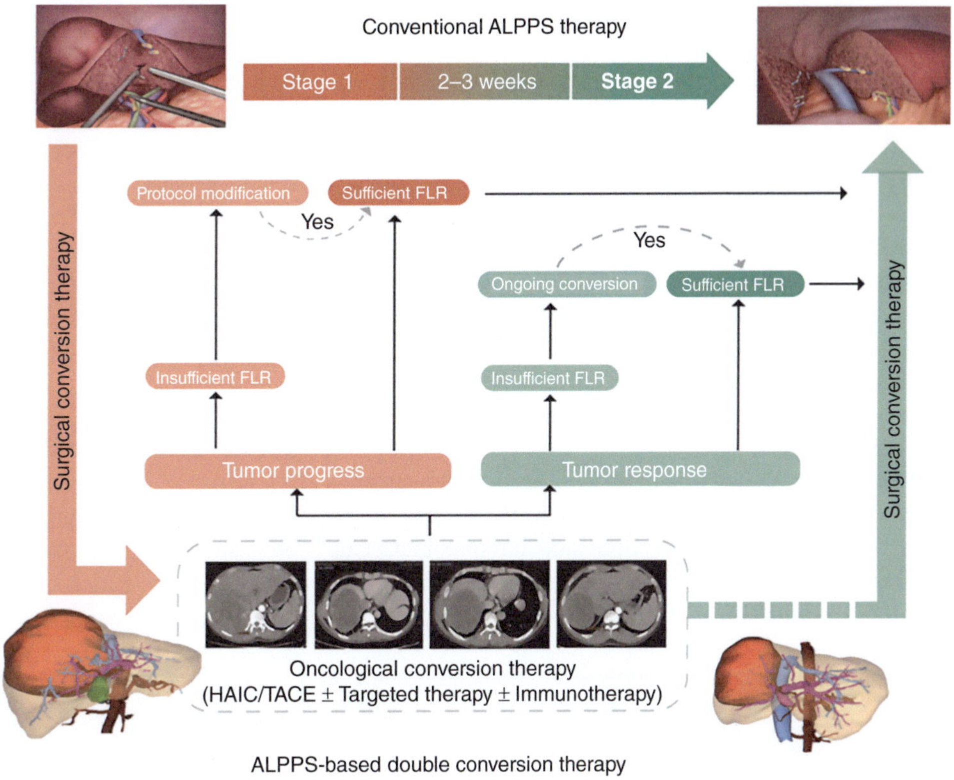

Fig. 18.2 Illustrative model shows the different routes for patients treated by conventional ALPPS or ALPPS-based dual-conversion therapy at our center. ALPPS indicates associating liver partition and portal vein ligation for staged hepatectomy; FLR indicates future liver remnant; HAIC indicates hepatic arterial infusion chemotherapy; TACE indicates transarterial chemoembolization

ticular, the advent of new-generation antiangiogenics such as lenvatinib, the application of immunotherapy, and the sequential combination of multiple treatments have significantly prolonged the survival of advanced HCC. For instance, immunotherapy alone achieved a disease control rate (DCR) of 56.6% and an objective response rate (ORR) of 17.3% [8]. Common combinations of targeted therapy + immunotherapy secured an ORR of 45.5% and a DCR of 81.8% [9], addressing previous difficulties in treating advanced HCC and creating more treatment choices. Additionally, HAIC plus targeted therapy and immunotherapy (triple therapy) achieved a median OS of 15.9–18 months, a DCR of 77.6–92.6%, and an ORR of 40–63% [10, 11]. Multidimensional combination, multimodal sequential treatment, and multidisciplinary collaboration compose the mainstream models of conversion therapy for HCC, converting some initially unresectable intermediate-to-advance stage cases into resectable disease, reducing the recurrence rate, and improving long-term survival.

Similarly, conversion therapy alone also faces a dilemma. First, there is a lack of clear guidelines for screening patients who may benefit from such a strategy, and a high ORR does not translate into a more prolonged survival. Second, the current resection rate after conversion is suboptimal, only around 15–30%. In addition to oncological factors, many cases are unresectable due to surgical factors, such as insufficient FLR and functional liver reserve. Third, drugs administered during conversion therapy can also cause liver damage, drug resistance, and tumor progression or metastasis, leading to an unresectable status.

To attain safer perioperative outcomes and longer OS, targeted therapy and immunotherapy are given to patients with insufficient FLR 2–3 weeks after stage 1 of ALPPS—portal vein branch ligation and parenchymal partition (classical stage 2 ALPPS of liver resection is proceeded in patients with adequate FLR). Four weeks later, TACE/HAIC is carried out per the patients' liver function and systemic condition. This strategy is continued for 3–6 cycles, with evaluation every 2 cycles. Stage 2 of ALPPS is performed to remove the affected liver when significant tumor remission, sufficient FLR, and desirable function are achieved (Fig. 18.2). This gives patients with insufficient FLR growth after stage 1 of conventional ALPPS the opportunity to transition to a state of low tumor burden and adequate FLR to complete stage 2 tumor resection, achieving the goal of dual conversion surgically and oncologically.

18.3 Issues That Need Attention in Dual Conversion for HCC

18.3.1 Target Patient Selection for Dual Conversion

The target HCC population of dual conversion is patients with insufficient FLR 2–3 weeks after the first stage of

ALPPS (Fig. 18.3). The patient in Fig. 18.3 is a typical case of successful dual conversion.

Figure 18.4 shows a liver cancer patient with a right portal vein tumor thrombus (CNLC-IIIa stage) and insufficient FLR. Patients with macrovascular invasion have a poor prognosis, with a median survival of merely about 6.9 months and a 1-year survival of only 12% [12]. In these patients, controlling the tumor thrombus from progressing to the main trunk and the contralateral side is the key to smooth, comprehensive treatment. Stage 1 of ALPPS involves PVL and liver partition to physically block the growth of tumor thrombus to the healthy side in this population. Combined with other treatments for downstaging, it enables a higher resection rate and survival rate.

Figure 18.5 shows a patient with hepatocellular carcinoma (HCC) with multiple tumor lesions (CNLC-IIa stage), with a primary tumor on the right side and oligometastatic foci on the left. In the case of insufficient FLR during simultaneous liver tumor resection, a dual-conversion treatment model can be adopted. This involves initial portal vein ligation on the side of the primary tumor and separation of the liver parenchyma between the left and right lobes, along with the resection of the foci on the left side. Two weeks after the stage 1 surgery, if the FLR proliferation has not yet met the requirements for resection, targeted therapy and immunotherapy combined with TACE/HAIC can be initiated. The primary tumor shrank, and the left liver lobe regenerated without de novo sub-lesions. Hepatectomy on the side of the primary lesion was then performed.

18.3.2 Selection of Surgical Timing

The surgical timing during dual-conversion therapy depends on simultaneous evaluation both surgically and oncologically.

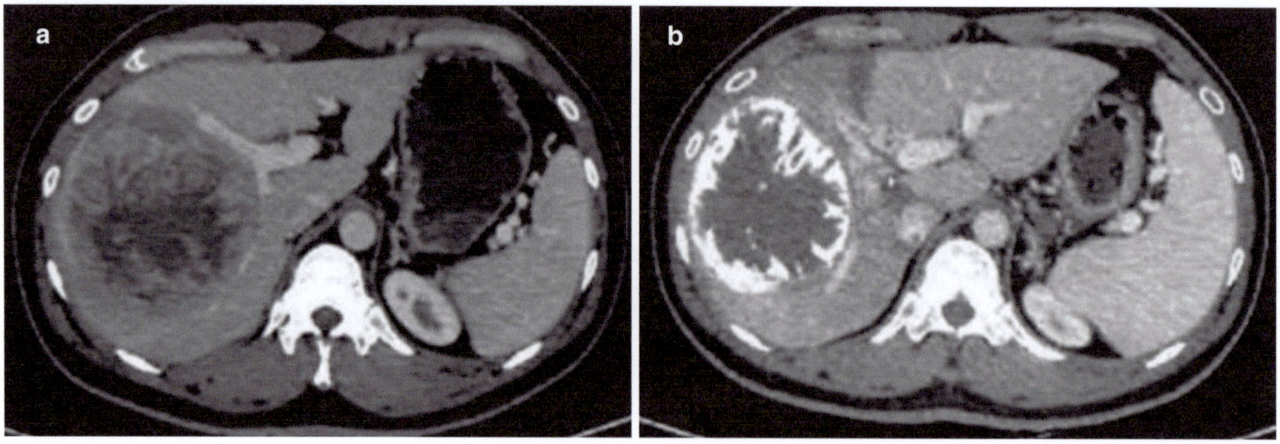

Fig. 18.3 A typical case of successful dual conversion. (**a**) Patient with a giant HCC tumor when initially diagnosed, FLR/SLV: 24%; (**b**) Two weeks after stage 1 of ALPPS, the FLR failed to reach the safe range for resection. After 20 weeks of dual-conversion therapy, the tumor shrank, its activity decreased, and the FLR/SLV was 48%

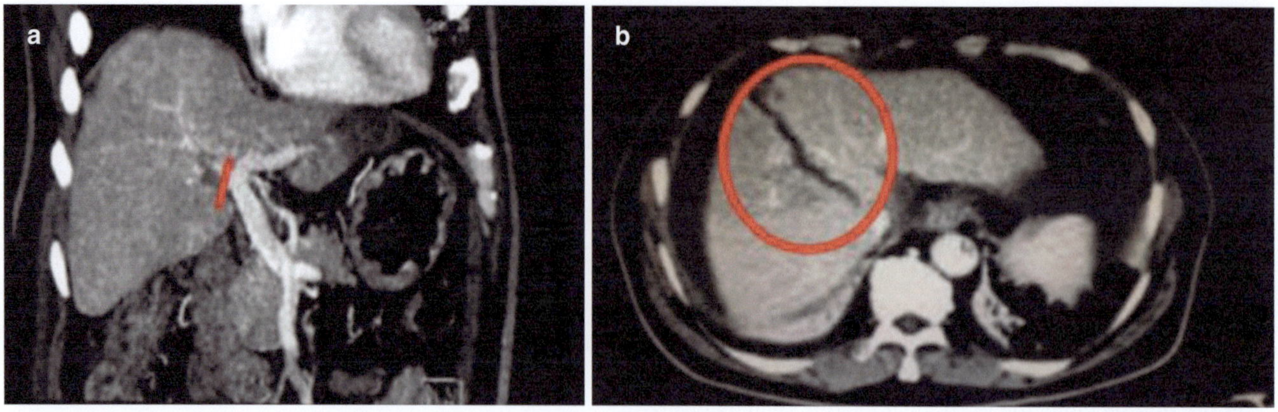

Fig. 18.4 Tumor thrombus in the right branch of the portal vein accompanied by insufficient left liver volume, ligation of the right branch of the portal vein (**a**) + liver parenchymal partition (**b**)

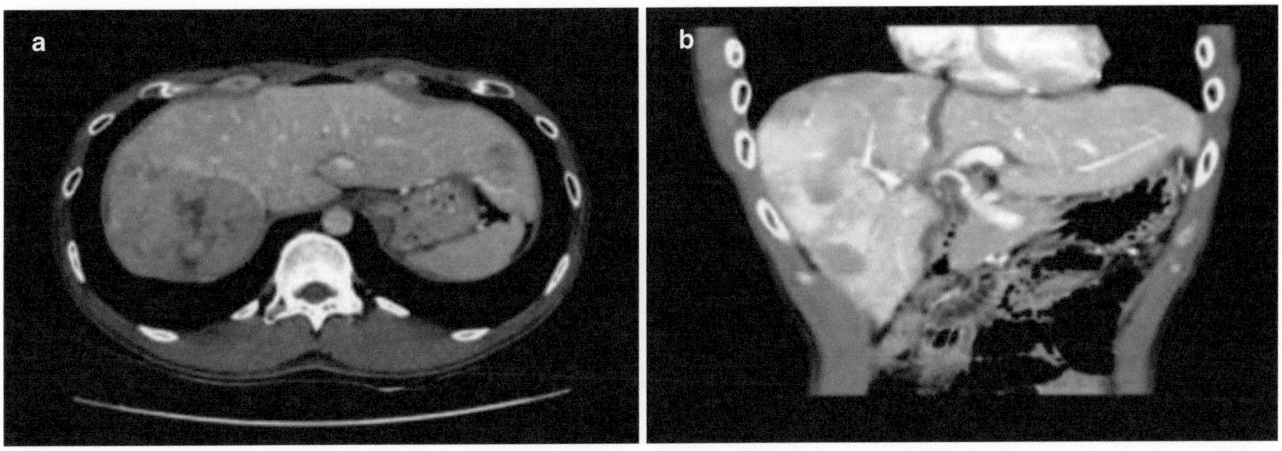

Fig. 18.5 A dual-conversion case with HCC oligometastatic on the reserved side. (**a**) Massive HCC in the right lobe combined with left oligometastasis. (**b**) Right portal vein ligation + parenchymal partition + left lobe lesion resection

After ALPPS stage 1, surgical safety is met if the FLR increases to more than 40% and the indocyanine green retention test (ICG-R15) drops to less than 10%. Under this circumstance, stage 2 surgery needs to be conducted as soon as possible to avoid the impact of targeted therapy and immunotherapy on liver function and tumor progression, leading to an unresectable status.

Patients whose FLR does not increase to a safe range 2–3 weeks after stage 1 can receive comprehensive oncological treatment and undergo regular surgical and oncological evaluations. If the surgical requirements are met, the operation needs to be performed as soon as possible to avoid delaying resection. Ideally, if the tumor meets the mRECIST criteria [13] of complete response/partial response/major pathological response, tumor thrombus regression and inactivation, the disappearance of metastases without distant metastasis, and oncological downstaging requirements are met. More prolonged survival may be achieved after surgical resection. Desirably, patients should be surgically and oncologically eligible for better mid- and long-term survival outcomes after resection. When they fail to meet desired surgical criteria, even if they are in oncological remission, stage 2 surgery cannot be performed, and systemic treatment must be continued until they are surgically qualified.

18.3.3 Preliminary Clinical Results of Dual-Conversion Therapy

Our center completed ALPPS on 56 HCC patients from 2013 to 2021. They were divided into the dual-conversion group and the simple ALPPS group based on the presence of dual-conversion techniques. Our results showed that the stage 2 resection rate of the dual-conversion group was 97%, higher than that of the other arm. The 1-year and 3-year survival rates were as high as 91.7% and 73.3%, respectively, also superior to the simple ALPPS group (77.1% and 47.5%, respectively), suggesting that dual conversion improved the post-conversion resection rate and short- and mid-term survival rates. Large-scale, multicenter studies are needed for further validation.

18.3.4 Safety and Improvement Strategies

The perioperative safety of ALPPS has always been a focus of attention in this field. The interval between the two stages of conventional open ALPPS is short, and patients have two surgical strikes in 2–3 weeks. Although the volume of the unaffected side can rapidly increase, there may be pathological proliferation caused by inflammation and injury, while functional liver units grow slowly. Therefore, this procedure resulted in high complication and mortality rates at the dawn of its development. Ways to improve its safety have also become a focus in clinical practices. With the advancement of ALPPS techniques and the expansion of indications, perioperative complications and mortality rates have been significantly reduced.

18.3.4.1 Minimally Invasive Stage 1/2 of ALPPS

With the development of surgical techniques and concepts, minimally invasive surgery, boasting the advantages of less trauma, faster recovery, and lower complication rate, has become the mainstream for certain procedures. However, there are few large-scale case reports for ALPPS in which both stages are conducted in a minimally invasive manner. Since our center performed the first case of laparoscopic ALPPS to treat a liver cancer patient on August 15, 2013, a total of 45 cases of laparoscopic ALPPS stage 1 and 25 cases of laparoscopic ALPPS stage 2 have been completed by the end of 2022. Only three cases suffered from severe complications after stage 1 and 2 after stage 2. Most complications occurred in the early years of laparoscopic ALPPS. In the mature era, there were no severe complications or perioperative deaths. These results are similar to those of an Italian multicenter study in which ALPPS cases in 12 hospitals were analyzed. The authors demonstrated that minimally invasive surgery had a shorter postoperative length of stay, a lower complication rate, and a lower mortality rate than open surgery [14]. It is recommended that centers with rich laparoscopic experience can perform this procedure routinely.

18.3.4.2 Damage Control

For patients with significant cirrhosis and poor liver function, the incidence of perioperative complications remains higher, and controlling surgical trauma is essential to achieve good postoperative recovery. Minimally invasive techniques are used to separate the left and right livers more thoroughly, but they also introduce risks of bleeding and bile leakage. If the patient's condition is not allowed, radiofrequency or microwave ablation can be applied to separate the liver for damage control (Fig. 18.6). Staged PVL can be combined to reduce the severe impact on liver function. Especially for patients with thicker portal vein branches on the affected side, 7# silk threads can ligate 50–70% of the blood flow from the portal vein intra-operatively. After the surgery, PVE can be supplemented under X-ray guidance, which reduces portal vein recanalization and ameliorates liver function protection, controlling ischemic necrosis and infection of the affected side.

For those who have undergone TACE/HAIC combined with targeted therapy and immunotherapy after stage 1 of ALPPS, the most significant risk in stage 2 remains the bile duct injury and stenosis in the confluence of the left and right hepatic ducts when dividing the hepatic pedicle of the affected side. Both stage 1 surgery and TACE/HAIC cause inflammation and thickening in the portal area. When dividing the right hepatic pedicle, try to dissociate the anterior and the posterior components, or use ICG fluorescence imaging to ensure the safety of bile duct confluence.

18.3.4.3 Monitoring and Treatment of Severe Adverse Events (SAE)

Serious adverse events mainly include hepatic insufficiency, immune-related hepatitis, immune-related pneumonitis, immune-related myocarditis, and other complications that are life-threatening, primarily associated with liver function damage, reduction of blood flow into the liver from the affected side, and immune response caused by systemic and local treatments. Although the incidence of SAE is low, it is severe and could threaten patients' lives at any time, influencing subsequent treatment. Therefore, during comprehensive treatment, it is essential to closely monitor symptoms, signs, and functions of the heart, liver, lung, and kidney, adjusting the treatment plan timely according to the severity of adverse events. For those with mild adverse events, dose reduction and liver-protecting medication should be initiated promptly. In case of severe events (grade 3 or above), the drug must be discontinued in time, and treatments such as liver protection, blood purification, immune regulation, and hormones must be given. When liver function normalizes, the treatment plan can be carried out.

18.3.5 Conversion Therapy for Liver Partition or Tumor Burden Reduction, Who Goes First?

With the advancement of systemic treatment in HCC, conversion therapy has gradually become an essential method for initially unresectable HCC. Studies have found that the post-conversion resection rate of targeted therapy and immunotherapy reached 42.4% [9]. Combining these two treatments with HAIC/TACE (triple therapy) achieved a median

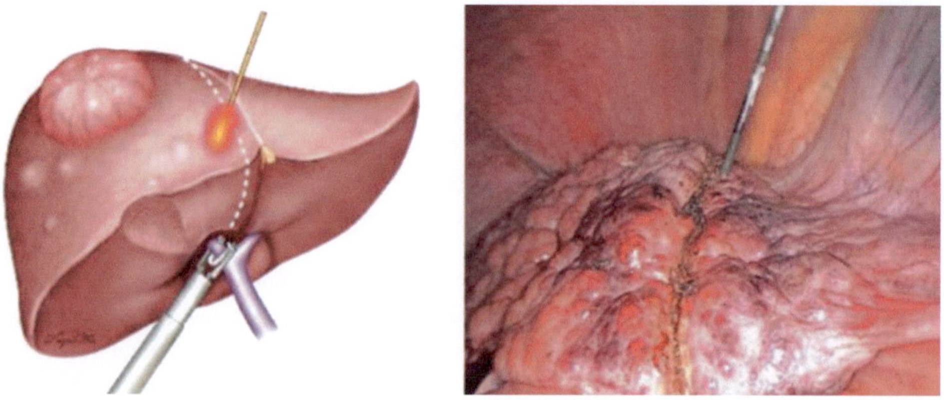

Fig. 18.6 A cirrhotic patient underwent laparoscopic right portal vein ligation + liver parenchymal partition using microwave ablation

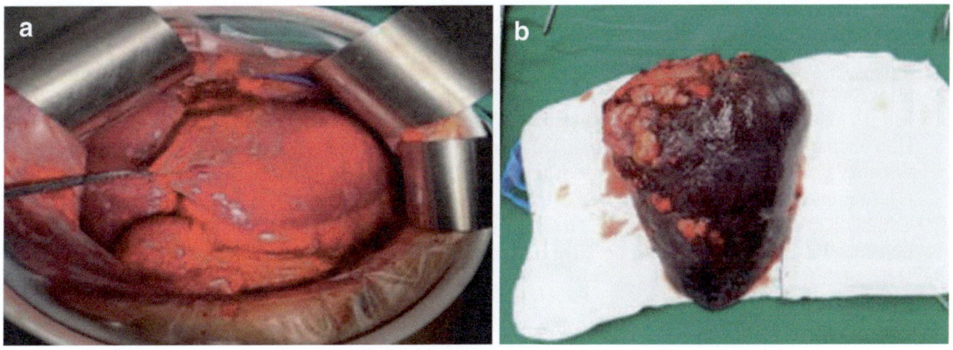

Fig. 18.7 The healthy component remains well-protected even if the tumor progresses on the affected side. (**a**) The patient underwent stage 2 of ALPPS 5 months after stage 1. (**b**) The tumor on the right side progressed, but the partitioned left side remained tumor-free, surviving for 7 years

OS of 15.9–18 months and a DCR as high as 83–92.6% [11, 15]. Hence, the choice between "dual conversion" and simple conversion is also one of the current focuses.

Based on existing research results, the success rate of resection after simple conversion is low, with tumor response rates between 30% and 50%. Therefore, its efficacy for a large number of cases remains unpredictable, and SAEs are not uncommon. For nonresponders, local progression, metastasis to the healthy side, and systemic metastasis may occur. In addition, comprehensive treatments may lead to damage to liver function. Stage 1 of ALPPS in dual conversion produces a physical blocking effect, especially for patients with combined portal vein branch cancer thrombus. It can prevent the tumor and cancer thrombus from invading and disseminating to the portal vein trunk and the healthy part. The healthy component remains well-protected even if the tumor progresses on the affected side (Fig. 18.7).

Moreover, while waiting for FLR growth, multidimensional combinations and multimodal sequential treatment measures could be gradually implemented. Both theories and practices suggest that it possesses the advantages of a safer and higher conversion rate, as well as more prolonged survival. Of course, more comprehensive application and further analysis of long-term effects are needed to confirm the clinical significance of dual conversion.

18.4 Prospects

Dual-conversion therapy is a comprehensive treatment model centered on ALPPS. For HCC patients with insufficient FLR 2 weeks after stage 1 of ALPPS, it provides them with the opportunity of radical resection. In the future, prospective, multicenter, large-scale studies are needed to better evaluate its safety and efficacy. At the same time, attention should also be paid to the effectiveness of systemic therapy and the prediction of hyper-progression and SAE. New serological markers and predictive immune response molecules are needed to better guide dual-conversion treatment in drug selection. In addition, we need to conduct basic research on the liver partition to explore its impact on the tumor immune microenvironment and microecology, offering more scientific evidence for the concept and techniques of dual conversion.

References

1. Benson AB, D'Angelica MI, Abbott DE, et al. Hepatobiliary cancers, version 2.2021, NCCN clinical practice guidelines in oncology [J]. J Natl Compr Cancer Netw. 2021;19(5):541–65.
2. Health China N. National guidelines for diagnosis and treatment of lung cancer 2022 in China (English version) [J]. Chin J Cancer Res. 2022;34(3):176–206.
3. Schnitzbauer AA, Lang SA, Goessmann H, et al. Right portal vein ligation combined with *in situ* splitting induces rapid left lateral liver lobe hypertrophy enabling 2-staged extended right hepatic resection in small-for-size settings [J]. Ann Surg. 2012;255(3):405–14.
4. Charalel RA, Sung J, Askin G, et al. Systematic reviews and meta-analyses of portal vein embolization, associated liver partition and portal vein ligation, and radiation lobectomy outcomes in hepatocellular carcinoma patients [J]. Curr Oncol Rep. 2021;23(11):135.
5. Wang Z, Peng YF, Hu JW, et al. Associating liver partition and portal vein ligation for staged hepatectomy for unresectable hepatitis B virus-related hepatocellular carcinoma: a single center study of 45 patients [J]. Ann Surg. 2020;271(3):534–41.
6. Chan A, Zhang WY, Chok K, et al. ALPPS versus portal vein embolization for hepatitis-related hepatocellular carcinoma: a changing paradigm in modulation of future liver remnant before major hepatectomy [J]. Ann Surg. 2021;273(5):957–65.
7. Sun HC, Zhou J, Wang Z, et al. Chinese expert consensus on conversion therapy for hepatocellular carcinoma (2021 edition) [J]. Hepatobiliary Surg Nutr. 2022;11(2):227–52.
8. Voutsadakis IA. PD-1 inhibitors monotherapy in hepatocellular carcinoma: meta-analysis and systematic review [J]. Hepatobiliary Pancreat Dis Int. 2019;18(6):505–10.
9. Zhang WW, Hu BY, Han J, et al. Preliminary report on the study of conversion therapy of advanced hepatocellular carcinoma combined PD-1 inhibitors with multi-target tyrosine kinase inhibitors [J]. Chin J Hepatobiliary Surg. 2020;26(12):947–8.

10. Mei J, Tang YH, Wei W, et al. Hepatic arterial infusion chemotherapy combined with PD-1 inhibitors plus lenvatinib versus PD-1 inhibitors plus lenvatinib for advanced hepatocellular carcinoma [J]. Front Oncol. 2021;11:618206.
11. Liu BJ, Gao S, Zhu X, et al. Real-world study of hepatic artery infusion chemotherapy combined with anti-PD-1 immunotherapy and tyrosine kinase inhibitors for advanced hepatocellular carcinoma [J]. Immunotherapy. 2021;13(17):1395–405.
12. Cabibbo G, Maida M, Genco C, et al. Natural history of untreatable hepatocellular carcinoma: a retrospective cohort study [J]. World J Hepatol. 2012;4(9):256–61.
13. Eisenhauer EA, Therasse P, Bogaerts J, et al. New response evaluation criteria in solid tumours: revised RECIST guideline (version 1.1) [J]. Eur J Cancer. 2009;45(2):228–47.
14. Serenari M, Ratti F, Zanello M, et al. Minimally invasive stage 1 to protect against the risk of liver failure: results from the hepatocellular carcinoma series of the associating liver partition and portal vein ligation for staged hepatectomy Italian registry [J]. J Laparoendosc Adv Surg Tech A. 2020;30(10):1082–9.
15. Mei J, Li SH, Li QJ, et al. Anti-PD-1 immunotherapy improves the efficacy of hepatic artery infusion chemotherapy in advanced hepatocellular carcinoma [J]. J Hepatocell Carcinoma. 2021;8:167–76.

19 Management of Complications of ALPPS

Zheng Wang and Lei Yu

Associating liver partition and portal vein ligation for staged hepatectomy (ALPPS) involves transecting the hepatic parenchyma and ligating the ipsilateral portal vein to induce the rapid hypertrophy of the contralateral future liver remnant (FLR) until an adequate volume is achieved. Following this, a two-stage hepatectomy of the ipsilateral lesion and liver is performed to prevent postoperative hepatic insufficiency or liver failure resulting from an inadequate FLR. Conventional hepatectomy requires preserving an adequate FLR to ensure postoperative safety. Therefore, conventional hepatectomy is unfeasible in cases where the FLR is insufficient because of the presence of multiple sporadic tumors or giant tumors. Thanks to its distinctive features, the ALPPS procedure overcomes the limitations of conventional hepatectomy, thereby expanding the indications for surgical treatment of liver tumors. Nonetheless, the ALPPS procedure entails high perioperative complication and mortality rates due to its aggressive nature, as evidenced by a reported perioperative complication rate of 68% in an early multicenter study [1]. As the ALPPS procedure becomes increasingly prevalent in clinical settings, major centers have amassed substantial expertise and achieved conceptual and technological improvements, e.g., improvements in indication selection, surgical procedures (e.g., refinement of hepatic transection techniques in stage 1 surgery, and introduction of minimally invasive techniques), and capture of timing for stage 2 surgery, providing a robust basis for lessening the incidence of perioperative complications associated with the ALPPS procedure. In addition, researchers from major centers become increasingly proficient in implementing ALPPS.

Almost three decades ago, Pierre et al. combined data from a substantial cohort of patients undergoing cholecystectomy ($n = 650$) and proposed a classification system for categorizing surgical complications into Grades I–IV, with a higher grade indicating greater severity and GradeIV complications signaling clinical death [2]. Subsequently, Dindo et al. modified the Clavien classification system by dividing postoperative complications into five grades (i.e., GradesI, II, IIIa, IIIb, IVa, IVb, and V), with a higher grade signifying greater severity and intensity of treatment indicated and GradeVcomplications representing clinical death. In addition, a study [3] conducted by Dindo et al. prospectively enrolled 6336 surgical patients from the center to validate the modified classification system, and the findings revealed that more than 90% of surgical patients were accurately classified into appropriate postoperative complication grades [3]. The resultant Clavien-Dindo classification of postoperative complications was essentially established. Due to its simple conceptual framework, ease of use, and high repeatability, the Clavien-Dindo classification is frequently employed for grading postoperative complications. The Clavien-Dindo classification of postoperative complications applies to the classification of complications following the ALPPS procedure.

While the ALPPS procedure diverges from conventional hepatectomy in terms of surgical procedures, it remains a liver-focused intervention. Despite sharing roughly identical types of postoperative complications with conventional hepatectomy, the ALPPS procedure exhibits distinct characteristics concerning the incidence of complications.

19.1 Bile Leakage

The International Study Group of Liver Surgery (ISGLS) defines post-liver surgery bile leakage as fluid with an elevated bilirubin level (at least 3 times higher than the serum bilirubin level measured at the same time) in the abdominal drainage or intra-abdominal fluid on or after postoperative day 3 or necessitating radiological intervention (i.e., interventional drainage) owing to abdominal bile collections or

Z. Wang (✉) · L. Yu
Zhongshan Hospital, Fudan University, Shanghai, China
e-mail: wang.zheng@zs-hospital.sh.cn

J. Zhou (ed.), *Associating Liver Partition and Portal Vein Ligation for Staged Hepatectomy (ALPPS)*,
https://doi.org/10.1007/978-981-96-7364-3_19

re-laparotomy due to biliary peritonitis. Furthermore, the ISGLS stratifies bile leakage into Grades A, B, and C. Grade A bile leakage may be detected solely through radiologic imaging and requires no clinical interventions, with abdominal drainage that persists for no more than 1 week. Grade A bile leakage typically features a sustained reduction in abdominal drainage volume and bilirubin concentration, potentially resulting in an extended hospital stay. Grade B bile leakage necessitates clinical interventions that do not involve re-laparotomy. Grade B bile leakage patients commonly experience accompanying clinical symptoms (e.g., pyrexia and abdominal discomfort) and generally need clinical interventions (e.g., antibiotic use and endoscopy- or imaging-guided drainage interventions). Some Grade B bile leakage patients may be discharged with a catheter, with a lengthened hospital stay. Grade C bile leakage, which is the most severe, requires a re-laparotomy for surgical suture for bile leakage and clearance of ascites, potentially followed by peritoneal lavage. Grade C bile leakage patients often experience accompanying severe clinical symptoms (e.g., severe abdominal pain, pyrexia, and signs of biliary peritonitis) and multiple organ failure and need admission to an intensive care unit (ICU) for treatment [4].

Following the ALPPS procedure, bile leakage occurs predominantly from the hepatic wound and secondarily from the hepatic duct near the porta hepatis, cystic duct stump, and T-tube site. An early study suggested that bile leakage was one of the most frequent complications following the ALPPS procedure. While the incidence rates of bile leakage differed among centers, the mean incidence of bile leakage was approximately 20% [5]. A large-cohort ($n = 501$) clinical retrospective study revealed that the ALPPS procedure, major hepatectomy, and choledochoenterostomy were significantly correlated with post-liver surgery bile leakage and that postoperative bile leakage was notably associated with surgical site infections (SSIs), postoperative liver failure, postoperative bleeding, and postoperative 90-day mortality [6]. Bile leakage following the ALPPS procedure occurs predominantly from the hepatic wound. Generally, surgeons may inject fat emulsion or methylene blue via the bile duct stump, and intraoperatively inspect the wound for bile leakage and repair any identified bile leakage (Figs. 19.1, 19.2, 19.3, and 19.4). In addition, the classic ALPPS procedure also entails transecting the hepatic parenchyma near the round ligament of the liver, resulting in parenchymal ischemia in segment IV and necrosis, bile leakage, and hemorrhage. In this regard, a scholar advocates resecting segment IV during the classic ALPPS procedure [7]. Precise anatomical resection, as well as meticulous and rigorous surgical operations, are essential for preventing bile leakage occurring from the large bile duct near the porta hepatis or the cystic duct stump. Bile leakage from the large bile duct is typically diagnosed with endoscopic retrograde cholangiopancreatography (ERCP). In

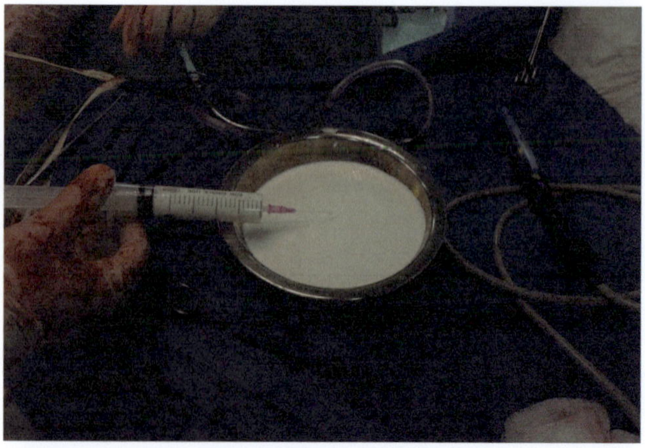

Fig. 19.1 Fat emulsion is intraoperatively prepared for inspecting the bile leakage from the hepatic wound

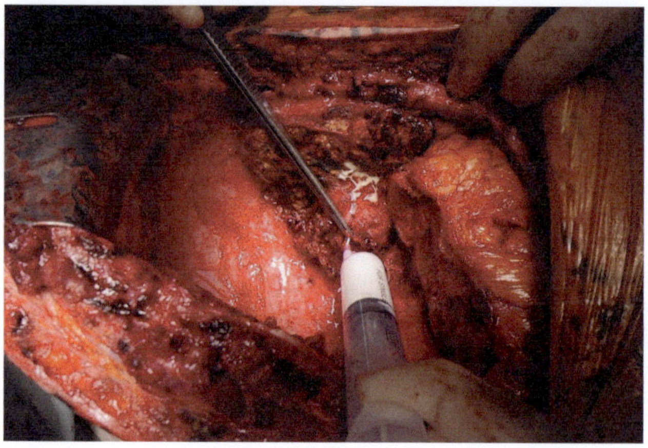

Fig. 19.2 Bile leakage is identified by intraoperatively injecting fat emulsion

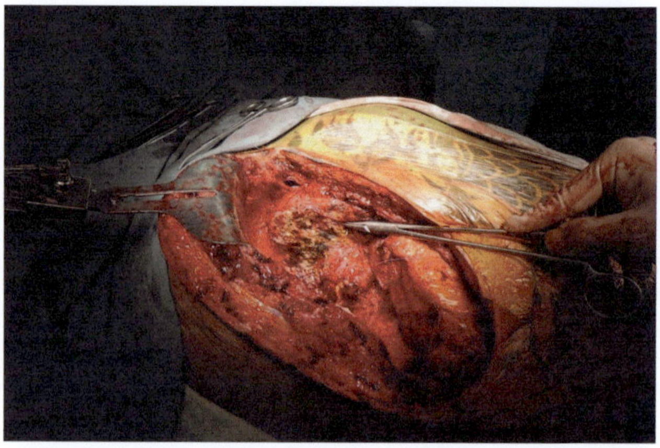

Fig. 19.3 The site of bile leakage is being sutured and ligated

some cases, Grade A postoperative bile leakage may be asymptomatic and is detected solely through abdominal drainage with an indwelling catheter (Figs. 19.5 and 19.6) or

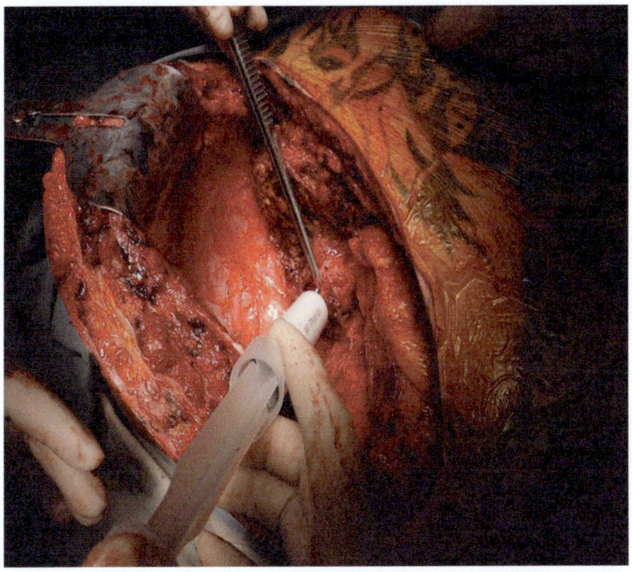

Fig. 19.4 Bile leakage from the hepatic wound disappears, as confirmed by reinspection with fat emulsion

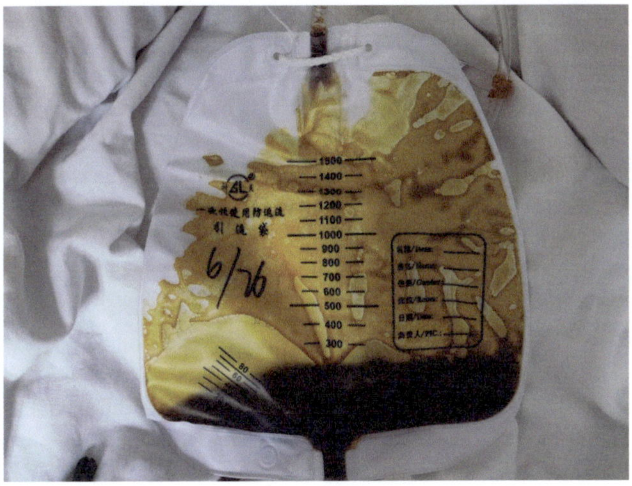

Fig. 19.5 Postoperative bile leakage drainage

cholangiography and requires no treatment. Grade B bile leakage from the large bile duct may be subjected to endoscopic nasobiliary drainage, and intra-abdominal bile may be drained with a percutaneous catheter [8]. Modified surgical procedures (e.g., partial hepatic parenchymal transection, tourniquet ALPPS procedure, and radiofrequency ablation or microwave ablation substituting for hepatic parenchymal transection) minimize the use of or supplant hepatic parenchymal transection to diminish the surgical wound, thereby mitigating the incidence of bile leakage following the stage 1 ALPPS procedure.

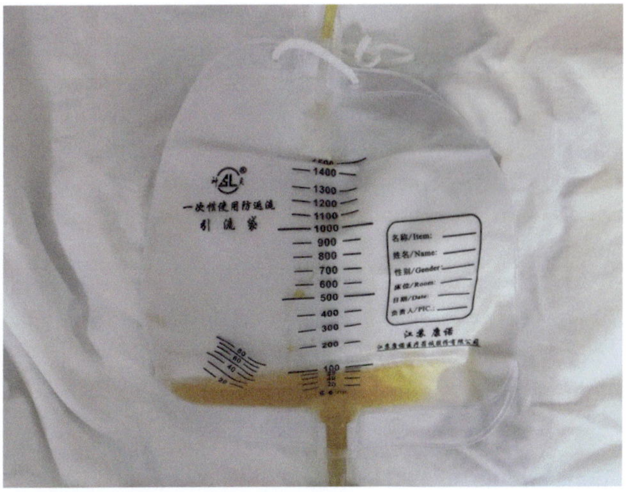

Fig. 19.6 Postoperative ascites drainage (without bile leakage)

19.2 Postoperative Hepatic Insufficiency

Hepatic insufficiency or liver failure following the ALPPS procedure, which is the complication garnering considerable attention from liver surgeons, represents a pivotal cause of near-term death following hepatectomy. The ISGLS defines postoperative hepatic insufficiency or liver failure as a postoperatively acquired deterioration in the ability of the liver (in patients with normal and abnormal liver function) to maintain its synthetic, excretory, and detoxifying functions, characterized by an increased international normalized ratio (INR) (or need of clotting factors to maintain normal INR) and hyperbilirubinemia (according to the normal cutoff levels defined by the local laboratory) on or after postoperative day 5 [9]. Specifically, postoperative hepatic insufficiency can be evaluated using the 50–50 criteria: prothrombin activity <50% and serum bilirubin >50 μmol/L on postoperative day 5 [10]. Postoperative hepatic insufficiency may be categorized into Grades A, B, and C. Grade A postoperative hepatic insufficiency is detected solely through routine postoperative examinations, is clinically asymptomatic, and does not require special clinical interventions; Grade B postoperative hepatic insufficiency manifests with clinical symptoms (e.g., ascites, weight gain, and mild respiratory insufficiency). Clinically, Grade B postoperative hepatic insufficiency patients commonly need non-invasive treatments (e.g., albumin supplementation, coagulation factor supplementation, diuretics, and noninvasive respiratory support) to facilitate recovery and may need admission to an ICU for treatment; Grade C postoperative hepatic insufficiency presents with overt clinical symptoms (e.g., large-volume ascites, generalized edema, hemodynamic instability, and advanced respiratory failure) and requires invasive procedures (e.g., hemodialysis, tracheal intubation and mechanical ventilation, extracorporeal liver support, and rescue hepatectomy or liver transplantation); in addition, Grade C postoperative hepatic insufficiency patients, who are in a critical clinical condition, should be monitored and treated in an ICU [9].

As patients undergoing the ALPPS procedure have an inadequate FLR volume following the direct resection of the diseased liver, inducing the hypertrophy of the contralateral liver following the stage 1 surgery is vital for increasing the FLR, facilitating complete tumor resection, postoperative liver function restoration, and physical rehabilitation. Following the ALPPS procedure, hepatic insufficiency is prevented through preoperative, intraoperative, and postoperative preventions and treatments.

19.2.1 Preoperative Evaluations and Preparations

Preserving an adequate functional liver volume following hepatectomy is essential for preventing postoperative hepatic insufficiency or liver failure. Various strategies, such as augmenting the FLR, diminishing the lesion size, and precisely delineating the resection margins, have been proposed and refined to enhance the safety of hepatectomy. The ALPPS procedure can induce rapid FLR hypertrophy within a short time frame, significantly broadening the spectrum of indications for hepatectomy. A report indicated that the perioperative mortality associated with the ALPPS procedure reached 9%, and the incidence of Clavien-Dindo Grade IIIa or higher complications following the ALPPS procedure soared to 40% [11]. A report showed that the mortality following the two-stage hepatectomy following portal vein embolization (PVE) was 3% [12], markedly lower than that following the ALPPS procedure. Therefore, adequate preoperative evaluations and preparations are imperative for patients slated for the ALPPS procedure, and inducing liver hypertrophy following the stage 1 ALPPS procedure to achieve an adequate liver volume is necessary for initiating the stage 2 ALPPS procedure. Generally, the FLR should be not less than 25% for a normal liver and not less than 40% for patients with underlying liver diseases [13]. The ALPPS procedure can induce rapid FLR hypertrophy within a brief period. A report revealed an FLR hypertrophy of 74% 1 week after the stage 1 ALPPS procedure. The liver cancer patients with a background of hepatitis B recruited at our center underwent stages 1 and 2 surgeries at an interval of 12 days, with a mean FLR hypertrophy of 56.8% [14]. A study revealed that while the ALPPS procedure induced FLR hypertrophy more rapidly than PVE, the hepatocytes, which proliferated as induced by the ALPPS procedure, exhibited an immature morphology [15]. Therefore, observing the outcomes of FLR hypertrophy in addition to the FLR hypertrophy rate is necessary. Liver disease patients commonly experience various types of liver damage. For instance, primary liver cancer patients typically present with comorbid chronic hepatitis B or hepatitis C, subsequently progressing to cirrhosis, colorectal liver metastasis (CRLM) patients often suffer from liver damage resulting from chemotherapy, and hilar cholangiocarcinoma patients frequently experience comorbid obstructive jaundice. The severity of a preoperative hepatic injury inversely correlates with liver regeneration capacity, surgical tolerability, and the likelihood of postoperative hepatic insufficiency or liver failure. Therefore, conducting adequate liver function evaluations and preoperative preparations, in addition to the precise preoperative evaluation of liver volume, is pivotal for preventing postoperative hepatic insufficiency or liver failure.

19.2.2 Measurement of FLR Volume

Conducting the precise preoperative measurement of liver volume and accurately estimating the FLR is essential for preparing for the ALPPS procedure. Clinically, color Doppler ultrasound, computed tomography (CT), and magnetic resonance imaging (MRI) examinations are routinely performed for radiological evaluations. These two-dimensional examinations offer imaging information of sections or cross-sections. Clinicians must mentally reconstruct organs and the three-dimensional morphology of lesions based on their experience and imagination, potentially resulting in significant errors. The advancement in computer technology has led to the widespread clinical adoption of three-dimensional visualization. Three-dimensional visualization contributes considerably to pre-liver surgery three-dimensional imaging, liver volume calculation, FLR estimation, and surgical planning. It is particularly instrumental in facilitating complex surgical procedures or surgical procedures involving extensive resection. Three-dimensional visualization allows the reconstruction of data based on objective imaging data, eliminating errors stemming from variations in clinicians' experiences. This notably improves standardization, accuracy, and individualization. Specifically, CT examinations and associated software are routinely conducted at our center before the ALPPS procedure for precise determination of the vascular course and precise measurement of the volume of each liver lobe, as well as the post-hepatectomy FLR. This aids in quantitatively evaluating the pre- and post-hepatectomy variations in the liver volume and precisely evaluating hepatic functional reserve, facilitating throughout and effective preoperative evaluations. Aside from the three-dimensional visualization of anatomical structures, effective surgical planning can be conducted based on lesion location and relationships with adjacent vessels, substantially augmenting surgical safety. At our center, measuring the standardized future liver volume is routinely performed before the ALPPS procedure. Multiple centers in China utilized three-dimensional visualization for surgical planning before the ALPPS procedure, yielding favorable outcomes. Compared to two-dimensional imaging, three-dimensional visualization provides superior guidance in safeguarding functional major vessels, bile ducts, and vessels within the FLR [16, 17]. Post-hepatectomy, the blood vessels supplying or draining the FLR may be transected, or the bile ducts surrounding the FLR may be damaged, rendering the functional liver volume lower than the actual liver volume. Therefore, employing technetium-99 imaging to measure the functional FLR volume before a two-stage hepatectomy offers significant guiding implications [18]. Nonetheless, the application value of technetium-99 imaging awaits further evaluation.

19.2.3 Measurement of Hepatic Functional Reserve

The ALPPS procedure induces the rapid hypertrophy of the contralateral liver in a short span, providing surgical opportunities for patients previously deemed ineligible for hepatectomy. Liver cancer patients undergoing the ALPPS procedure include patients with giant or multiple tumors, an inadequate FLR, and an inability to tolerate liver tumor resection. Primary liver cancer patients typically experience accompanying severe underlying liver diseases (e.g., cirrhosis), while metastatic liver cancer patients commonly undergo repeated or multiple cycles of chemotherapy, considerably heightening the risk associated with the ALPPS procedure. Therefore, evaluating hepatic functional reserve and precisely evaluating FLR is critical. The Child-Pugh score stands as the predominant scoring system for hepatic functional reserve in clinical settings, and its frequently employed clinical parameters (e.g., bilirubin, albumin, and prothrombin time) are indicative of immediate liver function, providing limited quantitative guidance for the ALPPS procedure. The model for end-stage liver disease (MELD) represents another prevalent scoring system for liver surgery. The MELD score, incorporating bilirubin, INR, creatinine, and etiology, can reflect the hepatic and systemic functions and is utilized to evaluate the prognosis following liver surgery [19]. A study suggested that a preoperative MELD score greater than 10 points is the foremost prognostic factor contributing to the postponement or even cancellation of stage 2 surgery [11]. Aside from preoperative scoring and liver volume measurement, the indocyanine green (ICG) excretion test is commonly employed to gauge hepatic functional reserve. While the monoethylglycinexylidide (MEGX) test and arterial ketone body ratio (AKBR) have been reported to showcase their values in evaluating hepatic functional reserve, they are not frequently utilized in routine clinical practice. The indocyanine green retention rate at 15 minutes (ICG-R15) is typically used to measure hepatic functional reserve. A recent study indicated that a semi-hepatic ICG-R15 of not more than 10% following stage 1 surgery is considered safe for conducting stage 2 surgery in two-stage hepatectomies, including the ALPPS procedure [20]. Generally, if a preoperative ICG-R15 is more than 20%, avoiding major hepatectomy is imperative for preventing postoperative hepatic insufficiency or liver failure [21]. It is noteworthy that the ICG excretion test should be utilized with caution or should be conducted following jaundice resolution, as the presence of evident jaundice may compromise its accuracy.

19.2.4 Preoperative Management of Jaundice

Preoperative jaundice is categorized as obstructive or nonobstructive. Obstructive jaundice typically results from a giant tumor compression of the porta hepatis, biliary obstruction associated with hilar cholangiocarcinoma, or biliary compression by metastatic or inflamed and enlarged lymph nodes. Biliary obstruction can lead to a notable increase in jaundice and hepatic insufficiency. A study confirmed that the preoperative total bilirubin level of more than 2.9 mg/mL increased post-hepatectomy mortality [22]. Conducting biliary drainage in the presence of a high preoperative total bilirubin level remains debated. A randomized controlled study indicated that routinely conducting biliary drainage elevated the risk of postoperative complications in pancreatic tumor patients [23]. The present indications for preoperative biliary drainage include: (a) treatment of cholangitis; (b) management of severe malnutrition and hypoproteinemia; (c) treatment of jaundice-induced liver or kidney failure; (d) prevention of a further deterioration of jaundice when the surgical procedure is postponed for any reason; (e) biliary drainage in patients with borderline resectable tumors, followed by post-recovery neoadjuvant therapy. The optimal duration for biliary drainage is not more than 14 days in patients undergoing biliary drainage [24]. Major hepatectomy should be approached with caution in nonobstructive jaundice patients if the preoperative bilirubin level is more than 40 μmol/L, as postoperative hepatic insufficiency is highly prevalent in such patients. Therefore, these patients should undergo hepatectomy after the bilirubin level returns to normal following drug therapy. The findings of a study associated with the ALPPS procedure revealed that biliary drainage rendered jaundiced patients with hilar cholangiocarcinoma eligible for the ALPPS procedure, leading to improved postoperative safety [25].

19.2.5 Strategies to Protect Liver Function During Surgery

The ALPPS procedure allows ligating the ipsilateral portal vein and transecting the hepatic parenchyma to induce contralateral liver hypertrophy. Achieving an adequate liver volume following contralateral liver hypertrophy is essential for initiating stage 2 surgery; in the presence of an adequate liver volume, the functional capacity of the liver may not increase concurrently with liver volume [26], potentially resulting in an elevated risk of postoperative hepatic insufficiency or liver failure. In such a scenario, the initial consideration should be to postpone stage 2 surgery to allow for liver hypertrophy and regeneration. An early study revealed that before stage 2 surgery, the future liver volumes (FLVs) were 30% and 40%, respectively, and that the incidence rates of postoperative liver failure were 31% and 16%, respectively [11]. Another study signaled that 1 week after stage 1 surgery, the FLR was more than 30%, and the kinetic growth rate (KGR) surpassed 6%, resulting in a low risk of postoperative hepatic insufficiency or liver failure [27]. Generally, an FLV greater than 40% is necessary for the stage 2 ALPPS procedure. If the FLV and KGR are less than 30% and less than 6%, respectively, allowing liver hypertrophy to achieve an adequate liver volume is essential for initiating stage 2 surgery. Radiologically evaluating liver function may be conducted for reference purposes if conditions permit. Our center has acquired extensive experience in managing inadequate liver hypertrophy following stage 1 surgery. Specifically, in the presence of insufficient liver hypertrophy following stage 1 surgery, trans-arterial embolization (TAE) may be performed to selectively embolize the right hepatic arterial branches supplying tumors, facilitating further hypertrophy of the contralateral liver [28].

During the classic ALPPS procedure, safeguarding the hepatic parenchymal function in segment IV is pivotal for mitigating the incidence of postoperative liver failure. A scholar indicates that avoiding liver injury and maintaining the patency of the blood supply channel, blood reflux channel, and biliary tract in segment IV can markedly lessen the incidence of postoperative hepatic insufficiency or liver failure [29]. In cases where a vascular injury is unavoidable due to factors (e.g., variations in the split location of hepatic parenchyma) or the anatomical locations of blood vessels (e.g., portal and hepatic veins), a scholar advocates resecting segment IV to prevent severe hepatic insufficiency or liver failure resulting from liver necrosis [30].

The ALPPS procedure inflicts considerable trauma on patients, as it is conducted in two stages within a brief time frame. The ALPPS procedure has been modified, with the original intention of minimizing surgical trauma while promoting liver hypertrophy to guarantee successful postoperative liver function restoration. The major modified procedures include partial ALPPS, tourniquet ALPPS, radiofrequency/microwave ablation-assisted ALPPS, and hybrid ALPPS procedures. Partial ALPPS procedure involves partially transecting the hepatic parenchyma while preserving the middle hepatic vein when feasible, along with ligating the ipsilateral portal vein branches in stage 1 surgery. Fernando et al. [31] reported that partial ALPPS procedure dramatically reduced postoperative complications and achieved near-zero mortality compared to the conventional ALPPS procedure in the presence of an identical increase in the liver volume following stage 1 surgery. A center reported that when a partial ALPPS procedure entailed transecting 50–80% of the hepatic parenchyma, liver hypertrophy of at least 50% following stage 1 surgery was achieved. Portal vein, hepatic vein, and bile duct system in segment IV tissues were preserved whenever possible, leading to a remarkably decreased risk of postoperative complications (e.g., hepatic insufficiency or liver failure) [32]. A scholar indicated that the conventional ALPPS procedure induced liver hypertrophy more rapidly than the partial ALPPS procedure [33]. Nonetheless, the partial ALPPS procedure remains a preferred modified surgical procedure. It is considered not inferior to the conventional ALPPS procedure in promoting liver regeneration, as it causes less trauma and a lower risk of postoperative hepatic insufficiency or liver failure. Tourniquet ALPPS procedure enables portal vein ligation with a tourniquet, which supplants hepatic parenchymal transection in conventional ALPPS procedure, at the Cantlie line where the liver parenchyma is planned to be transected in stage 1 surgery, and utilizes B-mode ultrasonography to intraoperatively confirm the absence of blood flow between bilateral hepatic parenchymal tissues. In addition, the tourniquet ALPPS procedure requires ligating the ipsilateral portal vein branches. The tourniquet ALPPS procedure offers multiple advantages, including short duration of stage 1 surgery, streamlined operations, minimal trauma, avoidance of the formation of two hepatic wounds, and absence of complications (e.g., bile leakage and bleeding) following stage 1 surgery. Nonetheless, the tourniquet ALPPS procedure may induce severe adhesion around the porta hepatis following stage 1 surgery, potentially heightening the complexity of stage 2 surgery and consequently elevating the risk of complications. With respect to liver hypertrophy following stage 1 surgery, the FLR hypertrophy was reported to be up to 189% 1 week after the tourniquet ALPPS procedure, with the mean FLR hypertrophy of 61% [34]. Radiofrequency/microwave ablation-assisted ALPPS procedure employs radiofrequency/microwave ablation, which serves as an alternative to the hepatic parenchymal transection in the conventional ALPPS procedure, to create necrotic and ischemic zones in the planned hepatic transection area in stage 1 surgery, along with the ligation of ipsilateral portal vein branches. A report on the treatment of CRLM patients with radiofrequency/

microwave ablation-assisted ALPPS procedure indicated that the mean FLR hypertrophy following stage 1 surgery was 62.3%, the incidence of postoperative complications was 20%, and that no perioperative deaths were observed [35]. Generally, radiofrequency/microwave ablation-assisted ALPPS procedure represents a viable modified surgical procedure, as it can circumvent the need for hepatic parenchymal transection in stage 1 surgery and effectively preserve the hepatic inflow and outflow tracts and biliary system; in addition, it can preclude the onset of postoperative complications (e.g., hepatic insufficiency or liver failure), as the hepatic parenchymal hypertrophy following stage 1 surgery is identical to that following conventional ALPPS procedure. As with the conventional ALPPS procedure, the hybrid ALPPS procedure utilizes hepatic parenchymal transection via the anterior approach in stage 1 surgery; however, it subsequently employs intraoperative or postoperative PVE instead of intraoperative portal vein ligation. The benefit of the hybrid ALPPS procedure lies in its capacity to diminish hilar adhesions resulting from surgical operations around the porta hepatis while effectively maintaining the "no-touch" principle in tumor management. A scholar reported that the FLR hypertrophies of 85.5% and 65.3% were achieved following stage 1 hybrid ALPPS procedure, respectively, which were not lower than those following the conventional ALPPS procedure, and that no major postoperative complications occurred [36]. The partial hepatic parenchymal transection combined with PVE (mini ALPPS procedure) [37], representing a further modification of the hybrid ALPPS procedure, streamlines stage 1 surgery with swift and straightforward operations, followed by extensive operations (e.g., further transection and resection of hepatic parenchyma and transection of portal vein branches) in stage 2 surgery.

The applications of the ALPPS procedure have increasingly been reported. Patients undergoing the conventional ALPPS procedure experience surgical trauma twice in a short time span. Introducing minimally invasive techniques to the ALPPS procedure aims to lessen surgical trauma and promote rapid recovery. Strategically, this can be achieved using minimally invasive techniques in stage 1 or 2 surgery or a two-stage surgery. A study, reporting the inaugural use of the laparoscopic ALPPS procedure, demonstrated that the completion rate of stage 2 laparoscopic ALPPS procedure was comparable to that of the conventional open ALPPS procedure, the perioperative incidence of Clavien-Dindo Grade IIIa, with higher complications and mortality was zero, and that the hospital stay following the laparoscopic ALPPS procedure was markedly shorter than that following open ALPPS [38]. Furthermore, modified ALPPS procedures (e.g., partial ALPPS and mini ALPPS procedures) may be performed using minimally invasive techniques (e.g., laparoscopy), further reducing postoperative complications (e.g., hepatic insufficiency or liver failure) upon achieving liver hypertrophy comparable to that following the conventional ALPPS procedure [39, 40].

During the ALPPS procedure, conventional surgical concepts and techniques may be utilized to decrease the risk of postoperative hepatic insufficiency or liver failure. The hepatic vascular control techniques can substantially promote postoperative liver function restoration. Nonetheless, employing hepatic vascular control techniques to minimize bleeding during hepatectomy is technically challenging in complex hepatectomies, including the ALPPS procedure. The conventional Pringle maneuver can interrupt the blood flow to the first porta hepatis. It may also occlude the inferior vena cava or hepatic veins if tumors are located adjacent to the second porta hepatis. Transecting the liver parenchyma and detaching portal vein branches are typically complex surgical operations demanding significant time. Prolonged or repeated periods of total hepatic vascular exclusion noticeably escalate the risk of hepatic ischemia-reperfusion injury. Patients with normal hepatic functional reserve experience normal recovery, whereas patients with comorbid severe cirrhosis face an elevated risk of postoperative hepatic insufficiency or liver failure. As such, sequentially occluding the first porta hepatis, shortening the duration of each occlusion, or partially occluding the porta hepatis may be considered for patients with comorbid cirrhosis. In addition, utilizing surgical instruments (e.g., high-pressure water jet system and bipolar electrocoagulation forceps) for precise hepatectomy may lead to diminished postoperative acute hepatic injuries and incidence of hepatic insufficiency or liver failure.

If tumors are located near or invade major contralateral blood vessels, the ALPPS procedure should be selected with caution. Suppose tumors are situated adjacent to the hepatic pedicle, main portal vein, or inferior vena cava. In that case, it is advisable to minimize surgical duration while performing meticulous operations to mitigate surgical trauma. Surgical procedures involving precise hepatic parenchymal transection without occlusion of hepatic blood flow should be preferably selected to minimize hepatic impairments.

The ALPPS procedure can be modified to safeguard the parenchymal blood flow and bile ducts in segment IV. However, maintaining the integrity and patency of the inflow and outflow tracts and biliary tracts in the FLR should intraoperatively receive enormous attention. Patients eligible for the ALPPS procedure typically possess multiple or giant tumors. In certain instances, complete tumor resection can inadvertently damage the surrounding contralateral hepatic parenchyma, eventually resulting in postoperative hepatic insufficiency or liver failure. In this regard, devoting considerable attention to and safeguarding the blood supply to the contralateral hepatic artery, portal vein, and hepatic vein, as well as the integrity of the bile duct system can evidently diminish the incidence of hepatic insufficiency or liver failure and biliary complications. In addition, moderately mobilizing perihepatic ligaments, as well as safeguarding potential vascular collateral circulations in perihepatic ligaments, aid in mitigating the incidence of postoperative liver failure.

19.2.6 Supplementary Measures

Irrespective of viral replication, hepatitis B virus surface antigen-positive patients should routinely undergo antiviral treatments (e.g., entecavir and tenofovir disoproxil fumarate) in order to ensure the effective preoperative control of hepatitis B virus replication and prevent exacerbated hepatic impairment resulting from increased viral replication induced by postoperative hypo-immunity. Liver tumor patients in China typically have a background of hepatitis B. Postoperative infection, bile leakage, bleeding, and fluid-electrolyte imbalance may become the predisposing factors for perioperative hepatic insufficiency or liver failure. Effective measures (e.g., enhanced infection control, adequate drainage, re-laparotomy for hemostasis, and correction of fluid-electrolyte and acid-base imbalances) should be implemented to lower the risk of postoperative hepatic insufficiency or liver failure.

19.3 Hemorrhage

Bleeding is one of the frequent complications following the ALPPS procedure [41], and its causes include intra-abdominal bleeding and coagulation disorders. Intra-abdominal hemorrhage typically occurs within 48 hours after stage 1 or stage 2 surgery. Intra-abdominal bleeding is attributable to three major causes: hemorrhage from the hepatic transection surface. It typically occurs after stage 1 surgery and arises from FLR congestion induced by portal vein ligation as well as the occlusion of collateral circulation of portal veins between hepatic lobes as a result of hepatic in situ splitting and intraoperative incomplete hemostasis. It results from improper operations for hepatic vein root, diaphragmatic injuries, or elevated pressure in the thoracic cavity and inferior vena cava, loosening, or detachment of vascular sutures. It is typically attributed to an increased pressure in the vena cava resulting from body movements (e.g., patient-turning procedures or severe cough). Intraoperative complete hemostasis and meticulous operations are paramount. Caution should be exercised to detect bleeding from the hepatic transection surface or hemorrhage anterior to the inferior vena cava. Additionally, any rise in blood pressure before abdominal closure should warrant thorough examination. Hemostatic membrane, gelfoam, and biogel are viable options for providing supplementary hemostasis on the hepatic transection surface [42]. Placing negative pressure drainage tubes below the right diaphragm and at the porta hepatis postoperatively is necessary for maintaining unobstructed drainage. Persistent bloody drainage may signal intra-abdominal thrombosis, obstructing abdominal cavity drainage to cause abdominal distension. Closely monitoring vital signs and infusing red blood cells, platelets, and plasma are typically recommended if a patient's blood pressure and pulse remain stable. Performing a re-laparotomy for hemostasis is recommended if blood loss exceeds 100 mL/h and persists for more than 8 hours.

The common causes of coagulation disorders following the ALPPS procedure include the following: (a) an inadequate FLR volume, liver failure following stage 1 surgery, particularly in the presence of comorbid cirrhosis; (b) intraoperative massive bleeding or blood transfusion of more than 4000 mL; and (c) severe postoperative infection, extensive depletion of coagulation factors and platelets. Perioperatively measuring the coagulation time, prothrombin time, platelet count, and fibrinogen level aids in diagnosing coagulation disorders. If necessary, the 3P examination may be conducted. Upon diagnosing coagulation disorders, it is imperative to discontinue the use of anticoagulants immediately, routinely expand circulating blood volume and administer fresh blood transfusions, and promptly administer fibrinogen, prothrombin complex, fresh platelets, and cryoprecipitates as necessary [43]. Conducting meticulous preoperative evaluations of the coagulation function is vital for preventing oozing bleeding from the surgical wound following the ALPPS procedure. Any coagulation function impairment can be ameliorated by infusing coagulation factors and plasma.

Persistent abdominal hemorrhage following the ALPPS procedure is emblematic of the need for a re-exploratory laparotomy. During exploratory laparotomy, attention should be directed to the presence of an intra-abdominal hematoma. Any hematoma identified should be completely cleared to prevent postoperative infections. This is followed by the meticulous inspection of bleeding from small blood vessels in the tissues surrounding the hematoma. In the absence of any obvious hematoma, it is imperative to detect bleeding from small blood vessels on the hepatic transection surface and surgical wounds, including those involving the omentum, adherent gastrointestinal wall, diaphragm, and perinephric fat capsule. The ALPPS procedure is associated with liver ischemia and necrosis resulting from the ALPPS procedure (e.g., segment IV in the classic ALPPS procedure). As such, intraoperatively resecting ischemic liver may be considered. The necessity to perform a re-exploratory laparotomy to detect delayed postoperative bleeding should be determined based on the specific circumstances. In case of the presence of any abdominal infection as well as the presence of any identified intra-abdominal hematoma as revealed by the postoperative examination, conducting an exploratory laparotomy assists in identifying hemostatic spots and clearing the source of infections, interrupting the vicious circle where infections and hemorrhage exacerbate each other. In case of postoperative bleeding resulting from coagulation insufficiency, the coagulation function should be corrected as described previously. In principle, a re-exploratory laparotomy should be approached with caution. It is noteworthy that in rare cases, bleeding from the hepatic transection surface stems from hepatic congestion caused by the occlusion of the venous reflux to the FLR tissues. As such, effectively managing reflux channels (e.g., left and middle hepatic veins) is crucial for maintaining the patency of the reflux to hepatic parenchyma during the ALPPS procedure. If preserving the middle hepatic vein is unfeasible, congested hepatic parenchyma (e.g., parenchyma in segment IV) may be resected as appropriate.

19.4 Infections

Infectious complications, which are major concerns following the ALPPS procedure, compromise the capture of surgical timing and perioperative prognosis. The rates of Clavien-Dindo Grade IIIa or higher infectious complications associated with hepatitis B-associated hepatocellular carcinoma (HCC) following stages 1 and 2 ALPPS procedures were 5.3% and 2.7%, respectively [44]. The rates of Clavien-Dindo Grade IIIa or higher and Clavien-Dindo Grade a or higher infectious complications associated with locally advanced intrahepatic cholangiocarcinoma (ICC) following stages 1 and 2 in the ALPPS procedures were 43.8% and 20.8%, respectively [41]. In a cohort (CRLM, 80.6%, 50/62; HCC, 4.8%, 3/62; hilar cholangiocarcinoma, 4.8%, 3/62; gallbladder cancer, 6.5%, 4/62; others, 3.3%, 2/62), the incidence rates of sepsis/infections (Clavien-Dindo grade was not mentioned) following stages 1 and 2 the ALPPS procedures were 17.7% and 18.6%, respectively [45].

Infections associated with the ALPPS procedure can be categorized into SSIs, respiratory infections, catheter-related bloodstream infections, and other types of infections. SSIs are strongly correlated with bile leakage. Grade C or higher bile leakages notably elevate the risks of deep-seated, superficial, and peri-organ SSIs [46]. The ALPPS procedure is more prone to inducing bile leakage compared to other hepatectomies [46]. Therefore, preventing bile leakage following the ALPPS procedure is essential for controlling SSIs. The long duration of the ALPPS procedure, diaphragmatic stimulation from liver surgery, and postoperative pain contribute to pleural effusion and atelectasis, which are the leading causes of lung infections [46]. Catheter-related bloodstream infections are strongly associated with the indwelling time of a catheter, aseptic operations, immunity, and health status. Given the substantial time and extensive interventions necessary for the ALPPS procedure, attention must be dedicated to other types of infections (e.g., catheter-related and drainage tube-related infections).

Preventing perioperative infections associated with the ALPPS procedure is paramount. Preoperatively, understanding the general conditions and comorbidities is crucial. Intraoperatively conducting meticulous operations, maintaining sterility, controlling surgical time and bleeding, and implementing respiratory management are critical. Postoperatively providing dynamic monitoring, adequate analgesia, nutritional support, sufficient drainage, and close observations is essential. The long-term (>4 days) postoperative prophylactic antibiotic use should be avoided to prevent SSIs and multidrug-resistant infections [47]. In case of infections, the causative factors should be promptly addressed, and the infections can be controlled using an appropriate anti-infective therapy combined with nutritional support therapy, offered in a full-dose and full-course manner.

The ipsilateral liver is prone to ischemia and necrosis following the stage 1 ALPPS procedure. Therefore, perihepatic effusion and infections are frequent complications. In the presence of a significant effusion of inflammatory substances and comorbid bile leakage from the hepatic wound, adequate drainage will be needed. An obstructed drainage tube can lead to inadequate drainage, potentially causing abdominal encapsulated effusion complicated by severe infections. This should be addressed with imaging-guided percutaneous drainage and an anti-infective therapy. In case of severe infections, attention should be drawn to the acid-base and fluid-electrolyte imbalances, which should be vigorously corrected. After stage 2 surgery, a small amount of bile leakage can spontaneously resolve following unobstructed drainage. If significant bile leakage persists over a long period, consideration may be given to placing a nasobiliary duct under ERCP to drain bile in vitro to facilitate healing. In case of bile leakage resulting from a severe bile duct injury, a re-laparotomy is typically needed. In addition, liver tumor patients typically experience comorbid cirrhosis and, therefore, are prone to develop pleural effusions and ascites. Obstructed drainage leads to infections, which are preferably treated with unobstructed drainage combined with antibiotic therapy. If subphrenic effusion complicated by infection is identified, the preferred treatment is percutaneous catheter drainage combined with antibiotic therapy. Inadequate drainage or an exacerbated infection during drainage suggests the need for exploratory surgery to identify the source of infection and establish unobstructed drainage channels.

19.5 Pleural Effusion

Pleural effusion, particularly right-sided pleural effusion, is highly prevalent following the ALPPS procedure. It is attributable to multiple factors, such as mobilization of perihepatic ligaments, lymphatic drainage, hypoproteinemia, large-volume ascites, and subphrenic effusion and infection. Currently, no effective preventive actions are available. Briefly, implementing preoperative evaluations and preparations for complex hepatectomies, individualized surgical protocols based on patients' conditions, and meticulous surgical operations are fundamental to preventing postoperative complications and achieving favorable outcomes. If patients present with large-volume pleural effusions along with symptoms (e.g., pyrexia, chest tightness, shortness of breath, and decreased oxygen saturation), thoracocentesis and catheter drainage will be needed. For patients with small-volume pleural effusions, the effusions will be absorbed and will resolve following conservative treatments (e.g., albumin supplementation).

19.6 Ascites

The underlying causes of ascites mirror those of pleural effusions. Following the ALPPS procedure, inflammatory responses, elevated portal vein pressures, and hepatic insufficiency are identified as the predisposing factors for postoperative ascites. Ascites are typically treated with supportive therapies (e.g., improvements in liver function, water and salt restriction, and diuretic therapy).

19.7 Gastrointestinal Hemorrhage

Gastrointestinal bleeding, which typically occurs within 3 months postoperatively, frequently arises from gastrointestinal ulcers induced by viral infection, bleeding resulting from portal hypertension, or other factors. Recurrent episodes of esophageal variceal bleeding following the ALPPS procedure are commonly associated with PVE. Hemorrhage from intestinal loops often manifests 1 week postoperatively and is typically self-limiting. Gastrointestinal hemorrhage following the ALPPS procedure should be positively diagnosed to determine the hemorrhagic site and the presence of other accompanying complications, such as hepatic insufficiency or intravascular thrombosis, commonly occurring in the portal vein. The hepatobiliary ultrasound examination in the emergency department aids in understanding the portal vein. A further endoscopic examination may be conducted. If esophageal bleeding is ruled out, gastric and duodenal hemorrhage should be detected to determine the hemorrhagic site. If the endoscopic examinations of the upper and lower digestive tracts fail to identify a hemorrhagic site, ^{99}TC-labeled red blood cell scintigraphy may be employed for a noninvasive diagnosis. If scintigraphy signals positive findings, visceral arteriography should be performed to provide a proven diagnosis, and vascular embolization may be performed to arrest hemorrhage. Gastrointestinal bleeding at any site may arise from opportunistic infections with pathogens (e.g., cytomegalovirus or lymphoproliferative disorders). Gastric and duodenal stress ulcers or ulcers caused by high doses of prednisone are prevalent. Pseudomembranous enteritis, resulting from persistent clostridial infections, can manifest with overt hemorrhage. Blood transfusion, coagulation factor supplementation, targeted antibiotic therapy, and judicious use of immunosuppressants may assist in controlling gastrointestinal hemorrhage. In severe cases, partial enterectomy or partial gastrectomy is needed.

References

1. Narita M, Oussoultzoglou E, Ikai I, et al. Right portal vein ligation combined with *in situ* splitting induces rapid left lateral liver lobe hypertrophy enabling 2-staged extended right hepatic resection in small-for-size settings [J]. Ann Surg. 2012;256(3):e7–8; author reply e16–e17.
2. Clavien PA, Sanabria JR, Strasberg SM. Proposed classification of complications of surgery with examples of utility in cholecystectomy [J]. Surgery. 1992;111(5):518–26.
3. Dindo D, Demartines N, Clavien PA. Classification of surgical complications: a new proposal with evaluation in a cohort of 6336 patients and results of a survey [J]. Ann Surg. 2004;240(2):205–13.
4. Koch M, Garden OJ, Padbury R, et al. Bile leakage after hepatobiliary and pancreatic surgery: a definition and grading of severity by the International Study Group of Liver Surgery [J]. Surgery. 2011;149(5):680–8.
5. Zhang GQ, Zhang ZW, Lau WY, et al. Associating liver partition and portal vein ligation for staged hepatectomy (ALPPS): a new strategy to increase resectability in liver surgery [J]. Int J Surg. 2014;12(5):437–41.
6. Spetzler VN, Schepers M, Pinnschmidt HO, et al. The incidence and severity of post-hepatectomy bile leaks is affected by surgical indications, preoperative chemotherapy, and surgical procedures [J]. Hepatobiliary Surg Nutr. 2019;8(2):101–10.
7. Andriani OC. Long-term results with associating liver partition and portal vein ligation for staged hepatectomy (ALPPS) [J]. Ann Surg. 2012;256(3):e5; author reply e16–e19.
8. Gholson CF, Zibari G, McDonald JC. Endoscopic diagnosis and management of biliary complications following orthotopic liver transplantation [J]. Dig Dis Sci. 1996;41(6):1045–53.
9. Rahbari NN, Garden OJ, Padbury R, et al. Posthepatectomy liver failure: a definition and grading by the International Study Group of Liver Surgery (ISGLS) [J]. Surgery. 2011;149(5):713–24.
10. Balzan S, Belghiti J, Farges O, et al. The "50-50 criteria" on postoperative day 5: an accurate predictor of liver failure and death after hepatectomy [J]. Ann Surg. 2005;242(6):824–8; discussion 828–829.
11. Schadde E, Raptis DA, Schnitzbauer AA, et al. Prediction of mortality after ALPPS stage 1: an analysis of 320 patients from the international ALPPS registry [J]. Ann Surg. 2015;262(5):780–5; discussion 785–786.

12. Lam VW, Laurence JM, Johnston E, et al. A systematic review of two-stage hepatectomy in patients with initially unresectable colorectal liver metastases [J]. HPB (Oxford). 2013;15(7):483–91.
13. Tucker ON, Heaton N. The 'small for size' liver syndrome [J]. Curr Opin Crit Care. 2005;11(2):150–5.
14. Wang Z, Peng YF, Hu JW, et al. Associating liver partition and portal vein ligation for staged hepatectomy for unresectable hepatitis B virus-related hepatocellular carcinoma: a single center study of 45 patients [J]. Ann Surg. 2020;271(3):534–41.
15. Matsuo K, Murakami T, Kawaguchi D, et al. Histologic features after surgery associating liver partition and portal vein ligation for staged hepatectomy versus those after hepatectomy with portal vein embolization [J]. Surgery. 2016;159(5):1289–98.
16. Tan K, Du XL, Chen A, et al. Application of preoperative accurate define of liver transection plane in ALPPS based on 3D visualization technology [J]. Chin J Hepatic Surg Electron Ed. 2020;9(2):158–63.
17. Hu ZG, Huang PB, Zhou ZY, et al. The application value of two-dimensional image technology and three-dimensional visualization technology in hepatocellular carcinoma treated by associating liver partition and portal vein ligation for staged hepatectomy: a preliminary study [J]. Zhonghua Wai Ke Za Zhi. 2016;54(9):686–91.
18. Rassam F, Olthof PB, van Lienden KP, et al. Comparison of functional and volumetric increase of the future remnant liver and postoperative outcomes after portal vein embolization and complete or partial associating liver partition and portal vein ligation for staged hepatectomy (ALPPS) [J]. Ann Transl Med. 2020;8(7):436.
19. Cucchetti A, Piscaglia F, Cescon M, et al. Conditional survival after hepatic resection for hepatocellular carcinoma in cirrhotic patients [J]. Clin Cancer Res. 2012;18(16):4397–405.
20. Yu TD, Ye XP, Wen Z, et al. Intraoperative indocyanine green retention test of left hemiliver in decision-making for patients with hepatocellular carcinoma undergoing right hepatectomy [J]. Front Surg. 2021;8:709017.
21. Clavien PA, Petrowsky H, DeOliveira ML, et al. Strategies for safer liver surgery and partial liver transplantation [J]. N Engl J Med. 2007;356(15):1545–59.
22. Farges O, Regimbeau JM, Fuks D, et al. Multicentre European study of preoperative biliary drainage for hilar cholangiocarcinoma [J]. Br J Surg. 2013;100(2):274–83.
23. van der Gaag NA, Rauws EA, van Eijck CH, et al. Preoperative biliary drainage for cancer of the head of the pancreas [J]. N Engl J Med. 2010;362(2):129–37.
24. Lai EC, Lau SH, Lau WY. The current status of preoperative biliary drainage for patients who receive pancreaticoduodenectomy for periampullary carcinoma: a comprehensive review [J]. Surgeon. 2014;12(5):290–6.
25. Balci D, Kirimker EO, Üstüner E, et al. Stage I-laparoscopy partial ALPPS procedure for perihilar cholangiocarcinoma [J]. J Surg Oncol. 2020;121(6):1022–6.
26. Olthof PB, Tomassini F, Huespe PE, et al. Hepatobiliary scintigraphy to evaluate liver function in associating liver partition and portal vein ligation for staged hepatectomy: liver volume overestimates liver function [J]. Surgery. 2017;162(4):775–83.
27. Kambakamba P, Stocker D, Reiner CS, et al. Liver kinetic growth rate predicts postoperative liver failure after ALPPS [J]. HPB (Oxford). 2016;18(10):800–5.
28. Peng YF, Wang Z, Qu XD, et al. Transcatheter arterial embolization-salvaged ALPPS, a novel ALPPS procedure especially for patients with hepatocellular carcinoma and severe fibrosis/cirrhosis [J]. Hepatobiliary Surg Nutr. 2022;11(4):504–14.
29. Nagorney DM. Commentary on "Can we improve the morbidity and mortality associated with the associating liver partition with portal vein ligation for staged hepatectomy (ALPPS) procedure in the management of colorectal liver metastases?" [J]. Surgery. 2015;157(2):202–3.
30. Tanaka K, Kikuchi Y, Kawaguchi D, et al. Modified ALPPS procedures avoiding division of portal pedicles [J]. Ann Surg. 2017;265(2):e14–20.
31. Alvarez FA, Ardiles V, de Santibañes M, et al. Associating liver partition and portal vein ligation for staged hepatectomy offers high oncological feasibility with adequate patient safety: a prospective study at a single center [J]. Ann Surg. 2015;261(4):723–32.
32. Petrowsky H, Györi G, de Oliveira M, et al. Is partial-ALPPS safer than ALPPS? A single-center experience [J]. Ann Surg. 2015;261(4):e90–2.
33. Chan ACY, Chok K, Dai JWC, et al. Impact of split completeness on future liver remnant hypertrophy in associating liver partition and portal vein ligation for staged hepatectomy (ALPPS) in hepatocellular carcinoma: complete-ALPPS versus partial-ALPPS [J]. Surgery. 2017;161(2):357–64.
34. Robles R, Parrilla P, López-Conesa A, et al. Tourniquet modification of the associating liver partition and portal ligation for staged hepatectomy procedure [J]. Br J Surg. 2014;101(9):1129–34; discussion 1134.
35. Gall TM, Sodergren MH, Frampton AE, et al. Radio-frequency-assisted liver partition with portal vein ligation (RALPP) for liver regeneration [J]. Ann Surg. 2015;261(2):e45–6.
36. Li J, Kantas A, Ittrich H, et al. Avoid "all-touch" by hybrid ALPPS to achieve oncological efficacy [J]. Ann Surg. 2016;263(1):e6–7.
37. de Santibañes E, Alvarez FA, Ardiles V, et al. Inverting the ALPPS paradigm by minimizing first stage impact: the mini-ALPPS technique [J]. Langenbeck's Arch Surg. 2016;401(4):557–63.
38. Machado MA, Makdissi FF, Surjan RC, et al. Transition from open to laparoscopic ALPPS for patients with very small FLR: the initial experience [J]. HPB (Oxford). 2017;19(1):59–66.
39. Pekolj J, Alvarez FA, Biagiola D, et al. Totally laparoscopic mini-ALPPS using a novel approach of laparoscopic-assisted transmesenteric portal vein embolization [J]. J Laparoendosc Adv Surg Tech A. 2018;28(10):1229–33.
40. Truant S, El Amrani M, Baillet C, et al. Laparoscopic partial ALPPS: much better than ALPPS! [J]. Ann Hepatol. 2019;18(1):269–73.
41. Li J, Moustafa M, Linecker M, et al. ALPPS for locally advanced intrahepatic cholangiocarcinoma: did aggressive surgery lead to the oncological benefit? An international multi-center study [J]. Ann Surg Oncol. 2020;27(5):1372–84.
42. Olthof PB, Rassam F, van Gulik TM. The use of a NHS-PEG coated, collagen-based sealant in a patient undergoing associating liver partition and portal vein ligation for staged hepatectomy (ALPPS) [J]. Int J Surg Case Rep. 2018;47:7–10.
43. Shan J, Quan F, Wuyun G, et al. Management of post-hepatectomy complications [J]. World J Gastroenterol. 2013;19(44):7983–91.
44. Li PP, Huang G, Jia NY, et al. Associating liver partition and portal vein ligation for staged hepatectomy versus sequential transarterial chemoembolization and portal vein embolization in staged hepatectomy for HBV-related hepatocellular carcinoma: a randomized comparative study [J]. Hepatobiliary Surg Nutr. 2022;11(1):38–51.
45. Truant S, Scatton O, Dokmak S, et al. Associating liver partition and portal vein ligation for staged hepatectomy (ALPPS): impact of the inter-stages course on morbi-mortality and implications for management [J]. Eur J Surg Oncol. 2015;41(5):674–82.
46. Cao Y, Jie B, Zheng SG, et al. Clinical analysis of perioperative complications of 26 cases of liver cancer after ALPPS [J]. J Third Mil Med Univ. 2019;41(15):1491–6.
47. Murtha-Lemekhova A, Fuchs J, Teroerde M, et al. Routine post-operative antibiotic prophylaxis offers no benefit after hepatectomy—a systematic review and meta-analysis [J]. Antibiotics. 2022;11(5):649.

Follow-Up Management and Prognosis

20

Xinrong Yang, Huichuan Sun, and Zhifeng Jiang

As a revolutionary surgical procedure in liver surgery in recent 10 years, associating liver partition and portal vein ligation for staged hepatectomy (ALPPS) ligatures the portal vein on the deportalized lobe (DL) of the liver and separates the liver tissue on the DL from the residual liver tissues at the same time, so that the healthy side can regenerate rapidly within 1–2 weeks. As the future liver remnant (FLR) grows enough, the DL can be removed in the second stage, which allows patients with liver cancer that could not be resected to regain the opportunity for radical resection. However, the surgical operation during ALPPS and the drastic change of microenvironment during the rapid liver regeneration may lead to high local recurrence and distant metastasis after ALPPS (the recurrence/metastasis rate within 1 year after surgery has been reported to be approximately 54.0% [1]), which affects the prognosis and quality of life of patients after ALPPS. This chapter summarizes the influence of ALPPS on tumor recurrence and metastasis and explores its prevention and treatment strategies based on the current research data and experience.

20.1 Factors Influencing Tumor Recurrence and Metastasis After ALPPS

ALPPS was initially developed by German professor Hans J. Schlitt in 2007. ALPPS was commented on and named by professors De Santibaese and Pierre-Alain Clavien in 2012, and the international registration system of ALPPS was established (www.alpps.org) in the same year [2]. While the application of ALPPS increased the surgical feasibility and resection rates for patients with colorectal liver metastases and primary liver cancer, reports were suggesting that ALPPS might potentially facilitate tumor metastasis and recurrence: 6 of 7 patients with colorectal cancer liver metastases (CRLM) had tumor recurrence within 8 months after ALPPS [3]. According to the retrospective data reported by Zhongshan Hospital affiliated to Fudan University, 17 of 38 patients successfully underwent the second-stage operation had tumor recurrence or metastasis after operation [4]. Albert Chan of Queen Mary Hospital in Hong Kong reported that 21 of 46 patients (45.7%) with hepatocellular carcinoma treated with ALPPS had tumor recurrence or metastasis [5].

Like other surgical operations, ALPPS may cause tumor cells to fall off or metastasize to other tissues [6]. At present, there are no clear conclusions about whether ALPPS promotes tumor recurrence or metastasis [7]. In the ALPPS stage 1, it is necessary to completely dissociate the liver, dissect the hilum of the liver, and block the part of the liver's blood flow with the liver partition, which will squeeze and stimulate the tumor and may lead to the spread of the tumor. At the same time, tumor-related factors, such as tumor size, number, differentiation, and vascular invasion, may also affect the occurrence of metastasis and recurrence after ALPPS [8, 9].

The change of immune system after ALPPS may also be one of the reasons for tumor metastasis and recurrence [10]. The immunity of cancer patients is generally suppressed, and such a state will be further aggravated by surgical strikes, resulting in the immune escape, proliferation, and invasion of residual tumor cells [11, 12]. E. Rebecca Longbottom and other researchers found that the level of IL-6 in patients after major surgery increased significantly, accompanied by a certain degree of immunosuppression [13]. Meanwhile, the activity of natural killer cells (NK cells) and the percentage of γδ-T cells in patients' peripheral blood are significantly reduced [13, 14]. Multiple factors in the perioperative period also affect the neuroendocrine response and immunity of patients, thus leading to postoperative tumor metastasis and recurrence [15], such as the use of analgesic drugs [16], intraoperative blood loss, and transfusion [17]. Therefore, factors including perioperative anesthetic drug selection,

X. Yang (✉) · H. Sun · Z. Jiang
Zhongshan Hospital, Fudan University, Shanghai, China
e-mail: yang.xinrong@zs-hospital.sh.cn

J. Zhou (ed.), *Associating Liver Partition and Portal Vein Ligation for Staged Hepatectomy (ALPPS)*,
https://doi.org/10.1007/978-981-96-7364-3_20

intraoperative bleeding and transfusion, surgical technique, selection of modified procedure, and the stress response of the patients may all lead to tumor metastasis and recurrence after ALPPS.

20.2 The Possible Molecular Mechanism of Tumor Metastasis and Recurrence After ALPPS

Tumor metastasis and recurrence after ALPPS adversely affect the surgical effect and the overall survival of patients, so it is crucial to find the fundamental mechanisms and related factors affecting metastasis and recurrence. According to the current research, the traumatic reaction of the liver parenchyma section can promote the release of interleukin, regeneration-related factors, and tumor necrosis factor from liver tissue after ALPPS stage 1. These cytokines are involved in the rapid regeneration of residual liver and play a significant role in tumor occurrence and progression [18, 19]. Studies have shown that the enhanced expression of IL-6 and TNF can significantly promote the genesis and progression of liver cancer [20]. Markus Reschke and others found that the activation of the EGFR signal can regulate the proliferation of hepatocytes and play a key role in the development and progression of liver cancer cells [21].

Tumor growth needs enough oxygen and essential nutrients; otherwise, the tumors will stagnate and necrosis [22]. After ALPPS stage 1, the hepatic portal venous blood flow changed significantly. Then, the portal blood flow of residual liver tissue increased, which inevitably supported the residual tumor lesions that were not cleared and provided conditions for the rapid growth of tumor cells [23, 24]. The liver tissue on the DL may be in a hypoxia state due to the decrease of blood flow after portal vein ligation, and hypoxia-related genes also play a significant role in tumor metastasis [25].

The liver is an important immune organ of the body. In the progression of ALPPS-induced liver regeneration, immune cells, as important non-parenchymal cells, are involved in the complex pathophysiological process in addition to liver parenchymal cells [26, 27]. Studies confirmed that the changes and disorders of immune cells and the liver immune microenvironment were closely related to the progression of tumors [28, 29]. The change of liver blood flow distribution and the inflammation caused by ALPPS stage 1 significantly changed the immune microenvironment of the liver, and the proportion of $CD4^+$ T cells, MAIT cells, NK cells, and B cells in the liver on the DL was significantly higher, which may further promote tumor metastasis [10]. Clinically, the indications of ALPPS mainly include metastatic liver cancer, primary liver cancer, hilar cholangiocarcinoma, and other malignant tumors. The related factors may promote tumor metastasis and recurrence after ALPPS. The research on the mechanism of CRLM mainly focuses on the tumor microenvironment. It has been reported that tumor-associated macrophages (TAMs) can enhance the invasion of colorectal cancer cells through the JAK2/STAT3 signaling pathway, thus promoting the occurrence of CRLM [30]. Cancer-associated fibroblasts (CAFs) can promote tumor progression and invasion by remodeling the extracellular matrix, secreting cytokines, and promoting angiogenesis [31]. Radical resection is the most essential treatment for patients with primary liver cancer to obtain long-term survival, while tumor metastasis and recurrence are the main factors relating to the poor prognosis of patients. The main components of tumor microenvironment and the key regulatory factors of tumor metastasis are the critical influencing factors of liver cancer recurrence, such as tumor-related immune cells (macrophages, Th1 cells, Th2 cells, Treg cells, etc.), tumor-related stromal cells (fibroblasts, etc.), osteopontin, related miRNAs (miR-219-5p, miR-122, etc.), angiogenesis-related factors (vascular endothelial growth factor, fibroblast growth factor, etc.), and Golgi-related proteins (epidermal growth factor receptors, etc.) [32–34]. Epithelial-mesenchymal transformation (EMT) is an essential biological process for tumor cells to acquire the ability of invasion and metastasis, and it is also an important factor affecting tumor metastasis [35]. T-lymphoma invasion and metastasis-inducing protein 2 (TIAM2) is related to the EMT process of tumor cells and can promote tumor metastasis in HCC [36]. Other proteins related to the EMT process (i.e., EMT-related protein Snail, etc.) can also promote or inhibit tumor metastasis in HCC [37, 38]. In addition, some non-coding RNA (miR-122), enzymes related to extracellular matrix degradation (MMP-2, MMP-9), and related signal pathways (Wnt signal pathway, PI3K-Akt signal pathway, etc.) are also associated with the process of liver cancer metastasis [39, 40]. Currently, it is inconclusive whether the dynamics of the local or systemic immune microenvironment during the ALPPS procedure are related to the occurrence of immune escape and postoperative relapse and metastasis. It is meaningful to further explore the dynamic changes of immune cell biofunction, distribution, and status during ALPPS, which is helpful to find out its influence on tumor metastasis and recurrence and to find relevant intervention strategies.

20.3 Prevention and Treatment of Tumor Metastasis and Recurrence After ALPPS

ALPPS is an effective radical treatment for liver metastases, primary liver cancer, and hilar cholangiocarcinoma. Postoperative tumor metastasis and recurrence directly affect the postoperative curative effect and prognosis of patients. ALPPS may cause tumor cells to fall off and spread. Therefore, some modified ALPPS operations suggest that liver tissue should not be separated as much as possible during the ALPPS stage 1, and the tumor should not be touched or squeezed during the operation to reduce the risk of postoperative recurrence [41, 42]. Meanwhile, biological anti-adhesion materials are used instead of plastic bags to wrap the hepatic lobe on the tumor side during operation, and the ALPPS operation is modified accordingly (microwave, ablation, tourniquet, and other methods for disconnection, laparoscopic technique, partial disconnection, etc.) to reduce postoperative tumor metastasis and recurrence [43, 44].

According to the *Guidelines for Diagnosis and Treatment of Primary Liver Cancer in China* issued by the National Health Commission in 2022, surgery is the main treatment for patients with primary liver cancer, supplemented by antitumor and comprehensive treatments, which can effectively prolong the survival time and reduce the possibility of metastasis and recurrence. Transcatheter arterial chemoembolization (TACE) is the most commonly used nonsurgical treatment for primary liver cancer. Preventive TACE treatment for patients with high recurrence after surgical resection (multiple tumors, patients with tumor thrombus and tumor diameter >5 cm) can reduce tumor recurrence and improve the clinical outcome of patients [45, 46]. Relevant studies show that targeted drugs can effectively reduce the tumor recurrence of patients with primary liver cancer after hepatectomy, thus prolonging the survival time of patients [47–49]. Huaier Granule can reduce the tumor recurrence of liver cancer patients after hepatectomy, thus prolonging their survival time [50]. The antiviral therapy of nucleoside analogues can reduce the tumor recurrence of liver cancer caused by chronic hepatitis B, and can control the progression of liver disease [51, 52]. Therefore, all these adjuvant treatments can be used to prevent tumor recurrence after ALPPS.

According to the guidelines for diagnosis and comprehensive treatment of CRLM [53], multiple surgical resections can be performed to resect the recurrent or the metastatic focus if the physical and liver conditions are permitted. Meanwhile, it has been confirmed that the postoperative survival rate of patients undergoing multiple resection operations can be the same as that of other patients. For patients who perform complete resection, postoperative adjuvant chemotherapy can effectively prevent liver metastases. For patients without preoperative chemotherapy or patients with chemotherapy within 6 months before surgery, hepatic arterial infusion chemotherapy after surgery is recommended. For patients who have undergone chemotherapy (or have combined usage of molecular targeted drugs) before surgery, adjuvant therapy should be considered as the first choice after surgery, if the treatment is appropriate and no contraindications exist.

Reoperation, local radiofrequency ablation, microwave ablation, radiotherapy, TACE, and liver transplantation can be considered treatments for intrahepatic recurrence after ALPPS. Active systemic antitumor therapy (targeted therapy, immunotherapy, etc.) can effectively prolong patients' overall survival. In conclusion, it is necessary to evaluate the patient's tolerance, sensitivity to treatment, and the volume of remaining functional liver and liver function to take individualized prevention and treatment measures for tumor metastasis or recurrence after ALPPS.

20.4 The Clinical Prognosis After ALPPS

In earlier times, the incidence of total complications after ALPPS was 16–64%, and the postoperative mortality rate reached 12–23%, among which about 50% of patients died of liver-related factors [54, 55]. With the gradual maturity and improvement in ALPPS technology, the incidence of complications and mortality has been gradually reduced, and the clinical application of ALPPS has been accepted [56].

Secondary liver cancer is one of the main indications of ALPPS. Erik Schadde et al. counted 202 patients who had undergone ALPPS in the international cooperation group of ALPPS, and 141 cases were CRLM, accounting for about 70%, in addition to 28 cases of primary liver cancer [57]. The retrospective data of 58 patients with CRLM recorded in London Health Science Center and Buenos Aires Hospital showed that the overall 1-, 2-, and 3-year survival rates were 93%, 66%, and 50%, respectively, and the median survival time was 36 months. The 1-, 2-, and 3-year recurrence-free survival rates were 50%, 16%, and 13%, respectively [58]. From January 2010 to June 2014, 17 ALPPS patients with CRLM in Paul Brouse Hospital in France had a median survival time of 37 months and a 2-year overall survival rate of 77%, which was significantly improved compared with the classic two-step hepatectomy patients in the same period [59]. In a comprehensive cohort study involving 510 patients with CRLM from 22 ALPPS centers over 10 years, the 90-day mortality rate was 4.9%, the median survival time was 39 months, and the median recurrence-free survival time was 15 months [60]. Tim Reese et al. reported that 6 of 30 ALPPS patients with CRLM had complications, and the 1-year survival rate of these patients was 87% [61]. Therefore, ALPPS can provide a satisfactory prognosis for patients with CRLM. Still, it is necessary to fully consider whether there are too many high-risk factors for poor prognosis before surgery, including the number of metastatic tumors ≥6, the remaining liver tumors in the healthy side ≥2, and the invasion of liver segments ≥6, which are also important factors affecting the prognosis of patients [62].

According to the retrospective study, Giammauro Berardi et al. reported that 28 primary liver cancer patients who underwent ALPPS survived after the first-stage operation, but 21.4% had complications. After the second-stage operation, 20 patients (69.2%) had complications, and three patients (11.5%) died. After a median follow-up of 18 months (7–35 months), the median survival time was 22 months, and the median disease-free survival time was 15 months [63]. Studies have shown that from 2002 to 2018, only one of the 46 primary liver cancer patients who underwent ALPPS failed to undergo resection (97.8% resection rate), and the 5-year survival rate was 46.8%. There was no significant difference in the 5-year survival rate of ALPPS patients compared with those who underwent portal vein embolization at the same time. Still, ALPPS had a higher surgical resection rate [5]. According to the retrospective analysis of 23 primary liver cancer patients who underwent ALPPS in the Department of Liver Surgery of the First Affiliated Hospital of Sun Yat-sen University from November 2013 to June 2018, the 90-day mortality rate of the patients was 13%. The 1-, 2-, and 5-year overall survival rates were 61.1%, 34.9%, and 8.7%, respectively. The 1-, 2-, and 5-year disease-free survival rates were 27.8%, 27.8%, and 0.0%, respectively [64]. According to the retrospective study reported by our center, from April 2013 to September 2017, 45 HCC patients underwent ALPPS, and 41 patients (91.1%) successfully completed the second-stage operation. Among the 45 patients who were followed up for 16 months, five patients (11.1%) died within 90 days. The 1- and 3-year overall survival rates of 45 patients were 64.2% and 60.2%, respectively. The 1- and 3-year disease-free survival rates were 47.6% and 43.9%, respectively. According to the propensity score matching (PSM), the survival rate of patients receiving ALPPS is significantly higher than that of their counterparts after TACE [4]. With more surgical experience and improved surgical techniques, the resection and survival rates of ALPPS surgery in our center have been significantly improved in the past 5 years for the treatment of primary or secondary hepatic carcinoma that cannot be removed by traditional surgery.

In conclusion, ALPPS brought the possibility of surgical treatment for patients who cannot receive surgical resection before. At the same time, the short-term and long-term overall survival rates and disease-free survival rates of CRLM or primary liver cancer patients undergoing ALPPS surgery are not inferior to those of other operations and are even better than these operations in some instances. Therefore, full consideration of the experience and condition of the medical center, the patient's condition, and surgical risks is necessary before the decision of ALPPS surgery. Furthermore, strict screening is also a meaningful way to ensure a good prognosis for patients after ALPPS and effectively reduce the incidence of postoperative complications and mortality. Before ALPPS stage 1, it is necessary to evaluate the patient's age, general state, liver function, operational tolerance, and underlying or chronic diseases according to different individual conditions. Before ALPPS stage 2, a careful assessment of preoperative liver volume and liver function is required to recognize the best candidates for ALPPS, which can significantly improve the overall prognosis of patients [65, 66].

20.5 Prospects

With improved surgical technique and perioperative management, clearer indications and contraindications, and enhanced screening conditions, ALPPS will be popularized for patients who cannot undergo traditional surgery. At the same time, it is necessary to clarify and explain the effect and mechanism of ALPPS on liver tumor metastasis and recurrence at the molecular level, which is helpful to further improve its curative effect. With the development of high-throughput sequencing, such as single-cell RNA sequencing and spatial transcriptomics, we can obtain and combine tissue single-cell transcriptional maps and spatial transcriptional maps to analyze more information at the single-cell level. Therefore, we can systematically understand and explore the composition, intercellular communication and interaction, and spatial distribution of specific cell subsets and functional molecules in liver tissue under physiological or pathological conditions. It provides a new perspective for further understanding the changes in the local liver immune microenvironment at ALPPS stages 1 and 2, the effect on the existing liver tumor, as well as the spread and implantation of residual tumor cells. Moreover, it also provides a new target and new aspect for the prevention and treatment of liver tumor metastasis and recurrence after ALPPS.

References

1. Schadde E, Ardiles V, Slankamenac K, et al. ALPPS offers a better chance of complete resection in patients with primarily unresectable liver tumors compared with conventional-staged hepatectomies: results of a multicenter analysis[J]. World J Surg. 2014;38(6):1510–9.
2. Schlitt HJ, Hackl C, Lang SA. 'In-situ split' liver resection/ALPPS – historical development and current practice[J]. Visc Med. 2017;33(6):408–12.
3. Oldhafer KJ, Donati M, Jenner RM, et al. ALPPS for patients with colorectal liver metastases: effective liver hypertrophy, but early tumor recurrence[J]. World J Surg. 2014;38(6):1504–9.
4. Wang Z, Peng YF, Hu JW, et al. Associating liver partition and portal vein ligation for staged hepatectomy for unresectable hepatitis B virus-related hepatocellular carcinoma: a single center study of 45 patients[J]. Ann Surg. 2020;271(3):534–41.
5. Chan A, Zhang WY, Chok K, et al. ALPPS versus portal vein embolization for hepatitis-related hepatocellular carcinoma: a changing paradigm in modulation of future liver remnant before major hepatectomy[J]. Ann Surg. 2021;273(5):957–65.
6. Benish M, Ben-Eliyahu S. Surgery as a double-edged sword: a clinically feasible approach to overcome the metastasis-promoting

effects of surgery by blunting stress and prostaglandin responses[J]. Cancers. 2010;2(4):1929–51.
7. Kikuchi Y, Hiroshima Y, Matsuo K, et al. Impact of associating liver partition and portal vein occlusion for staged hepatectomy on tumor growth in a mouse model of liver metastasis[J]. Eur J Surg Oncol. 2018;44(1):130–8.
8. Riddiough GE, Jalal Q, Perini MV, et al. Liver regeneration and liver metastasis[J]. Semin Cancer Biol. 2021;71:86–97.
9. Lee KT, Wang SN, Su RW, et al. Is wider surgical margin justified for better clinical outcomes in patients with resectable hepatocellular carcinoma?[J]. J Formos Med Assoc. 2012;111(3):160–70.
10. Anantha RV, Shaler CR, Meilleur CE, et al. The future liver remnant in patients undergoing the associating liver partition with portal vein ligation for staged hepatectomy (ALPPS) maintains the immunological components of a healthy organ[J]. Front Med. 2016;3:32.
11. Schellenberg AE, Moravan V, Christian F. A competing risk analysis of colorectal cancer recurrence after curative surgery[J]. BMC Gastroenterol. 2022;22(1):95.
12. Kim R. Effects of surgery and anesthetic choice on immunosuppression and cancer recurrence[J]. J Transl Med. 2018;16(1):8.
13. Longbottom ER, Torrance HD, Owen HC, et al. Features of postoperative immune suppression are reversible with interferon gamma and independent of interleukin-6 pathways[J]. Ann Surg. 2016;264(2):370–7.
14. Gryglewski A, Szczepanik M. The effect of surgical stress on postoperative Tαβ and Tγδ cell distribution[J]. Immunol Investig. 2017;46(5):481–9.
15. Gottschalk A, Sharma S, Ford J, et al. Review article: the role of the perioperative period in recurrence after cancer surgery[J]. Anesth Analg. 2010;110(6):1636–43.
16. Bharati SJ, Chowdhury T, Bergese SD, et al. Anesthetics impact on cancer recurrence: what do we know?[J]. J Cancer Res Ther. 2016;12(2):464–8.
17. Gupta R, Fuks D, Bourdeaux C, et al. Impact of intraoperative blood loss on the short-term outcomes of laparoscopic liver resection[J]. Surg Endosc. 2017;31(11):4451–7.
18. Langiewicz M, Schlegel A, Saponara E, et al. Hedgehog pathway mediates early acceleration of liver regeneration induced by a novel two-staged hepatectomy in mice[J]. J Hepatol. 2017;66(3):560–70.
19. Schlegel A, Lesurtel M, Melloul E, et al. ALPPS: from human to mice highlighting accelerated and novel mechanisms of liver regeneration[J]. Ann Surg. 2014;260(5):839–46.
20. Wullaert A, Heyninck K, Beyaert R. Mechanisms of crosstalk between TNF-induced NF-kappaB and JNK activation in hepatocytes[J]. Biochem Pharmacol. 2006;72(9):1090–101.
21. Reschke M, Ferby I, Stepniak E, et al. Mitogen-inducible gene-6 is a negative regulator of epidermal growth factor receptor signaling in hepatocytes and human hepatocellular carcinoma[J]. Hepatology. 2010;51(4):1383–90.
22. Wang CW, Liao YD, Qiu JL, et al. Transcatheter arterial chemoembolization alone or combined with ablation for recurrent intermediate-stage hepatocellular carcinoma: a propensity score matching study[J]. J Cancer Res Clin Oncol. 2020;146(10):2669–80.
23. Schadde E, Malagó M, Hernandez-Alejandro R, et al. Monosegment ALPPS hepatectomy: extending resectability by rapid hypertrophy[J]. Surgery. 2015;157(4):676–89.
24. Cai YL, Song PP, Tang W, et al. An updated systematic review of the evolution of ALPPS and evaluation of its advantages and disadvantages in accordance with current evidence[J]. Medicine. 2016;95(24):e3941.
25. Moy RH, Nguyen A, Loo JM, et al. Functional genetic screen identifies ITPR3/calcium/RELB axis as a driver of colorectal cancer metastatic liver colonization[J]. Dev Cell. 2022;57(9):1146–1159.e7.
26. Thorgersen EB, Barratt-Due A, Haugaa H, et al. The role of complement in liver injury, regeneration, and transplantation[J]. Hepatology. 2019;70(2):725–36.
27. Hu CX, Wu ZW, Li LJ. Mesenchymal stromal cells promote liver regeneration through regulation of immune cells[J]. Int J Biol Sci. 2020;16(5):893–903.
28. Sun YF, Wu L, Zhong Y, et al. Single-cell landscape of the ecosystem in early-relapse hepatocellular carcinoma[J]. Cell. 2021;184(2):404–421.e16.
29. Ma C, Han MJ, Heinrich B, et al. Gut microbiome-mediated bile acid metabolism regulates liver cancer *via* NKT cells[J]. Science. 2018;360(6391):eaan5931.
30. Wei C, Yang CG, Wang SY, et al. Crosstalk between cancer cells and tumor associated macrophages is required for mesenchymal circulating tumor cell-mediated colorectal cancer metastasis[J]. Mol Cancer. 2019;18(1):64.
31. Sahai E, Astsaturov I, Cukierman E, et al. A framework for advancing our understanding of cancer-associated fibroblasts[J]. Nat Rev Cancer. 2020;20(3):174–86.
32. Liu Y, Cao XT. Characteristics and significance of the premetastatic niche[J]. Cancer Cell. 2016;30(5):668–81.
33. Qin LX. Osteopontin is a promoter for hepatocellular carcinoma metastasis: a summary of 10 years of studies[J]. Front Med. 2014;8(1):24–32.
34. Liu YF, Zhang YL, Wang SH, et al. Prospero-related homeobox 1 drives angiogenesis of hepatocellular carcinoma through selectively activating interleukin-8 expression[J]. Hepatology. 2017;66(6):1894–909.
35. Zhao M, Ang L, Huang J, et al. MicroRNAs regulate the epithelial-mesenchymal transition and influence breast cancer invasion and metastasis[J]. Tumour Biol. 2017;39(2):1010428317691682.
36. Chen JS, Su IJ, Leu YW, et al. Expression of T-cell lymphoma invasion and metastasis 2 (TIAM2) promotes proliferation and invasion of liver cancer[J]. Int J Cancer. 2012;130(6):1302–13.
37. Sun TT, Wong N. Transforming growth factor-β-induced long noncoding RNA promotes liver cancer metastasis via RNA-RNA crosstalk[J]. Hepatology. 2015;61(2):722–4.
38. Tang B, Qi GY, Sun XY, et al. HOXA7 plays a critical role in metastasis of liver cancer associated with activation of Snail[J]. Mol Cancer. 2016;15(1):57.
39. Huang YK, Fan XG, Qiu F. TM4SF1 promotes proliferation, invasion, and metastasis in human liver cancer cells[J]. Int J Mol Sci. 2016;17(5):661.
40. Yin SY, Fan Y, Zhang HS, et al. Differential TGFβ pathway targeting by miR-122 in humans and mice affects liver cancer metastasis[J]. Nat Commun. 2016;7:11012.
41. Li J, Nashan B. Reply to: "Minimize the surgical damage at the stage-1 operation by combining hybrid ALPPS and nontotal parenchymal transection"[J]. Ann Surg. 2018;267(4):e82–3.
42. Li J, Kantas A, Ittrich H, et al. Avoid "all-touch" by hybrid ALPPS to achieve oncological efficacy[J]. Ann Surg. 2016;263(1):e6–7.
43. Vennarecci G, Grazi GL, Sperduti I, et al. ALPPS for primary and secondary liver tumors[J]. Int J Surg. 2016;30:38–44.
44. Edmondson MJ, Sodergren MH, Pucher PH, et al. Variations and adaptations of associated liver partition and portal vein ligation for staged hepatectomy (ALPPS): many routes to the summit[J]. Surgery. 2016;159(4):1058–72.
45. Wang Z, Ren ZG, Chen Y, et al. Adjuvant transarterial chemoembolization for HBV-related hepatocellular carcinoma after resection: a randomized controlled study[J]. Clin Cancer Res. 2018;24(9):2074–81.
46. Wei W, Jian PE, Li SH, et al. Adjuvant transcatheter arterial chemoembolization after curative resection for hepatocellular carcinoma patients with solitary tumor and microvascular invasion: a randomized clinical trial of efficacy and safety[J]. Cancer Commun. 2018;38(1):61.

47. Wang LM, Wang WH, Rong WQ, et al. Postoperative adjuvant treatment strategy for hepatocellular carcinoma with microvascular invasion: a non-randomized interventional clinical study[J]. BMC Cancer. 2020;20(1):614.
48. He X, Peng YR, Zhou ZY, et al. Immune checkpoint inhibitor-based systemic therapy shows remarkable curative effect in a hepatocellular carcinoma patient with intractable postoperative recurrence and metastases: a case report and literature review[J]. Front Oncol. 2022;12:784224.
49. Song TQ, Lang MR, Ren SH, et al. The past, present and future of conversion therapy for liver cancer[J]. Am J Cancer Res. 2021;11(10):4711–24.
50. Chen Q, Shu C, Laurence AD, et al. Effect of Huaier granule on recurrence after curative resection of HCC: a multicentre, randomised clinical trial[J]. Gut. 2018;67(11):2006–16.
51. Huang G, Li PP, Lau WY, et al. Antiviral therapy reduces hepatocellular carcinoma recurrence in patients with low HBV-DNA levels: a randomized controlled trial[J]. Ann Surg. 2018;268(6):943–54.
52. Huang G, Lau WY, Wang ZG, et al. Antiviral therapy improves postoperative survival in patients with hepatocellular carcinoma: a randomized controlled trial[J]. Ann Surg. 2015;261(1):56–66.
53. Chinese College of Surgeons, Section of Gastrointestinal Surgery, Branch of Surgery, Chinese Medical Association, Section of Colorectal Surgery, Branch of Surgery, Chinese Medical Association, et al. China guideline for diagnosis and comprehensive treatment of colorectal liver metastases (version 2020)[J]. Zhonghua Wei Chang Wai Ke Za Zhi. 2021;24(1):1–13.
54. Nadalin S, Capobianco I, Li J, et al. Indications and limits for associating liver partition and portal vein ligation for staged hepatectomy (ALPPS). Lessons learned from 15 cases at a single centre[J]. Z Gastroenterol. 2014;52(1):35–42.
55. Alvarez FA, Ardiles V, de Santibañes M, et al. Associating liver partition and portal vein ligation for staged hepatectomy offers high oncological feasibility with adequate patient safety: a prospective study at a single center[J]. Ann Surg. 2015;261(4):723–32.
56. Lang H, de Santibañes E, Schlitt HJ, et al. 10th anniversary of ALPPS-lessons learned and quo vadis[J]. Ann Surg. 2019;269(1):114–9.
57. Schadde E, Ardiles V, Robles-Campos R, et al. Early survival and safety of ALPPS: first report of the International ALPPS Registry[J]. Ann Surg. 2014;260(5):829–36; discussion 836–838.
58. Wanis KN, Ardiles V, Alvarez FA, et al. Intermediate-term survival and quality of life outcomes in patients with advanced colorectal liver metastases undergoing associating liver partition and portal vein ligation for staged hepatectomy[J]. Surgery. 2018;163(4):691–7.
59. Adam R, Imai K, Castro Benitez C, et al. Outcome after associating liver partition and portal vein ligation for staged hepatectomy and conventional two-stage hepatectomy for colorectal liver metastases[J]. Br J Surg. 2016;103(11):1521–9.
60. Petrowsky H, Linecker M, Raptis DA, et al. First long-term oncologic results of the ALPPS procedure in a large cohort of patients with colorectal liver metastases[J]. Ann Surg. 2020;272(5):793–800.
61. Reese T, Makridis G, Raptis D, et al. Repeated hepatectomy after ALPPS for recurrence of colorectal liver metastasis: the edge of limits?[J]. HPB. 2021;23(10):1488–95.
62. Olthof PB, Huiskens J, Wicherts DA, et al. Survival after associating liver partition and portal vein ligation for staged hepatectomy (ALPPS) for advanced colorectal liver metastases: a case-matched comparison with palliative systemic therapy[J]. Surgery. 2017;161(4):909–19.
63. Berardi G, Guglielmo N, Colasanti M, et al. Associating liver partition and portal vein ligation for staged hepatectomy (ALPPS) for advanced hepatocellular carcinoma with macrovascular invasion[J]. Updat Surg. 2022;74(3):927–36.
64. Ke LX, Shen R, Fan WZ, et al. The role of associating liver partition and portal vein ligation for staged hepatectomy in unresectable hepatitis B virus-related hepatocellular carcinoma[J]. Ann Transl Med. 2020;8(21):1402.
65. Sparrelid E. Reply to "Comment to Sparrelid, E. et al. Dynamic evaluation of liver volume and function in associating liver partition and portal vein ligation for staged hepatectomy. Journal of Gastrointestinal Surgery (2017)"[J]. J Gastrointest Surg. 2017;21(10):1756.
66. Buac S, Schadde E, Schnitzbauer AA, et al. The many faces of ALPPS: surgical indications and techniques among surgeons collaborating in the international registry[J]. HPB (Oxford). 2016;18(5):442–8.

21 Experimental Model of ALPPS

Feiyu Chen

21.1 Rodent ALPPS Model

21.1.1 Introduction to Experimental Animals

Experimental rodent models have garnered widespread adoption in the ever-evolving landscape of modern biomedicine. The frequently utilized experimental rodent models are experimental mice and rats. Experimental mice, artificially bred from wild house mice (Mus musculus) via a directional selection approach, have been bred into more than 500 independent inbred and outbred strains. In Europe, experimental rats, directionally bred from wild Rattus norvegicus, were first harnessed for experimental purposes. Based on a burgeoning body of research, researchers become increasingly proficient in understanding rodent liver anatomy [1]. Thanks to advancements in microsurgical techniques, experimental rodent models are increasingly utilized in liver-related research (e.g., liver regeneration, liver failure, liver transplantation, and liver tumor research) [2–4]. Given the role of the inflammatory response in ALPPS-induced liver regeneration [5], immunocompetent experimental rodents (e.g., BALB/c and C57BL mice, and Wistar, Spraque-Dawley, Lewis, and ACI rats) are typically employed in existing research.

21.1.2 Foundation of Liver Anatomy in Experimental Animals for ALPPS

Experimental rats and mice exhibit comparable hepatic anatomical structures [6], with the most pronounced distinction being the absence of a gallbladder in rats [7]. Based on hepatic morphology, the experimental rodent liver can be grossly stratified into the left lateral lobe, median lobe, right lobe, and caudate lobe. In addition, other classification systems of hepatic lobes are available [8]. The median lobe, comprising approximately 38% of the liver weight, is anchored by the falciform ligament to the diaphragm and abdominal wall and can be subdivided into the left median lobe and right median lobe by a hepatic fissure. The right lobe, occupying approximately 22% of the liver weight, is categorized into the superior right lobe and inferior right lobe by a horizontal fissure. The caudate lobe, constituting 8–10% of the liver weight, is classified into two parts. Specifically, the caudate process, representing 2–3% of the liver weight, surrounds the posterior wall of the inferior vena cava and connects the caudate lobe to the right lobe. The remaining portion of the caudate lobe is delineated into the anterior and posterior caudate lobe, with each lobe contributing to 4% of the liver weight. The anterior and posterior caudate lobes are located anterior to and posterior to the esophagus and stomach [1, 9]. The left lateral lobe, singular without hepatic fissures, is attached by a ligament to the diaphragm along its diaphragmatic surface (Fig. 21.1). Based on Couinaud classification of hepatic segments, the corresponding relationships between rodent and human liver segments are as follows: the caudate lobe corresponds to segments I and IX, the left lateral lobe corresponds to segment II, the left median lobe corresponds to segments III and IV, the right median lobe corresponds to segments V and VII and the inferior right lobe corresponds to segment VI, and the superior right lobe corresponds to segment VII [10].

In the rodent liver, the extrahepatic portal vein is positioned posterior to the hepatic artery and lateral to the bile duct. At the porta hepatis, the main portal vein sequentially gives off branches to the right lobe, caudate lobe, median lobe, and left lateral lobe (Fig. 21.1). The left lateral lobe, right lobe, and caudate lobe are fed by a main portal venous branch, whereas the median lobe is perfused by two portal venous branches. Immediately upon its origin, the portal venous branch supplying the right lobe bifurcates into two branches, with one branch feeding the superior right lobe and the other supplying the inferior right lobe. The portal

F. Chen (✉)
Zhongshan Hospital, Fudan University, Shanghai, China
e-mail: chenfy1992@126.com

J. Zhou (ed.), *Associating Liver Partition and Portal Vein Ligation for Staged Hepatectomy (ALPPS)*,
https://doi.org/10.1007/978-981-96-7364-3_21

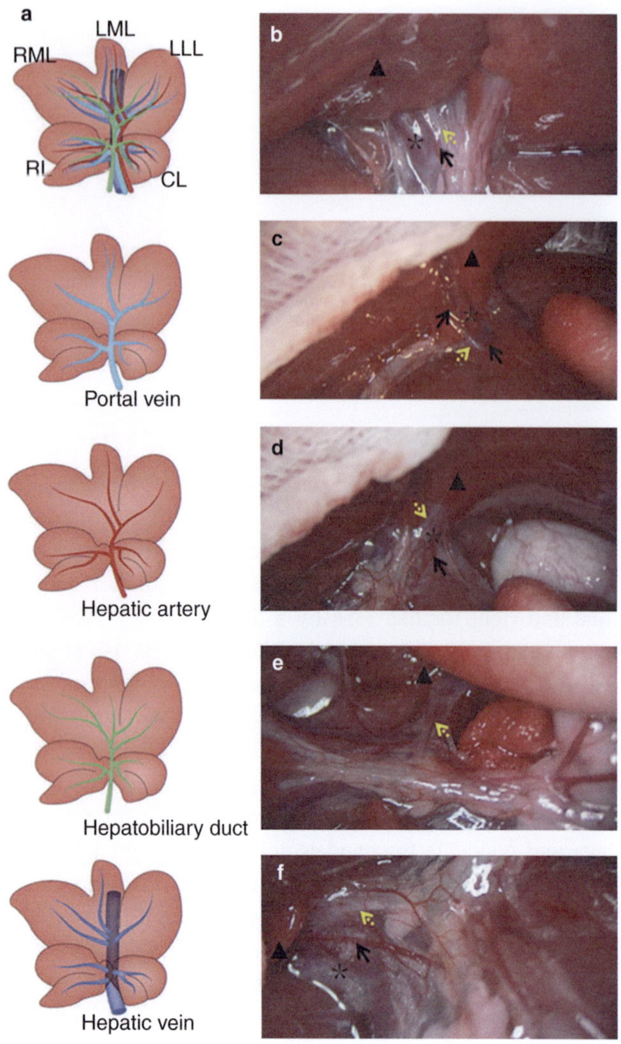

Fig. 21.1 Rodent liver anatomy. (**a**) Rodent liver structure (RML, right median lobe; LML, left median lobe; LLL, left lateral lobe; CL, caudate lobe; RL, right lobe). (**b–f**) Hepatic lobe structures at the porta hepatis, where **b** denotes the right median lobe, **c** denotes the left median lobe, **d** denotes the left lateral lobe, **e** denotes the caudate lobe, and **f** denotes the right lobe (the black triangle denotes the corresponding hepatic lobe, the asterisk denotes the portal vein, the black solid arrow denotes the hepatic artery, and the yellow dotted arrow denotes the hepatobiliary duct)

venous branch supplying the caudate lobe, situated posterior to the hepatic artery and bile duct, is notably short. Upon giving off branches to the right lobe and caudate lobe, the main portal vein bifurcates into two branches, with one branch supplying the right median lobe and the other traversing a short distance before further dividing into branches supplying the left lateral lobe and left median lobe.

The liver is perfused by the hepatic artery, originating from the common hepatic artery. The proper hepatic artery, typically located on the posterior surface of the portal vein, courses toward the porta hepatis, giving off branches anterior to the portal vein. The artery feeding each hepatic lobe is situated on the anterior surface of the portal vein and posterior to the bile duct. Upon giving off branches, the artery courses posterior to the hepatic duct, running parallel to the portal venous branch (Fig. 21.1). Specifically, the most prominent extrahepatic arterial branches are those supplying the right lobe and right median lobe (Fig. 21.1b, f). Aside from the four arterial branches feeding the main hepatic lobe, the hepatic artery gives rise to an inconspicuous branch (i.e., the hepatoesophageal artery supplying the inferior two-thirds of the esophagus) in the hepatic pedicle between the caudate lobe and the left lateral lobe. In addition, the left lateral lobe receives an accessory left hepatic artery arising from the left gastric artery and supplying the dorsal medial portion of the left lateral lobe.

The gallbladder is absent in rats. In rodents, the extrahepatic bile duct, formed from the confluence of the first-order branches from the respective hepatic lobe, courses along the surfaces of the hepatic arterial and portal venous branches (Fig. 21.1). Each hepatic lobe is typically drained by its bile duct, with occasional anatomical variations. For instance, the left lateral lobe can be drained via two biliary branches.

Generally, the superior right lobe and inferior right lobe drain into the inferior vena cava via a hepatic venous branch (Fig. 21.1a). The median lobe encompasses three principal hepatic veins (i.e., right hepatic vein, middle hepatic vein, and left median hepatic vein) responsible for draining the corresponding portions [10]. The left medial vein, which drains the left portion of the median lobe, can drain into the vena cava directly. Alternatively, the left medial vein can join with the left hepatic vein, which drains the left lateral lobe, to form a common trunk before draining into the superior vena cava. The two branches of the caudate lobe are drained by two major hepatic veins leading to the vena cava. In certain instances, these veins may converge into a common trunk. The caudate process empties into the intrahepatic vena cava via multiple venous tributaries.

The anatomical structure of the rodent liver stands in stark contrast to that of the human liver. Specifically, the mouse and rat livers are markedly lobulated, with each hepatic lobe boasting its portal venous and arterial supplies as well as an independent bile duct. In addition, all of the four lobes are connected to the inferior vena cava via a separate hepatic vein. To satisfy all eligibility criteria for the ALPPS procedure, the experimental rodent model for ALPPS must replicate the anatomy of hepatic structures and blood vessels in humans. In the rodent liver, only the median lobe exhibits circulatory patterns closely parallel to those observed in the human liver. The left median lobe or right median lobe possesses distinct portal venous and arterial branches as well as separate biliary structures (Fig. 21.1a). As with the human liver, the median lobe of the rodent liver demonstrates a venous reflux system comprising left, right, and middle hepatic veins. Furthermore, the left median lobe and right median lobe exhibit a broad parenchymal connection, allowing for the potential presence of portal venous collateral circulation. Partitioning the median lobe in the rodent liver aids in replicating the partition of the communicating branches between interlobar portal venous branches, resulting in partitioning the left and right hemilivers in humans undergoing the ALPPS procedure. Also, it assists in creating a sufficiently large transection plane to elicit an inflammatory response. Therefore, employing an experimental rodent model to replicate the ALPPS procedure in humans necessitates occluding the portal venous branches supplying the right lobe, caudate lobe, and LL, as well as disrupting the portal venous branch supplying one lobe within the median lobe (left median lobe or right median lobe) while designating the other lobe as the future liver remnant (FLR). As hepatectomy can induce liver regeneration [11], it is advisable to refrain from resecting additional hepatic lobes whenever feasible to provide a more precise and controlled model for ALPPS. Some noteworthy points occur during occlusion or ligation of the portal venous branch supplying the respective lobe. The hepatic artery feeding the right lobe typically accompanies the main portal venous branch closely. In this regard, caution should be exercised to avoid an accidental injury to the hepatic artery. Fortunately, the bile duct typically remains unaffected due to its long distance from the portal vein (Fig. 21.1f). The main portal venous branch perfusing the caudate lobe, situated directly posterior to the hepatic artery and bile duct, is invisible under direct vision, rendering portal vein ligation highly challenging (Fig. 21.1e). When the left median lobe is preserved as the FLR, the portal venous branch supplying the right median lobe, situated at a distance to the right of the hepatic artery and bile duct, can be straightforwardly ligated, as it exhibits an unobstructed course (Fig. 21.1b). When the right median lobe is designated as the FLR, the common trunk, formed by the confluence of the portal venous branches supplying the left lateral lobe and left median lobe, can be directly ligated via a straightforward operative approach (Fig. 21.1d). Ligating the portal venous branch supplying the left lateral lobe is regarded as the most technically demanding aspect, as the common trunk, formed by the confluence of the portal venous branches supplying the left lateral lobe and left median lobe, traverses a distance within the parenchyma of the left lateral lobe, giving rise to portal venous branches serving the left lateral lobe and left median lobe [9]. It is challenging to isolate the portal venous branch supplying the left lateral lobe from the hepatic parenchyma surrounded by a complex network of hepatic arteries and bile ducts (Figs. 21.1c and 21.2d). Moreover, ligating the portal venous branch feeding the left lateral lobe at a location excessively close to the confluence risks compromising the portal venous flow to the left median lobe. Furthermore, the anatomical proximity of the portal venous branch supplying the left lateral lobe to the left hepatic vein poses a heightened risk of an accidental injury to the hepatic or portal vein during dissection, potentially precipitating a catastrophic hemorrhagic event and subsequent animal death.

21.1.3 Surgical Procedure of Experimental Rodent ALPPS Model

Nearly 40 studies have reported 21 experimental rodent models for ALPPS (Table 21.1). In 2014, Yao et al. reported the first experimental rat model for ALPPS (Yao model) [12], in which the portal venous branches supplying the left median lobe, left lateral lobe, caudate lobe, and right lobe were ligated, followed by liver partition along the ischemic demarcation line in the median lobe, with the right median lobe preserved as the FLR. The Yao model involved preserving approximately 30% of the liver. In 2014, Schlegel et al. reported the first experimental mouse model for ALPPS (Schlegel model) [5], in which the portal venous branches feeding the right median lobe, caudate lobe, and right lobe were ligated, followed by resection of the left lateral lobe, with the left median lobe preserved as the FLR. The Schlegel model necessitated preserving approximately 10% of the liver. Subsequently, most of the experimental rodent models for ALPPS were slightly modified from the Yao and Schlegel models for use in experimental rats or mice [5, 12–28]. In 2019, Dili et al. reported an experimental rat model based on the post-extended hepatectomy volume (Dili model) [29]. The Dili model is comparable to the Schlegel model, with the left median lobe preserved as the FLR. Nonetheless, a key distinction lies in ligating the portal venous branch supplying the left lateral lobe while preserving the hepatic lobe in the Dili model. The Dili model entailed preserving approximately 10% of the liver. Due to its operational challenges, the Dili model has yet to be reported in mice [29, 30]. Aside from the above three models, Wei et al. developed a comparable experimental rat model based on the Yao model, in which the caudate lobe was resected [31]. In the model developed by García-Perez et al., the left median lobe and caudate lobe were preserved as the FLR [32]; however, preserving the caudate lobe as part of the FLR deviates from the principle of replicating human liver anatomy. Consequently, the model has been infrequently adopted by other researchers [32, 33]. Apart from experimental rodent models replicating the classic ALPPS procedure, experimental rodent models replicating the radiofrequency-assisted ALPPS (RALPPS) procedure have been reported [34, 35]. In addition, pathological factors (e.g., tumors, fatty liver, and cirrhosis) can be introduced into experimental rodent models [33, 36–41]. Shi et al. developed three experimental rodent models by comparing the impacts of various volumes of FLR values on liver regeneration [42]. Nonetheless, the FLR was

Table 21.1 Reported experimental rodent models for ALPPS

FLR	Hepatic lobectomy at stage 1	FLR proportion	Rodent species	Other factors	References
RML	–	30%	Rats	–	[12–22]
RML	–	30%	Mice	–	[23]
RML	–	30%	Rats	RALPPS	[34]
RML	–	30%	Rats	Drug-induced hepatic fibrosis	[39]
RML	–	30%	Rats	Partition inside the portal vein ligated Lobe	[43]
RML	–	30%	Rats	Physical rehabilitation	[44]
RML	–	30%	Mice	Drug-induced hepatic fibrosis	[45]
RML	CL	30%	Rats	–	[31]
RML	CL	30%	Rats	Nonalcoholic fatty liver disease	[38]
RML	CL	30%	Rats	Orthotopic tumor implantation	[41]
LML	LLL	10%	Mice	–	[5, 24–27]
LML	LLL	10%	Rats	–	[28]
LML	LLL	10%	Mice	Colorectal liver metastases	[36]
LML	LLL	10%	Rats	RALPPS	[35]
LML	–	10%	Rats	–	[29, 30]
LML + CL	–	20%	Rats	–	[32]
LML + CL	–	20%	Rats	Drug-induced hepatic fibrosis	[33]
LML + LLL + CL	–	50%	Rats	Colorectal liver metastases	[37]
LML + LLL + CL	–	50%	Rats	Drug-induced hepatic fibrosis	[40]
RML + RL + CL	–	60%	Mice	Colorectal liver metastases	[46]
CL/RL/RL + CL	LLL	10%/20%/30%	Rats	–	[42]

Note: *RALPPS* radiofrequency-assisted ALPPS

not situated in the median lobe in these models, rendering them unsuitable for replicating the ALPPS procedure. Other models are modified from the Yao, Schlegel, and Dili models, with certain debatable variations (i.e., the FLR is located outside the median lobe, or additional hepatic lobes are resected). Yao, Schlegel, and Dili models are detailed below.

21.1.3.1 Stage 1 ALPPS Procedure

Stage 1 ALPPS procedure involves portal vein ligation and liver partition (Fig. 21.2). Clinically, portal vein ligation redirects all portal venous flows to one side of the liver, resulting in an augmented risk of bleeding during liver partition. As such, patients undergoing the ALPPS procedure typically undergo liver partition, followed by portal vein ligation upon complete hemostasis on the hepatic transection plane. Differing from that in patients, hemorrhagic events can be effectively managed and controlled in experimental rodents undergoing the ALPPS procedure. Therefore, these rodents may undergo portal vein ligation as an initial step to aid in delineating the ischemic demarcation line.

1. Yao model (mice and rats, Fig. 21.3)

Liver mobilization: The liver should undergo complete mobilization. The falciform ligament and its associated round ligaments should be resected to mobilize the median lobe. The anterior caudate lobe is connected to the lesser curvature of the stomach via the hepatogastric ligament, while the posterior caudate lobe is connected to the duodenum via the hepatoduodenal ligament. Hepatogastric and hepatoduodenal ligaments adherent to Glisson's capsule should be mobilized and detached to expose the portal venous branch supplying the caudate lobe. Resecting the left triangular ligament, which connects the posterior aspect of the superior surface of the left lateral lobe to the diaphragm, may be necessary, particularly in the Schlegel or Dili model. It is noteworthy that the gallbladder should be simultaneously resected in mice.

Portal vein ligation: The portal venous branches supplying the left median lobe, left lateral lobe, caudate lobe, and right lobe should be ligated. Bypassing the accompanying artery is essential during ligation of the portal venous branch supplying the right lobe (Fig. 21.2b). Caution should be exercised to avoid an accidental injury to the artery, as the artery is sometimes intimately adherent to the superior surface of the portal venous branch supplying the right lobe. Following complete mobilization of the caudate lobe, the portal venous branch supplying the caudate lobe, situated directly beneath the hepatic artery and bile duct, necessitates careful retraction and exposure to facilitate its ligation, posing a tremendous challenge (Fig. 21.2c). Typically, we perform surgical maneuvers as follows: the curved micro-forceps are employed to access the posterior aspect of the portal vein, and the tail of the suture is clamped and retracted through the posterior aspect of the portal vein. Subsequently, the needle is passed through the spaces between the portal vein and the hepatic artery and bile duct, followed by ligation while bypassing the hepatic artery and bile duct. Ultimately, the common trunk, formed by the confluence of the portal

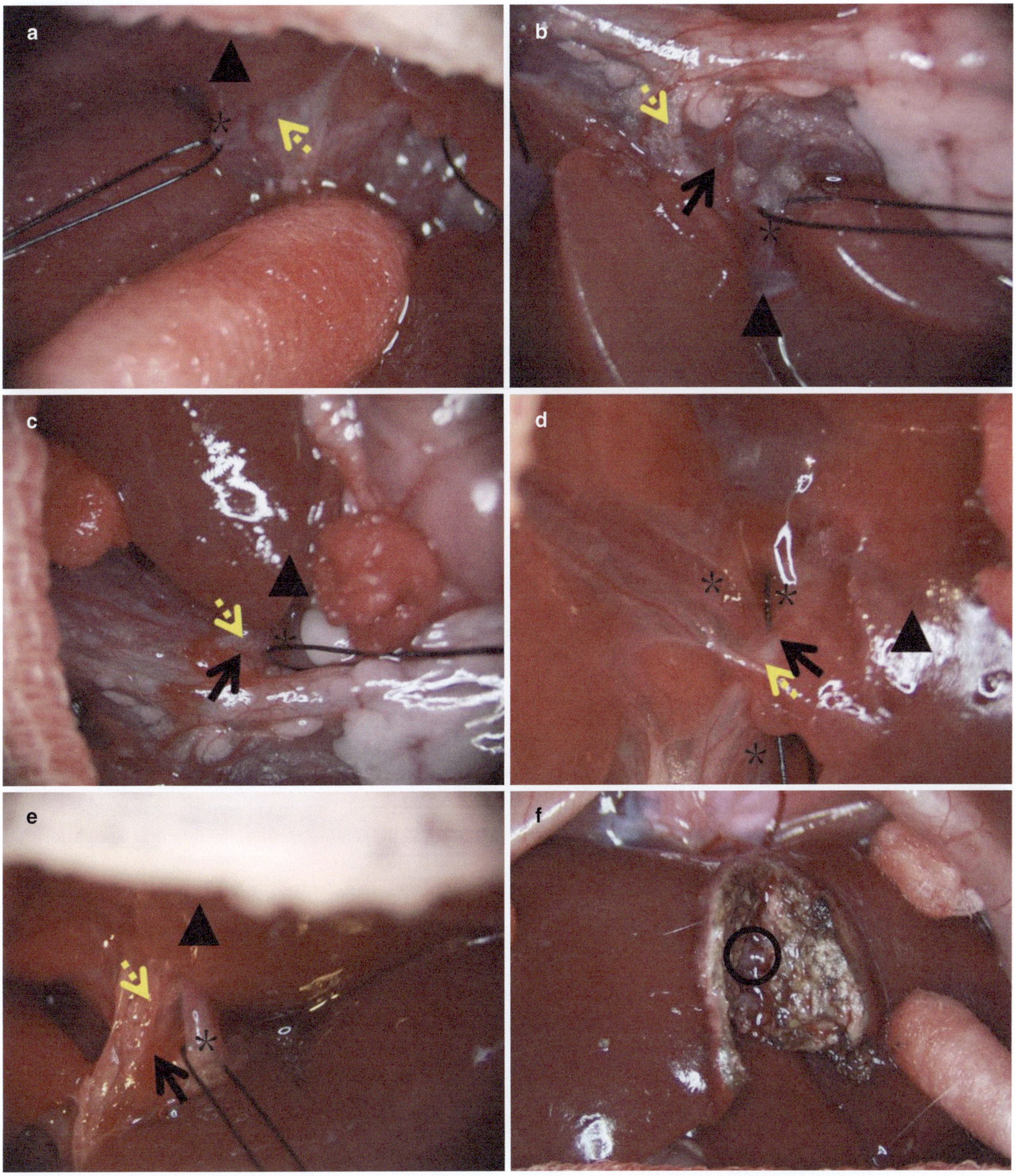

Fig. 21.2 Portal vein ligation and liver partition in stage 1 ALPPS procedure. (**a–e**) Denote the portal vein ligation in the corresponding hepatic lobes, where **a** denotes the right median lobe, **b** denotes the right lobe, **c** denotes the caudate lobe, **d** denotes the left lateral lobe, and **e** denotes the left portal vein (the black triangle denotes the corresponding hepatic lobe, the asterisk denotes the portal vein, the black solid arrow denotes the hepatic artery, and the yellow dotted arrow denotes the hepatobiliary duct). **f** denotes liver partition, and the black circle denotes that the liver partition extends to the hepatic vein surface and the hepatic vein remains intact

venous branches supplying the left median lobe and left lateral lobe, is ligated (Fig. 21.2e). Meanwhile, meticulous attention should be devoted to bypassing the accompanying accessory left hepatic artery. Prior to portal vein ligation, a suture with an appropriate thickness tailored for experimental rats or mice should be judiciously selected.

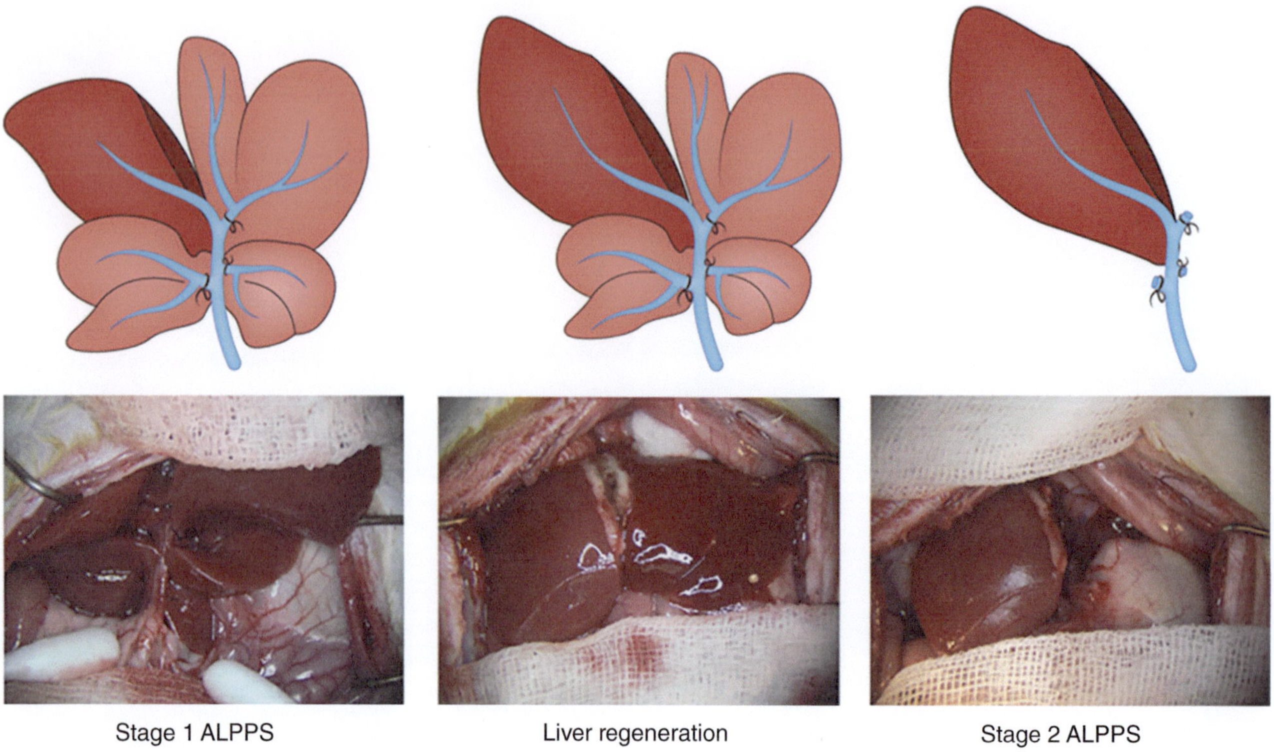

Fig. 21.3 Yao model for ALPPS. The images above depict the schematic diagram for the Yao model, while the images below showcase the surgical fields

Liver partition: Following portal vein ligation, the liver should be partitioned along the ischemic demarcation line identified in the median lobe (Fig. 21.2f). This can be accomplished by referencing the hepatic surgical maneuvers in humans, characterized by the utilization of electrosurgical devices to assist with precise resection, as well as the resection via the ligation of blood vessels (if any) to minimize bleeding. Typically, we perform surgical maneuvers as follows: the bipolar electrocoagulation forceps are utilized to dissect the corresponding parenchyma upon achieving complete hemostasis through electrocoagulation, thereby effectively controlling potential hemorrhage. According to our experience, employing gelfoam as an inter-positional material between the hepatic transection planes following liver partition aids in isolating bilateral liver remnants while further mitigating hemorrhage.

2. Schlegel model (mice and rats, Fig. 21.4): The Schlegel model entails ligating the portal venous branches feeding the right median lobe, caudate lobe, and right lobe, then resecting the left lateral lobe while preserving the left median lobe as the FLR. Liver mobilization and partition are performed as described previously.

Portal vein ligation: The portal venous branches perfusing the right median lobe, caudate lobe, and right lobe should be ligated. Specifically, the portal venous branches feeding the caudate and right lobe should be ligated by referencing the Yao model. The portal venous branch supplying the right median lobe, situated to the right of the hepatic artery and bile duct and displaying an unobstructed course, can be fully exposed with gentle traction, facilitating straightforward ligation (Fig. 21.2a).

Left lateral lobectomy: The left lateral lobectomy may be performed using circumferential ligation with a suture, with attention directed to ensuring that the circumferential ligation is not executed at an excessively proximal location to avoid compromising the portal venous flow to the left median lobe. Typically, we perform surgical maneuvers as follows: Vascular clamps are placed bilaterally on the left lateral lobe to secure the site of circumferential ligation and prevent the inadvertent slippage or dislodgement of the thread knot. Following resection, bipolar electrocoagulation forceps are utilized to achieve complete hemostasis. Additional hemostatic control can be attained by occluding the porta hepatis if necessary. As the portal venous branch supplying the left lateral lobe is situated adjacent to the hepatic vein, both the portal and hepatic veins must be securely and reliably tied with a well-placed knot, preventing uncontrollable hemorrhage resulting from inadvertent slippage or dislodgement of the thread knot following hepatectomy. Our experience signals that following left lateral lobectomy, inflammatory

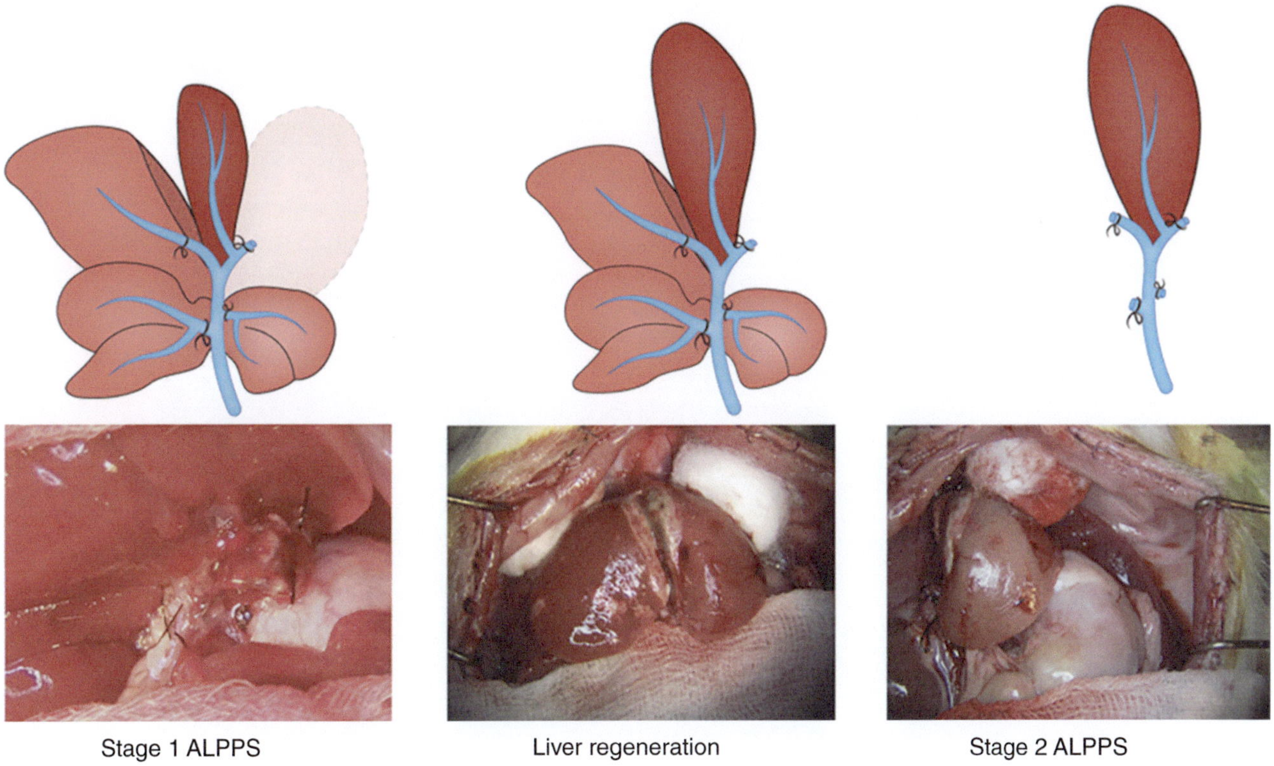

Fig. 21.4 Schlegel model for ALPPS. The image above depicts the schematic diagram for the Schlegel model, while the image below showcases the surgical fields

responses are noticeable on the hepatic transection plane, and that as the hepatic transection plane adheres to the left median lobe (FLR), it can trigger inflammatory responses in the corresponding area of the left median lobe (FLR) after closing the abdomen, potentially compromising liver regeneration (Fig. 21.5a). Therefore, we commonly apply a gelfoam to the hepatic transection plane following the left lateral lobectomy to isolate the left median lobe while achieving additional hemostasis.

3. Dili model (rats only, Fig. 21.6): The Dili model necessitates ligating the portal venous branches feeding the left lateral lobe, right median lobe, caudate lobe, and right lobe while preserving the left median lobe as the FLR. Liver mobilization and partition are performed as described previously.

Portal vein ligation: The portal venous branches supplying the left lateral lobe, right median lobe, caudate lobe, and right lobe should be ligated. Specifically, the portal venous branch supplying the left lateral lobe, intimately adherent to the accompanying hepatic artery and bile duct, traverses within the parenchyma of the left lateral lobe (Figs. 21.1c and 21.2d). The bile duct commonly exhibits variations with two distinct biliary branches, and the portal venous branch supplying the left lateral lobe is situated near the hepatic vein, rendering it challenging to completely dissect the corresponding structure. In addition, ligating the portal vein at a location excessively close to the confluence of the portal venous branches supplying the left lateral lobe and left median lobe risks compromising the portal venous flow to the left median lobe. Dili et al. employed the hydro-dissection technique, which harnesses the intrinsic tension properties of hydrodynamic forces, to dissect the corresponding structures in a layered fashion. Typically, we perform the following surgical maneuvers by referencing clinical surgical operations: the portal vein is meticulously dissected using a blunt dissection technique, followed by traction with a circumferential suture, with attention drawn to avoiding an inadvertent injury. Inflicting an inadvertent injury to or simultaneously ligating the hepatic artery and bile duct readily precipitates the necrosis of the left lateral lobe, resulting in model failure (Fig. 21.5d). During blunt dissection, assiduous attention must be devoted to the hepatic vein adjacent to the portal vein, as the hepatic vein in parenchyma is characterized by a thin-walled structure, rendering it exquisitely susceptible to an inadvertent iatrogenic injury. In addition to retracting the hepatic artery and bile duct, we retract the portal venous branch supplying the left median lobe at the site where the portal vein gives off branches to the left lateral lobe and the

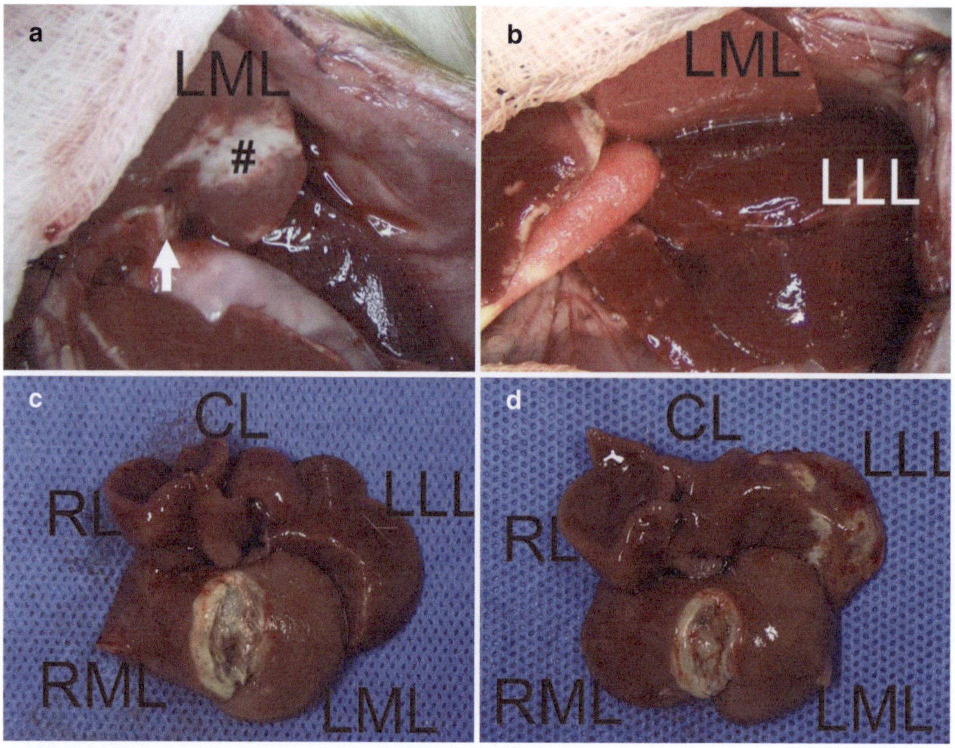

Fig. 21.5 Notes for the experimental rodent model for ALPPS. (**a**) On postoperative day 2 in the Schlegel model, an inflammatory response on the transection plane of the left lateral lobe precipitated the inflammatory necrosis in the corresponding location of the left median lobe (the hash denotes the inflammatory necrosis in the left median lobe, and the white arrow denotes the transection plane of the left lateral lobe); (**b**–**d**) Postoperative details of the left lateral lobe in the Dili model, where **b** denotes the surgical field on a postoperative day 2, indicating that the left lateral lobe was not necrotic; **c** denotes the whole liver procurement on a postoperative day 4; specifically, the left median lobe regenerated, the remaining lobes undergoing portal vein ligation did not regenerate, and the left lateral lobe was not necrotic; **d** denotes the whole liver procurement with an injury to the pedicle in the left lateral lobe on day 4 after first-stage surgery, suggesting that the left lateral lobe was partially necrotic and the model failed (RML, right median lobe; LML, left median lobe; LLL, left lateral lobe; CL, caudate lobe; RL, right lobe)

left median lobe. This aims to circumvent any potential compromise of the portal venous flow to the left median lobe during ligation of the portal venous branch supplying the left lateral lobe. To avoid compromising the portal venous flow to the left median lobe, it is advisable to prioritize managing the portal venous branch supplying the left lateral lobe during portal vein ligation, followed by subsequent operations upon confirmation of no deleterious impact on the left median lobe, as evidenced by the absence of the ischemic demarcation line in the median lobe.

21.1.3.2 Stage 2 ALPPS Procedure

During stage 2 surgery, all deportalized lobes need to be resected with the operative steps mirroring those employed during left lateral lobectomy. In areas with thick hepatic parenchyma, a stepwise resection approach can be used to ensure effective circumferential ligation. For instance, the right lobe can be resected by resecting the superior right lobe and inferior right lobe in a stepwise fashion to minimize bleeding.

21.1.4 Model Evaluation

Employing experimental rodents confers significant advantages. Experimental rodents are convenient and economical to maintain and breed and exhibit rapid reproduction and regeneration, facilitating massive data acquisition in a short span [6, 7]. In addition, experimental rodents offer a prominent advantage due to the extensive understanding of their physiological and anatomical structures and genomic profiles among researchers. Furthermore, the artificially inbred experimental rodents exhibit minimal genetic heterogeneity, facilitating the standardization of experiments and transgenic research endeavors [7]. The reagents utilized in experimental rodent-based research are readily accessible, facilitating the maintenance and execution of experimental rodent-based experiments. In animal experiments for ALPPS, experimental rodents also provide distinct advantages. The rapid regeneration and high metabolic rate in experimental rodents enable researchers to expedite their investigations. Experimental rodents exhibit rapid liver regeneration within

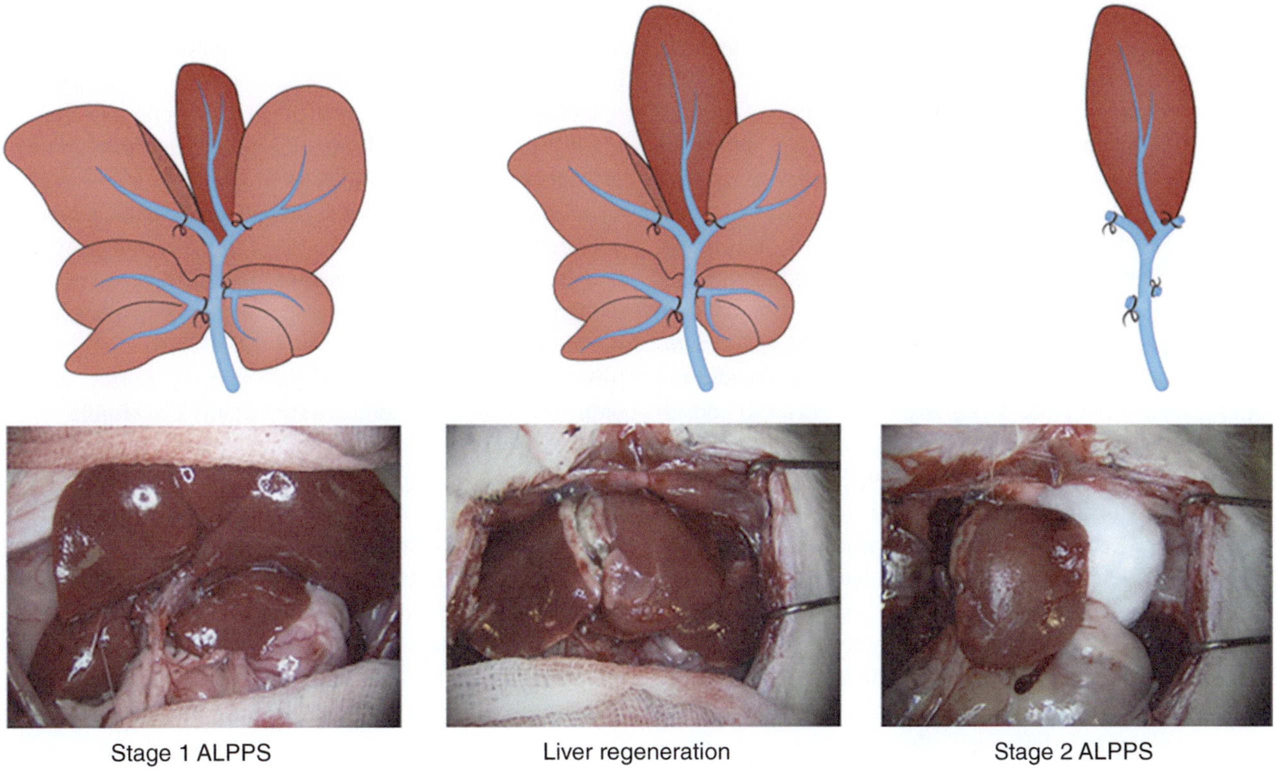

Fig. 21.6 Dili model for ALPPS. The image above depicts the schematic diagram for the Dili model, while the image below showcases the surgical fields

a brief time frame, allowing for the swift generation and collection of substantial data in the experimental rodent model for ALPPS. Fortunately, the median lobe in experimental rodents is uniquely supplied by two portal venous systems (Fig. 21.1), providing a natural anatomical framework for investigating ALPPS. More significantly, research findings indicate that the critical molecular components and gene-gene interactions driving liver regeneration and/or contributing to tumor development and progression exhibit evolutionary conservation; consequently, the experimental data obtained from investigating the impacts of ALPPS on liver regeneration and potential tumors can be extrapolated to larger experimental animals or human subjects [43, 44]. In addition, experimental rodents can be readily engineered to model pathological factors (e.g., cirrhosis and tumors), allowing for evaluating the impact of pathological hepatic parenchyma on ALPPS-induced liver regeneration as well as the potential risks contributing to tumor development and metastasis in the context of ALPPS-induced accelerated liver regeneration. Although experimental rodents differ considerably from humans concerning hepatic lobar structures and physiological and metabolic levels, experimental rodent models for ALPPS are essential for advancing liver research.

To date, numerous experimental rodent models have been reported. To evaluate multiple experimental rodent models and establish a foundation for selecting appropriate experimental rodent models for future research on ALPPS, we have comprehensively evaluated the Yao, Schlegel, and Dili models. A total of 77 experimental rats were experimentally selected for evaluation and were randomly euthanized on postoperative days 1, 2, 4, and 7. A total of 20 experimental rats were evenly distributed across each group, with five rats allocated for each designated time point. Experimental rats who died intraoperatively or before predetermined time points were excluded from the evaluation of liver regeneration. Experimental rats (n = 5) in the control group underwent baseline measurements following sham surgery. The evaluation focused on the challenges encountered during the stage 1 ALPPS procedure and the FLR hypertrophy and regeneration following the stage 1 ALPPS procedure.

We compared the three models based on surgery-related death, surgical duration, and blood loss to evaluate the challenges in model establishment. The findings of our study revealed that the overall mortality was 15.6% (12/72) in the experimental groups; specifically, the intraoperative or postoperative mortality was the highest in the Dili model group (Table 21.2). No operation-related deaths occurred in the Yao model group; two deaths (7%, 2/27) occurred in the Dili model group, and one death (4%, 1/24) occurred in the Schlegel model group. Accidental deaths occurring during the recovery from anesthesia up until the predetermined time of sample collection and euthanasia were considered postoperative. Dili model group accounted for the majority of postoperative deaths (5/9). The surgical duration was markedly more extended in the Dili model group as compared to the other two groups [one-way analysis of variance (ANOVA), $P < 0.0001$]. The mean surgical duration was 42.1 min in the Yao model group, 59.7 min in the Dili model group, and 49.0 min in the Schlegel model group (Table 21.2; Yao model group vs Dili model group, t-test, $P < 0.0001$; Yao model group vs Schlegel model group, t-test, $P = 0.0002$; Dili model group vs Schlegel model group, t-test, $P < 0.0001$). The intraoperative blood loss was estimated using the number of blood-soaked cotton balls. The three groups did not differ statistically (Table 21.2). The Dili model was considered the most complex because of its highest surgical mortality and most extended surgical duration. This is principally attributable to the anatomy of the portal vein in experimental rodents. In experimental rodents, the portal venous branches supplying the left median lobe and left lateral lobe converge into a common trunk. Nonetheless, the portal venous branch supplying the left lateral lobe typically traverses within the hepatic parenchyma, rendering it challenging to isolate the portal venous branch from the hepatic parenchyma surrounded by hepatic arteries and bile ducts. The key to establishing the Dili model is preserving the Glissonean pedicle leading to the left median lobe; however, precisely dissecting the pedicle requires considerable time. Failure to precisely dissect the pedicle may result in a compromised portal venous flow to the left median lobe upon ligation of the portal venous branch supplying the left lateral lobe. Furthermore, the anatomical proximity of the portal venous branch supplying the left lateral lobe to the hepatic vein poses a heightened risk of an inadvertent injury to the hepatic or portal vein during dissection, potentially precipitating a catastrophic hemorrhagic event and subsequent animal death. In contrast to establishing the Dili model, establishing the Schlegel model does not entail meticulously dissecting the portal venous branch supplying the left median lobe, as directly resecting the left lateral lobe does not compromise the venous flow to the left median lobe. Establishing the Yao model is straightforward and uncomplicated, as various portal venous branches awaiting ligation are structurally discernible.

FLR hypertrophy and hepatocellular proliferation rate are indicative of liver regeneration. In the control group (preoperative control), the mean left median lobe weight-to-body weight ratio was 0.004,9, whereas the mean right median lobe weight-to-body weight ratio was 0.009,6. FLR regeneration was observed in the three models (Fig. 21.7a). To simultaneously evaluate the hepatic hypertrophy rates across the three models, the liver regeneration rate was employed as the evaluative marker [(FLR weight ÷ body weight at the time of sampling) ÷ (mean FLR weight ÷ body weight in the control group) × 100 (%)]. The Schlegel model demonstrated enhanced regenerative capacity, particularly in the early stage of liver regeneration. On postoperative day 1, the liver regeneration rate was notably greater in the Schlegel model group as compared to the Yao model group ($P = 0.043$). On

Table 21.2 Surgical parameters in the experimental rodent model for ALPPS

Parameters	Yao model group	Dili model group	Schlegel model group	*P* value
No. of postoperative deaths	1	5	3	
No. of intraoperative deaths	0	2	1	
No. enrolled	20	20	20	
Preoperative body weight (g)	247.4 ± 10.2	249.1 ± 10.7	249.4 ± 11.1	0.818
Stage 1 ALPPS procedure				
Surgical duration (minutes)	42.1 ± 5.0	59.7 ± 7.0	49.0 ± 5.5	1.64×10^{-12}
Estimated blood loss (mL)	1.84 ± 1.3	1.3 ± 1.1	1.4 ± 1.1	0.351

Note: Data are expressed as mean ± standard deviation. Only enrolled experimental rodents were evaluated for the surgical duration and blood loss, while experimental rodents who died intraoperatively or postoperatively were evaluated for mortality only. The intraoperative blood loss was estimated using the number of blood-soaked cotton balls

Fig. 21.7 Postoperative liver regeneration in the three experimental rodent models for ALPPS. (**a**) Liver regeneration at various postoperative time points in the three experimental rodent models, the white arrow denotes the FLR. (**b**) Quantitative evaluation of liver regeneration based on FLR regeneration rate. (**c**) Quantitative evaluation of liver regeneration based on the relative KGR of the FLR volume. (**d**) Ki67 staining of the FLR at various postoperative time points in the three experimental rodent models. (**e**) Quantitative analysis of hepatocellular proliferation based on the proportion of Ki67-positive hepatocytes (* appended to Dili model group denotes t-test, Yao model group vs Dili model group, $P < 0.05$; * appended to Schlegel model group denotes t-test, Yao model group vs Schlegel model group, $P < 0.05$; ** appended to Schlegel model group denotes t-test, Dili model group vs Schlegel model group, $P < 0.05$. POD denotes postoperative day)

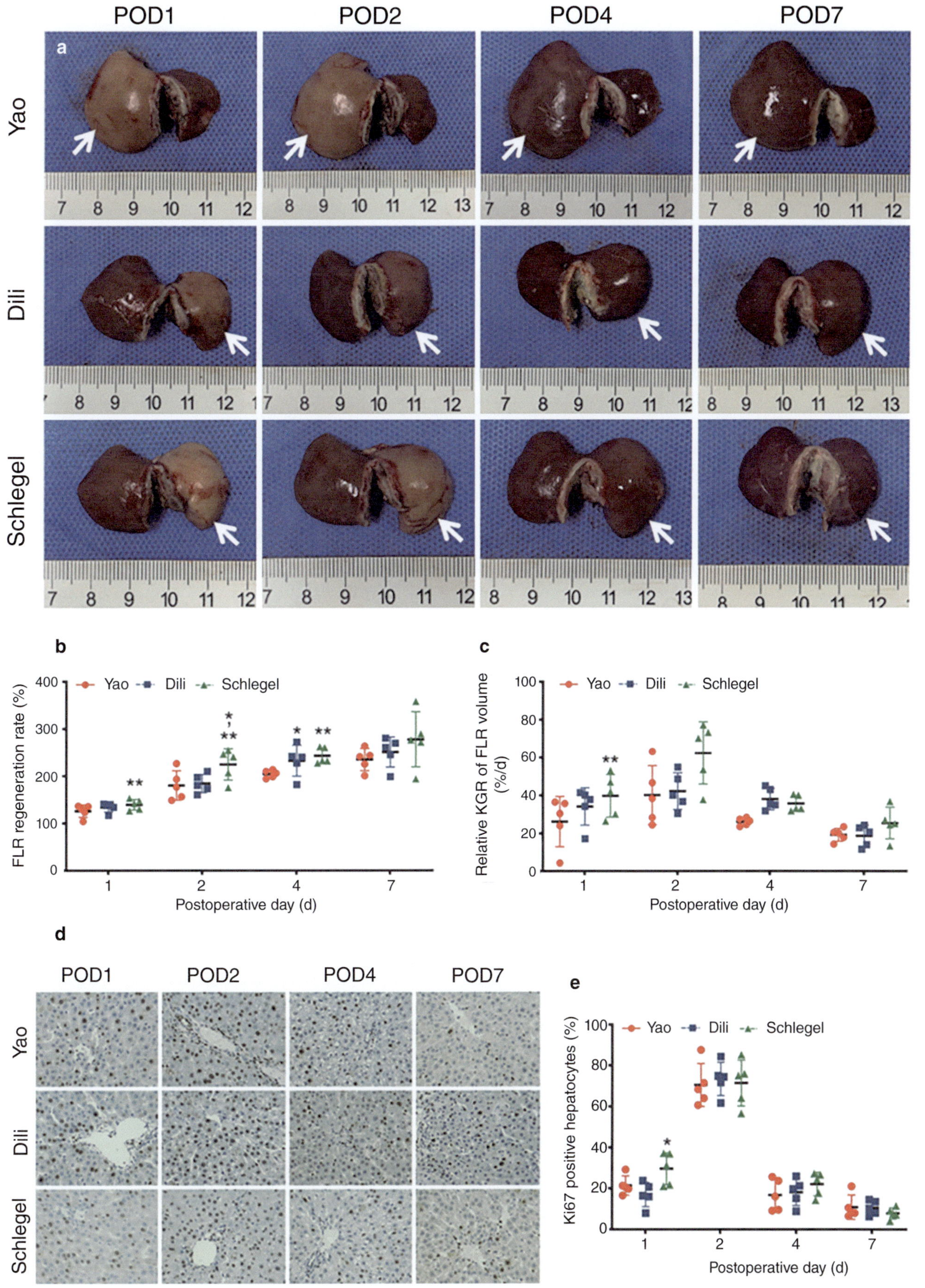

a
POD1
POD2
POD4
POD7
Yao
Dili
Schlegel
b
FLR regeneration rate (%)
Yao
Dili
Schlegel
Postoperative day (d)
c
Relative KGR of FLR volume (%/d)
Yao
Dili
Schlegel
Postoperative day (d)
d
POD1
POD2
POD4
POD7
Yao
Dili
Schlegel
e
Ki67 positive hepatocytes (%)
Yao
Dili
Schlegel
Postoperative day (d)

postoperative day 2, the liver regeneration rate was the highest in Schlegel model group, and the liver regeneration rates did not differ significantly between Yao and Dili model groups (Fig. 21.7b, postoperative day 2: Yao model vs Dili model, t-test, $P = 0.812$; Yao model vs Schlegel model, t-test, $P = 0.033$; Dili model vs Schlegel model, t-test, $P = 0.023$). On postoperative day 4, the liver regeneration rate was the lowest in the Yao model group (Fig. 21.7b, postoperative day 4: Yao model vs Dili model, t-test, $P = 0.002$; Yao model vs Schlegel model, t-test, $P = 0.0005$; Dili model vs Schlegel model, t-test, $P = 0.998$). The kinetic growth rate (KGR) analysis of the FLR volume revealed comparable outcomes across the three groups, with the Schlegel model group exhibiting a heightened propensity for enhanced regenerative capacity (Fig. 21.7c, postoperative day 2: Yao model vs Schlegel model, t test, $P = 0.042$; Dili model vs Schlegel model, t-test, $P = 0.055$). To further evaluate liver regeneration, we also compared the expressions of Kiel 67 (Ki67) across the three groups. The three groups exhibited the highest proportions of proliferating hepatocytes on postoperative day 2 as compared to any other time points (Fig. 21.7d, e). In addition, the proportion of proliferating hepatocytes in the Schlegel model group was apparently higher than that in the Dili model group on postoperative day 1; however, the three groups did not differ in terms of the proportion of proliferating hepatocytes at any other time points (Fig. 21.7d, e, postoperative day 1: Yao model vs Dili model, t-test, $P = 0.617$; Yao model vs Schlegel model, t-test, $P = 0.124$; Dili model vs Schlegel model, t-test, $P = 0.047$). Our findings revealed that the Yao and Dili model groups did not differ considerably concerning an increase in the FLR weight on postoperative days 1 and 2 and that the liver regeneration rate was lower in the Yao model group as compared to the Dili model group on postoperative day 4. This signified that the presence of an adequate FLR may lead to a compromise of ALPPS-induced liver regeneration in the Yao model. The Schlegel model exhibited enhanced regenerative capacity, indicating that the hepatectomy performed during the stage 1 ALPPS procedure inadvertently triggered a supplementary liver regeneration response, thereby introducing a research bias for ALPPS-induced liver regeneration.

While the three experimental rodent models for ALPPS effectively induced rapid liver regeneration, prudently selecting an appropriate experimental rodent model is crucial for investigating the mechanism of ALPPS. The Yao model cannot replicate the surgical scenario where the FLR is inadequate in humans, because the FLR mass is sufficient to support the survival of rats following resection of 70% of the liver [45], which does not correspond to clinical practice. During an investigation of the mechanism of ALPPS-induced liver regeneration, caution should be warranted with the utilization of the Schlegel model, as hepatectomy may inadvertently introduce additional confounding factors that could potentially promote liver regeneration. As such, employing the Dili model is recommended. During an investigation of the survival-sustaining mechanism following the ALPPS procedure, the Dili or Schlegel model should warrant consideration. Compared to the Schlegel model, the Dili model offers a more precise and controlled experimental paradigm within the realm of experimental rat models. Due to its operational challenges, the Dili model has yet to be reported for use in mice. Typically, patients undergoing ALPPS procedures present with a significant tumor burden and experience accompanying pathological hepatic parenchyma manifesting as cirrhosis or fatty liver degeneration.

Considering the reported FLR of more than 30% in the majority of tumor-bearing and cirrhotic rodent models for ALPPS [36, 38, 39], the Yao model seems to be the sole viable option when incorporating these factors into the experimental rodent model for ALPPS. The Schlegel and Dili models may suffer limitations in sustaining survival when the FLR falls below 10%, which awaits further investigation.

21.2 Porcine ALPPS Model

21.2.1 Introduction to Experimental Animals

The history of domestic pig usage in biomedical research extends back to the 1940s, and experimental pigs began to be extensively utilized from 1960 onwards [46]. More than 70 recognized purebred pig breeds are available, most predominantly used for production and consumption. Certain miniature pig breeds have gained prominence in biomedical research. Miniature pigs exhibit remarkable anatomical, physiological, and pathogenetic similarities to humans. The porcine genome, composed of 18 autosomes and 2 sex chromosomes, has been sequenced to demonstrate extensive homology to the human genome [47], rendering experimental pigs suitable for biomedical mechanism research. In addition, the cardiovascular system, kidneys, and digestive organs in experimental pigs mirror those in humans [48]. Consequently, experimental pigs are extensively employed within the realm of experimental surgery to fine-tune surgical techniques and validate novel experimental surgical treatments [49–51]. Experimental pigs have proven to be invaluable models in the field of hepatic surgery, particularly in the realms of liver transplantation, hepatectomy, and portal vein occlusion [52–54]. Aside from the above benefits, experimental pigs offer compelling advantages stemming from their compact size. Specifically, experimental pigs are more accessible to manipulate and breed and exhibit lower requirements for food and test substances than large experimental pigs. Due to factors (e.g., animal protection), experimental pigs are gaining preference over experimental dogs and nonhuman primates in the realm of life science research. The prominent experimental pig breeds beyond China include Göttingen minipigs, Minnesota minipigs, and Pitman-Moore miniature pigs. In contrast, the primary experimental pig breeds in China include Tibet minipigs, Xishuangbanna inbred minipigs, Guizhou minipigs, Guangxi Bama minipigs, and Wuzhishan minipigs.

21.2.2 Foundation of Liver Anatomy in Experimental Animals for ALPPS

Anatomical investigations into the gross structural composition of the experimental pig liver have revealed variability in the number of hepatic lobes, with the existing literature documenting the presence of four to six distinct hepatic lobes [55–57]. This variation may be attributed to differences among various experimental pig breeds. According to the recognized interstrain stable lobar classification system, the experimental pig liver can be delineated into five lobes, namely, left lateral lobe, left median lobe, right median lobe, right lateral lobe, and caudate lobe. In addition, the quadrate lobe has been reported (Fig. 21.8). While the lobar classification of the experimental pig liver remains a subject of ongoing debate, the hepatic segments of experimental pigs bear a striking resemblance to those of humans. Based on the Couinaud classification of hepatic segments and the characteristics of portal venous branches, the experimental pig liver can be categorized into eight hepatic segments clockwise [58, 59]. The nomenclature of hepatic segments in pigs closely aligns with that in humans: segment I, caudate lobe; segment II, the superior segment of the left lateral lobe; segment III, the inferior segment of the left lateral lobe; segment IV, left median lobe; segment V, the inferior segment of the right median lobe; segment VI, the inferior segment of the right lateral lobe; segment VII, the superior segment of the right lateral lobe; and segment VII, the superior segment of the right median lobe. Unlike the human liver, the experimental pig liver exhibits a prominently lobulated hepatic fissure, a profound notch along the round ligament fissure, and a well-demarcated Rex-Cantlie line.

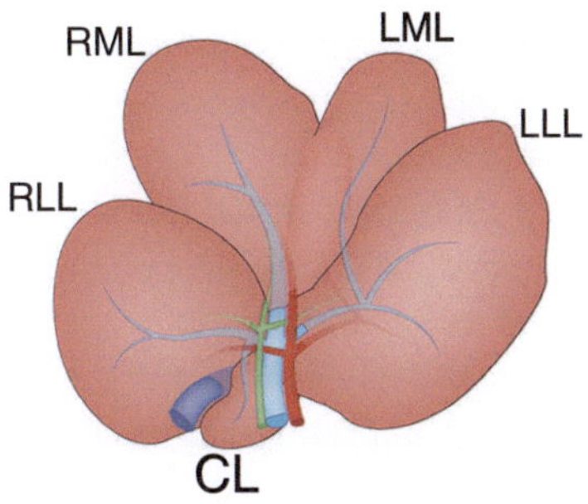

Fig. 21.8 Experimental pig liver structure. RML, right median lobe; RL, right lateral lobe; LML, left median lobe; LLL, left lateral lobe; CL, caudate lobe; light blue, portal vein; deep blue, inferior vena cava; red, artery; green, bile duct and gallbladder

The portal vein bifurcates into two main branches at the extrahepatic porta hepatis [60]. Typically, one or two communicating branches are present within the hepatic fissure between the right lateral lobe and the right median lobe, and no communicating branches are present between the left median lobe and the right median lobe. Consequently, the left and right hemilivers are completely isolated. Originating from the main portal vein, the right portal vein trifurcates into three branches, which supply segments I, VII, and VI, respectively. The main portal vein arches medially, giving rise to the middle branch toward the right median lobe, which supplies blood to segments V and VII. Upon originating from the main portal vein, the left portal vein traverses 2–3 cm within the parenchyma before bifurcating to supply blood to the left median lobe and the left lateral lobe. Specifically, the first branch, which supplies segment IV, gives rise to a branch that traverses the hepatic fissure to supply segment III. The second branch supplies segment II only.

In experimental pigs, the basin celiac artery arises from the abdominal aorta, and the basin celiac artery trifurcates into the main hepatic artery, left gastric artery, and splenic artery. Each hepatic lobe is supplied by a dedicated artery. The left hepatic artery bifurcates into the left medial and left lateral branches, supplying the corresponding hepatic lobe and gallbladder. The right hepatic artery bifurcates into the right medial and right lateral branches, supplying the right lobe [61]. Typically, three branches are situated anterior to the main portal vein. Among them, two branches, which supply the left lobe and the median lobe, respectively, are located at the median border of the porta hepatis, and they may further bifurcate before entering the hepatic parenchyma, resulting in the presence of three or four branches within the hepatic parenchyma. The main branch supplying the right lateral lobe typically traverses posterior to the portal vein, despite an accessory branch located anterior to the portal vein. The hepatic parenchymal artery invariably accompanies the portal vein and supplies the same hepatic segment as the portal vein.

The left and right hepatic ducts, which typically drain their respective halves of the liver, unite to form the common hepatic duct. Analogous to the human liver, the hepatic duct in the experimental pig liver accompanies the portal vein within the Glissonian sheath, resulting in a remarkably analogous segmental distribution pattern. The left hepatic duct, notably larger in diameter than the right hepatic duct, simultaneously drains the left median lobe and the left lateral lobe. The right hemiliver is drained by two dedicated hepatic ducts. The right anterior hepatic duct is small in diameter, drains the right median lobe, and converges with the common hepatic duct positioned medially to the middle branch of the portal vein. The right posterior hepatic duct, characterized by its large diameter, drains the right lateral lobe and caudate lobe. It typically converges with the right anterior hepatic duct to form a separate right hepatic duct. The right hepatic duct occasionally exhibits variations, as it may directly merge with the common hepatic duct or even drain into the left hepatic duct. The right posterior hepatic duct, originating from the right lateral lobe, traverses along the inferior surface of the left main portal vein and continues its course through the left side of the middle portal venous branch. Therefore, the right posterior hepatic duct is readily susceptible to an inadvertent injury during dissection and ligation of the left and middle portal venous branches or hepatic duct.

The hepatic vein divides into four main branches, originating directly from the inferior vena cava and draining the left lateral lobe, left median lobe, right median lobe, and right lateral lobe, respectively. The hepatic venous branches supplying the left lateral lobe and the median lobe frequently converge at the vena cava adjacent to the left hepatic fissure. The hepatic venous branch supplying the left lateral lobe encompasses several short branches draining segment II and a long branch draining segment III. The hepatic venous branch supplying the left median lobe drains the entire left median lobe (i.e., segment IV). The hepatic venous branch supplying the right median lobe is formed by the confluence of two branches that drain segments V and VII, respectively, and the site of the confluence is located at a long distance from the inferior vena cava. The right hepatic vein consists of short branches and a long branch, which drain segments VII and VI, respectively. The hepatic venous branch supplying segment I drains directly into the inferior vena cava. It is noteworthy that the inferior vena cava and hepatic vein converge within the hepatic parenchyma, underscoring the need for exercising caution during hepatectomy. The inferior vena cava and hepatic parenchymal vein, characterized by a thin-walled structure, are readily susceptible to an inadvertent iatrogenic injury.

When experimental pigs undergo the ALPPS procedure, a crucial consideration is the positioning of the porcine vena cava along the right side of the liver [60, 62]. In this regard, left-sided extended hepatectomy is the sole viable option in experimental pigs undergoing the ALPPS procedure. The inferior vena cava and hepatic parenchymal vein, characterized by a thin-walled structure, are exquisitely susceptible to an inadvertent iatrogenic injury in experimental pigs. Therefore, meticulously avoiding hemorrhage is necessary during liver partition. Caution should be exercised to circumvent an inadvertent compromise of the portal vein at the porta hepatis, as arteries traverse anterior to and posterior to the portal vein. In addition, the right posterior hepatic duct must be preserved, as it must drain bile from the right lateral lobe and caudate lobe. Due to its anatomical course, the right posterior hepatic duct must be meticulously dissected during portal vein ligation to prevent an inadvertent injury.

21.2.3 Operations of the ALPPS Procedure in Experimental Animals

The first experimental pig model for ALPPS, developed by Croome et al. and subsequently referred to as the Croome model, was reported in 2015 [63]. In the Croome model, the scope of portal vein ligation and the volume of hepatectomy were delineated predominantly by extrapolating from the previous model of experimental pigs with liver failure undergoing major hepatectomy [54, 64]. Specifically, the portal venous branches supplying the left lateral lobe left median lobe and right median lobe were ligated, the right posterior lobe was partially resected, and the liver was partitioned along the right lateral lobe and the right median lobe. The caudate lobe and a portion of the right posterior lobe were preserved as the FLR, representing 15–20% of the total liver volume. The operations of the ALPPS procedure in the experimental pig model are detailed below (Fig. 21.9).

21.2.3.1 Stage 1 ALPPS Procedure

The stage 1 ALPPS procedure in experimental pigs closely mirrors that in humans in clinical practice.

1. Liver mobilization: Isolating the ligament formed by the reflection of the peritoneal membrane between the diaphragmatic surface and the diaphragm is essential for complete liver mobilization. Following complete liver mobilization to safeguard the restoration of hepatic function, the hepatic lobe is lifted to fully expose the porta hepatis. Meanwhile, the gallbladder is resected.
2. Portal vein ligation: After meticulous dissection and isolation of the portal venous branches, particularly those situated at the confluence of the right median lobe and right posterior lobe, the surrounding connective tissues must be judiciously resected. Meanwhile, the hepatic arterial branch coursing anterior to the main portal vein becomes visible, necessitating utmost vigilance to avert an inadvertent iatrogenic injury. Completely mobilizing the portal venous branches as well as delineating the main portal vein and their branches supplying the left lateral lobe, left median lobe, and right median lobe, as well as the branches supplying the right posterior lobe and caudate lobe, is imperative, with the ligation line reserved for the former. At this juncture, the portal vein must not be completely ligated, as it may precipitate a redirection of the portal venous flow to the right posterior lobe, consequently augmenting the risk of intraoperative bleeding and detrimentally impacting the state of experimental animals during liver splitting. After the liver is completely split and partitioned and complete hemostasis is achieved, the portal venous branches should be ligated as planned.
3. Liver partition: Upon completion of the above preparations, the liver should be split and partitioned. The partition line should be delineated in the right posterior lobe,

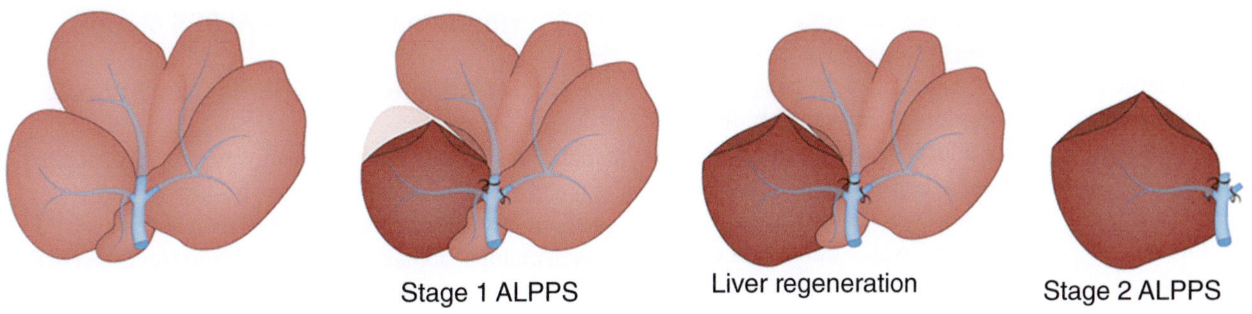

Fig. 21.9 ALPPS procedure in the Croome model

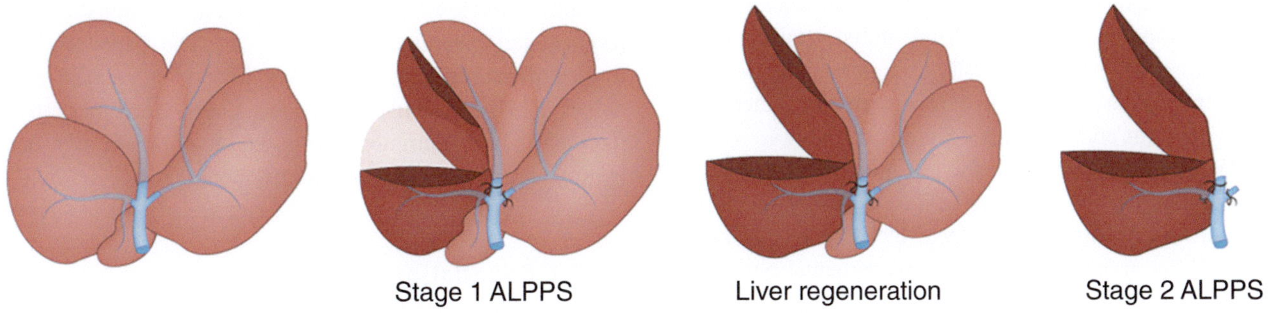

Fig. 21.10 ALPPS procedure in the Budai model

and then the hepatic parenchyma should be split along the partition line. The hepatic parenchyma may be split using a Cavitron ultrasonic surgical aspirator or a harmonic scalpel. During liver splitting, unwavering vigilance must be exercised to safeguard the integrity of the vena cava, thereby preventing massive hemorrhage. The hepatic transection plane follows the course of the hepatic vein, extending to the lateral border of the right median lobe. Then, it continues along the hepatic fissure, which is situated between the right median lobe and right lateral lobe, toward the left side of the caudate lobe. It is noteworthy that the inferior vena cava and hepatic parenchymal vein, characterized by a thin-walled structure, are readily susceptible to an inadvertent iatrogenic injury. In addition, partially resecting the right posterior lobe is necessary for preserving the post-extended hepatectomy FLR volume.

Upon completion of the aforementioned surgical maneuvers, the posterior aspect of the hilar plate can be further bluntly dissected utilizing right-angled dissecting forceps. This is followed by the judicious placement of a vascular annulus and an aseptic barrier at the porta hepatis and the hepatic venous confluence, thereby preventing adhesions during stage 2 surgery.

21.2.3.2 Stage 2 ALPPS Procedure

The adhesion formation occurs shortly after stage 1 ALPPS procedure in experimental pigs. Consequently, caution is exercised to dissect adhesion, which is vital before liver manipulation during the stage 2 ALPPS procedure. Prior to liver manipulation, the left-sided portal venous structures in the hepatoduodenal ligament must be completely mobilized to prevent adhesion formation and tearing or damaging the biliary tract. Upon complete adhesiolysis, the hepatic tissue should be resected with an endoscopic linear cutter stapler. If hemostatic reinforcement is deemed necessary, the continuous mattress suturing technique should be employed. This iterative process should be executed until complete liver resection and transection, with the FLR preserved (Fig. 21.9).

The Croome model has been subsequently applied by other researchers [65]. Budai et al. reported a model modified from the Croome model (Budai model). Specifically, they partitioned the liver along the midline of the right median lobe to preserve an adequate transection plane to partition the interlobar collateral circulatory pathways and elicit a robust inflammatory response. Their rationale stemmed from the hypothesis that the narrow transection plane delineated in the Croome model might prove insufficient to elicit a discernible inflammatory response. In addition, they judiciously resected two-thirds of the right posterior lobe to preserve an adequate FLR volume [66] (Fig. 21.10).

21.2.4 Model Evaluation

Compared to small experimental animals (experimental rodent models), large experimental animals more closely resemble humans in terms of body composition and metabolic rate. Consequently, the physiological and systemic impacts of surgical interventions on large experimental animals are more analogous to those experienced by humans. As such, large experimental animal models may yield more insightful and clinically translatable information during an investigation of the overall effects of a novel surgical intervention [67]. Due to the body size, the tissues and organs of large experimental animals are more amenable to frequent sampling and biopsy procedures, which inflict less damage on their major organs [64]. This renders large experimental animals more suitable for continuous dynamic research. Therefore, large experimental animals serve as indispensable animal models compared to small experimental animals. It merits emphasis that large experimental animals are characteristically devoid of standardized inbred strains, and the interindividual genetic diversity can potentially introduce confounding variables in fundamental research, necessitating meticulous consideration.

Regarding the experimental pig model for ALPPS, the hepatic parenchyma, characterized by a thin-walled venous structure, is readily susceptible to bleeding during hepatic parenchymal transection. Besides, experimental pigs exhibit a pronounced stress response and frequently struggle to tolerate blood loss, with mortality risks escalating when blood loss exceeds 500 mL. Consequently, bleeding must be rigorously managed during the ALPPS procedure. Achieving hepatic parenchymal transection without utilizing modern electrosurgical devices poses a formidable challenge. In addition, the hepatic vascular anatomy in experimental pigs deviates from that in humans. Specifically, the overtly lobulated experimental pig liver is devoid of interlobar portal venous collateral anastomoses, in stark contrast to the abundant interlobar portal venous collateral anastomoses present in the human liver. This anatomical structure, feature by significant collateral shunts between portally perfused and deportalized parts, is considered a contributing factor to inadequate liver regeneration following portal vein ligation or embolization and serves as a theoretical underpinning for liver partition in stage 1 ALPPS procedure. Therefore, the experimental pig models demonstrate limitations in accurately recapitulating the physiological alterations resulting from artificially partitioning the liver and resecting portal venous collateral circulatory pathways during the ALPPS procedure. Moreover, the branches of the portal vein and vena cava in the experimental pig liver are perpendicularly oriented, rendering it challenging to plan the hepatic transection plane. Left-sided extended hepatectomy remains the sole viable option as the vena cava runs along the right side of the liver. In humans, primary and secondary tumors frequently localize to the right hemiliver, necessitating right-sided hepatectomy during the ALPPS procedure. Furthermore, the anatomical structure of the experimental pig liver differs from that of the human liver, rendering experimental pigs unsuitable for preclinical training pertaining to the ALPPS procedure.

21.3 Nonhuman Primate ALPPS Model

21.3.1 Introduction to Experimental Animals

Nonhuman primates, predominantly monkeys, constitute pivotal experimental animals because of their shared biological similarities with humans. Apart from their widespread utilization in multiple domains (e.g., research on cranial nerve function, behavioral research, and viral and vaccine trials), nonhuman primates possess invaluable research potential within hepatic surgery. Aside from hepatitis virus research [68–70], nonhuman primates are principally utilized in liver transplantation research [71, 72] as well as research on hepatectomy and liver regeneration [73–76]. The frequently utilized experimental monkey breeds include macaques (e.g., rhesus monkey, Assamese macaque, stump-tailed macaque), marmosets (e.g., common marmoset, silvery marmoset, and pygmy marmoset), and cynomolgus monkeys.

21.3.2 Foundation of Liver Anatomy in Experimental Animals for ALPPS

While the gross anatomy of the nonhuman primate liver exhibits similarities to that of the human liver [77, 78], there remains a dearth of research on the fine-grained anatomical structure of the nonhuman primate liver. A researcher delineated the nonhuman primate liver into three primary lobes (i.e., median lobe, left lateral lobe, and right lateral lobe), with the caudate lobe positioned posteriorly, based on two prominent deep hepatic fissures on the hepatic surface [79]. The median lobe, the largest of the three primary lobes, is characterized by the falciform ligament and umbilical fissure on its surface, allowing for further subdivision into the left and right median lobes. The umbilical fissure extends to the porta hepatis on the visceral surface of the liver. The gallbladder is discernible along the right aspect of the umbilical fissure, extending from the midpoint of the gallbladder fossa to the right side of the inferior vena cava (main portal vein fissure) to further divide the right median lobe into two lobes (Fig. 21.11). The left lateral lobe, characterized by its thin and expansive trapezoidal shape, is tethered to the diaphragm via the left triangular ligament. On the visceral surface of the liver, a small protrusion is discernible in the vicinity of the porta hepatis, obscuring the left side of the porta hepatis and the gallbladder. Upon exposing the deep fissure delineating the median lobe from the left lateral lobe, it becomes evident that the left lateral lobe is connected to the remaining hepatic lobes solely through a remarkably attenuated parenchymal isthmus. This isthmic parenchyma harbors the vascular pedicle supplying the left lateral lobe, with the hepatic veins situated along the superior aspect of the parenchyma. The arterial branch courses

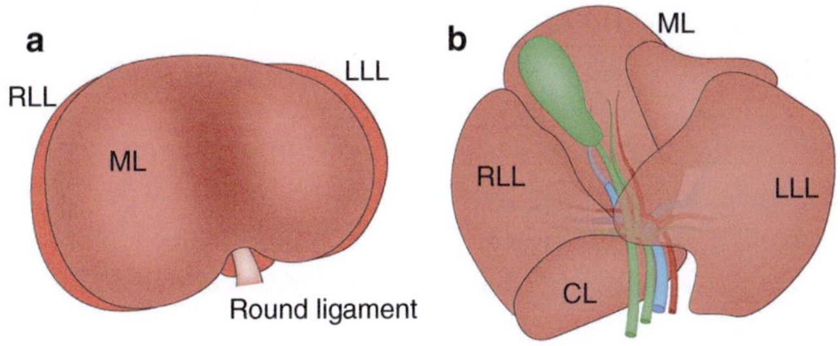

Fig. 21.11 Experimental monkey liver. (**a**) Ventral surface of the experimental monkey liver. (**b**) Lateral view of the experimental monkey liver (ML, median lobe; LLL, left lateral lobe; RLL, right lateral lobe; CL, caudate lobe; blue, portal vein; red, hepatic artery; green, hepatobiliary duct and gallbladder)

in close proximity to the inferior aspect of the portal venous branch, supplying the left lateral lobe. Nonetheless, the bile duct within the left lateral lobe remains indiscernible because of its compact size. Analogous to the left lateral lobe, the right lateral lobe is tethered to the diaphragm via the right triangular ligament. The right lateral lobe is connected to the remaining hepatic lobes via an attenuated parenchymal isthmus, with the vascular pedicle traversing within the isthmic parenchyma. The caudate lobe, exhibiting a rectangular configuration and entirety encapsulating the inferior vena cava, is contiguous with the right lateral lobe yet remains distinct from the left lateral lobe. Based on Couinaud classification of hepatic segments [58], the nonhuman primate liver can be classified into eight segments, with the following corresponding relationships: the caudate lobe corresponds to segment I; the left lateral lobe corresponds to segment II; the left median lobe corresponds to segment III; the left side of the main portal vein fissure in the right median lobe corresponds to segment IV; the right side of the main portal vein fissure in the right median lobe corresponds to segments V and VII; and the right lateral lobe corresponds to segments VI and VII.

Generally, the portal vein in nonhuman primates, closely resembling that in humans, typically bifurcates into two branches at the porta hepatis. The right portal vein is characterized by an exceptionally short common trunk, which then ramifies into anterior and posterior branches. Conversely, the left portal venous branch possesses an elongated extrahepatic segment (Fig. 21.11). Analogous to the portal vein in humans, the portal vein in nonhuman primates demonstrates anatomical variations classified as types I and II [79, 80].

The common hepatic artery courses anterior to the main portal vein, with the hepatic artery and its ramifications accompanying the corresponding portal venous branches. The hepatic arterial branches are situated at the same anatomical level as the confluence of the portal vein and bile duct. At the point of bifurcation of the portal vein, the common hepatic artery ramifies into two branches.

In nonhuman primates, the hepatic duct is situated along the right lateral aspect within the Glissonian pedicle. The confluence of the right and left hepatic ducts is located in close proximity to the porta hepatis. The common bile duct courses along the anterior right aspect of the main portal vein. The gallbladder is deeply embedded within the hepatic parenchyma, exhibiting an elongated and fusiform configuration and nestled within the gallbladder fossa beneath the median lobe. The cystic duct, which is remarkably elongated, establishes its junction with the common bile duct adjacent to the first part of the duodenum.

The hepatic vein comprises three primary branches (i.e., right, left, and middle hepatic veins) that drain into the suprahepatic inferior vena cava. The left hepatic vein is constituted by two branches, which drain the left lateral lobe and the left median lobe. Similarly, the right hepatic vein has two branches, which drain the right lateral lobe and right median lobe. The infrahepatic vena cava penetrates the hepatic parenchyma between the hepatic pedicle and the caudate lobe, becoming entirely encapsulated within the hepatic parenchyma.

The anatomical structures of the liver and porta hepatis in nonhuman primates bear a striking resemblance to those in humans. Consequently, the anatomical features in humans undergoing the ALPPS procedure can serve as a valuable reference for the anatomical features necessitating meticulous consideration in nonhuman primates undergoing the ALPPS procedure. Considering that the left lateral lobe and the right lateral lobe are connected to the median lobe solely through an attenuated parenchymal isthmus, successfully partitioning the liver, creating an adequate transection plane to modulate portal venous flow, and eliciting an appropriate inflammatory response mandate that the transection plane should be confined exclusively within the median lobe. Notably, the inferior vena cava is entirely encapsulated within the hepatic parenchyma. Therefore, utmost caution must be exercised to prevent an inadvertent injury to the inferior vena cava during liver partition in stage 1 ALPPS procedure and during hepatectomy in stage 2 ALPPS procedure.

21.3.3 Operations of the ALPPS Procedure in Experimental Animals

To date, no nonhuman primate models for ALPPS have been reported. Prior studies have substantiated the feasibility of hepatectomy in nonhuman primates [75, 76]. Consequently, our center explored the ALPPS procedure in rhesus macaques by establishing a rhesus monkey model for ALPPS. The surgical operations were meticulously executed by following the operative principles of the classic ALPPS procedure in clinical practice. Specifically, stage 1 surgery involved liver partition coupled with the ligation of the right portal venous branch. Following left-sided liver regeneration, stage 2 surgery commenced (Fig. 21.12).

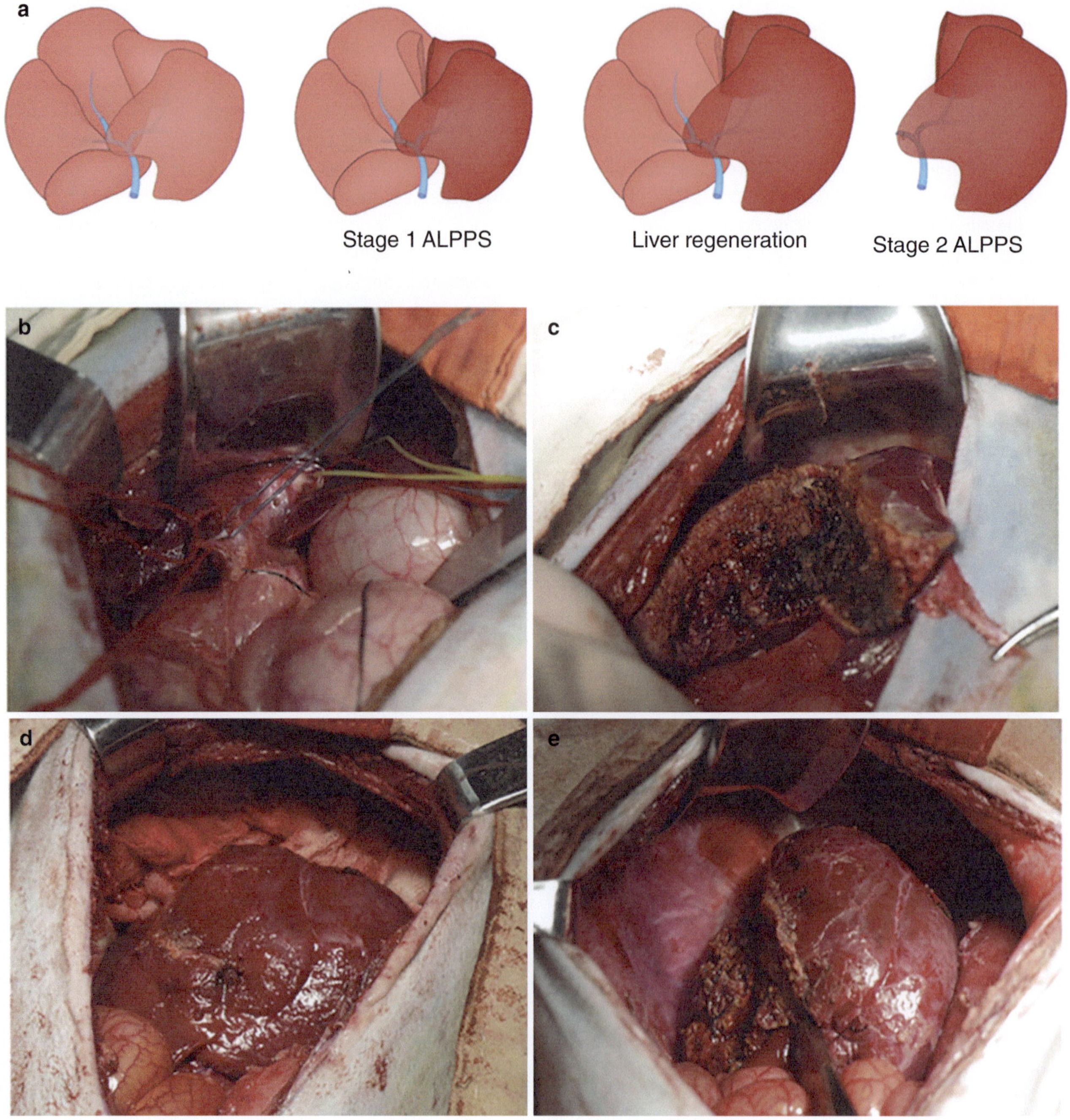

Fig. 21.12 ALPPS procedure in an experimental monkey model. (**a**) ALPPS procedure in experimental monkey model. (**b**) Anatomy of the porta hepatis in an experimental monkey model in first-stage ALPPS procedure (blue band, portal vein; red band, hepatic artery; yellow band, bile duct). (**c**) Liver partition in the experimental monkey model in first-stage ALPPS procedure. (**d**) Liver regeneration following first-stage ALPPS procedure; (**e**) After hepatectomy in an experimental monkey model in stage 2 ALPPS procedure

21.3.4 Model Evaluation

Despite the availability of multiple experimental animal species, nonhuman primates remain indispensable in experimental animal research. While experimental animals can serve as proxies for humans, interspecies variations frequently present formidable challenges in attaining anticipated outcomes during clinical validation and transformation of research findings [81–83]. In this regard, nonhuman primates emerge as a crucial complementary option and a valuable choice. Regarding the ALPPS procedure, nonhuman primates, exhibiting the closest physiological activities and anatomical structures to humans, can be employed to comprehensively investigate the mechanism of ALPPS-induced rapid liver regeneration based on localized microenvironmental or systemic alterations. In addition, they are more amenable to repeated sampling procedures because of their large body size, facilitating the evaluation of the entire liver regeneration process. Therefore, nonhuman primates represent invaluable animal models for investigating the ALPPS procedure. Nonetheless, the nonhuman primate models suffer limitations. In addition to intrinsic financial constraints and ethical considerations associated with nonhuman primate-based experiments, successfully implementing the ALPPS procedure in nonhuman primate models necessitates the involvement of highly experienced liver surgeons. Moreover, the limited availability of nonhuman primate strains, coupled with the intersubject variability, poses significant challenges in establishing a standardized process akin to the well-defined process employed for establishing experimental rodent models for ALPPS. Furthermore, experimentally associated reagents may not be readily accessible. The introduction of pathological factors (e.g., tumors or cirrhosis) into the nonhuman primate models is also impeded. Additionally, while nonhuman primates have been reported to be capable of tolerating hepatectomies involving the resection of up to 60% of the hepatic parenchyma [76], there is a paucity of reports investigating the post-extended hepatectomy volume in nonhuman primates. Therefore, further investigating the liver volumes in nonhuman primates undergoing liver partition in the first-stage ALPPS procedure and hepatectomy in stage 2 ALPPS procedure is imperative for simulating the clinical practice.

21.4 Sheep ALPPS Model

21.4.1 Introduction to Experimental Animals

In the realm of biomedical research, experimental sheep, which are commonly employed in immunological research, are frequently utilized as bioreactors. For instance, experimental sheep can be employed to prepare immune sera comparable to the whole sera from healthy individuals, and their red blood cells constitute primary test materials for the serological complement binding assay. As the assay is extensively performed to aid in diagnosing multiple diseases, experimental sheep represent crucial animal models for both instructional and practical purposes in microbiology and medical experimental testing. Furthermore, experimental sheep are well suited for physiological experiments, experimental surgical interventions, radiological observations of the liver, and surgical training purposes [84–86].

21.4.2 Foundation of Liver Anatomy in Experimental Animal for ALPPS

Compared to other domestic animals, domestic sheep exhibit noticeable similarities to humans with respect to hepatic gross morphology and vascular structure [85]. The sheep liver is not markedly lobulated, and lobulation necessitates the utilization of an anatomical surface landmark. According to the notch for the round ligament, the sheep liver can be demarcated into left and right lobes, situated on the left and right sides of the notch, respectively [87] (Fig. 21.13). Based on the gallbladder fossa, the sheep liver can be further split into the median lobe, situated between the notches for the round ligament. The median lobe can be stratified into the caudate lobe on the dorsal surface and the quadrate lobe on the ventral surface by the porta hepatis. The porta hepatis, through which the portal vein, hepatic artery, and hepatic nerve enter the liver and from which the hepatic duct and lymphatic vessel egress the liver, is situated on the central aspect of the visceral surface of the liver. Upon dissection of the porta hepatis, the bile duct, hepatic artery, and portal vein become discernible. As with the human liver, the sheep liver displays a remarkably analogous anatomical arrangement, wherein the portal vein is situated posteriorly, the common

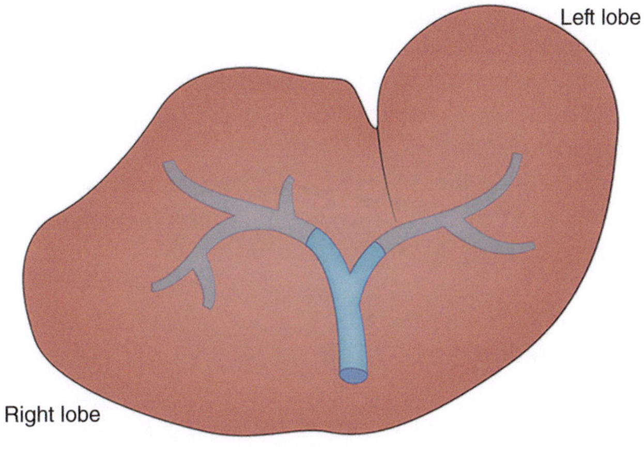

Fig. 21.13 Experimental sheep liver

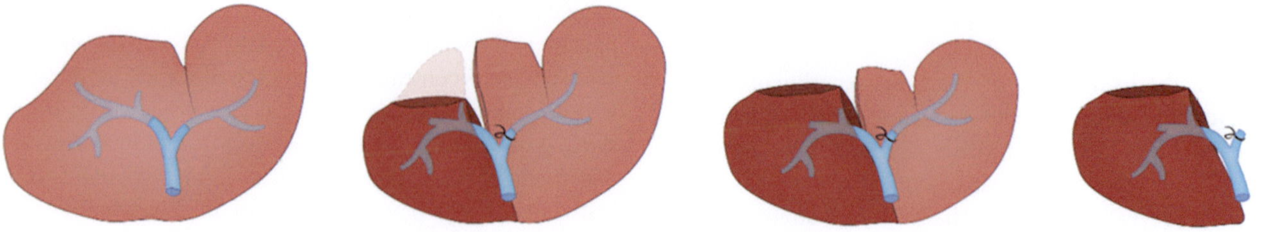

Fig. 21.14 ALPPS procedure in the experimental sheep model

hepatic artery is positioned anteriorly to the left, and the common bile duct is located anteriorly to the right. Typically, the bile duct, common hepatic artery, and portal vein extrahepatically bifurcate. The anatomical similarities between the sheep and human livers render experimental sheep ideal for hepatic surgical training [84] and for replicating the ALPPS procedure in humans. The sheep blood vessels, characterized by a thin-walled structure [88], are susceptible to inadvertent rupture during hepatic parenchymal transection. Furthermore, the staggered arrangement of parenchymal veins renders liver partition challenging.

21.4.3 Operations of the ALPPS Procedure in Experimental Animals

To date, only one experimental sheep model for ALPPS has been reported [66]. In the Budai model, the surgical procedure entailed the ligation of the portal venous branches supplying the median and left lobes, followed by the liver partition along the gallbladder bed. Finally, a small portion of the right lobe was judiciously resected to obtain a FLR volume constituting 20% of the total hepatic volume (Fig. 21.14).

It is noteworthy that sheep, which are ruminants, possess a highly developed digestive system, characterized by numerous organ cavities. Following the consumption and digestion of herbaceous plants, the gaseous byproducts will be generated. This can lead to a significant distension of the rumen, exerting substantial pressure on the adjacent liver and therefore posing significant challenges in dissecting the porta hepatis. Budai et al. [66] indicated the need for preoperative short-term starvation (12–16 h). Furthermore, the rumen can be evacuated by using acupuncture or inserting a stomach tube.

21.4.4 Model Evaluation

The experimental sheep model for ALPPS possesses the advantages and drawbacks inherent to large experimental animal models. Implementing the ALPPS procedure is feasible in experimental sheep [66]. Compared to other experimental animals, experimental sheep exhibit remarkable hepatic structural similarities to humans. Consequently, experimental sheep represent an alternative animal model for systematic research. The physiological relationships in experimental sheep diverge considerably from those in humans, rendering them unsuitable for investigating the mechanism of ALPPS-induced rapid liver regeneration. Nonetheless, experimental sheep demonstrate striking hepatic anatomical similarities to humans, rendering them suitable for preclinical hepatic surgical training on ALPPS.

21.5 Rabbit ALPPS Model

21.5.1 Introduction to Experimental Animals

The experimental rabbits, artificially bred from European wild rabbits (*Oryctolagus cuniculus*), emerge as one of the most ubiquitously utilized animal models in experimental biomedical research. In the realm of hepatic surgery, experimental rabbits are predominantly employed in research concerning portal vein embolization [89, 90] and also in hepatectomy [91]. The major experimental rabbit breeds include New Zealand rabbits, Japanese white rabbits, and Chinese white rabbits.

21.5.2 Foundation of Liver Anatomy in Experimental Animal for ALPPS

The experimental rabbit liver anatomy has been rarely reported. Existing research findings signal that the experimental rabbit liver can be broadly delineated into the left lobe, right lobe, and caudate lobe. Notably, the left lobe exhibits a conspicuous hepatic fissure, which divides the left lobe into the left lateral lobe and the left median lobe [90, 92, 93] (Fig. 21.15). In the human liver, the caudate lobe is intimately fused with its adjacent hepatic lobes, constituting a modest proportion of the total liver volume. In the experi-

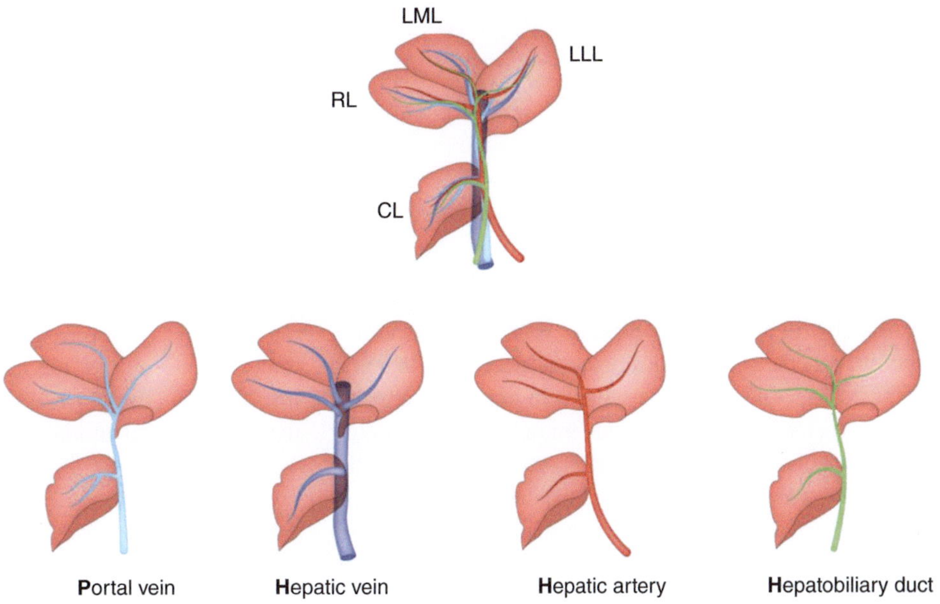

Fig. 21.15 Experimental rabbit liver. LML, left median lobe; LLL, left lateral lobe; CL, caudate lobe; RL, right lobe; light blue, portal vein; deep blue, hepatic vein and inferior vena cava; red, hepatic artery; green, hepatobiliary duct

mental rabbit liver, the caudate lobe is segregated from its adjacent hepatic lobes, comprising a considerable proportion of the total liver volume and frequently becoming twisted or contorted [94]. The portal venous branch supplying the caudate lobe emanates from the original portal vein. The original portal vein continues its course to form the main portal vein, which subsequently gives rise to the right and left portal veins supplying the right and left lobes, respectively. The left portal vein can further bifurcate to feed the left median lobe and the left lateral lobe [95] (Fig. 21.15). The bifurcation patterns and anatomical courses of the hepatic artery and hepatobiliary duct remain essentially consistent with those of the portal venous system [95]. The gallbladder is nestled within the gallbladder fossa, situated in the right lobe.

To mimic the human liver using the experimental rabbit model for ALPPS, the liver partition should be executed on the right lobe and left median lobe only. The right lobe and the left median lobe, interconnected by a broad expanse of contiguous hepatic parenchyma, are well suited for hepatic parenchymal partition. In addition, the hepatic parenchyma is supplied by two portal venous systems (i.e., the right portal vein and the portal venous branch supplying the left median lobe). This anatomical feature can mirror that of the human liver.

21.5.3 Operations of the ALPPS Procedure in Experimental Animals

The first experimental rabbit model for ALPPS was reported by Liao et al. in 2017 [96]. In this model, the left portal vein and portal venous branch supplying the caudate lobe were ligated, followed by liver partition between the right lobe and the left median lobe. The left median lobe and the left lateral lobe, which supplied the left portal vein, contribute 50% of the rabbit liver mass, and the caudate lobe represents 20% of the total rabbit liver volume. So, in their model, the FLR occupied approximately 30% of the total rabbit liver volume. In addition, VX2 is a stable tumor cell line derived from experimental rabbits, which has garnered widespread recognition as a robust platform for establishing xenograft tumor models in rabbits. The rabbit orthotopic VX2 liver cancer model has been proven to be feasible. The tumor-bearing rabbit model for ALPPS has been reported [97], where the tumor was transplanted into the left median lobe and the left portal vein was ligated, with the right lobe and caudate lobe preserved as the FLR.

During model establishment, the portal venous branch supplying the caudate lobe and the left portal vein were ligated, and an ischemic demarcation line emerged at the interface between the left median lobe and the right lobe. Upon delineation, the liver was partitioned along the ischemic demarcation line, extending to the anterior wall of the inferior vena cava (Fig. 21.16). The research team established the model by drawing upon extensive knowledge concerning the clinical classic ALPPS procedure. Specifically, the hepatic parenchyma was transected using a harmonic scalpel. For small blood vessels, hemostasis was achieved via bipolar electrocoagulation. For larger blood vessels, clamping and ligation were used to minimize bleeding to mitigate the risk of an excessive thermal injury. Furthermore, the postoperative transection plane was coated with a hemostatic agent to further control bleeding.

Concerning establishing an experimental rabbit model for ALPPS, the research team recommended (a) positioning the incision line slightly to the right of the ischemic demarcation

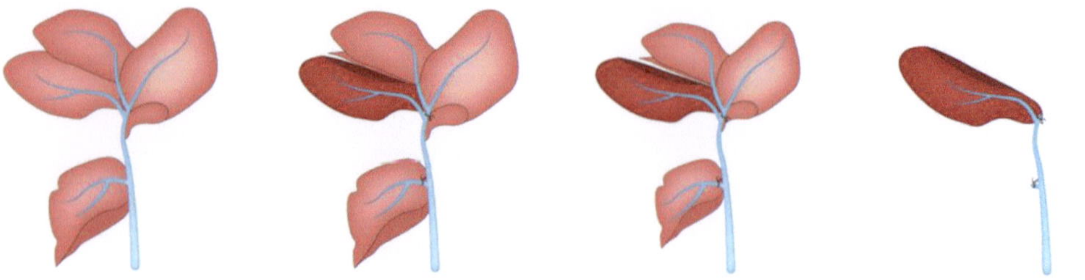

Fig. 21.16 ALPPS procedure in the experimental rabbit model

line, thereby bypassing the hepatic vein; (b) performing intermittent hepatic portal occlusion as necessary to minimize bleeding; (c) ligating the portal vein prior to liver partition to prevent a hepatic ischemia-reperfusion injury associated with intermittent hepatic portal occlusion in the hepatic lobe where the portal vein is slated for ligation; (d) employing an absorbable adhesion barrier between the hepatic transection plan to lessen the risk of adhesion formation.

Olthof et al. reported a comparable experimental rabbit model for ALPPS [98], wherein portal vein embolization and hepatic parenchymal transection were executed. In addition, they indicated that the reported model could replicate the mini-ALPPS procedure [99]. Nonetheless, this model suffers a significant limitation. Specifically, the portal vein embolization was performed along the main portal vein (i.e., embolization of the left and right lobes in the experimental rabbit liver). Thc hepatic parenchymal transection was performed in the left lateral lobe (i.e., hepatic parenchymal transection on the portal vein occlusion side), which deviates from the aforementioned modeling principles, clinical principles for ALPPS, and the mechanism of ALPPS-induced liver regeneration. Consequently, this model cannot serve as an ideal experimental rabbit model for ALPPS.

21.5.4 Model Evaluation

The experimental rabbit model for ALPPS presents multiple advantages. In contrast to large experimental animals (e.g., pigs and sheep), experimental rabbits are more accessible to breed and manipulate, more cost-effective, and more amenable to surgical procedures. Compared with small experimental animals (e.g., rodents), experimental rabbits demonstrate greater amenability to surgical interventions performed by surgeons without microsurgical experience. Nonetheless, the above advantages could be more compelling. For instance, the associated reagents for experimental rabbits are not as readily accessible as those for experimental rodents. While the volume concerning tolerable extended hepatectomy in experimental rabbits remains to be elucidated, experimental rabbits can tolerate portal vein embolization encompassing up to 80% of the portal venous system [98]. In the reported experimental rabbit model for ALPPS, the FLR was approximately 30%; however, whether the post-extended hepatectomy FLR volume has been attained warrants further investigation. Therefore, it is advisable to employ an alternative experimental animal model whenever feasible.

References

1. Martins PN, Neuhaus P. Surgical anatomy of the liver, hepatic vasculature and bile ducts in the rat[J]. Liver Int. 2007;27(3):384–92.
2. de Jong KP, Lont HE, Bijma AM, et al. The effect of partial hepatectomy on tumor growth in rats: *in vivo* and *in vitro* studies[J]. Hepatology. 1995;22(4 Pt 1):1263–72.
3. Rozga J, Jeppsson B, Bengmark S. Portal branch ligation in the rat. Reevaluation of a model[J]. Am J Pathol. 1986;125(2):300–8.
4. Pinto M, Herzberg H, Barnea A, et al. Effects of partial hepatectomy on the immune responses in mice[J]. Clin Immunol Immunopathol. 1987;42(1):123–32.
5. Schlegcl A, Lesurtel M, Melloul E, et al. ALPPS: from human to mice highlighting accelerated and novel mechanisms of liver regeneration[J]. Ann Surg. 2014;260(5):839–46.
6. Martins PNA, Theruvath TP, Neuhaus P. Rodent models of partial hepatectomies[J]. Liver Int. 2008;28(1):3–11.
7. Wei WW, Dirsch O, McLean AL, et al. Rodent models and imaging techniques to study liver regeneration[J]. Eur Surg Res. 2015;54(3–4):97–113.
8. Nikfarjam M, Malcontenti-Wilson C, Fanartzis M, et al. A model of partial hepatectomy in mice[J]. J Investig Surg. 2004;17(5):291–4.
9. Madrahimov N, Dirsch O, Broelsch C, et al. Marginal hepatectomy in the rat: from anatomy to surgery[J]. Ann Surg. 2006;244(1):89–98.
10. Kogure K, Ishizaki M, Nemoto M, et al. A comparative study of the anatomy of rat and human livers[J]. J Hepato-Biliary-Pancreat Surg. 1999;6(2):171–5.
11. Fausto N, Campbell JS, Riehle KJ. Liver regeneration[J]. J Hepatol. 2012;57(3):692–4.
12. Yao LB, Li CH, Ge XL, et al. Establishment of a rat model of portal vein ligation combined with *in situ* splitting[J]. PLoS One. 2014;9(8):e105511.
13. Almau Trenard HM, Moulin LE, Padín JM, et al. Development of an experimental model of portal vein ligation associated with parenchymal transection (ALPPS) in rats[J]. Cir Esp. 2014;92(10):676–81.
14. Dhar DK, Mohammad GH, Vyas S, et al. A novel rat model of liver regeneration: possible role of cytokine induced neutrophil chemoattractant-1 in augmented liver regeneration[J]. Ann Surg Innov Res. 2015;9:11.
15. Kawaguchi D, Hiroshima Y, Kikuchi Y, et al. Associating liver partition and portal vein occlusion, including venous congestion, induction in rats[J]. Anticancer Res. 2017;37(6):2919–25.
16. Schadde E, Hertl M, Breitenstein S, et al. Rat model of the associating liver partition and portal vein ligation for staged hepatectomy (ALPPS) procedure[J]. J Vis Exp. 2017;126:55895.

17. Tong YF, Meng N, Chen MQ, et al. Maturity of associating liver partition and portal vein ligation for staged hepatectomy-derived liver regeneration in a rat model[J]. World J Gastroenterol. 2018;24(10):1107–19.
18. Sheng RF, Wang HQ, Jin KP, et al. Histogram analyses of diffusion kurtosis indices and apparent diffusion coefficient in assessing liver regeneration after ALPPS and a comparative study with portal vein ligation[J]. J Magn Reson Imaging. 2018;47(3):729–36.
19. Budai A, Horváth G, Tretter L, et al. Mitochondrial function after associating liver partition and portal vein ligation for staged hepatectomy in an experimental model[J]. Br J Surg. 2019;106(1):120–31.
20. Colak D, Al-Harazi O, Mustafa OM, et al. RNA-Seq transcriptome profiling in three liver regeneration models in rats: comparative analysis of partial hepatectomy, ALLPS, and PVL[J]. Sci Rep. 2020;10(1):5213.
21. Dirscherl K, Schläpfer M, Roth Z'graggen B, et al. Hypoxia sensing by hepatic stellate cells leads to VEGF-dependent angiogenesis and may contribute to accelerated liver regeneration[J]. Sci Rep. 2020;10(1):4392.
22. Daradics N, Olthof PB, Budai A, et al. The role of farnesoid X receptor in accelerated liver regeneration in rats subjected to ALPPS[J]. Curr Oncol. 2021;28(6):5240–54.
23. Tong YF, Zhu YF, Cai XJ. The origin of newborn hepatocytes in associating liver partition and portal vein ligation for staged hepatectomy (ALPPS)-derived regeneration[J]. Hepatobiliary Surg Nutr. 2020;9(5):687–90.
24. Langiewicz M, Schlegel A, Saponara E, et al. Hedgehog pathway mediates early acceleration of liver regeneration induced by a novel two-staged hepatectomy in mice[J]. J Hepatol. 2017;66(3):560–70.
25. Langiewicz M, Graf R, Humar B, et al. JNK1 induces hedgehog signaling from stellate cells to accelerate liver regeneration in mice[J]. J Hepatol. 2018;69(3):666–75.
26. Borger P, Schneider M, Frick L, et al. Exploration of the transcriptional landscape of ALPPS reveals the pathways of accelerated liver regeneration[J]. Front Oncol. 2019;9:1206.
27. Zhao L, Dai CL, Gong Q. Changes of Endocan and its effect on hepatic stem cells during the rapid proliferation process of residual liver after ALPPS procedure[J]. Cell Biochem Funct. 2020;38(6):817–25.
28. Shi HW, Yang GC, Zheng TS, et al. A preliminary study of ALPPS procedure in a rat model[J]. Sci Rep. 2015;5:17567.
29. Dili A, Lebrun V, Bertrand C, et al. Associating liver partition and portal vein ligation for staged hepatectomy: establishment of an animal model with insufficient liver remnant[J]. Lab Investig. 2019;99(5):698–707.
30. Dili A, Bertrand C, Lebrun V, et al. Hypoxia protects the liver from Small For Size Syndrome: a lesson learned from the associated liver partition and portal vein ligation for staged hepatectomy (ALPPS) procedure in rats[J]. Am J Transplant. 2019;19(11):2979–90.
31. Wei WW, Zhang TJ, Zafarnia S, et al. Establishment of a rat model: associating liver partition with portal vein ligation for staged hepatectomy[J]. Surgery. 2016;159(5):1299–307.
32. García-Pérez R, Revilla-Nuin B, Martínez CM, et al. Associated liver partition and portal vein ligation (ALPPS) vs selective portal vein ligation (PVL) for staged hepatectomy in a rat model similar regenerative response?[J]. PLoS One. 2015;10(12):e0144096.
33. Zhang B, Meng FZ, Liu Y, et al. Inhibition of TGFβ1 accelerates regeneration of fibrotic rat liver elicited by a novel two-staged hepatectomy[J]. Theranostics. 2021;11(10):4743–58.
34. Andersen KJ, Knudsen AR, Jepsen BN, et al. A new technique for accelerated liver regeneration: an experimental study in rats[J]. Surgery. 2017;162(2):233–47.
35. Zhang WK, Zhu XW, Tang Y, et al. Kupffer cells depletion alters cytokine expression and delays liver regeneration after Radiofrequency-assisted Liver Partition with Portal Vein Ligation[J]. Mol Immunol. 2022;144:71–7.
36. Kambakamba P, Linecker M, Schneider M, et al. Impact of associating liver partition and portal vein ligation for staged hepatectomy (ALPPS) on growth of colorectal liver metastases[J]. Surgery. 2018;163(2):311–7.
37. García-Pérez R, Ferrer Fábrega J, Varona-Bosque A, et al. Role of Kupffer cells in the progression of CRC liver metastases after the first stage of ALPPS[J]. Sci Rep. 2018;8(1):8089.
38. Zhao JW, Xu HY, Li Y, et al. NAFLD induction delays postoperative liver regeneration of ALPPS in rats[J]. Dig Dis Sci. 2019;64(2):456–68.
39. Tong YF, Xu M, Wang YF, et al. Hepatic regeneration by associating liver partition and portal vein ligation for staged hepatectomy (ALPPS) is feasible but attenuated in rat liver with thioacetamide-induced fibrosis[J]. Surgery. 2019;165(2):345–52.
40. Yang XW, Yang C, Qiu YW, et al. A preliminary study of associating liver partition and portal vein ligation for staged hepatectomy in a rat model of liver cirrhosis[J]. Exp Ther Med. 2019;18(2):1203–11.
41. Zhao JW, Zhao WY, Xu HY, et al. Corosolic acid inhibits tumour growth without compromising associating liver partition and portal vein ligation-induced liver regeneration in rats[J]. Ann Med. 2022;54(1):1188–201.
42. Shi JH, Hammarström C, Grzyb K, et al. Experimental evaluation of liver regeneration patterns and liver function following ALPPS[J]. BJS Open. 2017;1(3):84–96.
43. Song GS, Sharma AD, Roll GR, et al. MicroRNAs control hepatocyte proliferation during liver regeneration[J]. Hepatology. 2010;51(5):1735–43.
44. Coban Z, Barton MC. Integrative genomics: liver regeneration and hepatocellular carcinoma[J]. J Cell Biochem. 2012;113(7):2179–84.
45. Mao SA, Glorioso JM, Nyberg SL. Liver regeneration[J]. Transl Res. 2014;163(4):352–62.
46. Bustad LK, McClellan RO. Swine in biomedical research[J]. Science. 1966;152(3728):1526–30.
47. Groenen MA, Archibald AL, Uenishi H, et al. Analyses of pig genomes provide insight into porcine demography and evolution[J]. Nature. 2012;491(7424):393–8.
48. Lossi L, D'Angelo L, De Girolamo P, et al. Anatomical features for an adequate choice of experimental animal model in biomedicine: II small laboratory rodents, rabbit, and pig[J]. Ann Anat. 2016;204:11–28.
49. Okada N, Mizuta K, Oshima M, et al. A novel split liver protocol using the subnormothermic oxygenated circuit system in a porcine model of a marginal donor procedure[J]. Transplant Proc. 2015;47(2):419–26.
50. Vogel T, Brockmann JG, Pigott D, et al. Successful transplantation of porcine liver grafts following 48-hour normothermic preservation[J]. PLoS One. 2017;12(11):e0188494.
51. Mylonas AI, Orfanos NF, Karmaniolou II, et al. The effects of hemorrhagic shock secondary to hepatectomy in a swine model[J]. J Surg Res. 2015;195(1):228–34.
52. Liska V, Treska V, Mirka H, et al. Tumour necrosis factor-alpha stimulates liver regeneration in porcine model of partial portal vein ligation[J]. Hepato-Gastroenterology. 2012;59(114):496–500.
53. Darnis B, Mohkam K, Schmitt Z, et al. Subtotal hepatectomy in swine for studying small-for-size syndrome and portal inflow modulation: is it reliable?[J]. HPB. 2015;17(10):881–8.
54. Pagano D, di Francesco F, Echeverri GJ, et al. Development of a standardized model for liver failure in pigs: anatomopathophysiologic findings after extended liver resection[J]. Transplant Proc. 2012;44(7):2029–32.
55. Bekheit M, Bucur PO, Wartenberg M, et al. Computerized tomography-based anatomic description of the porcine liver[J]. J Surg Res. 2017;210:223–30.
56. Junatas KL, Tonar Z, Kubíková T, et al. Stereological analysis of size and density of hepatocytes in the porcine liver[J]. J Anat. 2017;230(4):575–88.
57. Witter K, Tonar Z, Schöpper H. How many layers has the adventitia — structure of the arterial *Tunica externa* revisited[J]. Anat Histol Embryol. 2017;46(2):110–20.

58. Couinaud C. Liver lobes and segments: notes on the anatomical architecture and surgery of the liver[J]. Presse Med (1893). 1954;62(33):709–12.
59. Martins AC, Machado MAC, Ferraz AAB. Porcine liver: experimental model for the intra-hepatic glissonian approach[J]. Acta Cir Bras. 2008;23(2):204–7.
60. Court FG, Wemyss-Holden SA, Morrison CP, et al. Segmental nature of the porcine liver and its potential as a model for experimental partial hepatectomy[J]. Br J Surg. 2003;90(4):440–4.
61. Ntonas A, Katsourakis A, Galanis N, et al. Comparative anatomical study between the human and swine liver and its importance in xenotransplantation[J]. Cureus. 2020;12(7):e9411.
62. Kelly DM, Demetris AJ, Fung JJ, et al. Porcine partial liver transplantation: a novel model of the "small-for-size" liver graft[J]. Liver Transpl. 2004;10(2):253–63.
63. Croome KP, Mao SA, Glorioso JM, et al. Characterization of a porcine model for associating liver partition and portal vein ligation for a staged hepatectomy[J]. HPB (Oxford). 2015;17(12):1130–6.
64. Court FG, Laws PE, Morrison CP, et al. Subtotal hepatectomy: a porcine model for the study of liver regeneration[J]. J Surg Res. 2004;116(1):181–6.
65. Deal R, Frederiks C, Williams L, et al. Rapid liver hypertrophy after portal vein occlusion correlates with the degree of collateralization between lobes-a study in pigs[J]. J Gastrointest Surg. 2018;22(2):203–13.
66. Budai A, Fulop A, Hahn O, et al. Animal models for associating liver partition and portal vein ligation for staged hepatectomy (ALPPS): achievements and future perspectives[J]. Eur Surg Res. 2017;58(3–4):140–57.
67. Tuñón MJ, Alvarez M, Culebras JM, et al. An overview of animal models for investigating the pathogenesis and therapeutic strategies in acute hepatic failure[J]. World J Gastroenterol. 2009;15(25):3086–98.
68. Burwitz BJ, Zhou ZM, Li WH. Animal models for the study of human hepatitis B and D virus infection: new insights and progress[J]. Antivir Res. 2020;182:104898.
69. Thomas E, Liang TJ. Experimental models of hepatitis B and C—new insights and progress[J]. Nat Rev Gastroenterol Hepatol. 2016;13(6):362–74.
70. Wijaya RS, Read SA, Truong NR, et al. HBV vaccination and HBV infection induces HBV-specific natural killer cell memory[J]. Gut. 2021;70(2):357–69.
71. Cross-Najafi AA, Lopez K, Isidan A, et al. Current barriers to clinical liver xenotransplantation[J]. Front Immunol. 2022;13:827535.
72. Zhang XJ, Cheng X, Yan ZZ, et al. An ALOX12-12-HETE-GPR31 signaling axis is a key mediator of hepatic ischemia-reperfusion injury[J]. Nat Med. 2018;24(1):73–83.
73. Sheppard FR, Macko A, Fryer DM, et al. Development of a nonhuman primate (*Rhesus macaque*) model of uncontrolled traumatic liver hemorrhage[J]. Shock. 2015;44(Suppl 1):114–22.
74. Crossland RF, Mitchell A, Macko AR, et al. Rapid assessment of shock in a nonhuman primate model of uncontrolled hemorrhage: association of traditional and nontraditional vital signs to mortality risk[J]. J Trauma Acute Care Surg. 2016;80(4):610–6.
75. Gaglio PJ, Liu HF, Dash S, et al. Liver regeneration investigated in a non-human primate model (*Macaca mulatta*)[J]. J Hepatol. 2002;37(5):625–32.
76. Gaglio PJ, Baskin G, Bohm R Jr, et al. Partial hepatectomy and laparoscopic-guided liver biopsy in rhesus macaques (*Macaca mulatta*): novel approach for study of liver regeneration[J]. Comp Med. 2000;50(4):363–8.
77. Talcott MR, Dysko RC. Partial lobectomy *via* a ligature fracture technique: a method for multiple hepatic biopsies in nonhuman primates[J]. Lab Anim Sci. 1991;41(5):476–80.
78. Houssin D, Vigouroux C, Filipponi F, et al. One liver for two: an experimental study in Primates[J]. Transpl Int. 1988;1(4):201–4.
79. Vons C, Beaudoin S, Helmy N, et al. First description of the surgical anatomy of the cynomolgus monkey liver[J]. Am J Primatol. 2009;71(5):400–8.
80. Deshpande RR, Heaton ND, Rela M. Surgical anatomy of segmental liver transplantation[J]. Br J Surg. 2002;89(9):1078–88.
81. Zhang WH, Aida T, del Rosario RCH, et al. Multiplex precise base editing in cynomolgus monkeys[J]. Nat Commun. 2020;11(1):2325.
82. Seok J, Warren HS, Cuenca AG, et al. Genomic responses in mouse models poorly mimic human inflammatory diseases[J]. Proc Natl Acad Sci USA. 2013;110(9):3507–12.
83. Gundersen Y, Vaagenes P, Thrane I, et al. Response of circulating immune cells to major gunshot injury, haemorrhage, and acute surgery[J]. Injury. 2005;36(8):949–55.
84. Lang H, Junge A, Sitter H, et al. Experimental investigation of intraoperative ultrasound in anatomically precise liver resection[J]. J Investig Surg. 1995;8(4):253–61.
85. Teh SH, Hunter JG, Sheppard BC. A suitable animal model for laparoscopic hepatic resection training[J]. Surg Endosc. 2007;21(10):1738–44.
86. Stieger-Vanegas SM, McKenzie E. Abdominal imaging in small ruminants: liver, spleen, gastrointestinal tract, and lymph nodes[J]. Vet Clin North Am Food Anim Pract. 2021;37(1):55–74.
87. Douart C, Briand L, Betti E, et al. Temporal evolution of hepatic anatomy during gestation and growth in the sheep[J]. Anat Histol Embryol. 2015;44(1):22–36.
88. Kandeel A, Omar M, Mekkawy N, et al. Anatomical and ultrasonographic study of the stomach and liver in sheep and goats[J]. Iraqi J Vet Sci. 2009;23(Suppl II):181–91.
89. van den Esschert JW, van Lienden KP, de Graaf W, et al. Portal vein embolization induces more liver regeneration than portal vein ligation in a standardized rabbit model[J]. Surgery. 2011;149(3):378–85.
90. van den Esschert JW, van Lienden KP, Alles LK, et al. Liver regeneration after portal vein embolization using absorbable and permanent embolization materials in a rabbit model[J]. Ann Surg. 2012;255(2):311–8.
91. Fleig WE, Lehmann H, Wagner H, et al. Hepatic regenerative stimulator substance in the rabbit. Relation to liver regeneration after partial hepatectomy[J]. J Hepatol. 1986;3(1):19–26.
92. Urayama M, Ishiyama S, Kuzumaki T, et al. Change of liver function in hypertrophying lobe of rabbit liver after portal branch ligation[J]. J Surg Res. 1999;86(1):55–61.
93. Sakai Y, Ishiyama S, Tsukamoto M, et al. Effects of preoperative transcatheter portal embolization (TPE) on prevention of hepatic failure after massive hepatectomy[J]. Nihon Geka Gakkai Zasshi. 1992;93(7):716–22.
94. Weisbroth SH. Torsion of the caudate lobe of the liver in the domestic rabbit (*Oryctolagus*)[J]. Vet Pathol. 1975;12(1):13–5.
95. Seo TS, Oh JH, Lee DH, et al. Radiologic anatomy of the rabbit liver on hepatic venography, arteriography, portography, and cholangiography[J]. Investig Radiol. 2001;36(3):186–92.
96. Liao MH, Zhang T, Wang HC, et al. Rabbit model provides new insights in liver regeneration after transection with portal vein ligation[J]. J Surg Res. 2017;209:242–51.
97. Wang RF, Quan Z, Zheng TS, et al. Pathophysiological mechanisms of ALPPS: experimental model[J]. Br J Surg. 2022;109(6):510–9.
98. Olthof PB, Schadde E, van Lienden KP, et al. Hepatic parenchymal transection increases liver volume but not function after portal vein embolization in rabbits[J]. Surgery. 2017;162(4):732–41.
99. de Santibañes E, Alvarez FA, Ardiles V, et al. Inverting the ALPPS paradigm by minimizing first stage impact: the Mini-ALPPS technique[J]. Langenbeck's Arch Surg. 2016;401(4):557–63.

22 Mechanism of ALPPS

Xinrong Yang and Jiayan Yan

The liver is one of the most essential organs in the human body and the only organ with a capacity for regeneration. In homeostasis, most hepatocytes are in a highly differentiated state with weak proliferative capacity. In recent years, studies have shown that apart from factors such as partial hepatectomy, liver injuries, or liver transplantation, ALPPS can also enhance rapid liver regeneration, enabling the future liver remnant (FLR) to regenerate rapidly to its primary weight and volume to maintain the optimal liver weight-to-body weight ratio in the body [1–3]. Currently, the mechanisms underlying liver regeneration induced by ALPPS surgery are not fully understood, and this chapter will introduce its mechanisms and characteristics by combining other liver regeneration methods for comparison.

22.1 Pathophysiological Characteristics of Liver Regeneration

22.1.1 Models and Processes of Liver Regeneration

The liver possesses a robust regenerative capacity. Partial hepatectomy, liver injuries caused by chemical or biological factors, and bile duct ligation, among others, can stimulate liver regeneration to compensate for lost or functionally impaired liver tissue, ultimately restoring liver biological function. Liver regeneration involves a series of physiological and biochemical activities, including cell activation, dedifferentiation, cell proliferation and regulation, redifferentiation, and reconstruction of tissue structure and function [2, 3]. Microscopically, liver regeneration manifests as the proliferation of hepatocytes and cholangiocytes, accompanied by changes in the immune microenvironment within the liver tissue [2]. The liver regeneration process is artificially divided into three basic stages: initiation, proliferation, and termination [4]. Various cytokines and growth factors in the body regulate liver regeneration through different mechanisms. Tumor necrosis factor-alpha (TNF-α) and interleukin-6 (IL-6) can activate hepatocytes in the G0 phase, allowing them to enter the cell cycle under the influence of hepatocyte growth factor (HGF) and transforming growth factor-alpha (TGF-α). At the same time, the cyclin-dependent kinase (CDK) system stimulates hepatocytes into the DNA synthesis phase (S-phase). Apoptosis and transforming growth factor-beta (TGF-β) are involved in the termination of the regeneration process [4].

22.1.2 Basic Characteristics of ALPPS-Induced Liver Regeneration

ALPPS actively induces rapid regeneration of the target liver segment through the first stage of surgery, leading to a volume increase of 57–68% within 1–2 weeks to obtain an opportunity for surgery, which differs from traditional liver regeneration patterns [5, 6]. The critical feature of ALPPS is its rapid rate for induction of liver regeneration, with an FLR increase of 61–93% within 9–14 days, resulting in an average daily liver volume growth of 32 mL [7]. Similar to other liver regeneration models like partial hepatectomy, during the initial phase of ALPPS-induced liver regeneration (4 hours afterward), pathways involved in cell cycle, the HGF pathway, hypoxia pathways related to epithelial-mesenchymal transition, and interleukin-10 (IL-10) pathway are significantly upregulated [8]. Four hours after ALPPS, specific signaling pathways, including the insulin-like growth factor 1 receptor (IGF1R) signaling pathway (cell survival), integrin-linked kinase (ILK)

X. Yang (✉) · J. Yan
Zhongshan Hospital, Fudan University, Shanghai, China
e-mail: yang.xinrong@zs-hospital.sh.cn

J. Zhou (ed.), *Associating Liver Partition and Portal Vein Ligation for Staged Hepatectomy (ALPPS)*,
https://doi.org/10.1007/978-981-96-7364-3_22

signaling pathway (induced cell proliferation), and IL-10 pathway, are upregulated, while specific downregulated signaling pathways include interferon signaling pathway [8]. During the proliferation phase of ALPPS-induced liver regeneration (96 hours afterward), pathways related to cell proliferation, cell cycling, mitosis, and cell division were activated. At the same time, pathways involved in macrophage activation, ion transport, immune response, and lipid metabolism processes are significantly upregulated [9].

22.2 Pathophysiological Changes in Rapid Liver Regeneration Induced by ALPPS

22.2.1 Hemodynamic Changes After ALPPS Surgery

The main steps of ALPPS include portal vein ligation of the demoralized lobe (DL) and the liver partition of FLR and DL, which block the blood flow circulation between FLR and DL. ALPPS leads to dramatic changes in liver hemodynamics. Clinical observational studies have shown that after the first stage of ALPPS, the total portal vein blood flow of FLR sharply increases to 2.6 times the preoperative level. Subsequently, the portal vein blood flow gradually decreases, and by the second stage of ALPPS, it remains slightly higher than the preoperative level [10]. With the increase in portal vein blood flow and the decrease in hepatic artery blood flow in FLR, as well as the cutoff of portal vein blood flow and a significant increase in hepatic artery blood flow in DL, a hypoxic microenvironment is created in DL [11, 12]. Moreover, after the first stage of ALPPS, there is a positive correlation between portal vein blood flow and the volume growth of FLR [13].

It is believed that portal vein blood flow is one of the key factors influencing liver regeneration. Research based on extracorporeal cross-circulation indicates that liver regeneration results from the imbalance between portal vein blood flow factors and the number of residual hepatocytes [14]. ALPPS induces liver regeneration faster than portal vein ligation (PVL) or portal vein embolization (PVE), possibly because it divides the liver tissue between FLR and DL, disrupting the blood flow circulation between the two sides of the liver. Studies using a pig ALPPS model have shown that the speed of liver regeneration induced by ALPPS is inversely correlated with the number of collateral circulations between FLR and DL after portal vein ligation [15].

22.2.2 Pathophysiological Characteristics of ALPPS-Induced Liver Regeneration

22.2.2.1 Proliferation of Hepatocyte Induced by ALPPS

The most fundamental manifestation of liver regeneration is the increased number of hepatocytes. Various modes of inducing liver regeneration, such as partial hepatectomy, liver injury, and bile duct ligation, can lead to mitosis and increased numbers of hepatocytes, cholangiocytes, and immune cells, thereby resulting in liver volume growth. Recent studies using lineage tracing systems have shown that unlike hepatocyte proliferation in normal liver homeostasis and induced by bile duct ligation, which mainly occurs in the liver lobuleII zone (middle zone), hepatocyte proliferation induced by partial hepatectomy primarily occurs in the liver lobule I zone (portal triad zone) and II zone [16, 17]. ALPPS can induce a rapid increase in the volume of FLR [18, 19]. Pathological staining observations from our center further indicate that ALPPS-induced liver regeneration predominantly involves significant proliferation and increased numbers of cells in FLR, including hepatocytes and cholangiocytes (Fig. 22.1).

Dynamic studies based on rat ALPPS models in our center show an increase in hepatocyte volume in the early stages after first-stage ALPPS (1–2 days). The peak of hepatocyte proliferation occurs around 2 days after ALPPS. Subsequently, due to significant hepatocyte division, hepatocyte volume significantly decreases and gradually returns to pre-ALPPS levels. By 7 days after ALPPS, hepatocytes have mostly returned to a resting state. Furthermore, cholangiocyte proliferation slightly lags behind the peak of hepatocyte proliferation (Fig. 22.2).

22.2.2.2 Cell Maturity in ALPPS-Induced Liver Regeneration

Although ALPPS induces liver regeneration faster than PVE, the proliferating hepatocytes and cholangiocytes are relatively immature. Studies have shown that the proliferating hepatocytes induced by ALPPS exhibit characteristics of immaturity, with higher cell density, smaller volume, and glycogen enrichment [19–21]. Additionally, research has found downregulated expression of the multidrug resistance gene (MDR1) expression, incomplete development of bile canaliculi, and leaky tight junctions in FLR after ALPPS, indicating deficient bile canalicular-ductule networks and immaturity of the bile secretion system in FLR after ALPPS [20]. Comparison of transmission electron microscopy imaging of FLR after the first and second stages of ALPPS in our

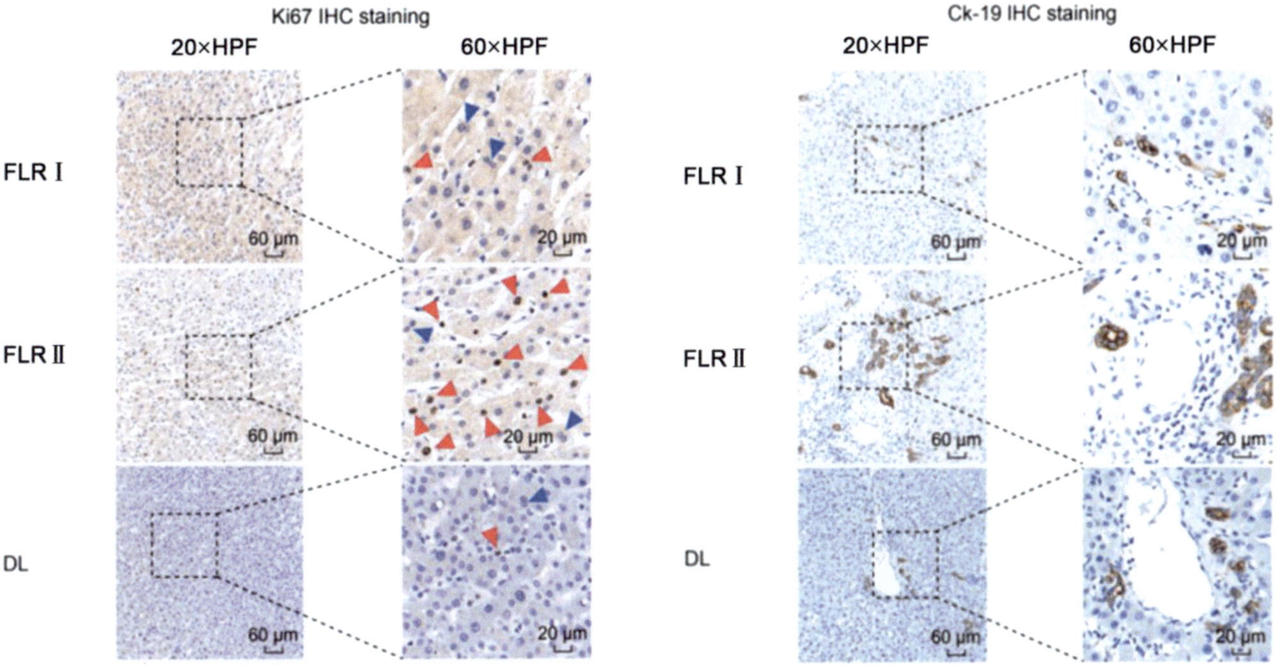

Fig. 22.1 Comparison of the number of proliferating hepatocytes and bile ducts before and after ALPPS surgery in humans

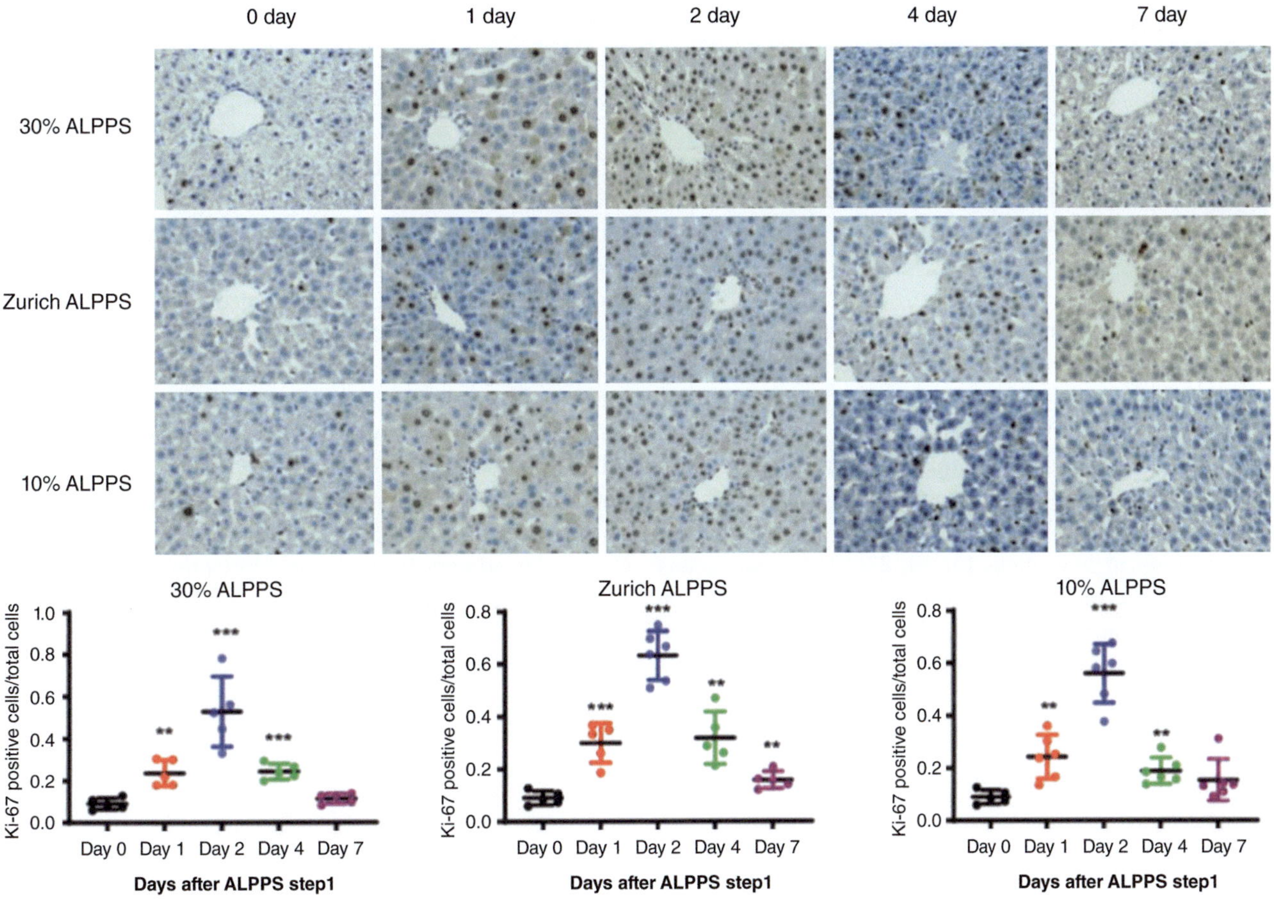

Fig. 22.2 Hepatocytes proliferation at different time points in three rat ALPPS models (Ki67 immunohistochemistry)

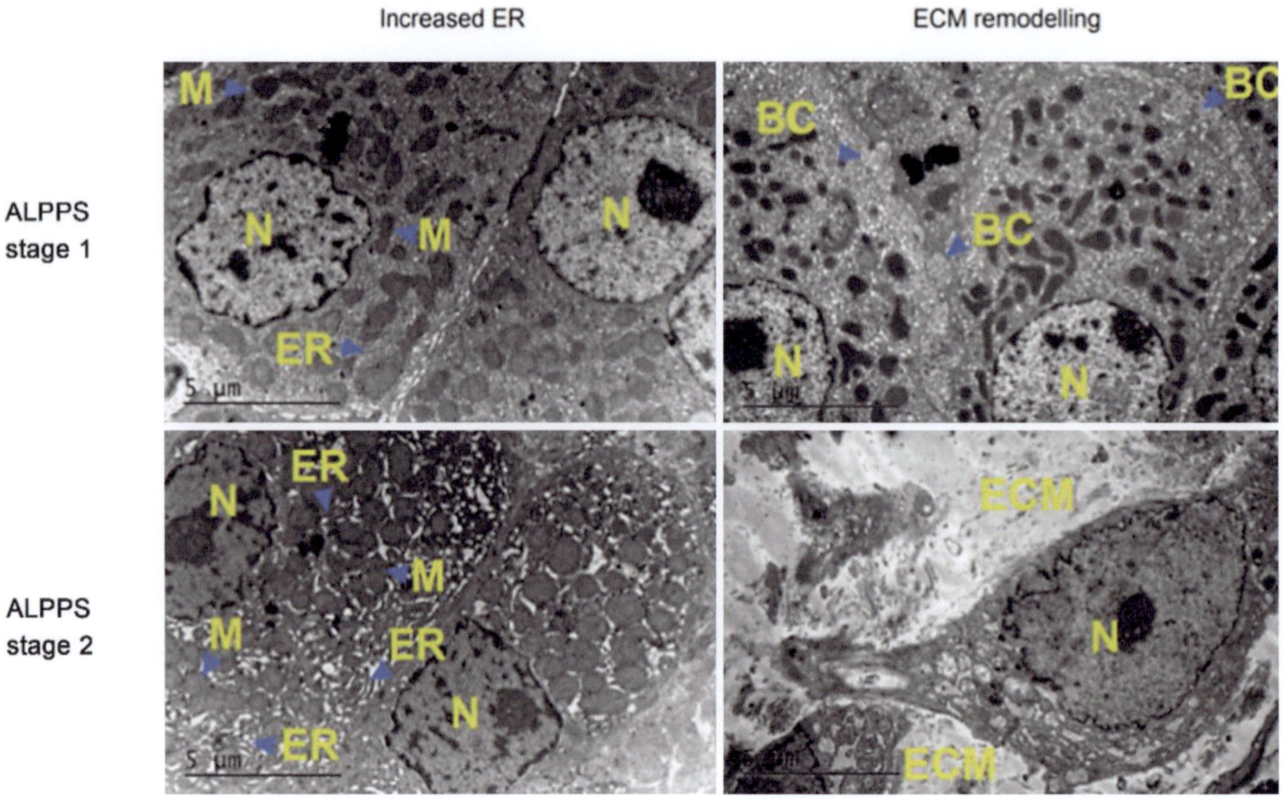

Fig. 22.3 Transmission electron microscopy images of FLR before and after ALPPS surgery in humans. M, mitochondria; N, nucleus; ER, endoplasmic reticulum; BC, bile canaliculi; ECM, extracellular matrix

center revealed distinct features of endoplasmic reticulum increase and extracellular matrix remodeling in FLR in the second stage of ALPPS (Fig. 22.3).

22.2.3 Clinical Factors Affecting Liver Regeneration During ALPPS Procedures

During the ALPPS procedure, there is still a certain rate of operation failure (4.0–8.9%), mainly related to the rate, extent, and function of liver regeneration, making it necessary to further optimize the surgical procedures and strict adherence to surgical indications [5, 10, 22]. The main factors influencing the rate of ALPPS-induced liver regeneration include age (over 60 years), degree of liver fibrosis or cirrhosis, and the presence of non-colorectal cancer liver metastases [23]. Primary liver cancer patients usually have a slower rate of liver growth due to concomitant cirrhosis compared to those without cirrhosis [5]. Studies in our center [5] have shown a significant negative correlation between the volume growth of FLR in ALPPS and the degree of liver fibrosis, with the time required to induce sufficient liver volume positively correlating to the degree of liver fibrosis (Fig. 22.4). Further mechanistic research suggests that blocking TGF-β1 can significantly accelerate the liver regeneration rate induced by ALPPS in livers with fibrosis [24, 25]. Studies indicate that patients with non-colorectal cancer liver metastases who undergo ALPPS have a poorer prognosis compared with those with primary liver cancer. Most primary liver tumor patients have underlying conditions, such as cholestasis or cirrhosis, leading to a slower rate of liver growth that may not meet the requirements for surgical resection [23].

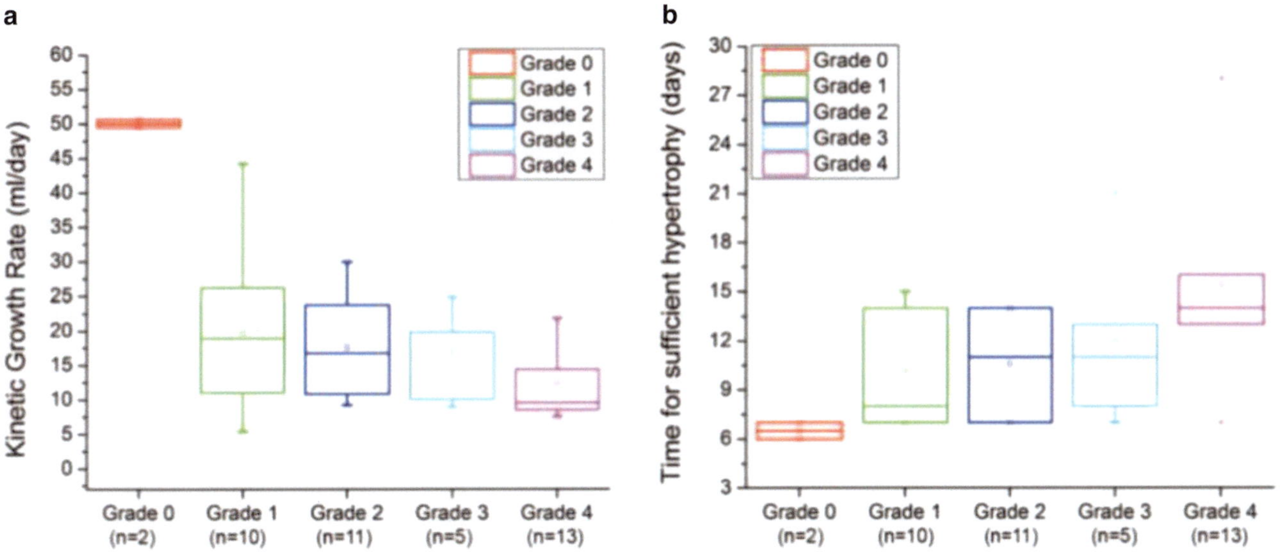

Fig. 22.4 Correlation between the volume increase of the contralateral liver and the degree of liver fibrosis in ALPPS. (This figure is reprinted with permission from the source of [5])

22.3 Molecular Mechanisms Related to ALPPS-Induced Rapid Liver Regeneration

22.3.1 Cytokines and Growth Factors in the Circulatory System

Liver regeneration is a complex physiological process involving interacting with different cells and releasing multiple cytokines and growth factors. During liver regeneration, the molecules involved in the regeneration of liver cell populations mainly include cytokines, growth factors, and related metabolic molecules [26]. Previous studies have shown that in the initiation phase of liver regeneration, factors such as tumor necrosis factor (TNF), IL-6, stem cell factor (SCF), and complement components C3a or C5a are involved [27–29]. Subsequently, the release of growth factors such as hepatocyte growth factor (HGF) and ligands of the epidermal growth factor receptor (EGFR) family drives the cell cycle process, promoting hepatocytes to enter into the G1 phase from the G0 phase [30, 31]. The metabolic demand increases during hepatocyte proliferation, and the application of branched-chain amino acids can promote hepatocyte proliferation [32].

Research indicates that the significant hemodynamic changes in the liver and the directly induced systemic inflammatory response following the first stage of ALPPS are the initiating factors for rapid liver regeneration [33]. Although the blood flow in the main portal vein decreases after the first stage of ALPPS, the blood flow and pressure in the portal vein of the remnant liver significantly increase, carrying more nutrients from the intestine to FLR, thereby promoting liver regeneration [34–37]. Studies combining liver specimens from ALPPS patients and animal models have shown that levels of cytokines and growth factors, such as IL-6, TNF, HGF, VEGF (vascular endothelial growth factor), and EGF (epidermal growth factor), are significantly elevated in FLR following ALPPS. Additionally, serum levels of factors such as IL-6 and HGF increase transiently [8, 9, 38, 39]. Serum factor analysis in ALPPS patients reveals that IL-6 levels are elevated significantly after the first stage of ALPPS and drop rapidly after the second stage; HGF levels increase significantly after the first stage, with the extent of increase correlating positively with the rate of liver growth [38]. In rat ALPPS model studies, cytokine microarray analysis of FLR also revealed that in the early stages of ALPPS (within 24 hours), the expression of cytokines such as CINC-1 (cytokine-induced neutrophil chemoattractant-1), IL-6, IL-2, IL-13, and MIP-1α (macrophage inflammatory protein-1α) in FLR significantly increased [38].

Another study indicates that the liver regeneration rate for ALPPS is similar to that of PVL and ablation-induced injury in other organs. The researchers suggested that the faster regeneration rate observed in ALPPS compared to PVL might be attributed to the additional surgical injury, which can also enhance liver regeneration by inducing injury in other organs [18]. Further research has shown that within the first few hours following ALPPS, the expression and secretion of Hedgehog molecules in hepatic stellate cells play a significant role in promoting rapid liver regeneration [40].

22.3.2 The Impact of Local Immune Inflammatory Microenvironment on Liver Regeneration

Accumulating evidence suggests that the liver is also a vital immune organ, and changes in its local immune microenvironment play an essential role in liver regeneration [37, 41, 42]. For example, in the context of partial hepatectomy, cell clusters such as macrophages, natural killer (NK) cells, natural killer T (NKT) cells, and dendritic cells (DCs) influence the liver regeneration process either directly by affecting hepatocytes or indirectly by releasing inflammatory factors [42]. The proliferation of CD68-positive Kupffer cells and the infiltration of CD11b-positive monocytes from the blood together form the F4/80^{+} Kupffer cell population. These cells influence hepatocytes through the production of mitogens such as macrophage-colony stimulating factor (M-CSF, derived from hepatic stellate cells) and granulocyte-macrophage colony-stimulating factor (GM-CSF), or producing IL-6, TNF, TGF-β1, and TNF-α via paracrine pathways, thereby affecting the liver regeneration process [4, 43–45].

Additionally, unlike partial hepatectomy or liver injury-induced regeneration, ALPPS can induce a hypoxic microenvironment in FLR, playing an essential role in promoting liver angiogenesis [8, 46, 47]. Clinical and animal model studies have shown that ALPPS induces liver regeneration faster than PVL. Further studies based on the ALPPS rat model have demonstrated that compared to PVL, the hypoxic state of the FLR is more aggravated. The hypoxic microenvironment in the remnant liver can significantly activate the VEGF-dependent angiogenesis pathway in hepatic stellate cells. In vivo use of hypoxia-inducing agents, such as dimethyloxalylglycine (DMOG), to maintain the stability of endogenous hypoxia-inducible factor α (HIF-α) molecules can significantly increase the rate of liver regeneration induced by PVL [46–48].

The liver regeneration process induced by ALPPS is a complex pathophysiological process involving the participation and interaction of parenchymal and non-parenchymal cells. Hepatocytes constitute approximately 60–80% of all liver cell populations, while non-parenchymal cells include endothelial cells, bile duct epithelial cells, and stellate cells, and approximately half of the non-parenchymal cell population are immune cells [42]. The activation of immune cells and the secretion of growth factors such as HGF and inflammatory factors like IL-6 play critical roles in the proliferation of liver cell subpopulations, including hepatocytes and cholangiocytes. Currently, there is a lack of comprehensive illustration of the dynamic changes in immune cells before and after ALPPS and their roles in liver regeneration, which requires further exploration. Emerging technologies such as single-cell RNA sequencing, spatial transcriptome sequencing, and multiplex immunofluorescence will provide new perspectives on the changes and roles of the immune microenvironment in liver regeneration induced by ALPPS.

22.4 Outlook

The rapid liver regeneration induced by ALPPS is a scientific phenomenon rooted in clinical practice. However, the exploration of the changes in the immune microenvironment and molecular mechanisms underlying ALPPS-induced rapid liver regeneration is yet to be comprehensive with systematic knowledge. High-throughput multi-omics technologies, including spatial transcriptomics, can provide detailed information and novel research perspectives on cellular component changes, spatial distribution, pathway regulation at the single-cell level, and tissue spatial transcription levels in the study of ALPPS-induced rapid liver regeneration. By exploring the mechanisms of ALPPS-induced rapid liver regeneration, the discovery of key cellular components and factors involved in the process are expected to be identified. If these key cellular components or factors can be successfully translated into clinical applications, it could further improve the success ratio and efficacy of ALPPS. Meanwhile, uncovering the mechanisms related to ALPPS-enhanced liver regeneration can provide new research directions for preventing and treating impaired liver function after routine partial hepatectomy, as well as offering novel ideals for the regeneration of hepatocytes and recovery of liver function in cases of acute liver injury [49].

References

1. Chan KS, Low JK, Shelat VG. Associated liver partition and portal vein ligation for staged hepatectomy: a review[J]. Transl Gastroenterol Hepatol. 2020;5:37.
2. Michalopoulos GK, Bhushan B. Liver regeneration: biological and pathological mechanisms and implications[J]. Nat Rev Gastroenterol Hepatol. 2021;18(1):40–55.
3. Forbes SJ, Newsome PN. Liver regeneration—mechanisms and models to clinical application[J]. Nat Rev Gastroenterol Hepatol. 2016;13(8):473–85.
4. Michalopoulos G. Liver regeneration[J]. J Cell Physiol. 2007;213(2):286–300.
5. Wang Z, Peng YF, Hu JW, et al. Associating liver partition and portal vein ligation for staged hepatectomy for unresectable hepatitis B virus-related hepatocellular carcinoma: a single center study of 45 patients[J]. Ann Surg. 2020;271(3):534–41.
6. Sandström P, Røsok BI, Sparrelid E, et al. ALPPS improves resectability compared with conventional two-stage hepatectomy in patients with advanced colorectal liver metastasis: results from a Scandinavian multicenter randomized controlled trial (LIGRO trial)[J]. Ann Surg. 2018;267(5):833–40.
7. Bertens KA, Hawel J, Lung K, et al. ALPPS: challenging the concept of unresectability—a systematic review[J]. Int J Surg. 2015;13:280–7.
8. Borger P, Schneider M, Frick L, et al. Exploration of the transcriptional landscape of ALPPS reveals the pathways of accelerated liver regeneration[J]. Front Oncol. 2019;9:1206.
9. Colak D, Al-Harazi O, Mustafa OM, et al. RNA-Seq transcriptome profiling in three liver regeneration models in rats: comparative analysis of partial hepatectomy, ALLPS, and PVL[J]. Sci Rep. 2020;10(1):5213.
10. Chan A, Zhang WY, Chok K, et al. ALPPS versus portal vein embolization for hepatitis-related hepatocellular carcinoma: a chang-

ing paradigm in modulation of future liver remnant before major hepatectomy[J]. Ann Surg. 2021;273(5):957–65.
11. Ogura Y, Hori T, El Moghazy WM, et al. Portal pressure <15 mmHg is a key for successful adult living donor liver transplantation utilizing smaller grafts than before[J]. Liver Transpl. 2010;16(6):718–28.
12. Yagi S, Iida T, Taniguchi K, et al. Impact of portal venous pressure on regeneration and graft damage after living-donor liver transplantation[J]. Liver Transpl. 2005;11(1):68–75.
13. Tomassini F, D'Asseler Y, Giglio MC, et al. Hemodynamic changes in ALPPS influence liver regeneration and function: results from a prospective study[J]. HPB (Oxford). 2019;21(5):557–65.
14. Michalopoulos GK, DeFrances MC. Liver regeneration[J]. Science. 1997;276(5309):60–6.
15. Deal R, Frederiks C, Williams L, et al. Rapid liver hypertrophy after portal vein occlusion correlates with the degree of collateralization between lobes-a study in pigs[J]. J Gastrointest Surg. 2018;22(2):203–13.
16. He LJ, Pu WJ, Liu XX, et al. Proliferation tracing reveals regional hepatocyte generation in liver homeostasis and repair[J]. Science. 2021;371(6532):eabc4346.
17. Wei YL, Wang YG, Jia YM, et al. Liver homeostasis is maintained by midlobular zone 2 hepatocytes[J]. Science. 2021;371(6532):eabb1625.
18. Schlegel A, Lesurtel M, Melloul E, et al. ALPPS: from human to mice highlighting accelerated and novel mechanisms of liver regeneration[J]. Ann Surg. 2014;260(5):839–46; discussion 846–847.
19. Tong YF, Meng N, Chen MQ, et al. Maturity of associating liver partition and portal vein ligation for staged hepatectomy-derived liver regeneration in a rat model[J]. World J Gastroenterol. 2018;24(10):1107–19.
20. Matsuo K, Hiroshima Y, Yamazaki K, et al. Immaturity of bile canalicular-ductule networks in the future liver remnant while associating liver partition and portal vein occlusion for staged hepatectomy (ALPPS)[J]. Ann Surg Oncol. 2017;24(9):2456–64.
21. Matsuo K, Murakami T, Kawaguchi D, et al. Histologic features after surgery associating liver partition and portal vein ligation for staged hepatectomy versus those after hepatectomy with portal vein embolization[J]. Surgery. 2016;159(5):1289–98.
22. Raptis DA, Linecker M, Kambakamba P, et al. Defining benchmark outcomes for ALPPS[J]. Ann Surg. 2019;270(5):835–41.
23. Schadde E, Ardiles V, Robles-Campos R, et al. Early survival and safety of ALPPS: first report of the International ALPPS Registry[J]. Ann Surg. 2014;260(5):829–36; discussion 836–838.
24. Tong YF, Xu M, Wang YF, et al. Hepatic regeneration by associating liver partition and portal vein ligation for staged hepatectomy (ALPPS) is feasible but attenuated in rat liver with thioacetamide-induced fibrosis[J]. Surgery. 2019;165(2):345–52.
25. Zhang B, Meng FZ, Liu Y, et al. Inhibition of TGFβ1 accelerates regeneration of fibrotic rat liver elicited by a novel two-staged hepatectomy[J]. Theranostics. 2021;11(10):4743–58.
26. Fausto N, Campbell J, Riehle K. Liver regeneration[J]. Hepatology. 2006;43(2 Suppl 1):S45–53.
27. Akerman P, Cote P, Yang SQ, et al. Antibodies to tumor necrosis factor-alpha inhibit liver regeneration after partial hepatectomy[J]. Am J Phys. 1992;263(4 Pt 1):G579–85.
28. Trautwein C, Rakemann T, Niehof M, et al. Acute-phase response factor, increased binding, and target gene transcription during liver regeneration[J]. Gastroenterology. 1996;110(6):1854–62.
29. Iwai M, Cui TX, Kitamura H, et al. Increased secretion of tumour necrosis factor and interleukin 6 from isolated, perfused liver of rats after partial hepatectomy[J]. Cytokine. 2001;13(1):60–4.
30. Madonna R, Cevik C, Nasser M, et al. Hepatocyte growth factor: molecular biomarker and player in cardioprotection and cardiovascular regeneration[J]. Thromb Haemost. 2012;107(4):656–61.
31. Böhm F, Köhler UA, Speicher T, et al. Regulation of liver regeneration by growth factors and cytokines[J]. EMBO Mol Med. 2010;2(8):294–305.
32. Tajiri K, Shimizu Y. Branched-chain amino acids in liver diseases[J]. World J Gastroenterol. 2013;19(43):7620–9.
33. Moris D, Vernadakis S, Papalampros A, et al. Mechanistic insights of rapid liver regeneration after associating liver partition and portal vein ligation for stage hepatectomy[J]. World J Gastroenterol. 2016;22(33):7613–24.
34. Schnitzbauer AA, Lang SA, Goessmann H, et al. Right portal vein ligation combined with in situ splitting induces rapid left lateral liver lobe hypertrophy enabling 2-staged extended right hepatic resection in small-for-size settings[J]. Ann Surg. 2012;255(3):405–14.
35. Lopez-Lopez V, Robles-Campos R, Brusadin R, et al. ALPPS for hepatocarcinoma under cirrhosis: a feasible alternative to portal vein embolization[J]. Ann Transl Med. 2019;7(22):691.
36. Lauber DT, Tihanyi DK, Czigány Z, et al. Liver regeneration after different degrees of portal vein ligation[J]. J Surg Res. 2016;203(2):451–8.
37. Thorgersen EB, Barratt-Due A, Haugaa H, et al. The role of complement in liver injury, regeneration, and transplantation[J]. Hepatology. 2019;70(2):725–36.
38. Sparrelid E, Johansson H, Gilg S, et al. Serial assessment of growth factors associated with liver regeneration in patients operated with associating liver partition and portal vein ligation for staged hepatectomy[J]. Eur Surg Res. 2018;59(1–2):72–82.
39. Alexandrino H, Rolo A, Teodoro JS, et al. Bioenergetic adaptations of the human liver in the ALPPS procedure—how liver regeneration correlates with mitochondrial energy status[J]. HPB (Oxford). 2017;19(12):1091–103.
40. Langiewicz M, Schlegel A, Saponara E, et al. Hedgehog pathway mediates early acceleration of liver regeneration induced by a novel two-staged hepatectomy in mice[J]. J Hepatol. 2017;66(3):560–70.
41. Racanelli V, Rehermann B. The liver as an immunological organ[J]. Hepatology. 2006;43(2 Suppl 1):S54–62.
42. Li N, Hua JL. Immune cells in liver regeneration[J]. Oncotarget. 2017;8(2):3628–39.
43. Ikarashi M, Nakashima H, Kinoshita M, et al. Distinct development and functions of resident and recruited liver Kupffer cells/macrophages[J]. J Leukoc Biol. 2013;94(6):1325–36.
44. Nishiyama K, Nakashima H, Ikarashi M, et al. Mouse CD11b+ Kupffer cells recruited from bone marrow accelerate liver regeneration after partial hepatectomy[J]. PLoS One. 2015;10(9):e0136774.
45. Michalopoulos GK. Principles of liver regeneration and growth homeostasis[J]. Compr Physiol. 2013;3(1):485–513.
46. Dili A, Bertrand C, Lebrun V, et al. Hypoxia protects the liver from small for size syndrome: a lesson learned from the associated liver partition and portal vein ligation for staged hepatectomy (ALPPS) procedure in rats[J]. Am J Transplant. 2019;19(11):2979–90.
47. Dirscherl K, Schläpfer M, Roth Z'graggen B, et al. Hypoxia sensing by hepatic stellate cells leads to VEGF-dependent angiogenesis and may contribute to accelerated liver regeneration[J]. Sci Rep. 2020;10(1):4392.
48. Schadde E, Tsatsaris C, Swiderska-Syn M, et al. Hypoxia of the growing liver accelerates regeneration[J]. Surgery. 2017;161(3):666–79.
49. Anantha RV, Shaler CR, Meilleur CE, et al. The future liver remnant in patients undergoing the associating liver partition with portal vein ligation for staged hepatectomy (ALPPS) maintains the immunological components of a healthy organ[J]. Front Med (Lausanne). 2016;3:32.

23 Future of ALPPS

Jian Zhou, Zheng Wang, and Guoming Shi

ALPPS is a breakthrough innovation in liver surgery in the past half-century, following liver transplantation and laparoscopic techniques. It offers curative hope for patients with liver cancer, who were previously considered inoperable, by potentially curing them with just one hospital admission in a short period. Overall, ALPPS is a complex procedure that has been developed thanks to the efforts of many surgeons.

Over the past 15 years, ALPPS has evolved mainly in the following ways:

(a) Utilizing minimally invasive approaches or techniques to reduce surgical trauma
(b) Modifying the surgical methods to expand the criteria for surgical indications
(c) Employing rescue ALPPS following the failure of portal vein embolization (PVE) or TAE–salvaged ALPPS (Zhou's ALPPS) following the failure of conventional ALPPS
(d) Adjusting surgical methods to improve postoperative outcomes, particularly for tumor prognosis

These advancements have made traditional ALPPS surgery more complex, although there are also attempts to simplify the surgical procedure. The ultimate goal remains to make ALPPS surgery safer, more effective, and standardized. In fact, mortality due to ALPPS surgery is no longer the primary concern. However, more rigorous and well-designed studies are still needed to evaluate the true value of modifications in ALPPS techniques. This evolution aligns precisely with the objective pattern of any new technique, from its learning stage to refinement, and eventual maturity, leading to widespread application for the benefit of patients.

Future research will focus on patients' long-term outcomes and quality of life after ALPPS surgery. Since the initiation of the first reported ALPPS procedure in Asia by the Hepatobiliary Surgery Department of Zhongshan Hospital, Fudan University, in 2013, several patients have achieved long-term tumor-free survival of over 8 years. In recent years, our understanding of embryogenesis, tumor biology, and liver regeneration has grown exponentially thanks to new technologies and concepts. Increasing evidence supports that many common biological processes and pathways are driving these complex phenomena. The liver's innate regenerative capacity makes extensive liver resection possible. However, the signals driving liver regeneration might also promote tumor progression, potentially creating a different microenvironment that reactivates dormant cancer cells. In the context of ALPPS, extreme liver resection is accompanied by increased portal vein blood flow and the release of numerous cytokines and inflammatory factors, altering signaling pathways that promote liver regeneration. This leads to changes in immune and stromal cells within the regenerating liver's microenvironment, potentially activating circulating tumor stem cells or residual cancer cells. ALPPS surgery generally completes liver regeneration and tumor resection within a short timeframe of 1–2 weeks. While there may be factors that simultaneously promote liver regeneration and tumor recurrence or metastasis, the short duration of these effects minimizes the potential for tumor spread or recurrence. Understanding the specific mechanisms involved will aid in developing corresponding anti-tumor interventions and selecting the best candidates for surgery, thereby informing future personalized surgical treatments for cancer.

ALPPS itself results from human innovation and the challenge of the unknown. It will continue to be refined and developed through ongoing clinical practice, mechanistic exploration, and translational medical research. The research outcomes from ALPPS are likely to improve the survival rates of patients with advanced liver cancer, enhance human liver function, and potentially contribute to prolonging human life, which is no longer a dream.

J. Zhou (✉) · Z. Wang · G. Shi
Zhongshan Hospital, Fudan University, Shanghai, China
e-mail: zhou.jian@zs-hospital.sh.cn

J. Zhou (ed.), *Associating Liver Partition and Portal Vein Ligation for Staged Hepatectomy (ALPPS)*,
https://doi.org/10.1007/978-981-96-7364-3_23

MIX
Papier aus verantwortungsvollen Quellen
Paper from responsible sources
FSC® C105338

If you have any concerns about our products,
you can contact us on
ProductSafety@springernature.com

In case Publisher is established outside the EU,
the EU authorized representative is:
Springer Nature Customer Service Center GmbH
Europaplatz 3, 69115 Heidelberg, Germany

Printed by Libri Plureos GmbH
in Hamburg, Germany